R. Benson

# *The* FAMILY PHYSICIAN

# *The* FAMILY PHYSICIAN

By

**DR. HERMAN POMERANZ**

Author of *Your Respiratory System, Health and Hygiene, First Aid, Child Care, Hernia,* etc.; Editor of *Every Woman's Standard Medical Guide,* etc.

and

**DR. IRVIN S. KOLL**

Director, Department of Health, Western Illinois State College; Former Head, Genito-Urinary Department, Chicago Post-Graduate School of Medicine, and Chief of Urology, Valley Forge Hospital; Author of *How to Stay Healthy,* etc.

NEW YORK

P. F. COLLIER AND SON CORP.

BY SPECIAL ARRANGEMENT WITH GREYSTONE PRESS

100 Sixth Avenue
New York 13, New York

## *Acknowledgments*

THE PUBLISHERS acknowledge a debt of gratitude to the following organizations and individuals for permission to use their specially prepared illustrations or other material in this volume: Alfred Feinberg, of Columbia University College of Physicians and Surgeons; National Foundation for Infantile Paralysis; National Tuberculosis Association; Standard Oil Company (New Jersey); National Safety Council; Dr. Herman N. Bundesen, President of the Chicago Board of Health, for his chart on when the baby will be born; the United States Army; Harry Berk, Time, Inc., and the New York State Civil Defense Commission, for the material on protection against the atomic bomb; Robert Latou Dickinson, David Loth, and the Planned Parenthood Federation; John Hancock Mutual Life Insurance Company; Johnson and Johnson Company; RKO-Radio Pictures, for scenes from their motion picture, "You Can Beat the A-Bomb"; Federal Food Service and Gerber's Baby Foods; National Organization for Public Health Nursing; Emerson Yorke Studio Pictures; Clark Kinnaird and King Features Syndicate; Helena Rubenstein, for several exercises, some featuring the "lithe-line"; Bonomo Associates; American Cancer Society; the National Film Board of Canada, for the scenes from psychological films it produced for the Mental Health Division of the Department of National Health and Welfare, Ottawa, Canada (films distributed in U. S. A. by McGraw-Hill)—and also the Board's Miss Janet Scellen; New York City Department of Health; Cleanliness Bureau; World Scope Encyclopedia; National Multiple Sclerosis Society; Atomic Energy Commission; International News Photos; Federal Security Agency, and others.



Manufactured in the United States of America

# *About This Book*

THIS book has been designed to provide a reliable and up-to-date answer to every question of health, hygiene, and medical care that is likely to arise in the average household. It gives you the essential facts about an enormous variety of medical problems—not only what causes them and their signs and symptoms, but also what you personally can do to prevent them. Practicing physicians and writers on health subjects with many years' experience, the authors have spared no effort to make this book as clear and understandable as possible.

A number of outstanding features mark this volume. First of all, it emphasizes what you can do yourself. The section on first aid covers practically every emergency you may be called upon to deal with before a doctor comes. Over and above this, you are given a wide range of safe and simple remedies you can readily use for the relief and cure of common ailments. These remedies are explained in full detail, with step-by-step advice on how to administer them. The section on home nursing is in itself a complete guide to the care of the sick in the home.

This book will prove valuable, too, because it describes at unusual length the medical treatment you can expect from your physician in a multitude of disorders. You are given helpful and enlightening facts about how the doctor proceeds—what medicines and methods he will use, and his reasons for using them. By showing you that there is nothing fearful or mysterious in your doctor's acts, this book should prove a source of reassurance and peace of mind. Moreover, with this information you will be better equipped to cooperate with your physician in achieving your common aim of lasting good health.

Among the health subjects of major interest explained here with this new approach are cancer and other tumors, disorders of the heart and circulation, allergies, change of life, arthritis and related disorders, menstrual troubles, sterility, diseases of the urinary system, digestive ailments, constipation, hygiene of the eye, ear, nose and throat, conduct of pregnancy, and hundreds of other health topics, both large and small. The fascinating story of the new "miracle drugs" is told here, and you are brought abreast of the most recent progress in medicine. You are given a basic picture of all the parts of your body and how they work—your glands, nervous system, reproductive organs, the mechanism by which you breathe, and other organs and body structures—so that you may better understand them and take the proper measures to keep them at the peak of good condition.

Exhaustive sections of this book are devoted to the health of the child, from birth to adolescence. You are told, step by step, how to care for the infant, from diapering right through food and formulas. The common troubles and diseases of infancy and childhood are discussed in full, and there is complete advice on problems of sleep, toilet-training, and other important aspects of child care. It should, of course, be clearly understood, in matters concerning children, and indeed in all matters of health, that no book can take the place of your doctor. Self-diagnosis is dangerous, except in the simplest ailments. Where home treatment is recommended, you will find full details in this volume, as well as instructions on how you can help your doctor to help you.

This book contains a thorough guide to eating for good health. It explains what you should know about foods, calories, vitamins, and minerals, and gives you diets and menus for losing or gaining weight. The food problems of the child, adult, elderly person, convalescent, and invalid are examined, and there are practical wholesome diets as well as special diets for diabetes, high blood pressure, ulcers. allergies, constipation, etc., etc.

The development of the atomic bomb and the possibility of its use against civilian populations has served to remind us that man's knowledge of science far exceeds his understanding of how to live at peace with his fellow man. Medicine has ever been concerned with the prevention of injury and ill health, and accordingly a section on protecting yourself against an atomic bomb has been included. At the end of this volume you will find a Dictionary of Common Medical Terms, which lists expressions you are likely to come across in daily life, with a concise explanation of what they mean. There is also an unusually complete and detailed Ready-Reference Index to help you to locate promptly any information in this book.

A large group of distinguished medical specialists and experts gave the authors the benefit of their experience and advice while this book was in preparation. The authors would like to thank them and all the others who gave freely of their time and their thought to make this volume a work of outstanding usefulness for the American home.

# CONTENTS

# *The* FAMILY PHYSICIAN

CHAPTER 1

# THE EYE AND EAR

**THE EYE: Eye-Strain . . . Nearsightedness . . . Farsightedness . . . Astigmatism . . . Aging of the Eyes . . . Foreign Bodies in the Eye . . . Black Eye . . . Styes . . . Twitching Eyelids . . . Wounds and Burns . . . Congestion of the Eyelids . . . Discharge . . . Conjunctivitis . . . Catarrhal Inflammation . . . Pink Eyes . . . Glaucoma . . . Diseases of the Optic Nerve . . . Trachoma . . . Color and Night Blindness . . . Crossed Eyes . . . Cataract . . . Cornea Disorders . . . Care of the Eyes, etc. THE EAR: Foreign Bodies in the Ear . . . Acute Inflammation . . . Earache . . . Mastoiditis . . . Deformed Ears . . . Impacted Wax . . . Otosclerosis . . . Hygiene of the Ear, Syringing It, etc.**

## EYE-STRAIN

***Symptoms of Eye-Strain.*** Headache is the most frequent symptom of eye-strain. It may be near the eyes, but there is no special characteristic which positively distinguishes an eye headache from other types of headache. The headache resulting from eye-strain may be in the forehead, temples, top or back of the head, or limited to one side. It frequently takes the form of a "sick headache," or migraine. It is perhaps more apt to appear after any unusual use of the eyes in reading, writing, watching the movies or television, sewing, riding, shopping, or sight-seeing, and going to the theater or a picture gallery. However, eye headache may appear without obvious cause.

Nausea and vomiting often accompany eye-strain, with or without headache, nervousness, sleeplessness, and dizziness. Sometimes there is also weakness of the eyes—lack of endurance for eye work, twitching of the eyelids, and tearing—as well as styes and inflammation of the lids.

***Treatment of Eye-Strain.*** The first essential in treatment of eye-strain is the wearing of proper glasses. It should be a rule, without exception, to consult an oculist—*never* an optician, whose proper job is to prepare lenses—for the selection of glasses. It is as foolish to have an optician test your eyes for glasses as it would be to seek medical treatment from a druggist. In order to determine the optical error in astigmatic and farsighted eyes, which may be the cause of the eye-strain, it is essential to put drops in the eyes to dilate the pupil and temporarily to paralyze the muscles that control the lens; also to use scientific instruments in the examination. All this can be properly undertaken, studied, and interpreted only by an oculist or eye specialist.

## NEARSIGHTEDNESS (MYOPIA)

***Causes and Symptoms of Nearsightedness.*** A myopic person is one who is unable to see distant objects distinctly because of the excessive length of his eyeball. The focus to which light rays are brought falls in front of the retina, the sensitive membrane of the eye that receives the image, instead of directly on it, as in the normal eye. This lengthening of the eyeball may be caused by weakness of its coats, perhaps as a result of malnutrition. Heredity is a major factor in producing this condition, and so is close work with the eyes.

***Treatment of Nearsightedness.*** Nearsightedness is corrected by wearing glasses which cause the light rays to diverge or separate before they enter the eyeball. A nearsighted person is given glasses with concave (hollow) lenses.

## FARSIGHTEDNESS (HYPEROPIA)

***Symptoms of Farsightedness.*** This is a congenital and common condition. In contrast to nearsightedness, the eyeball is shortened and the light rays are brought to a focus behind the retina, instead of on it. What causes this condition we do not know. Normal children are usually farsighted at birth, but later become less so.

If the condition is a minor one, or the person is advanced in years, vision for distance is usually good. A great many patients with farsightedness present no symptoms when they do no close work. However, the vision may be blurred, and there may be headaches as well as pain in the eyes.

***Treatment of Farsightedness.*** This condition is corrected through the use of convex lenses, which cause the light rays to converge or come together.

## ASTIGMATISM

***Causes and Symptoms of Astigmatism.*** This is caused by inequality of the outer surface of the front of the eyeball, the cornea, which admits light. In astigmatism, the front of the eyeball is not a regular sphere; it bulges out at parts of the curve, while the curvature is flattened or normal at other parts. Rays of light, in passing through the different parts of the astigmatic eye, are differently bent, so that along one line, rays may focus perfectly on the retina, while along another, the rays may focus on a point behind the retina. In this case the eye is made farsighted along one line, and is normal along the other. Or, again, the rays may be partly focused in front of the retina, and directly on the retina at another point.

As a result, a person with astigmatic vision who looks at a series of radiating lines sees some of the lines sharply focused, while others

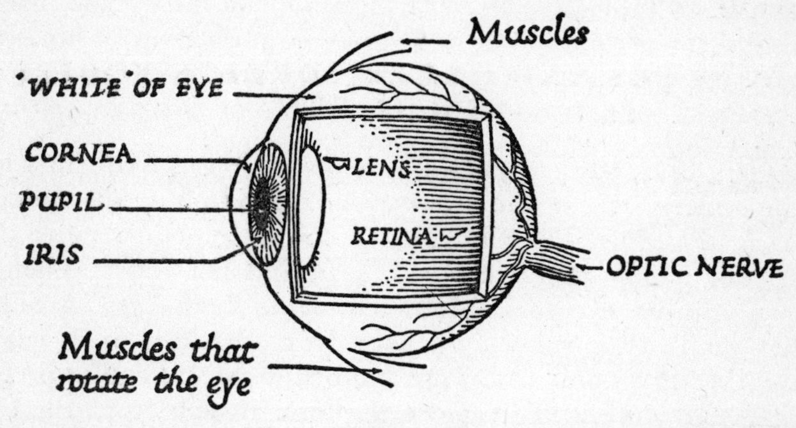


THE EYE

In this diagram, a "window" is cut in the side to show the interior. The cornea is the crystal-clear front of the eye. Behind it is the iris, the colored part, which changes in size to make the central opening, the pupil, larger or smaller. Just behind the iris is the lens, which is changed in shape by a ring of muscle that surrounds it. The flattening or rounding of the lens focuses the incoming picture upon the sensitive inner lining, the retina, at the back of the eye. The optic nerve carries the "picture" to the brain.

are blurred because they are focused either in front of, or behind, the retina, and not on it, as they should properly be. Besides this abnormality of vision, there may be nervousness and headaches, and the eyes may be painful during continued close work.

***Treatment of Astigmatism.*** This error in the curvature of the cornea is corrected by wearing appropiate glasses.

## AGING OF THE EYES (PRESBYOPIA)

***Causes and Symptoms of Presbyopia.*** One of the commonest causes of eye-strain is old age of the eyes (presbyopia). After reaching the age of forty, many persons are compelled to hold books and newspapers farther and farther away from the eyes in order to focus properly, and require an increasing amount of light for reading. This is due to a change in the ability of the eye to accommodate, or adjust for looking at objects at different distances. The lens of the eye undergoes a process of hardening all through life, and somewhere between the ages of forty and forty-five the range of accommodation becomes progressively smaller. As this hardening proceeds, objects at close range become more and more difficult to see distinctly.

***Treatment of Presbyopia.*** Properly prescribed glasses are the answer to the problem.

## CINDERS AND OTHER FOREIGN BODIES IN THE EYE

Cinders, dust, ashes or small fragments of objects frequently lodge on the undersurface of the upper eyelid, less often on the surface of the eyeball and the lower lid. Before you attempt to remove them, wash your hands thoroughly with soap and hot water. Then rub your uninjured eye to produce tearing in both eyes. Avoid the natural tendency to rub the eye with the cinder in it. Such action is harmful. It serves only to irritate and bruise the eye and to press the foreign body deeper. To remove the foreign body, turn the eyelid lining outward in the following manner: Grasp the lashes of the upper eyelid, pulling away from the eyeball and downward over the lower lid; a quick release of the lower lid will then often dislodge the annoying particle. If you have been successful, procure an eye-cup and use a boric acid solution (4 per cent) or salt water (one teaspoonful of table salt to a pint of clean water) to wash the affected eye.

If unsuccessful in removing the object from your eyelid or eye, ask someone to help you. Sit in a good light, and tilt your head backward. Your helper stands behind you. If the foreign body seems to be on the lower eyelid, he will pull the lid downward while you glance upward. If he sees the offending object, he should brush it away gently with sterile cotton on a toothpick.

If the foreign body is on the upper lid, the volunteer assistant should turn the lid inside out. You look downward while he grasps the edge of the lid with the thumb and index finger of one hand, placing a padded match or padded toothpick (or the end of the index finger or thumb of the left hand) horizontally across the center of the lid. Drawing the lid forward and upward turns the eyelid inside out and discloses the particle of matter so that it can be brushed away gently with sterile cotton. If this fails, place a drop or two of boric acid solution in the eye and consult a physician.

## BLACK EYE

To relieve this bruised condition, it is necessary to reduce the swelling. This can be done by applying to the closed lid, every three minutes, squares of iced white cotton or linen, four-fold and about as large as a silver dollar. The cold compresses should not be permitted to overlap the nose.

## BLEEDING IN THE EYE

Bleeding occurring under the membrane lining the inner surface of the lids and covering the outer surface of the eyeball (conjunctiva) may be caused by blows, or other injury to the eye due to violent coughing or straining. Dark-red spots which may appear in the white of the eyeball, slightly raised above the surface, are little blood clots under the conjunctival membrane. No special trouble results, and there is nothing to be done except to wait until the blood is absorbed, which generally occurs in a few days. If spots persist, or if there is no history of injury—consult a physician.

## STYES

***Causes of Styes.*** A stye is a small abscess at the margin of the lid, involving the roots of the eyelashes. It is often very painful and tends to recur. It is often found when there is poor vision, eye-strain, or impaired health.

***Treatment of Styes.*** At the beginning of infection apply yellow oxide of mercury along the margin of the eyelid. If this is not effective, use hot boric acid compresses (half a teaspoonful of the acid to a cup of boiled water), to hasten the stye's "coming to a head." When it opens spontaneously, wipe the pus clear with moist cotton. When styes recur frequently it is well to have the eyes examined and to have a general physical check-up.

## TWITCHING EYELIDS

Tremor of the eyelids is commonly caused by eye-strain, and vision should be corrected by the use of glasses. The condition is sometimes due to physical or mental fatigue, or both. The lids are, in effect, the windshield wipers of the eyes, and their function must be kept normal in order to protect the eyes.

## WOUNDS AND BURNS ABOUT THE EYES

***Treatment of Wounds and Burns.*** Slight wounds of the inner surface of the eyelids close readily, without stitching, if boric-acid solution (ten grains to each ounce of water) is dropped into the eye four times daily. Because of the excellent protection afforded by its socket, the eye usually escapes injury. However, burns of the inner surface of the lids may follow contact with hot water, hot ashes, lime, acids, or molten metals. If an eye burn is caused by a chemical, a physician must be called. In the meantime, put your face in a bowl of warm water and open and close your eyes under the water.

## CONGESTION OF THE EYELIDS

***Causes and Treatment of Congestion.*** This may be caused by smoke or dust in the atmosphere, or by various foreign bodies in the eye. It is also frequently the result of eye-strain due to far- or nearsightedness, astigmatism, or muscular weakness, and these should be corrected by glasses. Excessive glare of light (as in the case of firemen), excessive reading, and reading in a poor light, also may produce irritation of the lids. Also, the germs which cause a "cold in the head" often reach the eyes through the tear ducts, which connect the inner corners of the eyes with the nose.

When there is a sensation as of sand in the eyes, with itching and burning, the condition is best treated by an oculist.

## EYE DISCHARGE IN CHILDREN

If an infant has a sore eye with discharge, the child should be held in the lap, with its head backward and inclined toward the side of the sore eye, so that in washing the affected eye, there is no danger that discharge from the sore eye will flow into the sound one. Boric acid may then be dropped from a medicine dropper, or applied upon a little wad of absorbent cotton, to the inner corner of the eye, while the eyelids are held apart. If the symptoms do not disappear soon, consult a physician.

## CONJUNCTIVITIS ("SORE EYES")

The conjunctiva consists of the inner surface of the lids, the coating of the front of the eyeball, and the fold between the two. Any of these parts may become infected.

*Symptoms of "Sore Eyes."* Just around the lashes, on the margins of the lids, a slight redness and inflammation frequently occur. The lashes tend to fall out, and little scales collect on the margins of the lids. The cause is often found to be general weakness, or eyestrain from working in a bad light. The underlying cause may also be defective sight, and should then be relieved by suitable eye glasses.

*Treatment of "Sore Eyes."* The best home treatment is to remove the scales by bathing the lids two or three times a day with warm sodium bicarbonate solution, then to apply yellow oxide of mercury along the margin of the lids.

## CATARRHAL INFLAMMATION OF THE EYES

*Symptoms of Inflammation.* In this disorder there is a discharge which sticks the lids together during the night. Their inner surface is much reddened, the blood vessels in the lining membrane are greatly enlarged, and the lids are slightly swollen. The redness may extend to the eyeball and give it a bloodshot appearance, but there is no interference with sight other than momentary blurring caused by the discharge. Occasionally there is very severe pain, as if a cinder had suddenly fallen into the eye. This symptom may occur at night and awaken the patient, and may be the reason for his first consulting a physician.

One eye is commonly affected twenty-four to thirty-six hours before the other. A sense of discomfort is felt about the eyes, and often there is a burning, with constant watering, the tears containing flakes of white discharge. When the discharge is a copious, creamy pus or "matter," associated with great swelling of the lids and pain on exposure to light, the cause is usually a germ, and there is the grave danger that the eyesight will be lost unless an eye specialist is consulted. Early treatment, however, is of great value, and until a physician can be seen, the measures recommended below should be followed most conscientiously; by this means, the sight may be saved.

*The Condition Is Contagious.* All forms of severe inflammation of the lids are contagious (especially the above-mentioned variety) and can be spread by means of the discharge on towels, handkerchiefs, soap, wash basins, etc.

***Treatment of Conjunctivitis.*** Penicillin injected by a physician is healing, as a rule. Aureomycin also quickly controls the infection.

Iced compresses should be applied for fifteen minutes four times daily, and irrigations with boric acid solution are helpful.

## CONJUNCTIVITIS IN THE NEWBORN

This dangerous variety of inflammation of the eye is not rare in the newborn. Infants whose eyes are red immediately after birth should receive proper attention, or blindness for life will be the result. This can be avoided by dropping a 1 per cent argyrol solution into the eyes immediately after birth.

The essential rules are: (1) As soon as a child is born, see that its eyes are carefully wiped and gently washed with boric acid, and the drops instilled; (2) if the child's eyes become inflamed, consult a physician immediately; (3) do not apply a poultice to the eyes when there is any discharge; (4) when moist heat is required, apply lint wrung out of hot boric acid solution.

## "PINK EYE"

***Symptoms of "Pink Eye."*** This is an acute contagious variety of catarrhal conjunctivitis, occurring, as a rule, in the spring and autumn. The infection is caused by a germ. The eyelids become red, swollen, and painful.

***Treatment of "Pink Eye."*** It is best to avoid strong light, and to use dark glasses for the duration of the condition. Iced compresses should be applied for fifteen minutes to an hour, three times a day. The eye should be irrigated several times a day with a solution of boric acid.

## GLAUCOMA

***Causes of Glaucoma.*** Glaucoma is a disease of the eye that demands quick recognition and prompt treatment; otherwise blindness occurs. It is caused by some obstruction in the channels through which the fluid formed in the eye ordinarily escapes; as the fluid accumulates, the tension of the eye increases, the eyeball becomes more or less hard, and, in a very short time, the back pressure acting on the retina destroys its function, and blindness follows.

Glaucoma usually occurs without apparent cause.

***Symptoms of Glaucoma.*** The attacks may be acute or chronic. In the acute form, the eye is red and vision is very dim. Pain in the head is present. The patient frequently vomits, and the disease is often mistaken for a "sick headache." Another very common and most important symptom is that a light, such as a candle flame, seems to be surrounded by a halo of colored lights or "rainbows." (It should be stressed that whenever a patient past middle age complains of this sensation, even if it is unassociated with other symptoms, it is wise to consult an oculist.) The pupil is usually larger in the affected eye than in the other, and when a strong light is thrown on the pupil, it contracts very slowly.

***Treatment of Glaucoma.*** Drugs are used successfully in the treatment of glaucoma. However, in many cases the only safe treatment for glaucoma is an operation.

## DISEASES OF THE OPTIC NERVE

When this nerve, which is part of the retina, becomes diseased—when it deteriorates or shrinks so that its vitality is diminished—blindness follows. Various serious infections bring this about, especially the third stage of syphilis. Tumors may involve the retina, or the retina may become detached. If the disease is detected at an early stage, it may be possible to prevent serious damage to the sight.

## TRACHOMA

***Symptoms of Trachoma.*** Trachoma (granular conjunctivitis) is a chronic form of contagious conjunctivitis. It is a serious affliction because of its grave complications, which often end in partial or complete blindness. Sometimes there are no symptoms for a long time. In general, the patient complains of tearing, pain and burning of the eyes from looking at the light (photophobia), pain, visual disturbances, and a feeling that foreign bodies are in the eye.

***Treatment of Trachoma.*** Whether mild or severe, this condition urgently requires the attention of an oculist. The sulfonamides are remarkably effective in their action against trachoma.

## "BLIND SPOTS"

***Color Blindness.*** The explanation of color vision is still largely a matter of speculation, but it is a fact that color blindness dating from birth occurs in from 3 to 5 per cent of men, and in only 0.3 per cent of women. Color blindness usually affects both eyes, and is often hereditary. In other respects the eyes are normal. It is incurable; but it is possible to develop some color sense if training is begun early. Acquired color blindness is often found as a symptom of disease of the retina and optic nerve.

***Night Blindness.*** In this condition sight is deficient at night or in a dim light. One of the causes is shrinkage of the optic nerve. Lack of vitamin A may also be responsible for this condition, in which case it must be added to the diet in abundance.

## SQUINT

***Causes and Symptoms of Squint.*** A squint occurs when the axes or central lines of both eyes are not parallel, so that an observer looking at the "squinter" sees one eye turned inward or outward as the case may be. In some cases the squint affects the eyes alternately, but eventually settles in one eye, and the squinting eye often becomes useless. Double vision occurs because, with both eyes looking at an object (the eyes not being in the same axis), the image is formed on different parts of the retina in each eye. This is the case where the squint is in an adult, owing to paralysis; but the instinct of the young leads them to ignore one of the images in one eye, and thus after months or years, the eye becomes almost blind.

***Squint in Children.*** The cause of squinting in young children is usually defective action of the eye muscles, especially if associated with weakness. As a rule, if the child is farsighted, the eye turns outward. If children are provided with glasses which correct their defects of vision, a great many of them cease to squint.

***Treatment of Squint.*** (1) correction of refractive errors by the use of glasses, (2) exercise of the squinting eye by shutting off the unaffected eye, (3) training, with the use of instruments for viewing or observing, (4) surgical operation.

## CROSSED EYES

***Causes and Symptoms of Crossed Eyes.*** Crossed eyes, which are often found when a child is very young, are produced by defective eyesight. Also, muscles control the movements of the eyeballs, turning them inward or outward, and a weakness of some of these muscles will make the eyeballs tend to turn in one direction or the other.

In some persons the eyes are crossed when they are fixed on objects close at hand. In others, they are crossed all the time.

***Treatment of Crossed Eyes.*** Glasses fitted by an oculist provide help, and so do exercises which the oculist will prescribe. If these exercises are to be effective, they must be carried out faithfully over a long period of time. Regular visits to the oculist provide a check on the patient's progress. In some cases, operations, which are relatively simple, are required to correct the condition.

## CATARACT

***Causes and Symptoms of Cataract.*** Cataract is a clouding of the lens of the eye, interfering with the transmission of light. The lens, normally as transparent as glass, becomes more or less like opal.

The disease is predominantly one of old people, in whom sight gradually fails. It is, in this case, known as senile cataract, and is rare before the age of fifty. It often affects one eye more than the other.

There is a congenital variety in which there are numerous "milk dots" in the lens substance, especially near the periphery or outer boundary, but it has no great importance.

Cataract frequently occurs when there is diabetes or an accident involving the eye.

***Treatment of Cataract.*** The majority of patients require surgery, to remove the opaque lens.

## CORNEA DISORDERS

***Conical Cornea.*** The central part of the cornea may have a greater curvature in one part than in some other, a condition which results, as previously mentioned, in astigmatism, or it may be so thin and weak that it gradually bulges forward to produce a condition known as conical cornea. This causes defective sight and usually involves both eyes.

***Injuries to the Cornea.*** When the cornea is inflamed it usually produces fear of light, pain, tearing, sudden closure of the lids caused by involuntary muscular contractions, and impairment of vision.

Severe injuries to the cornea usually heal by scar tissue, and not by a renewal of the same clear corneal tissue. Since this scar tissue is opaque and whitish, differing from corneal tissue, it can be readily understood how even a slight wound of the cornea may cause serious impairment of sight.

***Ulcers of the Cornea.*** These may be produced by injuries. The chief symptom is dread of light, and young children sometimes screw up the lids so that it becomes necessary to give them an anesthetic in order to examine the eyes. Penicillin is used in ointment form, applied on the inner surface of the eyelid.

***Corneal Transplantation.*** It is now possible to take corneal tissue quickly from a person who has just died, and graft it into the defective cornea of another person to provide a clear window, thus lessening actual or impending blindness. The tissues are transported in special containers to eye-banks, from which they are flown to hospitals where the transplantation operations are to be carried out. The tissue must be used within thirty-six hours of death.

***Eye-banks.*** Eye-banks for the restoration of sight have been established in a number of cities. In Boston, the bank is at 243 Charles Street; in New Orleans, at 621 Hutchinson Memorial Building; and in New York City, at 210 East 64th Street. The eye-bank has been set up in order to make available to hospitals and surgeons who are qualified to perform the corneal transplantation operation a supply of fresh or preserved corneal tissue, wherever and whenever needed, and to encourage and extend, by teaching and research, the knowledge and skill required to perform the operation.

## CARE OF THE EYES

Many of our eye defects can be prevented by proper lighting and intelligent eye care. For close work such as reading and writing, light should come from slightly above and behind the shoulder and should illuminate the reading or writing surface clearly. The source of light must be a steady one, for artificial lights that waver and flutter are harmful to the eyes. The distance between the book or work and the eyes should be about fourteen inches.

Books printed in extremely small type or on poor paper are harmful to the eyes. Reading in bed is not objectionable if the positions of the light and the body are correct, and the eyes look down upon the page. When using the eyes steadily, glance away occasionally to rest the eye muscles. No one should read or do close work when drowsy or physically tired.

***Getting Glasses.*** Indispensable to the proper care of the eyes are regular eye examinations. These are especially necessary if a person has persistent headaches, or holds a book for reading closer than twelve inches. Other warning signals are styes, blurred vision, or eye irritation. When you discover any of these conditions, consult the oculist. The oculist, as we have said elsewhere, is a physician who does more than merely examine the eyes for glasses. He examines the eyes with reference to the general condition of the body. If he finds glasses are required, have the lenses ground by an optician, or maker of lenses, whom he recommends. Do not go to an optometrist to determine whether or not you need glasses. The optometrist only measures visual powers. He finds eye defects, but does not attempt to diagnose the condition of the eye in regard to general health. It must be kept in mind that a disease in the body itself may be the cause of your eye trouble, and only an oculist or ophthalmologist is fully qualified to diagnose and treat such a condition.

***Protecting the Child's Eyes.*** From early childhood the eyes should be carefully cleansed of any sticky secretion, and the lashes freed from all particles of conjunctival secretion that stick to them, by morning and evening bathing with a warmed saturated solution of boric acid. Children should be protected from all toys or articles with sharp edges or points which can possibly injure the eyes. Almost needless to say, every child should have a careful eye examination before beginning school, and regular ones thereafter, and be fitted with glasses if necessary.

***Colored Glasses.*** Tinted glasses are helpful in extremely bright sunlight. Otherwise, for normal eyes, there generally is no need for them. In recent years, however, the prescribing of colored or tinted glasses has had an enormous vogue. They are worn constantly, in and out of doors, often with the idea that they keep certain harmful light rays from entering the eye. This is overdone. Neither daylight nor ordinary sources of artificial light contain radiations which are harmful to the healthy eye, either in kind or in degree. Diseased eyes, however, may require protection even from rays due to ordinary light sources; under these circumstances, glasses of a neutral shade are best.

***Care of Glasses.*** It is essential for good sight that glasses should not only be optically correct—they should also be kept bright and free from scratches. Therefore, never place the lenses downward on a surface when you take off your spectacles, but let them rest on the rim and the ear pieces. This will effectually preserve the glasses and prevent much annoyance and expense. For active children who wear glasses, there is available a remarkably durable lens which will not shatter nor splinter.

The "bridge" of the frame (the part between the glasses) should fit the bridge of the nose. If it causes any irritation, don't make it unsightly by wrapping wool or cotton around it, but take it back to the optician; and don't be satisfied until the fault in fitting has been corrected.

If the frames are of steel, an occasional application of a little vaseline will prevent their rusting from perspiration and moisture. If the lenses become dirty and greasy, wash them in warm, strong soda and water, or with ammonia.

Protective "goggles" that are worn during an inflammation of the eye should be well washed with strong ammonia and water, then placed in a solution of carbolic acid (one part of acid to twenty parts of water) for some hours. Afterwards, rub a little vaseline on the rims.

### How to Avoid Eye Infections

1. Above all, keep in good physical condition.
2. Wash your face and hands several times daily and keep your fingernails clean; never touch your face with your hands unless they are absolutely clean.
3. Have your own towel and handkerchiefs, and don't let anyone else use them, particularly a person with infected eyes. Boil your handkerchiefs before adding them to the general laundry.
4. Do not permit your clothing or bedclothes to become soiled with the discharges from your eyes.
5. Do not sleep with persons having sore eyes, nor use the bedclothes that have been used by them.

### Eye Irrigations

***How to Give Irrigations.*** The following equipment should be at hand: one basin for boric acid solution, another for hot water; rubber irrigating bulbs; sterile cotton; towel; thermometer; "pus basin"; paper bag for waste. Solution, bulbs, and basin must be sterile.

Scrub hands with care, using brush, soap and hot water. Put the basin for solution into a bowl of hot water to keep it at the requisite temperature (100° F.). Request the patient to lie down, one pillow supporting his head.

Place towel over the head and along the side of the affected eye. First cleanse the area about the eye with damp cotton; then tilt the head to the side to be treated, and adjust the second basin under the

# Your Eyes Are Precious

## EYES SHOULD BE EXAMINED REGULARLY

The examination of the eyes is just as vital as that of other parts of the body. Periodically, you should have your vision checked by an oculist, a specialist in eye troubles.

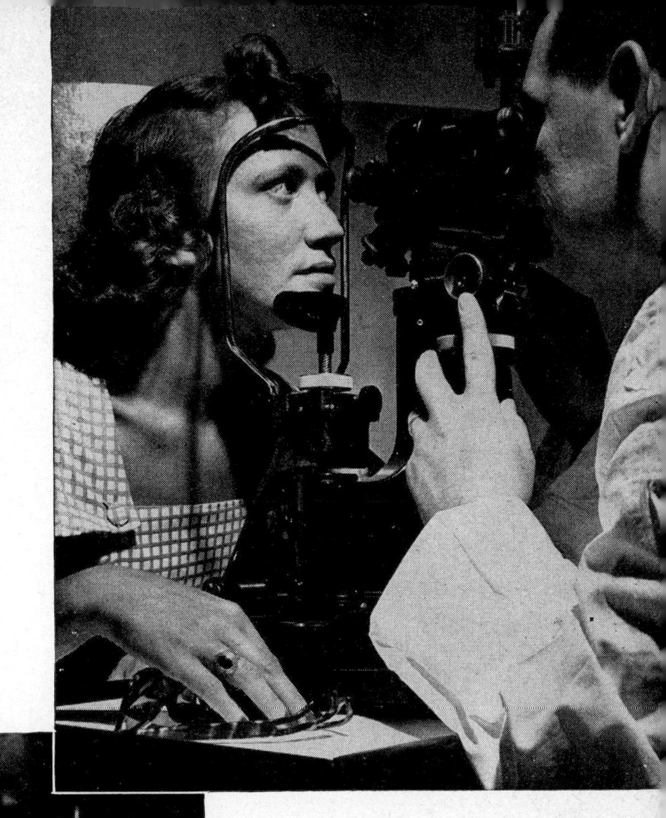

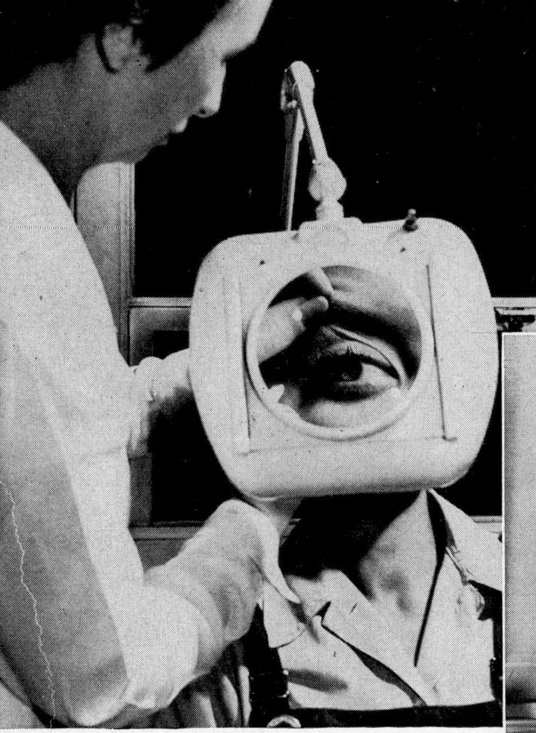

## MAGNIFYING THE EYE

If a foreign body is difficult to remove, see a doctor. To locate matter embedded in the eye, oculists use magnifiers like the one shown.

## HANDLE THE EYE WITH CARE

Hands must be clean, instruments must be sterile. Eye should not be rubbed.

## VALUABLE WEAPON

Radioactive materials, prepared by Atomic Energy Commission, are gaining importance in war on disease. Role of radioactive iodine is shown on chart.

U. S. Atomic Energy Commission

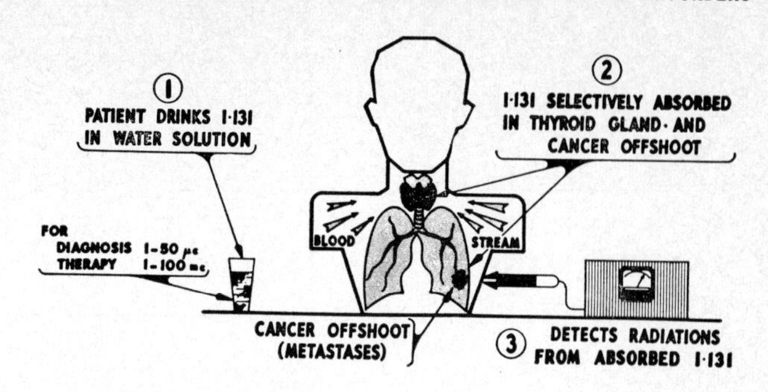


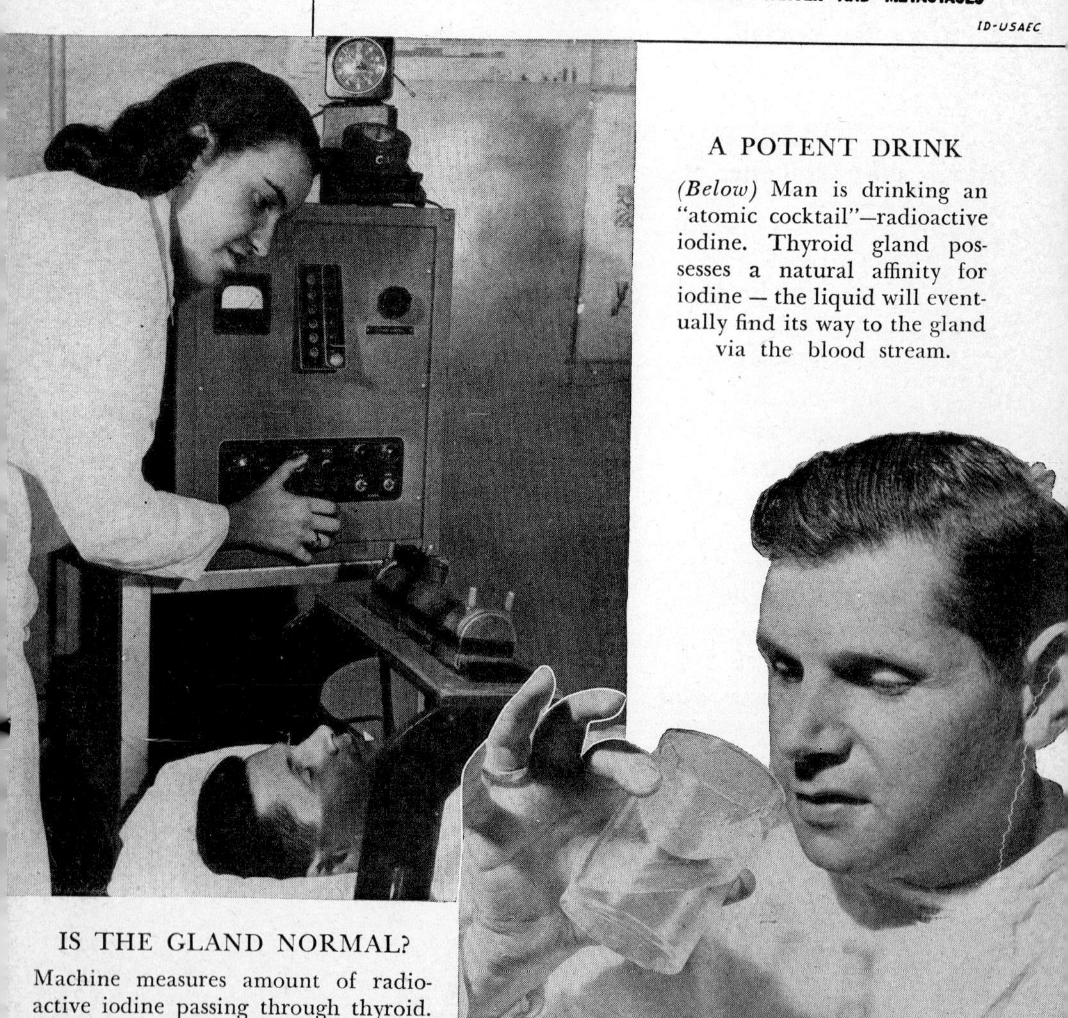

## A POTENT DRINK

*(Below)* Man is drinking an "atomic cocktail"—radioactive iodine. Thyroid gland possesses a natural affinity for iodine — the liquid will eventually find its way to the gland via the blood stream.

## IS THE GLAND NORMAL?

Machine measures amount of radioactive iodine passing through thyroid. This tells whether gland is healthy.

eye to catch the fluid. Test the temperature of the solution. Separate the lids with thumb and forefinger. Fill the bulb. Let the solution flow slowly and not forcibly over the eyeball, and irrigate it in a direction toward the temple. Don't permit the solution to drip over the bridge of the nose. Dry the lids with cotton, gently removing any discharge that may remain. Wipe the face around the eyes with damp cotton.

### Eye Drops

***How to Use Eye Drops.*** The patient lies in bed, with one pillow supporting his head. The shoulders are placed so that the head tilts backward. Wipe pus or other discharge away from the eye with sterile cotton moistened in sterilized water or solution. Draw the upper lid away from the eyeball. Request the patient to look downward, and drop the exact number of drops of solution under the upper lid. Don't touch the eyeball. Request the patient to close the eye in order to wash the eyeball. Wipe away dripping solution and tears with sterile cotton dampened with boiled water.

### Eye Ointments

Have the patient lie flat in bed, without pillows. Place the required amount of ointment on the tip of a sterile applicator. Draw the lid away from the eyeball, and the applicator along the margin of the lid. Direct application of the ointment can be made by placing it on the lining of the lower lid, closing the eye, and then gently massaging the eyelids and eyeball.

### Eye Compresses (Hot)

Scrub your hands before and after treatment. Prepare solution (2 per cent boric acid in sterile water). Have the patient lying down, and lubricate the area around the affected eye with sterile vaseline. Remove the compresses from hot solution (not too hot); wring them dry by twisting. Lay a pad gently on the eyelid. After removing the first, follow with a second moist pad. Continue treatment, alternating pads, for fifteen to twenty minutes.

### Eye Compresses (Cold)

Scrub your hands, as above. If discharge is present, use a compress only once. Use a firm but gentle touch, avoiding pressure on the eyeballs. Treatments should last not longer than twenty minutes, one hour apart. Have a tray covered with a clean towel, a half-dozen oval pads (2 x 1½ inches), dressings, bowl of ice (cover ice with gauze), face towel, cotton balls, solution, paper bag, safety pins, kidney-shaped basin if there is a discharge.

Place the patient at the edge of the bed, lying on his back. Remove all pillows except one, unless the patient has difficulty in breathing. Attach the paper bag to the bedside with a safety pin. Place a towel across the chest, and use clean cotton moistened in solution to remove any eye discharge present. Fold a compress once, moisten with solution, place on ice, and when thoroughly chilled, place on the eye. Change the compress every half-minute, and oftener if the patient has high temperature. Dry the eye and face.

## CHIEF SYMPTOMS OF EAR DISEASE

***Deafness.*** The most common symptom of ear disease is impaired hearing, which may vary from a degree so slight as to escape the patient's attention, to complete loss of hearing. Sudden deafness may be caused by a plug of wax in the ear canal or acute inflammation of the middle ear. Gradual deafness occurs in otosclerosis, which is discussed later in this chapter.

***Discharge.*** This is often a symptom of trouble in the middle ear. The pus in chronic middle-ear conditions is usually foul.

***Pain.*** This symptom may have varied causes. When the pain is caused by an inflammatory condition in the external ear, such as a boil, it is increased by pulling the external ear, by pressure in front of the ear, or by chewing. The pain of middle-ear inflammation is aggravated by any act such as sneezing, blowing the nose, or yawning. In inflammation of the mastoid bone, the pain is experienced back of the ear and is usually increased by pressure over the painful area. Pain in the ear caused by an ailment in another part of the body (for example, the teeth or face) is sometimes deceiving. The most common source is a decaying lower molar, an impacted wisdom tooth, or facial neuralgia.

***Noises in the Ear.*** This symptom is common, and may be the only one present in ear disease. It is also sometimes noted in valvular disease of the heart. What it means must be determined by a physician.

***Dizziness (Vertigo).*** This symptom is common in ear disease, but is equally noticeable in blood pressure changes and in diseases of the nervous system.

## FOREIGN BODIES IN THE EXTERNAL EAR CANAL

Avoid force or roughness in attempts to remove any object which has passed into the ear canal, or has been placed there. If gentle means for its removal are not successful, the patient should wait until the

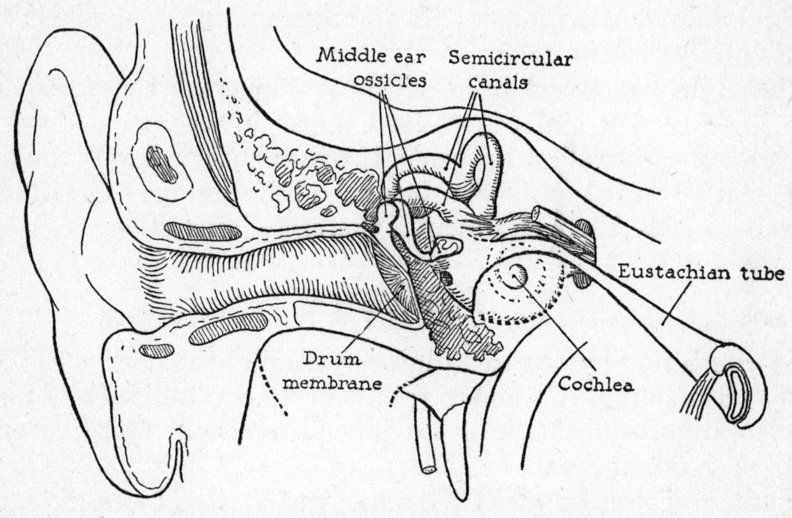


OUR HEARING APPARATUS

The visible part of the ear is only a small portion of the whole. From it a canal about an inch long extends into the head. A tight membrane, called the eardrum, is stretched across the deep end of the canal. Behind the drum is the middle ear chamber, in which there are the three tiny bones of hearing (ossicles). From the middle ear chamber, the Eustachian tube leads to the side of the throat. Deeper in the head is the inner ear. One part of it is called the cochlea. In it, the end of the nerve of hearing receives sounds from the outside.

services of a physician can be obtained. Such instruments as hairpins, roughly used, may set up serious complications and cause lasting injury.

Never use fluids if the foreign body is a dried pea or bean; it will swell, induce extreme pain, and be difficult to remove.

## ACUTE INFLAMMATION OF THE EARDRUM

***Causes and Symptoms of Acute Inflammation.*** This condition is caused by an acute infection of the middle ear. It is most common in infants and young children, especially after a cold. It also occurs as a complication of scarlet fever, measles, whooping cough and diphtheria. During the course of one of these diseases a child suddenly begins to complain of earache, or screams in distress, and there is a rise in temperature.

***Treatment of Acute Inflammation.*** In the early stages it is permissible to apply dry heat and to instill warm glycerin into the ear. If there is no quick lessening of pain and temperature, a physician must be consulted without delay.

When infection passes from the throat along the Eustachian tube to the middle ear, and pus collects there, it becomes necessary to pierce the drum to allow drainage. If treatment is delayed, the membrane may rupture spontaneously, or the infection may spread to the mastoid air cells. Early treatment is therefore imperative.

## EARACHE

Earache is usually due to an inflammation of the middle ear. This inflammation either subsides or results in the accumulation of inflammatory products until the drum is ruptured and discharge occurs from the external canal.

***Causes and Prevention of Earache.*** Any source of chronic catarrh of the nose or throat, such as enlarged and diseased tonsils, or adenoids in children, or nasal obstruction, favors the growth of germs. Germ-carrying fluid or secretions from the back of the nose may be forced up into the Eustachian tube, and thus into the middle ear, starting an inflammation there. The use of the nasal douche, the sniffing of water into the nose, violent blowing of the nose to get rid of secretion or fluid, or the use of the post-nasal syringe—all may be responsible for the beginning of an inflammation.

Swimming on the back, diving, and surf bathing also may endanger the ear, as cold water is forcibly driven not only into the external auditory canal, but—what is more frequently a source of damage—into the Eustachian tube through the nose or throat. In such cases plugging the nose with cotton would be of more value than plugging the external ear canal, as is commonly practiced. If water has entered the Eustachian tube, blowing the nose merely aggravates the trouble. The best plan is to do nothing, but trust that the water will drain out, and if pain ensues, treat it as recommended below.

Water in the ears is sometimes removed by jumping about on one foot with the troublesome ear held downward; and if the water is in the external canal, it may be wiped out gently with cotton securely wound on the end of a match.

To avoid inflammation of the ear, in the treatment of catarrh of the nose or throat, use only a spray from an atomizer. The solution may be made of common table salt.

***Symptoms of Middle-Ear Inflammation.*** In adults, the pain is severe, often excruciating. It may be felt over the temple, over the sides and back of the head and neck, and even in the lower teeth, as well as in the ear itself. This pain is increased by blowing the nose, coughing, and stooping. There is considerable tenderness on pressing the skin in front of the ear passage.

In infants there may be little evidence of pain in the ear, but they are apt to be fretful, to refuse food, and to cry out in their sleep. They often lie with the affected ear resting on the hand. Dullness, fever, chills and convulsions are not uncommon in children. On the other hand, after some slight illness, it is not infrequent for discharge from the ear to be the first sign which calls attention of the parent or nurse to the source of the illness.

***Dangers of Middle-Ear Inflammation.*** Although earache or middle-ear inflammation is common, its dangers are not fully appreciated. Common after-effects of acute inflammation are perforation of the eardrum and chronic discharge from the ear.

***Treatment of Earache.*** If the condition is an early one, you can warm glycerin slightly and instill several drops into the ear canal a few times each day. Dry heat, in the form of an electric pad, applied to the external ear, gives temporary relief. In case of severe or persistent earache, consult your physician.

## MASTOIDITIS

***Causes and Symptoms of Mastoiditis.*** The mastoid bone behind the ear sometimes becomes infected in the course of an ear infection. When this happens, there is a sudden fever, and there is pain behind the ear. Redness, tenderness, and swelling there are soon evident. If there has been an ear discharge, it may suddenly decrease in amount or cease altogether.

Mastoiditis demands prompt attention, because the mastoid bone is located near the brain, and is also closely connected with the jugular vein and the blood, which can also become infected.

***Treatment of Mastoiditis.*** Formerly, infections of the mastoid bone almost invariably required surgery. Nowadays, however, with the use of the sulfa drugs or penicillin early in the disease, the progress of infection may be stopped. But when the infection cannot be controlled by the use of drugs, it is necessary to remove the diseased part of the mastoid, by a relatively uncomplicated operation.

## DEFORMED EARS

Various congenital and acquired deformities of the external ear are corrected by plastic surgery. Children with markedly protruding ears, for example, are now physically and psychologically benefited through reconstructive surgery. A small piece of cartilage is removed from behind the ear, and the ears are set back against the head at the proper angle, thus improving the general appearance of the child.

## IMPACTED WAX

***Causes of Impacted Wax.*** The canal of the healthy ear needs no particular cleansing. One of the functions of the wax secreted by the glands there is to serve as a sticky protection against entrance of dust. The wax carries to the exit the accumulated material, the flow being maintained by the movement of the jaw. When this natural cleansing mechanism is defective, an accumulation of wax occurs, and hearing may be imperfect.

***Removing Impacted Wax.*** The ear is syringed with a lukewarm solution of bicarbonate of soda until the plug of wax comes away. When the wax is hard, considerable difficulty may be experienced in removing it; in these cases, especially if there is pain, a solution of bicarbonate of soda is dropped in several times before syringing, or a half eye-dropperful of peroxide of hydrogen may first be dropped into the ear to loosen the wax.

## INFLAMMATION OF THE EAR OPENING

The lining of the canal sometimes becomes inflamed, especially when it is scratched with a pin, hairpin, or toothpick. The symptoms are redness and swelling of the skin which lines the canal, and a thin discharge. The pain is often excruciating. It is increased by moving the jaw, as in chewing, and also by pulling the flap of the ear.

Hot compresses, applied according to your doctor's directions, may be necessary to relieve this condition.

## OTOSCLEROSIS

***Causes and Symptoms of Otosclerosis.*** The cause of otosclerosis is unknown. In this condition the patient hears subjective noises of various kinds—hissing, rushing noises, roaring, etc. A bony growth slowly closes the tiny window around the stirrup, a bone in the inner ear, and vibrations cannot reach the inner ear fluid. The auditory nerve inside is unaffected. There is gradual loss of hearing in both ears.

***Treatment of Otosclerosis.*** For persons afflicted with this kind of deafness, there is hope from an ear operation called the "fenestration operation." A new opening is drilled above the old window, and a small piece of cartilage taken from the outer ear is shaped and placed in the new opening. This serves as a new stirrup capable of transmitting sound vibrations to the inner ear.

## HYGIENE OF THE EAR

The following measures are helpful in the avoidance of ear infections:

1. Prevent, as far as possible, all infections of the nose and throat.
2. With children, especially, prevent, as far as possible, the communicable diseases of childhood, such as measles, scarlet fever, diphtheria, and whooping cough. These are frequently complicated by middle-ear disease, which may result in deafness or even in death.
3. Adenoids should be removed. When the adenoid tissue near the opening of the Eustachian tube becomes large and infected, it causes deafness by shutting off this opening, partly or completely.
4. Avoid diving in cold salt water. In all diving, the pressure of the water may force infectious material up the Eustachian tube. This is particularly true in salt-water diving, probably because the salt water clears the mucus from the nose and throat and opens the ventilating tube. Too much exposure to cold also causes ear disturbances at times.
5. Carefully remove excess wax from the ear canal. The wax that is secreted in the ear canal is a normal and useful product, but at times it increases to excess and requires removal to restore hearing. Do not use hairpins or other hard objects.
6. At the first sign of ear trouble, see a doctor.

Careful attention to the ear must be maintained throughout a head cold, an attack of croup, whooping cough, measles, or scarlet fever in infants and older children.

### How to Syringe the Ear

The ear may be syringed only under the instructions of a physician. Sterile salt-water solution of boric acid, warmed to a comfortable temperature (98° or 100° F.) should be used for syringing.

### How to Place Medicated Drops in the Ear

Among the drugs most commonly used for introduction into the ear canal are carbolized glycerin, peroxide of hydrogen in solution, and menthol in glycerin. The patient bends his head to one side, with the affected ear uppermost. The external ear is pulled upward and backward to straighten the ear canal, and about ten drops are instilled into the opening with a sterilized eye dropper. After the lapse of about five minutes the fluid is permitted to escape and the ear is dried.

CHAPTER 2

# THE NOSE, THROAT, AND MOUTH

**THE NOSE: Sinus Infection . . . Foreign Bodies in the Nose . . . Wounds . . . Inflammation of the Nostrils . . . Obstructions and Deformities . . . Nose Bleeds . . . Colds . . . Dry Nasal Catarrh . . . Allergy . . . Hay Fever . . . Polyps, etc. THE MOUTH: Mouth-Breathing . . . Inflammation of the Tongue and Mouth . . . "Cold Sores" . . . Thrush . . . Pyorrhea . . . Aveolar Abscess . . . Toothache . . . Halitosis . . . Mouth Hygiene . . . Diseases of the Lips, etc. THE THROAT: Foreign Bodies in the Throat . . . Bleeding . . . Tonsillitis . . . Adenoids . . . Pharyngitis . . . Chronic Post-Nasal Discharge . . . Septic Sore Throat . . . Quinsy . . . Trench Mouth . . . Ludwig's Angina . . . Laryngitis . . . False Croup . . . Diseases and Hygiene of the Larynx.**

## SINUS INFECTION

***Causes of Sinus Infection.*** The nasal sinuses are hollow spaces in the skull connected directly with the nasal cavity. There are eight sinuses, four on each side. They are connected with each other. These spaces are covered by an extension of the nasal mucous lining, which is moist and well-supplied with blood vessels. Infection anywhere in the nasal mucous membrane proper is likely to extend into these air spaces. Consequently, there is danger that in the course of a severe head cold the infection will involve the sinuses. Sinusitis due to an allergy is very similar to that due to bacterial infections.

In children, the great predisposing factor is the diet. It is presumed by some authorities that diets deficient in fat-soluble vitamins predispose to the infection. Cod-liver oil, therefore, is helpful in preventing sinus infection.

***Symptoms of Sinus Infection.*** Sinus disease may be limited to one air space, or it may involve two or three, or the whole group on both sides, at the same time or at different times. The symptoms vary in degree depending upon the variety and severity of the infection, the particular sinus or sinuses and the size of the area affected, and the amount of drainage or opportunity for the discharge to be gotten rid of.

The main symptoms of sinus disease are nasal obstruction and a profuse discharge of pus and mucus from the nose. Other annoying symptoms are sneezing, itching of the nose, dryness and ulceration.

When the normal opening of a sinus becomes blocked, the symptoms become more intense, because of the pressure of the fluid that is not drained off. Nasal obstruction may be almost complete. If the frontal sinus is involved, there is more or less frontal headache. A throbbing or bursting feeling over the eyebrows is a frequent complaint. The nasal discharge is more or less constant, especially in the morning. When the infection invades the sinus within the cheekbone, pain in the face and eye are often excruciating. There is headache and a burning sensation in the cheek.

***Diagnosis of Sinus Infection.*** The diagnosis of sinus disease is made by examination of the nose, X-rays, and passing light through the affected area, as well as by the symptoms. Sinus disease should be considered if a cold lasts longer than a fortnight, particularly where there are fever, pain, chills, swelling, etc.

***Treatment of Sinus Infection.*** Certain general principles hold good in the treatment. The maintenance of an even temperature in the sick room is always best. Unless fever is present, confinement to bed is not always necessary. The medical treatment of acute infection of the sinuses is that of any local inflammatory condition within the nose. Heat should be applied, preferably with an electric pad. Penicillin and the sulfonamides may be used to control the infection. These can be obtained only by doctor's prescription. Drugs for the relief of pain are frequently required. The best drug for this purpose is empirin. This is harmless. It can be taken as often as one tablet every two to three hours over a period of one or two days. Ephedrine sprays and warm irrigations (given gently, without force) are beneficial.

The vitamin C intake should be maintained at a high point. The diet depends upon the general condition of the patient. After the acute inflammation subsides, any deformities inside the nose which interfere with breathing or drainage should be corrected, by surgery if necessary.

## FOREIGN BODIES IN THE NOSE

These may obstruct the nasal passages by their presence as well as by the secondary irritation which they cause. They are most likely to be found in children whose curiosity often takes the form of pushing objects into the nostrils or ears. The objects most frequently inserted are small articles used in their games—such as pencil erasers, buttons, pebbles, beads, peas, beans, etc. If the right hand was used, the foreign body will usually be found on the floor of the right nasal cavity against the outer wall.

If the foreign object has been in the nose for a long time, a persistent discharge, sometimes bloody and ill-smelling is noticeable.

The treatment, obviously, is removal of the object, preferably with an object that curves at the end. If there is difficulty, consult a doctor.

## WOUNDS OF THE NOSE

When the wound is a simple one, clean it by washing it with tincture of green soap and water. Cold compresses may be applied to

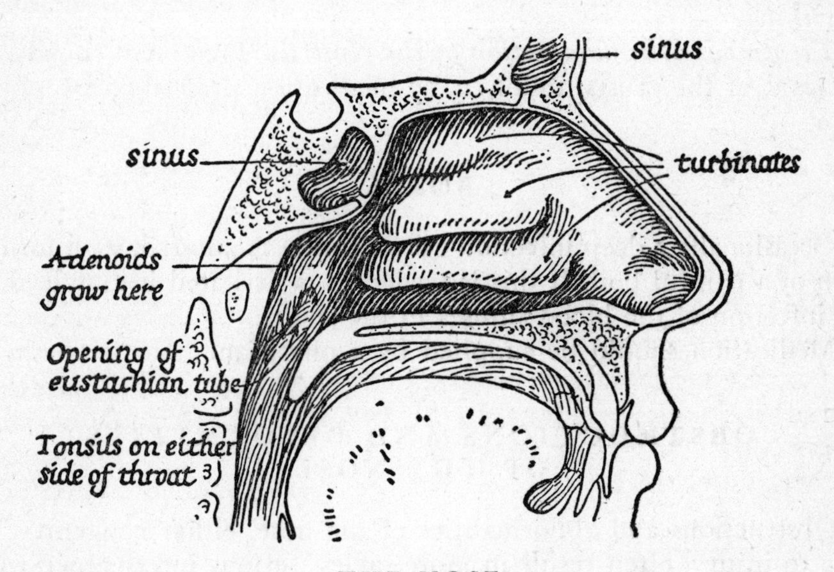


THE NOSE

The nasal cavity is divided throughout by a flat partition, called the septum, extending from the point of the nose to the back of the throat. Each half of the passage has three shelf-like projections, called the turbinates, extending inward from the cheeks toward the middle partition. Above the nasal passages (near the eyes), and in back of the passages, and at the sides (under the cheek bones) are three sets of cells in the skull bone itself. These are called sinuses. They lighten the weight of the skull bone, they help to warm the air we breathe in, and they give resonance to the voice.

stop the bleeding, and small compresses of cotton inserted into the nose to stop oozing from within. When it dries, bring the edges of the wound together with adhesive strips, and then cover with cotton and collodion. Remove the dressing after twenty-four hours, and apply a new one.

Ragged wounds which extend deeply over a large surface require special medical attention, as there is likely to be an associated injury inside the nose. The wound should be dusted with one of the sulfonamide powders. If the wound is contaminated with soil, tetanus antitoxin should be given.

## INFLAMMATION OF THE NOSTRILS

***Cause and Symptoms.*** This is often the result of a prolonged nasal discharge, which causes redness, chafing, and splitting of the skin in and around the nostril. Crusts which form may obstruct nasal breathing.

***Treatment of Inflammation of the Nostrils.*** Treatment consists in removal of the crusts, followed by medication prescribed by physician.

## BOILS

Occasionally a deep infection occurs inside the nostril, with formation of a painful boil. If this is neglected or irritated it may lead to an infection of the blood sinuses in the skull.

Medication should be supplied by a physician.

## OBSTRUCTIONS AND DEFORMITIES OF THE NOSE

Obstructions and abnormalities of the nose, either congenital or due to injury, often result in more or less serious interference with breathing and the necessary conditioning of air passing through the nose. This interference may bring on a chain of physical and mental ills. The senses of taste and smell may be impaired. There may be sinus trouble, and lung disease later on.

For example, in older children, obstruction may prevent the normal development of the face, palate, and jaws. The eventual result of prolonged interference is that the normal development of the child's chest may be retarded; the chest becomes flat and the shoulders rounded.

Incidentally, the degree of obstruction of the nose in infants and older children can sometimes be determined by holding a small piece of cotton wool under the nostrils and observing whether or not it moves in the air current from the nose.

***Distorted Septum.*** A cause of nasal obstruction of varying degree is the broken, bent, or misshapen septum. This condition is commonly caused by injury—a broken nose, for example—or a child may be born with the disability.

The distorted septum may, in turn, cause enlargement of the turbinates. These swell and further increase the nasal obstruction. When the condition becomes chronic, the turbinates, through prolonged irritation, finally remain enlarged and press on the septum, blocking the incoming air current.

An abnormally long nose, a nose with a twisted tip, a depressed nose, and deformed nasal cartilages all may interfere with proper breathing. These deformities deflect the course of the air currents. Spurs or slight projections on the septum and other irregularities in structure which may not cause marked obstruction may still turn aside the air currents in such a way as to make normal breathing through the nose difficult.

Obstruction of the nasal air passages may also be caused by foreign bodies, by tumors, by polyps, by fracture of the turbinates or of the nasal bones or cartilages, by hemorrhage, or by catarrh (chronic inflammation of the membranes of the nose) with sticky secretions, and by excessive blood in the mucous membrane.

***How Obstruction Varies.*** There may be a sense of blockage on one side of the nose, or an obstruction that is felt on alternate sides. This is particularly noticeable when a person lies down. If only one nasal passage is obstructed, the consequences are usually not serious, although ear infections may result. Mouth breathing occurs when the passages on both sides of the nose are completely barred. Infants find difficulty in sucking milk or in taking in other food, and there is the constant danger of drawing in some foreign substance. Older persons, however, learn to adapt to this condition so that they have little difficulty in eating and breathing at the same time.

***Treatment.*** Any abnormality or deformity of the nose calls for prompt treatment. Often this consists of minor surgery, either inside or outside the nose, or both. The remedy is complete. If the nose is ugly, as well as dangerous to the health, plastic surgery will make it attractive.

## NOSE BLEEDS

Bleeding from the nose may be due to a great number of causes, the chief of which are injury, accident or surgery. When bleeding follows injury, it usually stops after a short time. Spontaneous bleeding may occur at any age.

***Nose Bleed in Infants and Children.*** Ordinarily, nose bleed is caused by local irritation or congestion, a blow, a fall on the nose, or irritation of the mucous membrane induced by picking the nose. A foreign body is sometimes the cause of recurrent bleeding. Nasal diphtheria, polyps, and adenoids may also be the cause of nasal bleeding in infants.

Nose bleed is a much more common symptom in older children. The condition may be an early symptom of many diseases, such as typhoid, pneumonia, scarlet fever, measles, and other infectious diseases. Frequently it is an early symptom of rheumatic fever or congenital syphilis. Certain blood diseases may be the cause.

***Nose Bleed in the Old.*** In people with high blood pressure, nasal bleeding is often a safety valve. However, *recurrent* nose bleeding, in those past middle age, should be thoroughly investigated—particularly if it is accompanied by one-sided obstruction—because the symptoms may indicate malignant tumors within the nose.

***Treatment of Nose Bleed.*** In the treatment of slight or moderate nose bleed, the patient should in all instances immediately be made to lie down. Ice may be applied over the nose or at the back of the neck. Turn the patient sideways. Pinch the nose with the finger and thumb for a few minutes. This will cause a clot to form and block the bleeding blood vessel.

Slight hemorrhage may be treated first by searching for the bleeding point. This is usually in the front part of the nasal septum. After the bleeding point has been found, moisten a cotton plug with adrenalin chloride in a 1:1000 solution, which can be obtained at any drug store. Place it against the bleeding point and let it remain for a few minutes. After the bleeding stops, the patient should be cautioned against forcibly blowing his nose.

In severe hemorrhage a physician should be called.

## THE COMMON COLD

Someone has labeled the common cold "Public Malady No. 1." The common cold is indeed the commonest of all diseases of the respiratory system. It is an acute inflammation of the nasal mucous membranes, marked by signs and symptoms throughout the body. It frequently has temporary or lasting complications.

Popularly, any infection and acute inflammation of the upper respiratory system is called a cold. It must be kept in mind, however, that almost all of the communicable diseases of infancy and childhood—for example, measles, scarlet fever, whooping cough, diphtheria, and tonsillitis—may at first show symptoms suggestive of a cold. Everyone knows that sneezing spells may usher in a cold in the head, hay fever, or infectious childhood diseases. Sinus infections, particularly during their flare-ups, are likely to be referred to as colds. Allergy to foods and to various inhalants may produce the symptoms of a cold because of changed tension of the blood vessels of the nose.

***The Cold Virus.*** The common cold is primarily caused by what is known as a filterable virus. This agent of infectious disease, chemical or living, is so small that it cannot be discovered by ordinary microscopic means. Since it can pass through certain filters it is called filterable. The virus is highly contagious and is spread by coughing, sneezing or kissing.

When a cold virus infects the lining of the nose it weakens the natural defenses by interfering with the activity of the cilia and the secretion of mucus. Bacteria then have a favorable environment. They induce sneezing, nasal obstruction, nasal discharge, headache, temperature, and a sense of fatigue. The nasal infection sometimes spreads. It may spread up into the sinuses or downward into the throat or lungs, or both. It may spread into the Eustachian tube to the middle ear, carrying a potential injury to hearing, to the mastoid bone and even to the lining membranes of the brain, thereby causing meningitis. While the common cold *per se* is rarely a cause of death it may bring on such serious infections as pneumonia.

***Conditions Favoring the Common Cold.*** Infections of the respiratory system are more common in winter than in summer. This is perhaps due to the fact that people are more likely to stay indoors during cold weather and are therefore in closer contact with each other. This favors the distribution of disease germs.

Almost every susceptible person who is in immediate contact with an infected person will contract the disease. The immunity gained is ordinarily of short duration; consequently it is possible for one individual to have a number of attacks of the infection each year. Another reason why the common cold is so prevalent is its relative mildness. The disease as a rule is so mild that infected persons often continue at their usual occupations, thus spreading the infection to others.

***Chills and Drafts.*** Colds are usually attributed to a chill because they are frequently ushered in by a sensation of being chilly. Actually, there is no scientific proof that exposure to chills and drafts causes colds in healthy persons who have not been exposed to infection. It is known, for example, that those exposed to arctic conditions, such as sailors and fishermen, do not readily catch colds and pneumonia.

Epidemics of colds are most common when atmospheric humidity is great, and the temperature is cool but variable; when the weather is raw, with thawing snow and sleet; or winds blow with cold rain, and the ground is wet and cold. However, cold dry weather and strong dry winds do not provide favorable conditions for epidemics of infections of the upper respiratory system.

***Bad Ventilation.*** Bad ventilation is a common predisposing cause. It produces lowered resistance in the nasal and respiratory membranes, which is not so likely to occur in persons living open-air lives. Bad weather, as previously stated, drives or keeps people indoors. Windows are kept shut, and infection is thus spread. People in passing suddenly from overheated rooms into cold air put a strain on the functions of the respiratory mucous membranes.

In general the predisposing factors in the case of the common cold are physical fatigue, damp clothing, sudden changes in atmospheric pressure, poor ventilation, nasal obstruction, susceptibility, and certain occupations.

***Cold Symptoms.*** The onset of a common cold is usually sudden. There is a sensation of dryness, burning and itching in the nose and nasal pharynx, and sometimes in the larynx, with hoarseness, even loss of voice, and a dry spasmodic cough. The sense of nasal stuffiness compels breathing through the mouth. Bodily symptoms are usually confined to headache, generalized pains in the limbs, especially the knees, and a general feeling of illness, with more or less fever. Within twelve to twenty-four hours the initial suppression of nasal secretion gives place to a profuse watery flow, with sniffling and sneezing. Smell, taste and hearing are impaired in varying degrees.

***Cold Symptoms in Children.*** Infections of the nose and throat, or those of the rest of the upper respiratory tract, are extremely common during childhood. They are a common factor in the production of many of the minor, and some of the major, diseases of infancy and childhood. Infants incubating the common cold are fretful and sleepy. An initial vomiting is often alarming to the mother or nurse. There is fever, accompanied by headache and loss of appetite. Older children complain of pain in the throat and in the chest. Nose breathing is obstructed. There is a profuse, watery discharge at the nostrils, and at first a dry cough.

***Cold Complications.*** In children there are many complications, as previously stated, and many consequences of the common cold. In adults, perhaps the most frequent after-effect is acute ear trouble, sometimes going on to abscess formation. The nasal sinuses are usually more or less involved in all colds. Laryngitis, broncho-pneumonia, infection and swelling of the glands in the neck, acute tonsillitis, abscess around the tonsil or in the wall of the throat, and acute rheumatic fever are not infrequent complications.

***Cold Prevention.*** The best method of prevention is to avoid contact with infected persons and to stay away from crowded places. Surgical removal or correction of conditions which predispose to acute respiratory disease is frequently helpful. These include infected tonsils, infected sinuses, enlarged adenoids, and the various causes of nasal obstruction, such as deformities, deflected septums, enlarged turbinates, spurs and polyps.

***Cold Treatment.*** There is actually no sure way to cure a cold. The principal treatment consists of relieving the local discomfort. Aspirins are helpful, and the bowels should be moved regularly. Rest plays an important part in raising the resistance, and so does a well-balanced diet. Fruit juices and water should be drunk in abundance. When the larynx is involved, absolute rest of the voice is essential.

If an infant or older child has a cold, he should be put to bed with a hot water bottle. The room should be warm, and hot baths and hot drinks, as well as alkalis, are helpful.

***Antihistamine Drugs for Colds.*** Many people assert that the use of antihistamine drugs—as for example, benadryl, pyribenzamine, and chlortrimeton—in small doses for a short period of time is effective in the treatment of colds. It is declared that the cold can be avoided or controlled if a few doses are taken beginning within an hour or two after the appearance of the first symptoms. However, this is still an unsettled subject, and it must be remembered that some persons experience ill effects from taking the antihistamine drugs.

## CHRONIC RHINITIS

***Causes and Symptoms of Chronic Rhinitis.*** Chronic inflammation of the membrane lining the nose is common. It is usually caused by long-standing attacks of the common cold, especially among workers constantly exposed to dusty or damp atmospheres and other irritants. The main symptoms are nasal obstruction and change in the character of the secretions, which ordinarily become thick and scanty. There is usually deflection or deformity of the nasal septum, with impairment of the senses of smell and taste. Mouth breathing due to nasal obstruction becomes more or less constant, especially at night. The patient complains of dryness of the mouth and throat. Coughing, sneezing, and alteration of the tone of the voice are common symptoms.

***Treatment of Chronic Rhinitis.*** Treatment is largely a matter of removing excess tissue, and restoring unimpeded nasal breathing.

## DRY NASAL CATARRH

***Causes and Symptoms.*** Disease may cause progressive wasting away of the mucous membrane of the nose and throat, and sometimes of the underlying bone. This is usually disclosed through extensive formation of crusts, discharge of a sticky secretion, and excessive width of the nasal airways. Often there is a repellent odor. Causes are both local and general. Sometimes surgical injury is responsible. The disease often extends into the larynx and to the middle ear. The sense of smell, in time, is completely lost because of the destruction of the cells of the lining of the nose and obstruction of the nose cavities by foul, greenish crusts and excessive secretion.

***Treatment of Dry Nasal Catarrh.*** Various treatments are used for the disease, but an actual cure is rare.

## NASAL ALLERGY (ALLERGIC RHINITIS)

***Causes of Nasal Allergy.*** Of the many factors which are responsible for nasal allergy, the following are the most common: drugs, food, pollens, cosmetics, linens, silks, dust, dander from horses and dogs, furs, feathers and hair, local irritation, heat stimuli, deficiency of blood calcium, intestinal toxemia, glandular disturbances, certain phenomena of climate, and any other agents which produce allergies.

As a cause of respiratory allergy, ordinary house dust is generally considered of basic importance. Next are such specific factors as may be present in feathers, cotton, wool, kapok, etc. Of secondary influence are certain occupational and environmental dusts, such as the dust in grain elevators and stables. Some authorities consider dusts to be the cause of respiratory allergy in 90 per cent of patients.

Among foods that cause attacks of nasal allergy, melons, for example, and strawberries, raspberries, cucumbers, and cherries are commonly responsible. Often the same variety of reaction occurs from eating crab, lobster, or other shellfish; and sometimes from pork, as well as from a number of common foods which are not well tolerated.

***How Allergies are Classified.*** Stated simply, nasal allergy or allergic rhinitis may be divided into three varieties: (1) seasonal; (2) perennial, with positive skin tests; (3) perennial, with negative skin tests.

In seasonal allergic rhinitis, symptoms are caused by the breathing in of pollen. They are limited to the seasons when the specific plant to which the patient is sensitive pollinates.

In perennial allergic rhinitis, a person shows all the signs and symptoms common to the seasonal variety, but these are felt all year round, constantly or in repeated attacks, and are brought on by sensitivity to a number of substances in the air or in food. The group of people afflicted throughout the year usually give positive skin tests showing that an allergy is present.

The perennial allergic rhinitis group that give negative skin tests possess a definite immunity. In a large proportion of cases, those in the first two groups give clear evidence of a hereditary tendency and reveal other signs and symptoms of allergy (asthma, for instance); those in the third group generally present only nasal symptoms.

***Symptoms of Nasal Allergy.*** The person who suffers from this variety of rhinitis appears to have a constant head cold. Spells of sneezing on arising in the morning are followed by a profuse watery nasal discharge. There is obstruction to nasal breathing, a dull headache, and a feeling in the ears as though the ear canals were blocked with cotton wool. Speech is nasal, as if uttered through the nose. The condition is often associated with asthma. These symptoms vary considerably in different persons, both in degree and duration.

The common cold is always present as a possibility, and may temporarily hide the signs and symptoms of allergy. Repeated observations may therefore be necessary to determine the precise nature of the infection. For an accurate diagnosis, the following factors must be kept in mind: (1) the nasal, sinus, and bronchial symptoms; (2) conditions discovered on examination of the nose; (3) composition of nasal and bronchial secretions; (4) information obtained by X-ray examination; (5) bacteriologic data; and (6) skin tests. Nasal allergy is common in children, and the attacks of sneezing and nasal obstruction may lead to the diagnosis of an infectious cold. It must be remembered, however, that infection and allergy may occur at the same time.

***Treatment of Nasal Allergy.*** In general, the treatment is the same as for hay fever, which follows.

## HAY FEVER

This is a condition, not purely nasal, in which a person shows excessive sensitiveness to the pollen or germ cells of the male plant of certain flowers and trees, and especially to grasses. Hay fever is primarily a seasonal, summer or fall, disease, which occurs most often in young adults and children. It may be associated with a neurotic tendency. Heredity appears to play a part. It is often considered a form of nasal allergy. In hay fever victims, the mucous membrane lining of the nose and upper respiratory system has a particularly high degree of sensitivity.

***Varieties of Hay Fever.*** There are two common varieties of hay fever: that of early summer, brought about by an allergy to June grass and timothy; and the more frequent autumnal form produced by sensitiveness to ragweed, or a combination of ragweed and other pollens.

In the Eastern part of the United States, three varieties of seasonal hay fever occur. (1) The spring form begins at the end of March or early in April and extends to the end of May. It is caused almost exclusively by pollens from trees, especially oak, hickory, maple, birch, and elm. (2) The second, or summer, variety beginning at the end of May and extending to the middle of July, is ordinarily caused by the pollen of grasses. The important pollens in this group are redtop, timothy, June grass, orchard grass, sweet vernal, and plantain. (3) The third, or fall, variety begins in the middle of August and continues until frost. The pollen of the ragweed is mainly responsible for this group.

***Results of Hay Fever.*** Children and adults who have suffered from perennial nasal allergy during early childhood often show nasal depressions which make the nose unduly prominent, a V-shaped palate, and marked overriding of the teeth. A child with nasal allergy frequently becomes a nose-rubber or a nose-wrinkler, or both, because of uncomfortable itching of the nasal mucous membrane. If such a habit begins in early life and continues over a period of years the result is often a distorted nose. This effect upon the features, however, is quite different from that caused by adenoids, with the characteristic pinched appearance of the nose, the prominence of the upper incisor teeth, and the abnormal mouth and lower jaw.

***Treatment of Hay Fever.*** Treatment includes: elimination of the cause or causes and desensitization. If the particular substances causing the allergy can be discovered, they should be avoided, whenever possible. A change of residence to a pollen-free area, filtered-air rooms, air-conditioned living quarters, and an ocean voyage are all helpful for the relief of symptoms. If this is not practical, the process called desensitization should be carried out. There are two plans of treatment: the preseasonal and the perennial or all-year-round plan. In both, small doses of the sensitizing agents are injected.

A number of drugs (especially benadryl and pyribenzamine, both of which may be taken internally in tablet form) have been found effective in many allergic conditions. However, these drugs are not panaceas, and frequently cause unpleasant after-effects, such as marked dizziness and groggyness. A single application of pyribenzamine nasal solution from a fine-spray atomizer often brings quick relief from allergic nasal congestion. Relief is obtained for a number of hours or days but the effect is not lasting.

There is no particular locality in which the patient suffering from the spring or summer variety of hay fever may be certain of complete relief, except on the ocean. Patients suffering from the autumnal variety can avoid the attacks in the White Mountains, in Florida, on the coast of Maine, in California, or in Europe.

## NASAL POLYPS

Nasal polyps are projecting masses of swollen mucous membrane. They form slowly; consequently they are usually found in adult life. Varying greatly in size and number, they appear as grayish and gelatinous tumors.

***Symptoms of Nasal Polyps.*** The main symptoms are those caused by nasal obstruction. Many sufferers complain that their symptoms vary with the humidity in the air. The pressure of polyps against the septum may produce severe neuralgia, especially across the bridge of the nose and above or below the eyes. Loss of the sense of smell is a frequent symptom.

***Treatment of Polyps.*** The treatment consists of early recognition of the condition and surgical removal of the mass or masses. A polyp that is not treated tends to grow gradually larger.

## RHINOPHYMA

***Cause and Symptoms of Rhinophyma.*** This is also called "potato nose" and "whisky nose"—though addiction to alcohol has no relation to the disease. Early in the disease, the blood vessels become dilated, with a resultant increase in the blood supply. This causes an overproduction of connective tissue, which in the course of time produces lumpy areas, leaving the nose swollen. The cause is unknown. This condition is much more common in men than in women and appears usually in middle or later life.

***Treatment of Rhinophyma.*** Plastic surgery is, in general, the only way to treat rhinophyma effectively, once it is well developed.

## HYGIENE OF THE NOSE

The mucous membrane of the nose is particularly sensitive to atmospheric changes. Temperature, humidity, prevailing winds, sunshine, and dust—all have their specific effects. For this reason change of climate is frequently adequate treatment in nose disorders.

Exposure of the body to sunlight or to other forms of light is also of benefit, as is keeping up one's general physical condition. Those who work in the open air are in the main remarkably free from respiratory disease. It is obvious, therefore, that these diseases are the result of indoor life, of overheated surroundings, and infections from "carriers" of various types of germs.

Many industrial occupations cause disease of the respiratory system. Those who suffer from constant colds should in general avoid certain occupations which involve harmful dusts—for example, file cutting, glass and metal grinding and polishing, stone cutting, painting, paper-hanging, woodworking, typesetting, gilding, etc.

***Protecting Children Against Colds.*** Prevention of the common cold should begin at birth. In infants, because of the shape and character of their nasal cavities, infections are not easily confined to one area. There is therefore great risk of spread to the bronchial tubes. The child should be protected from colds, especially during the first few months. Even before that, prenatal treatment should be given to a mother suffering from a persistent infection of the upper air passages. If she has a cold, while she is nursing her infant or attending to it, she should wear a mask or a folded handkerchief over her nose and mouth. Visitors suffering from colds should be excluded. Children should be taught the value of fresh air.

Overdressing should be avoided. One should keep in mind the possible danger arising from a so-called common cold, which may be a forerunner of pneumonia and other serious complications. Tonsils and adenoids, if diseased, should be removed. Rooms should not be heated above 70°F., and a humidity of 40 per cent is desirable.

***How to Blow the Nose.*** Children must be taught how to blow the nose. They should be instructed, first of all, never to blow too forcibly; to blow down one nostril (with the mouth open), while the other is held tightly closed. The process is then reversed. Most people blow their noses improperly, and in this way ear infection is often caused.

## NOSE DROPS AND NASAL IRRIGATIONS

There are any number of medicines used for nasal conditions. Some are useful, and others are not. They may even be actually harmful. They include medicines to contract the blood vessels in the nose, medicines to dilate them, silver preparations, antiseptics, oils, volatile inhalants, and vaccines. The use of nose drops and sprays for the relief of nasal diseases has become widespread. Many contain a harmful oily base. Use nose drops only with great caution. Do not buy any such medicaments unless they are recommended by your physician.

***How to Administer Nose Drops to an Infant.*** Hold the infant on your lap, with his head low. A few minutes after the drops have been inserted with a dropper, turn the child face downward to permit the nasal contents to flow from the nostrils. In this procedure the solution does not enter the throat and is not breathed into the lungs. The drops should be non-oily. Mineral oil is irritating to the lining of the respiratory system. When it is instilled in the nose, it often gets down into the lung, and in infants or in the elderly may cause a certain variety of pneumonia.

***How to Use Nose Drops with Older Children.*** Have the child lie on his side, with his head low. A pillow under the shoulder makes it easier. The drops are inserted with a dropper. The child then lies on his abdomen, and in this way drainage of the nasal contents is assured.

***How to Use Nose Drops for Adults.*** One of two methods may be used. In the first, the drops are instilled while the patient lies on his back, with his head well extended over the edge of the bed. In the other, the patient lies on the side with the head extended toward the lower shoulder as far as possible. The solution is dropped into the lower part of the nostril and permitted to remain for a few moments.

***Care Must Be Exercised.*** Salt-water and other lotions should be used with the greatest caution. No forcible syringing should ever be done in the nose, because the fluid used may be forced beyond the nose into the sinuses and the Eustachian tube, with disastrous results.

Too frequent use of antiseptics injures the nasal lining. An antiseptic strong enough to sterilize the nasal cavity is too strong for this lining membrane. Plain water, on the other hand, must never be used. The only case in which douching is justifiable is in a type of inflammation of the lining of the nose called atrophic. Douching is then necessary for the removal of ill-smelling crusts. The cilia are already destroyed in this disease, and douching can therefore do no harm.

## HOW TO USE STEAM INHALATIONS AND SPRAYS

Steam inhalations are helpful in many acute infections in the nose and throat. Pour a pint of steaming, but not boiling, water into a vaporizer, and add a teaspoonful of medication. Compound tincture of benzoin is helpful, or a few drops of a 20-30 per cent solution of menthol. A special inhaler may be used, with a thermometer to mark the correct temperature of the water, which should be 140°F. The water should be left standing for a few minutes before adding the medicine. When the solution is gently steaming, the patient applies his mouth not too close to the nozzle and inhales the vaporized medication for a minute or two, having previously protected his eyes with a towel or cloth.

***How to Spray the Nose.*** Wash the atomizer with warm water and soap. Use a bottle brush to clean it. Place in cool water and bring the water to a boil for ten minutes. Cool the atomizer and fill it half full with the solution prescribed by your physician. Then spray the nose for a fraction of a minute.

## MOUTH-BREATHING

***Causes of Mouth-Breathing.*** In children, the most important disorder producing mouth-breathing is enlargement of the glandular tissue or adenoids in the back of the nose. They often block the air passage in these areas so completely that breathing through the nose becomes difficult. Associated with this condition are enlarged tonsils. Inflammation of these organs often occurs during the course of contagious diseases, such as scarlet fever, measles, or diphtheria; probably, also, it is induced by constant exposure to a germ-laden atmosphere, as in the case of children herded together in crowded tenements.

The adenoids cannot be readily seen because of their position, but we can be reasonably sure of their inflammation in children when we find symptoms resulting from mouth-breathing. The surgeon finds the adenoids by putting his finger up back of the roof of the patient's mouth, where they may be felt as a soft mass filling the back of the nasal passages, or he can view them with a throat mirror.

Other less common causes of mouth-breathing, seen in adults as well as children, are deviations of the nasal septum, swelling of the mucous membrane covering certain bones in the nose, and polyps (growths arising from the surface of a mucous membrane and attached to it by a stalk-like process).

***Deviations of the Septum.*** Deviations of the septum are displacements of the partition dividing the two nasal cavities, so that the cavities are more or less obstructed. This condition may be brought on by blows on the nose received in accidents such as are common in childhood. The resulting deformity leads in time to further obstruction in the nose. This brings over-filling of the blood vessels in the walls of the nasal passages. Continued congestion is followed by increased thickness of the lining mucous membrane, making the entrance of air still more difficult.

***Symptoms of Mouth-Breathing.*** Mouth-breathing is more noticeable during sleep, when snoring is common. The breathing is of a snorting character, with prolonged pauses. Children suffering from enlarged tonsils and adenoids are often backward in their studies. They appear dull and stupid, and are often cross and sullen. The mouth remains open, and the lower lip is rolled down and prominent. The nose has a pinched aspect. The roof of the mouth is high.

***Effects of Mouth-Breathing.*** Because the air that is breathed in through the mouth is not first warmed, moistened, and cleared of dust by passing through the nose, but goes almost directly into the windpipe, constant colds, chronic catarrh of the throat, laryngitis, or bronchitis may result. The constant irritation of the throat also weakens natural resistance against such diseases as acute tonsillitis, scarlet fever, and diphtheria. But these are not the only ailments to which the mouth-breather is liable, for earache and deafness may follow because of obstruction of the Eustachian tubes.

Deformity of the chest is another result, the common form being the "pigeon breast," where the breastbone is unduly prominent. The voice is altered so that the patient, as the saying goes, "talks through the nose," although, in fact, nasal resonance is reduced.

In this condition stuttering is common. Obstruction of the nose may lead to poor nutrition, and hence children with adenoids and enlarged tonsils are apt to be puny and weak.

***Treatment of Mouth-Breathing.*** The treatment in all examples of obstruction of the nose is purely surgical: removal of the adenoid growths, enlarged tonsils, or polyps; straightening of the displaced nasal septum, or treatment of the thickened mucous lining obstructing the air passages in the nose. These operations are not dangerous if skillfully performed, and should in general be carried out, even in the case of delicate children. The after-treatment is important. The patient should have a simple, generous diet (plenty of milk, bread and butter, green vegetables and fresh meat), with avoidance of pastries, sweets, fried food, pork, salt fish, salt meats, root vegetables, such as parsnips, turnips, carrots and beets, and tea and coffee. Plenty of fresh air, vitamin D, daily sponging with cold water while the patient stands in warm water, followed by vigorous rubbing, will all assist in return to health.

## INFLAMMATION OF THE TONGUE

In inflammation of the tongue and mouth caused by deficiency of nicotinic acid (vitamin B group), the tip and sides of the tongue are fiery red and swollen, and ulcers form on the tongue and lining of the mouth. Nicotinic acid may be given by mouth.

## ULCERATION OF THE TONGUE

This may be caused by decaying or uneven teeth, tuberculous and syphilitic ulcers and hard cancerous ulcers. It requires prompt treatment by a doctor.

## EPULIS

This is a small, soft tumor of the gum which commonly grows opposite the roots of decayed teeth. Treatment consists of removal of the growth by a physician or dentist.

## INFLAMMATION OF THE MOUTH (SIMPLE)

This is a catarrhal inflammation of the lining of the mouth. It occurs most commonly when the first teeth are coming in.

The physician will treat the inside of the child's mouth. It and the nursing bottle and nipple must all be kept clean. The bowels should be kept open. For older persons, any druggist can make up an alkaline mouth wash such as sodium borate, one drachm; glycerin, two drachms; rose water added to two ounces, to be used every two hours.

## FEVER SORES ("COLD SORES")

These sores usually appear at the junction of the mucous membrane and skin at the corner of the lips, but may occur anywhere around the mouth or elsewhere. They have various causes—colds, indigestion, or fever. They appear first as eruptions containing fluid, which later turn into sores. As a rule the condition heals spontaneously. An application of 5 per cent solution of silver nitrate hastens the healing process.

## APHTHOUS INFLAMMATION OF THE MOUTH

***Cause and Symptoms of Aphthous Inflammation.*** Children from six to eighteen months are most commonly affected. The causes are uncleanliness, improper food, teething, digestive disturbances and general malnutrition. The condition usually begins with fever, and the child refuses to eat. Spots occur on the lips and gums and in the mouth, but especially about the tip of the tongue.

***Treatment of Aphthous Inflammation.*** Treatment consists of the application of a mild antiseptic several times a day. A 1 per cent solution of potassium chlorate may be used, or Lugol's solution (iodine) diluted with four parts of water.

## THRUSH

***Symptoms of Thrush.*** This is a fungus infection of the mouth, found in children. It appears as if patches of milk are left stuck to the cheeks, tongue and roof of the mouth, and these patches are not easily removed. The mouth is sore. Want of cleanliness in feeding children is the chief cause.

***Treatment of Thrush.*** If the patient is a nursing infant, the mother's nipple must be kept clean. The areas in the mouth should be touched twice daily with a 1 per cent solution of gentian violet, with absorbent cotton wound tightly on a toothpick. The mouth should be cleansed several times a day, especially after feeding. For the child that is old enough to use a mouth wash, a good one can be made up by the druggist, consisting of boroglycerin, and sodium sulphite, one drachm to one ounce of water. Cod-liver oil should be given. For a child of six months, give one-half teaspoonful once or twice daily.

## GANGRENOUS SORE MOUTH

Badly fed children, especially after an acute fever such as measles, may reveal a gangrenous sore mouth. A large rapidly spreading ulcer may be formed inside the cheek. The condition requires very strenuous treatment by a physician.

## GEOGRAPHIC TONGUE

As the term denotes, geographic outlines are noticable on the entire tongue. There are no symptoms, as a rule, and all that is required is a mild antiseptic mouth wash.

## "FUR" ON THE TONGUE

"Fur" on the tongue is a symptom, rather than a disorder in itself. The appearance of the tongue varies in different persons. There can be a chronic "furred" tongue in normal health, and a clean tongue is not always indicative of normal stomach and intestinal functions. The appearance of the tongue may change because of digestive disturbances in the stomach, fever, local conditions (i.e., mouth-breathing), sprue (a deficiency disease), pernicious anemia, and ulcerations of the mouth. The main changes in the appearance of the tongue, besides the presence of "fur," are dryness and darkness.

"Fur" is formed usually during sleep by matter which accumulates on the papillae (small nipple-like elevations) of the tongue. "Fur" does not form on an infant's tongue, due to the absence of certain papillae.

## PYORRHEA

***Causes and Symptoms of Pyorrhea.*** What precisely causes pyorrhea is unknown, but poor nutrition is believed to be a factor. The gums become soft and puffy. They bleed easily. Pus collects between the gums and the teeth, and eventually loosens the teeth. The roots of the teeth become decayed. On removal, they sometimes reveal a "pus pocket."

***Treatment of Pyorrhea.*** The local condition must be treated by squeezing out the pus frequently and applying antiseptics and astringents. Hydrogen peroxide is used as a local application. Regular massage of the gums is of help. Calcium and vitamin D should be taken, with plenty of raw fruits and salads. However, frequently the teeth must be removed, as the disease, if untreated, may be followed by rheumatism, kidney trouble, or other disorders.

## ALVEOLAR ABSCESS

***Cause and Symptoms of Alveolar Abscess.*** This condition is sometimes incorrectly called "ulcerated tooth." An alveolar abscess begins as an inflammation in the socket of a tooth and, if near its deepest part, causes great pain. This is because there is an accumulation of pus which can neither escape nor expand the unyielding bony wall of the socket. There may be no cavity in the tooth, but the tooth is usually dead, or its nerve is dying, and the tooth loses its natural color. An "ulcerated tooth" often projects beyond the surrounding teeth and so gives pain in chewing.

***How to Avoid an Abscess.*** For a local inflammation of the gum, which is likely to end in the formation of an abscess, water, as hot as can be comfortably borne, should be held in the mouth in the area of the tooth, and the process repeated for as long a time as possible. Then the patient should lie with the painful side of the face on a hot-water bag or electric pad. Inflammation may subside under this treatment, owing to disappearance of the infection, or to the escape of minute amounts of pus through a small opening in the gum. If the inflammation continues, pain becomes intense and throbbing, and the gum and face swell. After several days of distress, the bony socket loosens the tooth and pus makes its exit.

***Treatment of Abscess.*** Serious results sometimes follow permitting nature alone to work a cure. Obviously, pulling the tooth is the most effective way of relieving the condition and avoiding serious consequences. Under all circumstances where teeth and gums are involved, it is wisest to consult a dentist.

## TOOTHACHE

When there is a cavity in an aching tooth it should be cleaned of food, and a little wad of cotton wool wrapped on a toothpick may be used to wipe the cavity dry. Then the cavity should be loosely packed, by means of a toothpick or one prong of a hairpin, with a small piece of absorbent cotton rolled between the fingers and saturated preferably with oil of cloves, or with spirits of camphor. This is only a temporary remedy. Visit your dentist promptly and have the tooth attended to.

## HALITOSIS

***Causes of Halitosis.*** Halitosis means unpleasant breath. The causes include indigestion and constipation, inflammation of the mouth, and pyorrhea of the gums. Sometimes it is a result of shrinking of the internal lining of the nose, chronic tonsillitis, or respiratory diseases, such as grave bronchitis and gangrene of the lung. Also, tobacco, garlic, onions, and certain drugs may affect the breath.

***Treatment of Halitosis.*** The treatment obviously depends on correct diagnosis and removal of the cause. It is insufficient to use mouth washes in most cases if the cause is more than transient. The effectiveness of mouth washes is limited to a few minutes, and then the basic bad odor returns.

## MOUTH HYGIENE

Mouth hygiene, particularly the care of the teeth and gums, is absolutely necessary for maintaining good health. However, it is not, as a rule, necessary—in fact it is unwise—to cleanse an infant's mouth. The delicate lining is often injured by attempts at cleansing.

***Mouth Washes.*** Unless there is some local disease of the mouth or throat, gargling and mouth washing are useless, except for the removal of food particles. No solution *in strength which tissues can bear* will disinfect the mouth and throat in its entirety. A good mouth wash consists of equal parts of lemon juice and soda water, or peroxide of hydrogen, one part to three parts of water.

## DENTAL HYGIENE

***Importance of Diet for Good Teeth.*** Since teeth are formed from materials furnished by food, good nutrition is important in the formation of sound teeth. The diet must provide adequate amounts of: calcium and phosphorus, the basic minerals from which teeth are formed; vitamin D, which aids in the utilization of these minerals; vitamin B, which controls the formation of enamel; and vitamin C, for the formation of dentine. Good diet is especially important in infancy, childhood, and pregnancy.

***Cleansing Foods.*** Fruit acids are cleansing. They prevent the formation of tartar. They are cleansers of the tongue and the mucous membrane of the mouth and throat. The juice of fruit is most effective in its cleansing action at the end of a meal.

***Cleaning the Teeth.*** Teeth should be brushed soon after food is eaten. The bristles of the tooth brush should not be too stiff, and should be of unequal lengths so as to reach the innermost crevices of the teeth. Tooth powders and pastes may be used, but the main reliance should be on brushing. Some powders, if constantly used, may destroy the enamel. An excellent tooth cleanser is a mixture of one part each of baking soda (sodium bicarbonate) and ordinary table salt. Regular examinations by a dentist at least twice a year and following the dentist's advice are indispensable if you want to have good teeth.

## DISEASES OF THE LIPS

***Paleness of the Lips.*** While not a disease, this is suggestive of anemia and other constitutional diseases.

***Inflamed Lips.*** The lips may become inflamed and dry due to exposure to cold, wind, drugs, sun, or cosmetics. Zinc oxide ointment gives relief, but the cause must be avoided.

***Perleche.*** This infectious disease of children is recognizable when small white patches form, or blister, at the corners of the mouth. In time painful fissures form. Treatment usually consists of correcting faulty mouth hygiene, administering riboflavin (vitamin B complex) in adequate dosage when a nutritional factor is present, and local application of a 2 per cent watery solution of gentian violet.

## FOREIGN BODIES IN THE THROAT

Fishbones and other small bones are apt to be caught in the tissues around the tonsil, at the base of the tongue, or in the back wall of the pharynx. Even a very small fishbone in such a location may cause a fair amount of pain and irritation in swallowing.

A child may swallow a coin, which then lies transversely, or a large lump of food may block the throat and cause pressure on the larynx or trachea.

Large foreign bodies, such as a denture, a bone, or a coin, stuck fast in the throat and larynx, may remain behind the larynx and cause pain or difficulty in swallowing until they are removed. It is important not to neglect the condition merely because the first symptoms subside.

***How to Remove Foreign Bodies from the Throat.*** An ordinary method of getting rid of small fishbones, etc., is to chew a mouthful of hard crusts of bread, and then to swallow them with a large gulp of water. If this does not succeed, and if the obstruction still remains, it may be advisable to bring on vomiting. A pinch of salt in peppered water, or syrup of ipecac, will produce vomiting, and the upward rush of matter from the stomach may clear the throat.

***Dislodging Large Foreign Bodies.*** The sizable body may be removed by putting a finger into the pharynx to the back of the throat and getting hold of the obstruction. If this is not effective, a physician's help is required. Diagnosis of a foreign body in the air or food passages includes physical and X-ray studies, followed by examination with special instruments which give a direct view of the larynx. One of these, called the esophagoscope, is often used in the extraction of foreign bodies. In extremely urgent instances, it is sometimes necessary to cut into the windpipe to save the patient's life.

## BLEEDING FROM THE THROAT

What appears to be bleeding from the throat is often, actually, bleeding from the lungs due to tuberculosis. Bleeding may also arise in the gums, the larynx, the nasopharynx, the nose, the windpipe, or the esophagus. When the bleeding is actually in the pharynx itself, it may be a symptom of syphilitic ulceration or malignant disease. Sometimes, in a victim of gout, an enlarged vein in the pharynx may have ruptured. On the other hand, there may be no local condition to account for the bleeding, but a blood disease such as hemophilia,

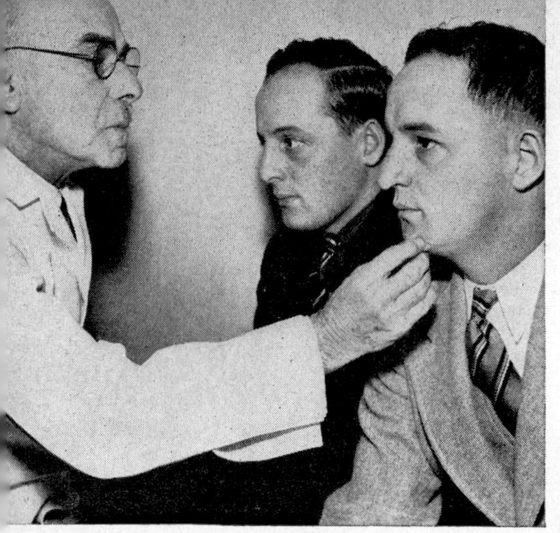

# Plastic Surgery

THEIR NOSES DO NOT MATCH

*(Left)* Plastic surgeon examines noses of twin brothers. One had nose injured by baseball, wants it remodeled to resemble brother's.

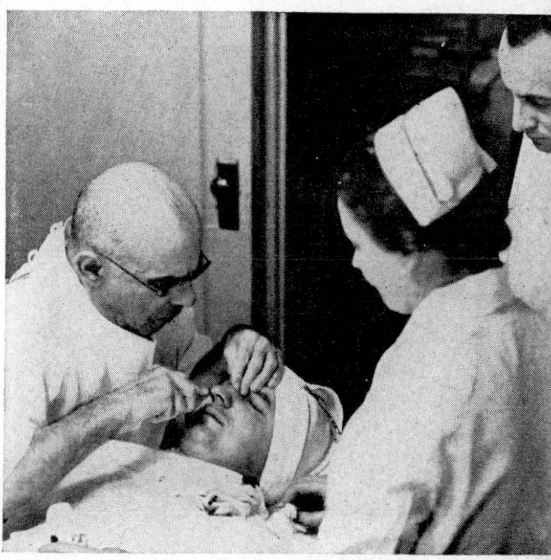

PLASTIC SURGEON AT WORK

During operation, brother with intact nose stands by, serving as model for surgeon restoring damaged nose of twin. Branch of plastic surgery dealing with noses is called rhinoplasty.

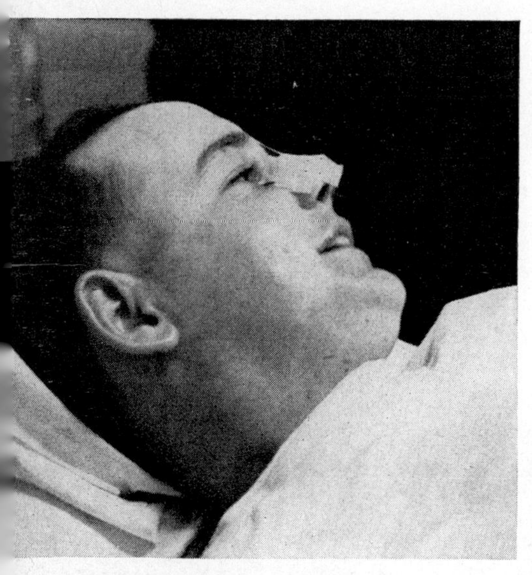

OPERATION COMPLETED

Even under protecting plaster, it is clear that deformed nose has been corrected, operation is a success. Surgery is quick

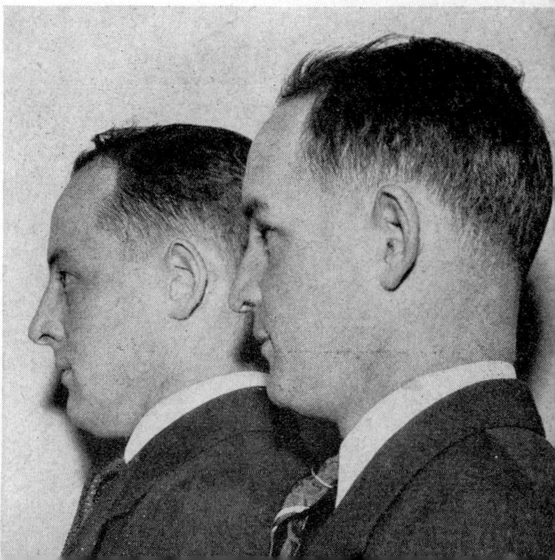

TWINS LOOK ALIKE AGAIN

In modern plastic surgery, not only nose, but eyebrows, eyelids, ears, lips, and, in fact, practically whole face can be rebuilt. Disfiguring scars and defects resulting from war wounds or accidents can be readily repaired, leaving hardly a trace. Excess breast tissue or excess fat may also be removed this way.

## CHILD'S TEETH NEED CARE

Many parents neglect decay in child's first set of teeth because they are not permanent. But decayed teeth are painful, may cause jaw infection. Dentist should make checkup twice a year.

## INCUBATOR BABY

*(Below)* Modern incubator has openings in side, so baby can be cared for without being removed. Temperature, humidity, oxygen supply are carefully controlled. Baby weighing under 5½ pounds is considered premature, even if full term by mother's reckoning.

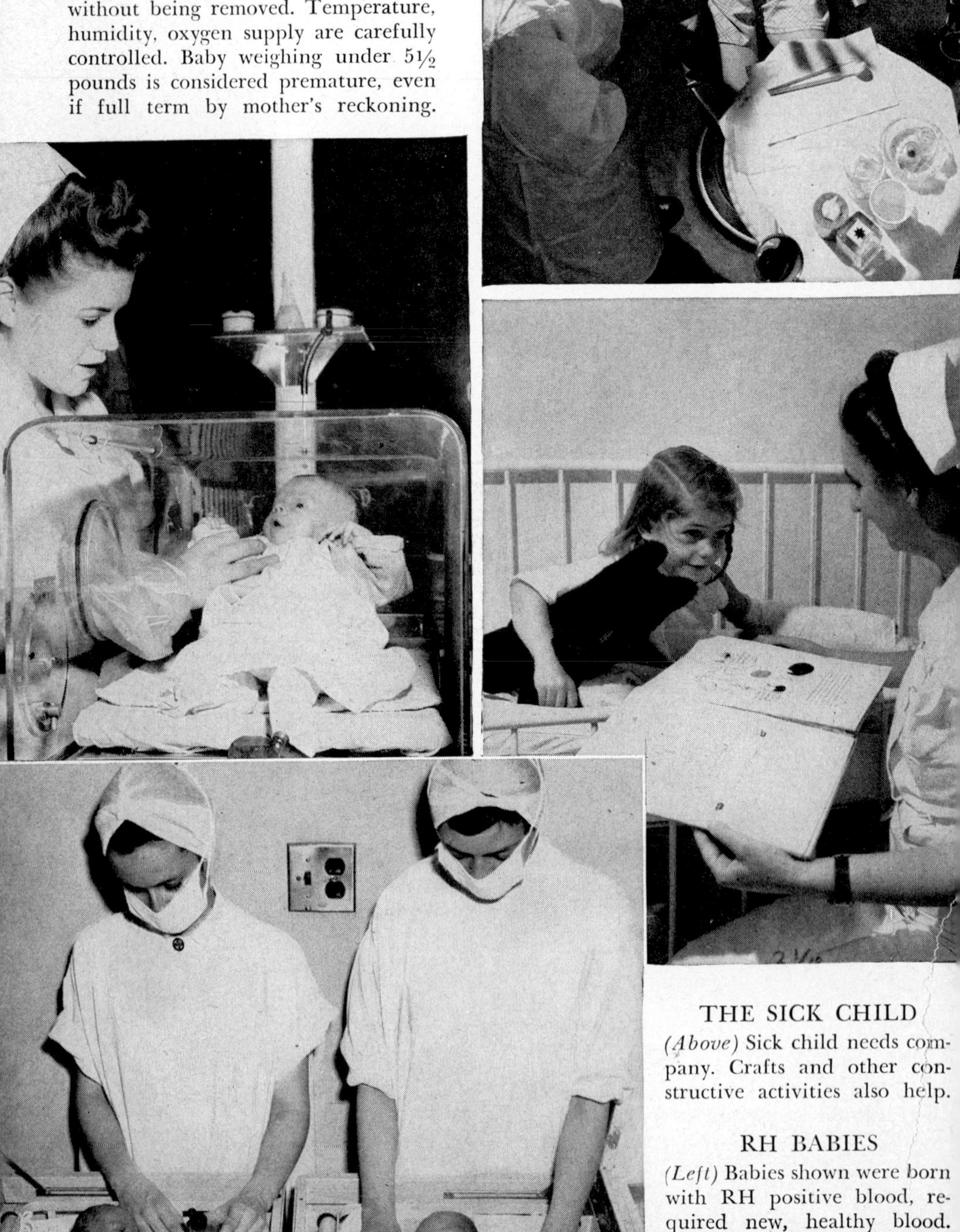

## THE SICK CHILD

*(Above)* Sick child needs company. Crafts and other constructive activities also help.

## RH BABIES

*(Left)* Babies shown were born with RH positive blood, required new, healthy blood.

pernicious anemia, or leukemia may be responsible for the attack. In any event, a physician must be consulted without delay.

## TONSILLITIS

***Causes of Tonsillitis.*** Tonsillitis in an inflammation of the tonsils which can be caused by many different germs. There are two forms of the disease, acute and chronic. In severe cases, tonsillitis can have serious results. It may lead to rheumatic fever, pneumonia, arthritis, ear infection, or other disorders.

Lowered resistance favors an infection of the tonsils.

***Symptoms of Tonsillitis.*** Enlarged tonsils are not in themselves a symptom of tonsillitis. However, in tonsillitis, there is swelling of the tonsils and a sore throat, making it hard to swallow. White spots appear on the tonsils. The lymphatic glands are enlarged. Mild fever, restlessness, and general discomfort are present. There is an increase in the pulse rate. If a gray or greenish membrane appears in the throat and on the tonsils, this is a symptom of diphtheria, and urgent action is called for.

***Treatment of Tonsillitis.*** Rest in bed is required. Ice bags may be applied to the throat. Gargling with a mild warm salt water or baking soda solution is helpful. The diet should be light, with ample liquids. The physician will prescribe medicines to aid in controlling the infection. However, if the condition is a chronic one, removal of the tonsils is essential.

The operation is avoided when the patient is very young, and, indeed, is rarely necessary in children under three years of age. It should be avoided, too, during epidemics of contagious or infectious diseases; in the presence of serious blood and lung diseases, especially tuberculosis; when there is a throat abscess; and in cases of diabetes, hardening of the arteries (arteriosclerosis), or thyroid gland disease.

## ADENOIDS

***Causes of Adenoids.*** Children are not born with adenoids although some authorities claim they are. These enlargements of lymphoid tissue begin to form early in life, and are a common trouble in childhood. In most children, some degree of enlargement is always present. Excessive enlargement, sufficient to induce symptoms, frequently follows one of the acute infectious fevers—for example, scarlet fever, measles, or diphtheria. Serious adenoid trouble is rare before the third year.

Adenoid enlargement is relatively uncommon in adults. Climate is an important factor; adenoid enlargement occurs more often in a cold, damp atmosphere than in a hot, dry climate.

***Symptoms of Adenoids.*** The symptoms vary according to the degree of adenoid enlargement. In severe examples, a characteristic picture—the adenoid face—is noted. This is the result of persistent mouth-breathing caused by nasal obstruction, a condition which gives a child a dull facial expression, an open mouth, a pinched nose, and a deep toneless voice. The child with adenoids sleeps restlessly and snores. He is tired and listless in the morning, and is an indifferent student at school. His appetite is poor and he remains undernourished.

In some children the chief symptoms are ear complications. In many, deafness is the result of enlarged adenoids. The condition varies somewhat with the weather, and is worse when the child is suffering from a cold. Nose bleeding is common in children with enlarged adenoids. A chain of small glands can nearly always be felt in the neck.

The most common effect is a tendency to repeated colds. The mouth breathing is responsible for laryngitis and bronchitis. The nasal obstruction causes a chain of symptoms including headache, mental depression, and a listless state. Some children, unable to breathe with food in the mouth, swallow food hurriedly; others, having difficulty in chewing, take only small mouthfuls.

***Treatment of Adenoids.*** Adenoids should be surgically removed. Such operations are often remarkably beneficial. Even after well-performed adenoid removals, however, there is a definite tendency to recurrences in some children. When this lymphoid tissue becomes re-infected (as it usually does), it often causes repeated, and later chronic, inflammations of the respiratory tract.

## PHARYNGITIS

This is the common variety of sore throat, especially in measles, scarlet fever, and influenza. In syphilis, it is an early manifestation of the disease.

***Symptoms of Pharyngitis.*** An attack begins with a sense of chilliness, slight rise in temperature, headache, pains in the limbs and back, and a sensation of rawness in the throat which sometimes amounts to actual pain. Cough may be present, and there is a varying degree of pain on swallowing. If the inflammation extends to the larynx, the voice becomes hoarse.

***Chronic Pharyngitis.*** This occurs most frequently in persons who use the voice a great deal; it may also follow excessive use of tobacco. An irritating, hawking cough is often present, especially in the morning. Tobacco should be given up and all irritating food must be avoided.

***Treatment of Pharyngitis.*** The patient should go to bed after a hot bath, and take two to three tablets of aspirin, one hour apart. Another remedy, if taken early in the disease, is two tablets of sulfadiazine, with two 5-grain tablets of bicarbonate of soda. Repeat in two hours. Drink a full glass of water with each dose. This medication will often check a severe sore throat, which usually is a forerunner of a cold. It is valueless unless taken as soon as the first symptom is noted. Teaspoonful doses of very mild solutions of bicarbonate of soda, a very light diet, and orange juice are helpful. A teaspoonful of bicarbonate of soda in a glass of hot water makes a soothing spray. Gargles and throat paints are of little value, but lozenges or pastilles of penicillin are highly effective in infections of the throat and mouth.

## CHRONIC POST-NASAL DISCHARGE

***Causes of the Discharge.*** This common condition is sometimes caused by sinus trouble. There is a large amount of secreting tissue in the space at the back of the nose (post-nasal), and a variable amount of mucus therefore normally flows from the sinuses and the nasal mucous membrane. Under disease conditions, it may become sticky, or full of pus. Chronic inflammation may extend from the nose to the space behind it. The disease is also aggravated by obstruction in the nose, or it may be a sign of nasal sinus infection.

***Symptoms of Chronic Post-Nasal Discharge.*** The chief symptom, besides the discharge, is a sense of blockage at the back of the nose, and there is in consequence a constant attempt to clear the throat. Fever usually accompanies the acute stage of infectious disease in the throat.

***Treatment of Chronic Post-Nasal Discharge.*** This disorder should be cared for by a physician, who will determine the cause and provide the treatment required.

## SEPTIC SORE THROAT

***Causes of Septic Sore Throat.*** Streptococcic sore throat is an acute infection of the tonsils and pharynx, usually appearing in epidemic form. It is ordinarily traceable to milk or some other outside factor, and streptococci bacteria are the fundamental cause. If untreated, the disease usually has a high mortality. In the numbers of persons infected, it heads the list of milk-borne diseases in the United States. Most of the outbreaks occur in small communities where raw milk is consumed.

***Symptoms of Septic Sore Throat.*** The infection usually begins suddenly, with fever, dull pain on swallowing, general aching, headache, and at times nausea. The patient is gravely ill. The tonsils are red and covered with spots, or occasionally with gray patches. The disease lasts about a week or ten days. The most frequent complications are enlarged glands of the neck, infection of the middle ear, and extension of the infection to the lungs.

***Treatment of Septic Sore Throat.*** Treatment is preventive, to get rid of the symptoms, and specific for the disease. The use of vaccines and serums is often of great value. Moderate doses of blood sera from patients who are convalescing from various streptococcic infections, properly checked, or blood transfusions from such donors have proved highly valuable. One of the drugs of the sulfa group is remarkably effective.

## ABSCESS IN BACK OF THE THROAT

This infection usually appears in childhood and occurs in the lymphoid tissue in the back wall of the throat. There is fever, pain on swallowing and shortness of breath. The mouth is kept open and the head backward; a soft mass is seen in the middle of the back wall of the throat. The glands of the neck are enlarged. This is a serious condition and a doctor must be called at once.

## QUINSY

***Causes of Quinsy.*** Quinsy is a peritonsillitis—that is, an inflammation of the tissues around the tonsil. The swelling of these tissues pushes the tonsil out into the throat, but the tonsil itself is little affected. Quinsy also involves the surrounding structures of the throat, and usually causes an abscess. It often occurs in those subject to rheumatism and gout, and may recur.

***Symptoms of Quinsy.*** Quinsy is characterized by much greater pain in the throat and in swallowing than is the case in tonsillitis, and the temperature is often higher—sometimes 104° to 105°F. On inspection, one or both tonsils can be seen to be enlarged and crowded into the mid-throat area owing to swelling of the neighboring parts. The tonsils may almost block the entrance to the throat. The voice is thick and indistinct, the glands in the side of the neck become swollen, the neck is sore and stiff, and because of pain, the mouth can be only partly opened. For the same reason, the patient can swallow neither solid nor liquid food. The secretion of saliva is increased, but is not swallowed on account of the pain produced by the act. There is much pain and distress.

Having reached this stage, the inflammation usually goes on to form abscesses. After five to ten days from the beginning of the attack, the pus finds its way to the surface of the tonsil, and breaks into the mouth, to the great relief of the patient. Then the symptoms quickly subside.

***Quinsy and Tonsillitis.*** Quinsy differs from tonsillitis in the following respects: the swelling affects also the immediate surrounding area of the throat; there are no white spots on the tonsil unless the infection begins as ordinary tonsillitis; there is even greater pain on swallowing; and finally, in most instances, abscesses are formed near the tonsil.

***Complications of Quinsy.*** Quinsy itself is rarely a dangerous disease; yet, occasionally, it leads to so much obstruction in the throat that it may cause death from suffocation unless a surgeon opens the throat and inserts a tube.

***Treatment of Quinsy.*** The bowels must be kept open. A gargle of potassium chlorate or potassium permanganate may be used. Two tablets of aspirin, three times a day, should be given until the temperature falls. Hot salt-water solution makes a comforting gargle. This can be alternated at intervals of two hours by gargles or irrigations of iced milk. Ice-collars are comforting to patients with any inflammation of the tonsils.

Sulfadiazene prescribed by the physician is very effective in this condition. In extremely severe examples of the disease, penicillin may be given by mouth or injected into the muscles.

No first-aid treatment should be attempted. The abscess must be opened by a physician.

## TUMORS OF THE PHARYNX

***Symptoms of Pharynx Tumors.*** Throat tumors may be of the malignant or the non-malignant variety. The malignant or cancerous forms of throat tumor, often beginning in the tonsil, are particularly dangerous, since there is sometimes no noticeable symptom in the throat other than slight difficulty in swallowing. Throat tumor causes obstruction to nose breathing, and is often accompanied by some bleeding, usually not severe. There may be ulceration, with some discharge. There is great production of saliva, thick speech, and difficulty in opening the jaws and moving the tongue. The Eustachian tube is usually obstructed, causing impaired hearing, as well as pain and noises in the ears. The neck glands are involved early. Microscopic examination of a piece of the tumor tissue should be made early for diagnosis.

***Benign Tumors.*** In the non-malignant variety, the outstanding symptoms usually are bleeding and obstruction, with the secondary ear symptoms of deafness, noises in the ears, inflammation of the middle-ear and mastoiditis. The tumors are painless.

***Treatment of Pharynx Tumors.*** Treatment must be by a physician. Surgery may be performed, if not too difficult. X-ray and radium treatment are recommended for cancerous tumors.

## TUBERCULOSIS OF THE PHARYNX

***Symptoms of Pharynx Tuberculosis.*** Tuberculosis, a disease caused by tubercle germs, affects the throat less frequently than it affects any other part of the respiratory system. Primary tuberculosis of the tonsils, however, is not rare. Tuberculosis sometimes acutely attacks the throat in association with its attack on the lungs. On the throat or palate, there are minute gray or yellow tubercles, which rapidly break down into shallow ulcers. It is an extremely painful disorder. There is great distress, especially in swallowing and producing saliva, accompanied by throaty speech and rapid loss of weight.

***Treatment of Pharynx Tuberculosis.*** If the tonsils are diseased, they are removed. Various measures are adopted, depending on the part of the throat affected. The general health must be restored, as in all kinds of tuberculosis.

## VINCENT'S ANGINA (TRENCH MOUTH)

***Cause and Symptoms of Vincent's Angina.*** Vincent's angina is an infection of the throat which begins as a deep ulceration of the tonsils and extends as a false membrane (resembling that in diphtheria) to the surrounding parts. The gums, tooth sockets, bronchial mucous membrane, and even other parts of the body may be attacked. The disease may be mistaken for diphtheria, syphilis, and other infections. Its precise cause has not been identified.

The patient complains of a sore throat affecting one or both sides. The mouth has an unpleasant odor. As a rule, there are no other bodily symptoms. On examination a deep, dirty gray ulcer is found on one or both tonsils. These ulcers may also be found elsewhere on the mouth. Microscopic examination of a throat swab reveals Vincent's organisms, usually in a pure state.

***Treatment of Vincent's Angina.*** The gums must receive appropriate medical and dental treatment. Crystalline penicillin is the most beneficial drug. Mouth washes or irrigations with 1 part in 3,000 of potassium permanganate, or perborate of soda, or hydrogen peroxide are beneficial. The contagious nature of the disease must be kept in mind and care taken to prevent its spread.

## LUDWIG'S ANGINA

This is a term applied to a variety of infection which involves the area below the jaw. It is usually caused by the streptococcus, and may be secondary to some infection in the throat. There is great swelling, hardening of the local tissues, pain and tenderness in the tissues of the neck, with high fever and severe constitutional symptoms. The disease should be treated only by a physician.

## GENERAL HYGIENE OF THE THROAT

The normal mouth is always alkaline in reaction and must be maintained in that state. When the mouth is infected, the mouth and throat surfaces are generally acid, and the mucus there becomes thick and sticky, clogging the lining and failing in its normal protective, lubricating function.

One of the best ways of keeping the mouth and throat alkaline is to rinse the mouth and gargle the throat with warm alkaline solution—

a level teaspoonful of bicarbonate of soda, for example, dissolved in a glass of warm water.

Dry conditions of the throat are often induced by infection in the mouth. For the prevention of throat ailments, it is therefore most important to attend to cleansing of the teeth. In fact, the care of the throat largely depends upon that of the teeth.

Another source of infection of the throat is the diseased tonsil. Troublesome tonsil conditions should be brought to the attention of your physician. He will advise you whether or not to have your tonsils removed. Tonsils appear to play a roll in maintaining good health and they should not be taken out without excellent reason, as was the custom some years ago.

Prolonged over-exertion of the voice often results in various annoying throat conditions. Avoid irritating your throat by using the voice too much. Give it frequent rest, and use sprays and gargles regularly if your profession requires you to do considerable speaking or singing.

Excess of common salt in food is also harmful to the throat, as is the use of over-hot food, which causes scalding, congestion, and other injuries. After repeated and prolonged injury from heat, the mucous lining of the throat becomes dry and insensitive. Tobacco smoke, likewise, has a severely drying effect on the lining of the throat. This varies in different people, depending partly on the thickness of the throat lining. When your throat is dry or irritated from smoking, this is a signal to cut down on tobacco consumption. Chew gum instead, if you find it hard to do without tobacco.

***Disinfectants.*** Disinfection of the air with triethylene glycol vapors has been introduced for prevention of acute respiratory diseases. Bacteria-killing concentrations of this vapor are odorless, tasteless, non-irritating, non-toxic, invisible and have no harmful effect on walls, fabrics, books or other objects in the treated area. The presence of even tiny amounts of vaporized triethylene glycol under controlled conditions is deadly for the common respiratory bacteria, as well as for the viruses of influenza, parrot disease (psittacosis) and other diseases.

## HOW TO TREAT THE THROAT

***Painting the Throat.*** This procedure is old-fashioned and has been largely discarded.

***How to Have a Patient Gargle.*** Throat gargles are not of much help for infected throats. A gargle may be used for cleansing, as follows: Prepare the solution. Use a tube if the solution contains any drug which will stain the teeth, as, for example, iodine. Remove the pillows so that the patient lies flat. Put a towel under his head, and ask him to turn his head. Have him take a large mouthful and gargle, and permit the solution to run into a basin which is held tightly at the side of the mouth.

***How to Spray the Throat.*** To spray the throat, the helper stands in front of the patient, but a little to one side. When the patient has opened his mouth wide, insert the nozzle of the spray well into the mouth, pointing and pressing the roof of the tongue downward. While the patient breathes in deeply or says "ah," work the rubber bellows. Repeat this as often as is necessary. The solutions used for spraying are boric acid, hydrogen peroxide, sodium bicarbonate and penicillin.

***How to Irrigate the Throat.*** The irrigation should be warm or hot. Tell the patient to open his mouth and hold his breath while the irrigation is carried out. Cover the bed and patient with rubber sheeting. Fold a towel over the edge of the rubber which comes close to the neck. The patient's head and shoulders may be raised with pillows, or he may be lying down on a single pillow. He holds his head over the basin in front or at the side so that the water from his mouth will run into the basin and not onto the bed. Raise the rubber bag or can twelve inches above his head. First let water run into the basin to remove any cold solution from the tube. Control the flow by pinching the tube.

***How to Steam the Throat.*** Electric vaporizers can be bought at drug stores. In an emergency—croup, for example—take the small child, wrapped in a blanket, into the bathroom. Close the doors and windows. Turn on the hot water. The moist air will give the child some relief. If this brings no relief, fill a tea kettle with water. Place it on the stove or on an electric heater, with the nozzle of the kettle toward the patient. Be careful not to have it too close. To keep the steam confined to the bed-area, place an open umbrella over the child's head and make a tent over it with a sheet. Instead of the umbrella, the bottom of a large, open, heavy paper bag may be pushed over the nozzle of the kettle.

Penicillin may be given by inhalation. A special inhaler is used, and the "mist" is inhaled every two hours during the day. The vaporization is effected by oxygen and takes about fifteen minutes.

***How to Examine a Child's Throat.*** If a child refuses to allow examination of the throat, some coercion may be necessary. The most satisfactory method is for the nurse to place the child on one knee, imprisoning the child's legs with her own. She then places one arm around the child's body, pinioning his arms, while with the other arm and hand she steadies the head against her shoulder. The mother holds the child's nose, in this way forcing him to open his mouth to take a breath; a tongue depressor or clean spoon is then quickly introduced and the throat is examined.

## HARSHNESS OF VOICE IN AN INFANT

Always an alarming symptom, this is sometimes a sign that the child's life is in danger. The condition may be either spasmodic or persistent. The spasmodic variety occurs in disorders characterized by the fact that they begin suddenly, and are accompanied by a bluish tinge of the skin and lips, with respiratory distress. The most common cause is the drawing of a foreign body into the larynx. A physician's attention is urgently required.

A variation of the spasmodic type in infants is "laryngismus stridulus," or false croup. This is seldom dangerous, if cared for properly. The child is asleep, apparently well, when respiration becomes suddenly "crowing" and then is arrested; the face, flushed at first, becomes bluish. But the spasm relaxes, the child makes a loud, harsh breathing sound, and then quickly, in a crying spell, becomes normal.

***Persistent Harshness.*** Persistent harshness in an infant's voice is sometimes congenital. It is usually present at birth, when it is described as "clucking," "crowing," or "croaking." The infant is not distressed, nor does it turn bluish. As the child grows older, the noise increases in intensity. Sometimes, however, after the sixth or eighth month, the noise noticeably decreases, and eventually disappears.

## LARYNGITIS

***Causes of Acute Laryngitis.*** The causes of acute laryngitis—acute inflammation of the larynx—are general infections of the upper respiratory tract, such as colds; over-use of the voice; mechanical and chemical irritation; and infection from diseased tissue nearby, such as infected tonsils or adenoids. Infections carried in by the blood stream, and acute infectious diseases, such as scarlet fever, measles, chickenpox, smallpox, diphtheria and influenza, as well as various inflammatory skin diseases, may also be responsible for this condition.

Acute infections of the influenza variety often involve different parts of the respiratory system at various times. One year, the nose and sinuses may be most frequently involved; another year, the ears or the larynx. Acute laryngitis is common after tonsils have been removed and before the local defense mechanism of the individual has become adjusted to the changed conditions.

***Symptoms of Acute Laryngitis.*** The first symptoms of acute laryngitis are mild fever, chilly sensations, discomfort in the throat, and

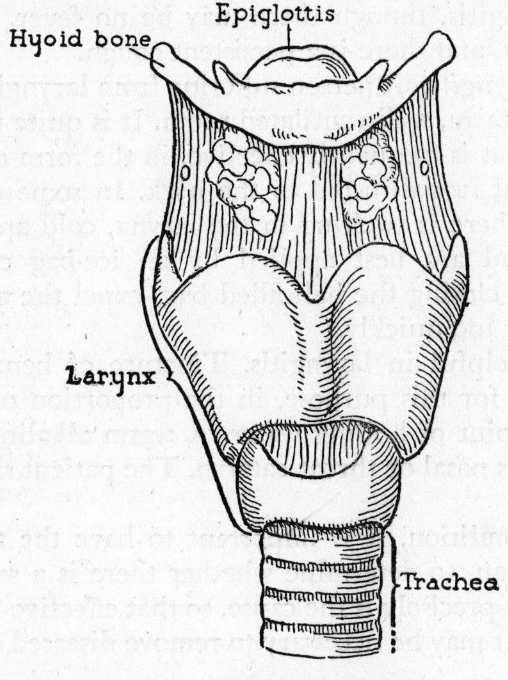


THE LARYNX

hoarseness. There may be pain in the larynx and tenderness around it, sometimes complete loss of voice, and a painful cough, with some expectoration, and pain on swallowing. When it is a secondary condition, caused by an extension downward of an infection from the nose, or upward of an infection from the windpipe, the symptoms are those of the disease from which it starts. Treatment of any contributing disease must not be overlooked.

***Causes of Chronic Laryngitis.*** Chronic laryngitis may result from repeated attacks of acute laryngitis, as well as from the effects of obstruction of the nose, excessive use of alcohol or tobacco, excessive use of the voice, and faulty voice production, especially when catarrhal laryngitis is present. Dust, hay fever, and asthma are often the factors responsible. In children, the larynx may be the site of a number of chronic disorders indicated by hoarseness, harshness of voice or obstructive shortness of breath. Chronic laryngitis is nearly always present when there is a condition of tuberculosis of the larynx as well as lupus, syphilis, paralysis of the vocal cords, and tumors. It demands immediate attention.

***Symptoms of Chronic Laryngitis.*** The symptoms often resemble those of acute laryngitis, though there may be no fever. Mucus is present in the throat, and there is a persistent cough.

***Treatment of Laryngitis.*** A person suffering from laryngitis should remain in bed in a warm, well-ventilated room. It is quite important to rest the voice. Heat is frequently effective, in the form of an electric pad, or infra-red rays directed to the neck. In some cases, and particularly where there is swelling in the larynx, cold applications give more relief and are best applied by an ice-bag containing crushed ice. (Before closing the half-filled bag, expel the air so that the ice will not melt too quickly.)

Inhalations are helpful in laryngitis. Tincture of benzoin compound may be used for this purpose, in the proportion of one-half teaspoonful to one pint of boiling water. A warm alkaline spray is comforting if there is nasal or throat catarrh. The patient should not smoke.

In the chronic condition, it is important to have the throat examined by a physician, to determine whether there is a serious disease present, or what precisely is the cause, so that effective treatment can be undertaken. It may be necessary to remove diseased structures from the throat.

## NODULAR LARYNGITIS (SINGER'S NODES)

***Causes and Symptoms of Nodular Laryngitis.*** This variety of chronic laryngitis is brought on by faulty use of the voice. After the nodes (knotlike swellings) are formed, hoarseness is persistent; sometimes they develop in a few days, following excessive use of the voice, and may disappear rapidly after an enforced voice rest. This difficulty may be due entirely to weakness of the muscles concerned in voice production, and the attendant hoarseness may be mistaken for chronic laryngitis. The two conditions may occur at the same time.

***Treatment of Nodular Laryngitis.*** In addition to the elimination of factors causing the irritation, such as exposure to fumes, tobacco, and alcohol, treatment of nodular laryngitis calls for training in the proper use of voice, periods of silence, and frequent inhalations of steam. It is always best, of course, to consult a physician.

## FALSE CROUP

***Causes of False Croup.*** This variety of laryngitis occurs chiefly in young children from two to eight years of age, especially in conjunction with influenza, measles, scarlet fever, chickenpox and smallpox.

***Symptoms of False Croup.*** The symptoms are more severe and alarming in children than in adults. In some ways they resemble those of true croup, and it should be made certain that the condition is not true croup, or diphtheria. (See Diphtheria, Index.) The child during the day may have a slight rise in temperature and a cough. During sleep he suddenly awakens, with noisy breathing and a harshness in the voice. At first the child is restless and cries, and respiration becomes labored. Hoarseness increases, and the cough may be described as "crowing" or "hacking." There is usually shortness of breath. The attacks may last for only a few minutes, or continue for several hours, and they may vary from a mild form to one of impending suffocation. Simple spasmodic croup is rarely fatal, but when an attack has once occurred, similar ones are to be expected.

***Treatment of False Croup.*** Treatment includes raising the child's lowered resistance. Cod-liver oil should be given every day, plenty of fresh fruit and green vegetables, milk, cheese, fresh meat, eggs, and the other elements of a protective diet. Vaporizing the air in the child's room helps.

## TUBERCULOSIS OF THE LARYNX

***Causes of Tuberculosis of the Larynx.*** Tuberculosis is the most common specific disease of the larynx. It is one of the most important, because discovering its presence there may make certain a diagnosis of lung tuberculosis in a person with suggestive symptoms. Primary infection of the larynx by the tubercle bacillus does not occur. It is always secondary to tuberculosis of the lungs. However, it is a serious complication, since the involvement of the larynx doubles the seriousness of the lung condition. This emphasizes the great importance of early examination of the larynx, where there are symptoms indicative of tuberculosis of the lungs. It is not uncommon to find syphilis associated with tuberculosis.

In most persons with tuberculosis of the larynx both lungs are affected. The voice box appears to become involved when the infection is carried there by the blood.

***Symptoms of Tuberculosis of the Larynx.*** Tuberculosis of the larynx may be present without producing symptoms that can be referred directly to the organ. In the early stage of the disease, the voice may not show any change. Later, however, the most frequent indication is found in the quality of the voice. The hoarseness, slight at first, grows progressively worse, and the voice reveals a soft huskiness. The hoarseness is frequently a morning complaint, and should always be suggestive of the disease; as should, also, passing or persistent loss of voice.

With advancing ulceration in the larynx, pain on swallowing becomes a distressing feature of the disease. Dryness of the throat in the morning is most common, and is usually caused by sputum adhering to the larynx. There is therefore a constant desire to clear the throat. Cough is often present, but this is due rather to the lung infection than to that of the larynx. With the advance of the lung trouble, the coughing spells are associated with agonizing pain.

Sometimes, in tuberculosis of the lungs, the symptoms in the larynx precede other signs or symptoms of the disease. Temperature is variable. Pain and tenderness over the larynx are felt, especially where the cartilages are involved. Pain on swallowing, or difficulty in doing so, follows even in the absence of ulceration. The final result of the illness depends on the variety, site, extent, depth, age, and progress of the damage.

***Treatment of Tuberculosis of the Larynx.*** Treatment consists largely of attention to the primary disease and to the general health of the patient. The condition of the larynx is largely influenced by the lung disease, and the course of the two is likely to be parallel. Any improvement in the lung condition is therefore likely to be followed by a similar change in that of the larynx. Remarkable results are obtained with the use of streptomycin in tuberculosis of the larynx, the windpipe, and the lungs. However, drugs are not substitutes for institutional or surgical treatment of tuberculosis.

## CANCER OF THE LARYNX

It is generally accepted among physicians that if there is persistent hoarseness of two or more weeks' duration, cancer, tuberculosis, or syphilis may be present, and the patient should be examined with this in mind.

Cancer of the larynx is much more common in men than in women. It is estimated that 4 per cent of all malignant tumors occur in the larynx. Any long-continued irritation may cause the slow development of what is at first a painless growth. In the majority of cases this naturally means that by the time the tumor is first discovered, its area is already extensive. As it continues to grow, the functions of the larynx are affected.

***Symptoms of Cancer of the Larynx.*** The early symptoms of cancer of the larynx vary greatly because they depend on the size, variety and situation of the growth. A small malignant nodule on a cord causes hoarseness that is easily noticed, whereas such a growth can reach a larger size in one of the folds of the larynx before causing sufficient symptoms to attract attention. Any persistent discomfort in the throat, or hoarseness which lasts more than three weeks, particularly in a person over forty-five years of age, urgently demands an examination of the larynx.

***Treatment of Cancer of the Larynx.*** More than 80 per cent of patients with beginning vocal cord cancer can be cured by early surgical operation. Early cancer within the larynx, if treated promptly, offers a better chance of recovery than any other internal cancer in the human body. Surgery shows the best statistical results, but there are patients for whom X-ray or radium treatment is preferable to surgery.

***Speech Devices After Removal of Larynx.*** After the larynx is removed by surgery, the two essentials for production of normal voice are gone—the vocal folds and the moving current of air flowing past them into the mouth. Several artificial devices are in use by which the patient whose larynx has been removed produces a form of speech through vibration and articulation. Speech specialists have also worked out devices so that victims of cancer of the larynx no longer have to depend on artificial aids. It has become possible to develop a substitute voice by using other parts of the body, such as the esophagus, in place of the larynx.

## BENIGN TUMORS OF THE LARYNX

***Symptoms of Benign Tumors.*** A benign tumor in the larynx may be without symptoms. On the other hand, benign tumors which cause hoarseness occur in both children and adults. In children they are usually papillomas, small mucous membrane growths, like corns, which involve both cords. In adults (especially among males) fibromas or fibroid tumors are found in the form of small polyps with pedicles (growths with stem-like supports). The majority of these tumors are small and so do not obstruct respiration. Occasionally, however, spasm may result from irritation, with temporary difficulty in breathing, and harshness of voice.

***Treatment of Benign Tumors.*** Some tumors, particularly those that cause no symptoms, demand no treatment. However, even these must be watched, since they may later grow, or change in nature. When the tumor is troublesome, it must be removed.

## FOREIGN BODIES IN THE LARYNX

Lodging of foreign bodies in the larynx usually occurs during swallowing. The accident is not uncommon among children. Substances which are frequently stuck in the larynx may be large objects which stick in the entrance and cause sudden suffocation. Or they may be flat or irregular objects which adhere to the walls of the larynx. Small smooth objects, such as peanuts, may drop into the windpipe.

***Symptoms.*** Foreign bodies in the larynx produce one or more of the following symptoms: hoarseness, a croupy cough, harshness of voice, wheezing, shortness of breath, a bluish discoloration of the skin from lack of oxygen, hemorrhage from the throat, and loss of voice.

***Treatment of Foreign Bodies in the Larynx.*** Prompt removal of the object is urgent, because suffocation may occur at any instant. Also, infection sets in rapidly. The removal can be accomplished only by a physician with the use of special instruments.

## INJURIES OF THE LARYNX

The larynx may suffer several different kinds of injury—bruises (contusions), wounds, and fractures—all of which require the prompt attention of a physician, if complications, which may be serious, are to be avoided.

***Contusions.*** Bruises lead to pain on speaking and swallowing; to hoarseness, and in some cases to loss of voice; to shortness of breath, and to suffocation.

***Wounds.*** Incised wounds of the larynx (from cuts or gashes) are likely to occur as a result of highway or railway accidents; in most cases they are inflicted by broken glass. Larynx injuries of this kind also occur frequently in attempts at suicide.

***Fractures.*** Injuries of this type, to bones and cartilages, result in pain, tenderness, and swelling. In the larynx they often interfere more or less with breathing, speaking, chewing, and swallowing. There may be bleeding from the throat. Air in the tissues of the neck, a very serious complication, is likely to occur.

***Direct Injury to the Larynx.*** To a large extent the larynx is protected from injury by the lower jaw and the front wall of the chest; also by the elasticity of the way it is suspended in the neck. The vocal cords are so placed that they are rarely damaged, but hemorrhage in one cord may occur as a result of blows on the neck. Simple, direct injuries to the larynx are frequently caused by falls, or by motor or airplane crashes. Usually, the result is a fracture of the thyroid cartilage. This is not, as a rule, of serious import. However, if the fracture is that of another, namely the cricoid cartilage, it is dangerous in the extreme, because later breathing may be obstructed. The windpipe must then be opened as a life-saving measure. Compound fracture of the larynx is most serious because of the danger of infection, particularly to the cartilages.

***Indirect Larynx Injury.*** Effects on the larynx may be produced by various wounds on the neck, in which the vagus nerve is injured or compressed by a large blood clot. The effect noted is paralysis of the nerve supplying the vocal cord, with consequent disturbance of speech.

## SWELLING OF THE LARYNX

***Causes of Swelling of the Larynx.*** Non-inflammatory swelling of the larynx may be caused by general bodily disease, such as nephritis (inflammation of the kidneys), by traumatic laryngitis (caused by an injury); as a complication of infectious disease; or by large doses of potassium iodide. It is usually brought about, however, by an extension of acute infection of the larynx. Also, the cause may be such mechanical factors as compression by external scars and tumors causing blockage of the veins; tumors in the neck or in the chest; or enlargement of parts of the wall of an artery.

***Symptoms of Swelling of the Larynx.*** The symptoms are extreme hoarseness and progressive difficulty in breathing.

***Treatment of Swelling of the Larynx.*** A physican should be consulted. In severe cases an emergency operation (tracheotomy) may be required to open the windpipe so that the patient will not become asphyxiated.

## ABSCESS OF THE LARYNX

***Causes of Abscess.*** Many abscesses of the larynx are caused by injuries which result from swallowing a foreign body. After the pain has subsided, there is an interval of relative comfort; then infection follows, and the patient suffers pain on swallowing, as well as occasional shortness of breath. Tuberculous as well as syphilitic infection of the cartilages of the larynx sometimes results in the formation of an abscess. Infections following influenza, scarlet fever, and erysipelas may be complicated by the development of an abscess. In infants, abscess of the larynx is rare. When it does occur, scarlet fever is usually the cause.

In the past, an abscess of the larynx ordinarily occurred as a complication of typhoid fever, but in the course of years this has notably decreased.

***Symptoms of Abscess.*** When the abscess is fully developed, pain may be present, or there may be mere tenderness on pressure. Hoarseness is invariably noted, but it may not be severe. Sometimes only the epiglottis is involved.

***Treatment of Abscess.*** Under all circumstances a specialist (laryngologist) must be consulted at once. Treatment with penicillin is begun as soon as possible. The abscess must be opened. Early opening of the windpipe is indicated when shortness of breath is even a mild symptom. The use of steam inhalations is helpful.

## LOSS OF VOICE

Functional loss of voice is a relatively common condition, usually noted in women. As a rule it comes on suddenly as a result of a cold or of anxiety. The voice is either completely gone or reduced to a whisper. The patient should abstain from talking in order to rest the larynx, and a physician should be consulted if the condition persists.

Loss of voice is also caused by acute catarrhal laryngitis, swelling within the larynx, diphtheria, or paralysis of the larynx. Treatment depends upon the disease. Early laryngitis in syphilis may be relatively free of symptoms; later, a gradually increasing hoarseness is noted and the voice becomes raucous. There may be pain, a hacking cough, severe shortness of breath, and a foul odor from the mouth. Penicillin is widely used for the treatment of syphilis. (The subject is treated more fully under the heading of Syphilis: see Index.)

## ULCERS OF THE LARYNX

The ulcers most frequently found are those resulting from Vincent's infection. The disease begins, like catarrhal laryngitis, with slight hoarseness. Swallowing is often disturbed because of simultaneous involvement of the pharynx. The voice becomes muffled and sometimes croupy. Breathing and swallowing are difficult and painful. The treatment depends on the specific cause of the disease.

## ALLERGY OF THE LARYNX

Allergy of the larynx may occur separately, or when other parts of the respiratory system are involved. It may also be noted with other signs of allergy, such as skin signs—urticaria and eczema, for instance—and may be caused by hypersensitivity to foods, chemicals and inhalants. The symptoms—difficulty of breathing, loss of voice or harshness of voice—often come on so suddenly and alarmingly that prompt diagnosis and adequate treatment, as for other allergies, are imperative in order to prevent a fatal issue.

## HYGIENE OF THE LARYNX

It is urgent that any hoarseness of a few weeks' duration be promptly investigated to be sure that a possible cancer of the larynx is not permitted to reach an advanced stage.

A normally functioning nose, as has been shown, is all-important in the proper functioning of the larynx, since air passing through the nose on the way to the speech-box is there filtered, warmed and moistened. Any condition in the nose that prevents this natural air-conditioning tends to damage the vocal cords.

Too spacious nasal passages may be equally harmful. This condition results from a disease called atrophic rhinitis, or from operative procedures which have been inexpert or too extensive. In both cases, the destruction of normal mucous membrane permits dusty, unmoistened air to be breathed in and sets up irritation or infection in the larynx and windpipe.

Proper hygiene of the larynx naturally includes correct use of the voice in speaking and in singing, which means avoiding strain. In industry the use of masks often prevents disease of the larynx.

## HOW TO GIVE INHALATIONS FOR THE LARYNX

Fill an inhaler (or tea kettle) half full of boiling water and let the patient inhale the steam. If an inhaler or vaporizer is used, turn the spout toward the patient, being careful to have it far enough away so that there is no danger of burning or scalding. Drugs, such as tincture of benzoin or menthol, may be added to the water, as required.

Good dry inhalants are formalin, pine oil, oil of eucalyptus, or guaiacol. They may be dropped in small amounts on lint and inhaled, or sprinkled on cotton wool contained in a small face-mask.

A good inhalant mixture (for acute laryngitis, for example), is the following: creosote, three teaspoonfuls; glycerin, three teaspoonfuls; water, add up to three-fourths teacupful. A teaspoonful is added to a pint of boiling water and the steam is inhaled for five minutes. Electric vaporizers can be bought at drug stores.

By means of an aerosol apparatus, a fine suspension of a solid or liquid in a gas can be used for the direct administration of medicines to the larynx, as well as to the nose, sinuses and bronchi. The aerosol is formed by the passage of a gas through the medication, in an inhaler operated by hand, or by oxygen supplied from a tank. Penicillin is used in the spray.

CHAPTER 3

# THE LUNGS AND BRONCHIAL TUBES

**The Respiratory System and How It Works . . . Chief Symptoms of Lung Disease . . . Acute Bronchitis . . . Chronic Bronchitis . . . Lobar Pneumonia . . . Bronchopneumonia . . . Primary Atypical Pneumonia . . . Tuberculosis . . . Miliary Tuberculosis . . . Chronic Tuberculosis . . . Asthma . . . Emphysema . . . Pleurisy . . . Empyema . . . Foreign Bodies in the Bronchi . . . Influenza . . . Bronchiectasis . . . Pneumoconiosis . . . Plumonary Embolism.**

THE LUNGS and bronchial tubes are important parts of the respiratory tract. The respiratory tract is the mechanism by which we breathe. It supplies oxygen and removes carbon dioxide. It regulates chemical changes in the blood. It helps control body temperature, and it also excretes water. Its most important parts are the nose, the sinuses, the upper nose-throat cavity, the larynx or voice-box, and the trachea or windpipe, as well as the bronchial tubes and the lungs. The bronchial tubes are the subdivisions of the windpipe inside the lungs.

The respiratory tract has a moist, sensitive lining, called mucous membrane. This membrane contains cells with hair-like processes called cilia which act like little brooms in sweeping upward toward the mouth any dirt which may have been breathed in. In this way they keep the respiratory tract clean.

***The Useful Cough.*** If the ciliated cells are unable to clear the respiratory tract, another mechanism goes into action—coughing. Coughing is one of the many protective reflex mechanisms with which the body is equipped. Coughing serves the useful purpose of helping us to get rid of dust, mucus, blood, pus, or other matter irritating the respiratory passages.

***The Lungs.*** The highly elastic lungs are two irregular, air-containing organs resting on the diaphragm or midriff. They occupy most of the chest cavity, being separated from each other by the heart and great blood vessels. Their work consists essentially in taking in oxygen for the vital processes of the body, and exhaling carbon dioxide, one of the waste products of body metabolism. The right lung is divided into an upper, a middle, and a lower lobe; the left lung has only an upper and a lower lobe. The pleura is the watertight and airtight covering of the lung.

***Rate of Respiration.*** The usual rate of respiration (breathing) in the adult is roughly sixteen to eighteen respirations per minute, but this number is subject to great variations. It is increased by muscular exertion, higher body temperature, and during excitement. In women the rate is higher by two to four a minute, because of the relatively smaller size of the body. The rate also varies with age; at birth, it is forty to fifty a minute; at five years, about twenty-five a minute; at fifteen years, about twenty a minute; at thirty years, about sixteen a minute. The rate is influenced also by the position of the body: reclining, thirteen a minute; sitting, eighteen a minute; standing, twenty-two a minute.

## CHIEF SYMPTOMS OF LUNG DISEASE

***Cough.*** Cough is almost always present in disorders of the lungs and bronchi (bronchial tubes); also, in some heart and blood vessel diseases. It is, as we have said, a protective reflex symptom, usually induced by changes in the mucous membrane of the windpipe and bronchial tubes, or caused by the presence of foreign matter or excess mucus.

***Hemorrhage.*** The most common causes of blood spitting are tuberculosis of the lungs, certain heart conditions, bronchiectasis (infected dilated bronchial tubes), and cancer of the lungs. It may occur in many other constitutional and lung disorders.

Severe coughing from "swallowing the wrong way" may bring up blood-tinged sputum. This type of cough results when food particles get under the epiglottis instead of over it. The epiglottis is the covering of the larynx (vocal box). It protects the windpipe from food particles, except on occasion when the swallowing of a mouthful of food is accompanied by a deep breath or a laugh.

***Sputum.*** The nature of the lung disease can frequently be determined by the nature of the sputum (phlegm)—by its amount, color, consistency, bacteria, and foreign matter. Rarely, fatal lung diseases may be present without expectoration or cough.

***Fever.*** Fever, in various lung diseases, may be regular or irregular in degree and duration.

***Emaciation and Weakness.*** These are symptoms of a great many lung diseases, but particularly of tuberculosis. It generally occurs late in the course of cancer of the lung.

***Pain.*** Pain in the chest is not common in lung disease, except where there is an acute inflammation of the pleura (cover of the lung), or pressure by tumors and other growths touching upon near-by organs, nerves, or blood vessels. There may be extensive lung disease without even the mildest pain.

***Disturbances of Breathing.*** Shortness of breath is one of the outstanding symptoms of lung disease—for example, asthma, pneumonia, and emphysema (stretching of the air sacs of the lungs)—but it is also significant in diseases of the heart and blood vessels.

## ACUTE BRONCHITIS

***Causes of Acute Bronchitis.*** Acute bronchitis is a sudden inflammation of the bronchial tubes and usually the trachea as well, of short duration. Its most usual origin is from the downward extension of a common cold—"the cold settling in the chest." It may, however, be due to a variety of viruses and bacteria. Frequently, in children, recurrent bronchitis is caused by allergy rather than infection. An acute bronchitis may be a part of a specific disease such as whooping cough or measles. Asthmatic persons are more prone to develop bronchitis. Infections of the sinuses, tonsils and adenoids; chilling; exposure to irritating dusts and gases; debilitating diseases—all may predispose to its occcurrence.

***Symptoms of Acute Bronchitis.*** A head cold most commonly precedes the symptoms. Fever, low-grade, may be present. Some degree of hoarseness is usual due to involvement of the larynx. There is a tightness and rawness experienced beneath the breast bone. Malaise and muscular aching occur. The characteristic feature is a disturbing cough—at first dry, hard and painful, and finally becoming loose. Sleep is often interrupted by coughing spells. As a rule recovery occurs in about a week.

***Treatment of Bronchitis.*** A patient suffering from acute bronchitis has a potentially serious disease. Put him to bed in a warm, well-ventilated room, and keep him there until acute symptoms have subsided. The treatment in general is that of the common cold. Give plenty of warm fluids and fruit juices. A soft diet is allowable. Steam inhalations from an open pan or, better, an electric vaporizer are comforting. A teaspoonful of tincture of benzoin may be added to a quart of boiling water. A mustard plaster over the breast bone often relieves the tight feeling there. If this is used, it must be carefully watched so that the skin does not blister. A cough syrup such as elixir of terpin hydrate with codeine is useful—a teaspoonful every three to four hours for an adult. Aspirin is helpful for muscular aching and slight fever. The new antihistaminic drugs tend to dry secretions and prevent loosening of the cough. They should not be used.

***Complications.*** Acute bronchitis may be complicated by pneumonia, usually bronchopneumonia, especially in children. Danger signals are increase in fever, shortness of breath and severe pain in the side of the chest made worse by cough and deep breathing. In severe cases and in those with complications the physician may use the "sulfa drugs," penicillin, or one of the other new antibiotic drugs.

The oxygen tent should be used if breathing becomes difficult. Private homes can get a supply of oxygen cylinders with the tent. The physician in charge usually advises this additional treatment.

## CHRONIC BRONCHITIS

This is a variety of bronchitis sometimes called "the winter cough of the aged." The disease is characterized by constant or recurring attacks of cough and expectoration over a long period and is usually accompanied by a certain degree of emphysema, or stretching of the air sacs of the lung.

***Causes of Chronic Bronchitis.*** Often this disease is secondary to some other disorder such as chronic infection in the tonsils and sinuses, congestion of the lungs due to heart weakness, and bronchial asthma. It may arise from the continued inhalation of irritating dust, especially dust containing silica. Especially in younger children chronic bronchitis may arise from allergic cause, and the origin is frequently overlooked because asthma does not always accompany it. Certainly excessive use of alcohol and tobacco may be aggravating factors if not causative. Of course some cases are simply the result of repeated attacks of acute bronchitis in those who are low in resistance to respiratory infections.

***Symptoms of Chronic Bronchitis.*** Persistent cough with the production of more or less purulent sputum is common to all persons afflicted with this disease. Gradually shortness of breath on exertion is noted. This is chiefly due to the developing emphysema rather than the bronchitis itself.

***Why Diagnosis Is Important.*** Many cases of pulmonary tuberculosis, cancer of the lungs, and bronchiectasis masquerade as simple chronic bronchitis. In the case of tuberculosis, not only the welfare and future life of the patient hinges on its discovery but also the health of his family and of other persons who come in immediate contact with him. Sputum must always be examined and X-ray study made of the lungs.

***Treatment of Chronic Bronchitis.*** If sinusitis, chronic tonsillitis, heart disease, dust exposure, bronchial asthma, or allergic irritation are producing the bronchitis, these conditions must be treated primarily. Tobacco should be given up. Many physicians recommend whiskey or brandy as an important part of treatment. Diet and rest should be ample to raise the general resistance. If the origin is that of repeated attacks of acute bronchitis, vaccines may raise the resistive powers to infection. If feasible, moving to a dry warm climate may be of remarkable benefit. Medications are frequently prescribed which liquefy the thick tenacious sputum and thus aid in its expulsion. Cough syrups which suppress cough may do harm in excessive use by reducing useful cough.

Although penicillin and other new drugs used in infectious disease may be of great aid in controlling an acute flare-up in symptoms, their use in the chronic condition is for the most part disappointing.

## THE PNEUMONIAS

Pneumonia is an acute infection of the lungs. It is characterized by an inflammatory discharge in one or more lobes.

***Kinds of Pneumonia.*** Pneumonia is classified in three general groups: lobar pneumonia, usually caused by the pneumococcal germs, and with a characteristic set of symptoms; bronchopneumonia, also caused by bacteria, but with a more treacherous beginning, and a more irregular course than the first variety; pneumonia for which no identifiable bacterial cause can be found (primary atypical pneumonia).

***Conditions Favoring Pneumonia.*** Many factors serve to promote the infections, notably economic, physical, and psychic conditions which lead to lowered vitality and dimenished physical resistance. Lowered resistance produced by colds, influenza, measles, scarlet fever, exposure, chilling or other causes may make it easy for the germs to gain headway. Examination of the chest at intervals reveals the various stages of the disease. The X-ray and sputum examinations are of primary importance in diagnosis and treatment.

### Lobar Pneumonia

Lobar pneumonia is an acute disease associated with inflammatory changes in the lung, causing, also, in most casts an inflammation of the cover of the lung (pleurisy). The infection usually travels along the respiratory tract. The disease was commonly fatal in the past.

Pneumonia is more frequent during the winter months than in the summer. Young children, elderly persons, and alcoholics are more prone to contract the disease, and it is more frequent in men than in women. The mortality is greatest in the extreme age groups, and it is higher in women than in men. The death rate is higher in the lower-income brackets, where lack of early medical attention, poor food, and poor housing are contributory factors.

***The Pneumococcus.*** The exciting causes in adults, in the vast majority of cases, are virulent strains of the pneumococcal bacteria. They may be associated with other germs, notably the streptococcus and the influenza bacillus.

***Symptoms of Lobar Pneumonia.*** Lobar pneumonia has a typical course although there may be, frequently, variations. The disease usually begins suddenly with a chill. Characteristically the temperature rises rapidly and may reach 104° or 105° F. The patient appears ill, and, in breathing, ordinarily experiences severe pain over the involved area, together with a short, dry, hacking cough. Very rarely cough may be absent throughout the disease. The respirations are rapid and shallow, with a corresponding increase in the pulse rate. There is a grunt on breathing out, and the normal rhythm of breathing is reversed so that the pause which ordinarily takes place after exhaling now occurs after inhaling.

The sputum, as a rule, is sticky and scanty, and characteristically has a rust-brown color. Blueness of the face and lips (cyanosis) may be most pronounced in the first few days.

The white blood cells are usually greatly increased in number (leucocytosis). If this condition is absent, it has a serious meaning.

The fever, as a rule, is high and continuous. In 60 to 75 per cent of patients the decline in fever is by crisis, which ordinarily consists of a progressive fall from a high level to subnormal, in from twelve to eighteen hours. The other symptoms cease simultaneously. This usually occurs in the fifth to ninth day of the disease. Lobar pneumonia is one of the few infectious diseases which end in this manner. The change in the patient's general condition is dramatic. From being restless, wakeful, or delirious and short of breath, the patient falls into a quiet and prolonged sleep. He awakens refreshed and with easier breathing. The cough becomes loose and the pulse slower. The crisis is almost always accompanied by profuse sweating. There may appear, at times, a false crisis in which there is only a temporary fall in the elevated temperature and without the abatement of the other symptoms.

***Complications of Lobar Pneumonia.*** A "dry" pleurisy is so frequently an accompaniment of this form of pneumonia that it is to be considered a part of the disease rather than a complication. Sometimes fluid accumulates in the pleural cavity (space between the lung and chest wall). This may clear up by itself or require tapping. The most serious common complication is empyema, a collection of pus in the pleural cavity. This complication is now infrequent with modern treatment. Other complications such as lung abscess, meningitis, inflammation of the heart valves and covering of the heart (pericarditis) and arthritis are extremely rare.

***Treatment of Lobar Pneumonia.*** Before recent years lobar pneumonia used to carry a mortality rate as high as 30 to 35 per cent. The first treatment advance was that of specific sera. Serum treatment was technically difficult, expensive, and gave rise to rather frequent serious reactions. It is now almost entirely discarded. The sulfonamide drugs (sulfa drugs) are highly efficacious in this disease. The most frequently used are sulfadiazine and sulfamerazine. Penicillin works as well but is probably no better in the uncomplicated case. It is now used often, especially since modified injectable forms which prolong its action over a period of twenty-four to forty-eight hours are now readily available. This permits treatment at home, whereas this was not feasible when the original solutions were used, which had to be injected every three to four hours. Aureomycin is another recent treatment. In difficult cases where old age or other disease is present, hospital treatment is imperative.

During the acute stages of the disease a liquid diet is generally prescribed. For the average adult three quarts of fluid per day may be given. Milk may not be well tolerated. Morphine or codeine is frequently given for pain. Attention to the bowels is necessary especially when these drugs are used, as they tend to be constipating. Occasionally the chest is bound or strapped for the relief of pleural pain. In the hospital, when rapid pulse rate, excessive shortness of breath or cyanosis appears, oxygen may be given by nasal tube, mask, or oxygen tent. A very ill patient may be given fluids by vein. The physician observes the patient for side reactions to the drugs used. Skin rashes, changes in the blood cell counts, and decrease in kidney function may infrequently occur with the sulfa drugs. The latter possibility makes intake of fluid important and the amount of urine produced should be measured daily while taking these drugs. Any sign of decrease in urine output or skin rash should be promptly reported to the physician. Skin rash is the most important side-reaction of penicillin. It does not affect the blood or kidney function.

The advance in the treatment of lobar pneumonia is one of the most thrilling accomplishments of modern-day medicine. The mortality rate of this disease has been greatly reduced.

### Bronchopneumonia

***Causes of Bronchopneumonia.*** Bronchopneumonia is an acute disease in which there is inflammation of the smaller bronchial tubes, with patches of lung tissue, irregularly distributed, surrounding the tubes. Thus it is a scattered process in contrast to lobar pneumonia, in which an entire lobe or more than one lobe is involved. Bronchopneumonia is usually secondary to measles, influenza, whooping cough, or a common bronchitis. It frequently occurs in children and in the elderly with debilitating disease. Pneumococci, streptococci, staphylococci, and the influenzal bacillus are frequent bacterial causes. In small children, under two, it may occur as a primary affliction. It is usually then caused by pneumococci.

***Symptoms of Bronchopneumonia.*** In small children the disease runs a course much like lobar pneumonia. In the other cases it has a slow, irregular onset with fever, cough and shortness of breath gradually growing worse. Temperature does not fall by crisis but abates gradually when recovery occurs.

***Treatment of Bronchopneumonia.*** The general treatment is the same as that of lobar pneumonia. The sulfonamides and penicillin are most frequently used in drug treatment. Some organisms are not affected by these, such as the influenzal bacillus, and then streptomycin may be of service.

### Primary Atypical Pneumonia

***Causes of Primary Atypical Pneumonia.*** This is commonly known as "virus pneumonia." It presents an involvement of the smaller bronchial tubes and patches of lung tissue similar to that in bronchopneumonia. However, bacteria are not a cause. Probably the condition is caused by a variety of viruses—organisms too small to be seen under the microscope. In some few types the virus has been identified.

***Symptoms of Primary Atypical Pneumonia.*** The disease starts slowly, resembling a cold. Then a harassing dry cough, difficult to control, is a common outstanding complaint. Headache may be distressing. Fever may not be so high and the patient not appear so ill as in the other pneumonias. Pleural pain is not common. The course may last for two to three weeks and the patient then has a slow convalescence. Fatalities are rare and they occur usually when the patient has some other serious disease such as a heart condition.

***Treatment of Primary Atypical Pneumonia.*** Until recently no specific treatment was available since the disorder was not affected by penicillin or the sulfa drugs. Now aureomycin seems to show a definite curative effect on virus pneumonia—greatly shortening the course and period of convalescence.

## TUBERCULOSIS (CONSUMPTION)

Amazing progress has been made in the prevention and cure of tuberculosis. One of the most prevalent of infectious diseases, it affects not only man but also many of the lower animals. Moreover, it attacks all the tissues and organs of the body, so that physicians refer to tuberculosis of the lungs, tuberculosis of the bones and joints, tuberculosis of the kidneys, etc. No complete immunity, either natural or artificial, is obtainable in the human being, although specific resistance is increased by previous mild infections.

The most prevalent form of tuberculosis is that of the lungs which, with its direct complications, causes about 90 per cent of the fatalities from this disease. It is also the most important from the viewpoint of preventive medicine and public health, for it is mainly through the lung form that the disease is spread. Formerly, a great number of infections, especially among children, were caused by drinking the raw milk of tuberculous cows, but that source of infection is now virtually eliminated in the United States. The great source of spread, now, is the coughing and expectorating tuberculous victim himself. The danger lies in the infected human sputum.

***Who Gets Tuberculosis.*** Many of us adults, as high or higher than 50 per cent, have at some time in our lives been infected with tubercle bacilli. However, because of most persons' resistance, a much smaller number have symptoms of the disease. The fact that the majority of infected persons never develop obvious disease indicates that although man is extremely susceptible to tuberculosis he also possesses or is capable of developing a high degree of resistance to the disease.

### Factors Predisposing to Tuberculous Disease

There can be no tuberculosis without the presence of, and infection by, the tubercle bacillus, the cause of the disease. However, there are modifying factors, some poorly understood, which favor or protect against frank disease once the bacillus has gained entrance into our bodies by inhalation of infected particles of sputum.

Probably there is an inherited natural resistance to tuberculosis in some and an inherited lack of resistance or hereditary predisposition to tuberculosis in others. Some dispute the existence of this factor.

During adolescence there is a greater susceptibility in girls than boys to tuberculosis. Race has a bearing on liability to the disease. The Jews possess a relatively high resistance while Negroes have a great proneness to develop tuberculosis.

Poverty, overcrowded living conditions, and poor diet undoubtedly contribute their weight in lowering natural resistance to the tubercle bacillus.

Occupation has a bearing. The death toll is much greater in unskilled industrial workers than, for instance, in professional workers. This may be due to poor economic circumstances rather than directly to the type of job. Exposure to dust containing silica, however, such as in quartz mining, sandblasting, and stone cutting, renders one increasingly liable to tuberculosis.

Other conditions and diseases may favor the development of tuberculous disease. Pregnancy may worsen its course. Young diabetics are prone to acquire tuberculosis, less so now than in the days before insulin. Alcoholism favors susceptibility. Overindulgence in tobacco seems to have no bearing on the initiation of the disease. Measles, influenza, and whooping cough have a bad effect in young children. Fatigue from overwork or loss of sleep has a detrimental influence.

Recently some investigators have stressed emotional disturbances and psychic strain as occurring frequently in persons just preceding the development of symptoms from the disease.

***Mortality Rate in Tuberculosis.*** There has been a striking and steady decline in deaths due to tuberculosis in recent years. In 1900 in the United States the disease caused 202 deaths per 100,000 population. This had dropped to 49 deaths per 100,000 population in 1936 and in 1948 was still lower, 30 deaths per 100,000 population. Despite this decline it still remains the leading cause of death in young men and women between adolescence and their middle thirties.

### The Two Types of Tuberculous Infection

When tubercle bacilli are breathed into the lung in sufficient number a small "spot" develops in the lung tissue as a result of the infection. The germs spread by way of the lymphatic vessels (small channels which drain tissue juice) to the lymph glands surrounding the windpipe and main bronchial tubes. ("Kernels" which appear in the armpit and neck with infection of the hands and neck, respectively, are swollen lymph glands.) These glands enlarge and become inflamed but usually stop the infection from spreading further. This is called *primary tuberculosis, first infection tuberculosis,* or *"childhood tuberculosis."* The child or adult (if he has never been infected before) may show no symptoms. Sometimes he may be slightly irritable, prone to fatigue and appear generally not up to par. Failure to gain weight, slight fever, and some cough may be noticed. Symptoms, if present, may last only several weeks to months. Almost always the "spot" grows smaller and the lymph glands return to more or less normal size. Rarely one of the acute forms of tuberculosis or progressive disease in the glands develops. One sign of the infection appears and does remain. The tuberculin test (to be discussed later) becomes positive.

In a person *previously infected,* tubercle bacilli cause a different course of events. This may come about in two ways. Resistance may be lowered and germs lying quiet and dormant from the first arrested infection may light up in activity. Or contact with a tuberculous individual may bring about re-infection from without. Now the baccilli do not tend to spread by the lymphatics (spread is resisted) but locally where the germs appear there is more violent inflammation than with the first infection. Death of tissue and the appearance of cavities may occur. The body has changed in its reaction to the tubercle bacillus so that on one hand resistance to distant spread is increased (immunity), but locally more destructive action by the germ takes place (hypersensitivity or allergy of tuberculosis). This is the re-infection or adult type of tubercular infection.

### The Different Forms of Re-Infection Tuberculosis

Acute forms of tuberculous disease may arise by themselves or complicate a chronic process. Usually they arise from re-infection from within the lungs. An infected gland can break into or invade a bronchial tube; infected sputum may be inhaled in an undiseased part of the lung; a disease spot may invade and feed bacilli into a blood vessel. There may result a tuberculous bronchopneumonia or a tuberculous lobar pneumonia. These have a short onset and severe symptoms. They resemble in symptoms the common pneumonias but their course is protracted and they do not respond to the ordinary antipneumonic drugs. They are sometimes called "galloping consumption."

***Miliary Tuberculosis.*** This is an acute form of the disease, seen most frequently in young children. The bacilli are spread through the body by invasion of a blood vessel. Numerous "spots" (tubercles) occur in the lungs, liver, spleen, kidneys, coverings of the brain and spinal cord (meningitis) and elsewhere. Fever, rapid loss of weight and strength occur. Shortness of breath and cough develop. Until recently this form was fatal in six to eight weeks.

***Chronic Forms of Tuberculosis.*** These are by far the most common forms of re-infection tuberculosis. Two main kinds of reaction of lung tissue to the infection occur: "Soft" lesions (a lesion is an area of inflammation or injury), in which serum and various white blood cells form the principal constituents; "hard" or productive lesions, in which tissue cells make up the spot. "Soft" lesions may clear up rather rapidly or grow rapidly worse. "Hard" lesions tend to change more slowly but their centers may liquefy and cavities result. The signs and symptoms of chronic tuberculosis and its course in the individual are dependent on the varying amounts of intermixture of these two types of tissue reaction since neither appears in pure form.

***Symptoms of Chronic Tuberculosis of the Lungs.*** A feeling of fatigue or loss of energy is almost always present. Loss of weight may occur early or may not be remarkable. Fever usually occurs somewhat later. It may be slight and is most apt to be noticed in late afternoon or early evening. The pulse tends to be moderately accelerated. Decrease in appetite is a rather frequent complaint. Decrease in amount of menstrual flow or cessation of menstrual periods is common in young women and girls. Irritability and excess nervous tension are prominent in some persons. Cough is not an outstanding early symptom. Later it is more noticeable and varying amounts of sputum are produced. When even a small cavity forms, the spitting of blood may take place. Some have estimated that this takes place in over half the patients in the first year or so of the disease. Shortness of breath is not a symptom unless far advanced disease or some complication is present.

# Science *vs.* Tuberculosis

## TESTING FOR TUBERCULOSIS

The nurse is making a scratch test for tuberculosis. TB, one of ten top killers in this country, takes about 80,000 lives each year. To avoid it, you must get plenty of fresh air, sunlight, and rest, and eat good food. Disease is associated with poor hygiene.

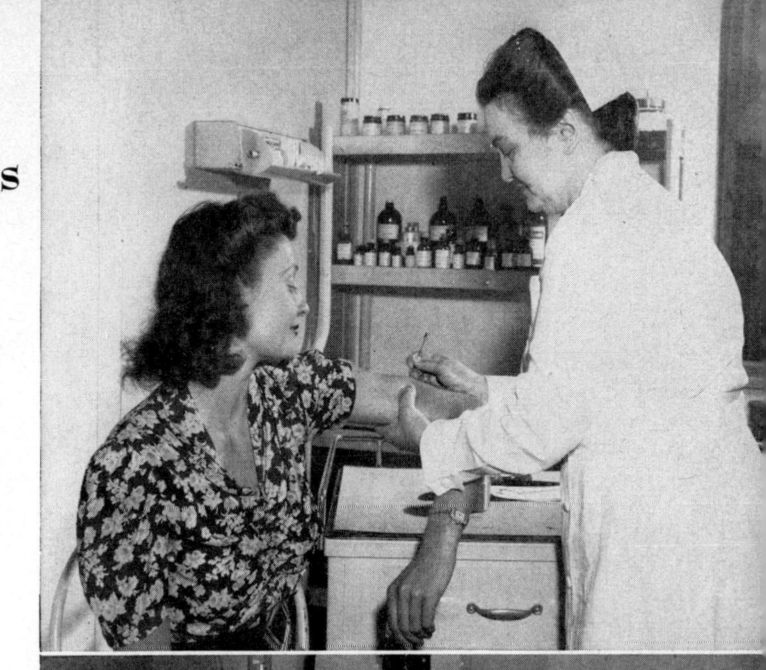

## HOW TO DETECT TB EARLY

X-ray examination makes possible an early diagnosis of tuberculosis, when it is more easily controlled. Everyone should have a chest X-ray regularly.

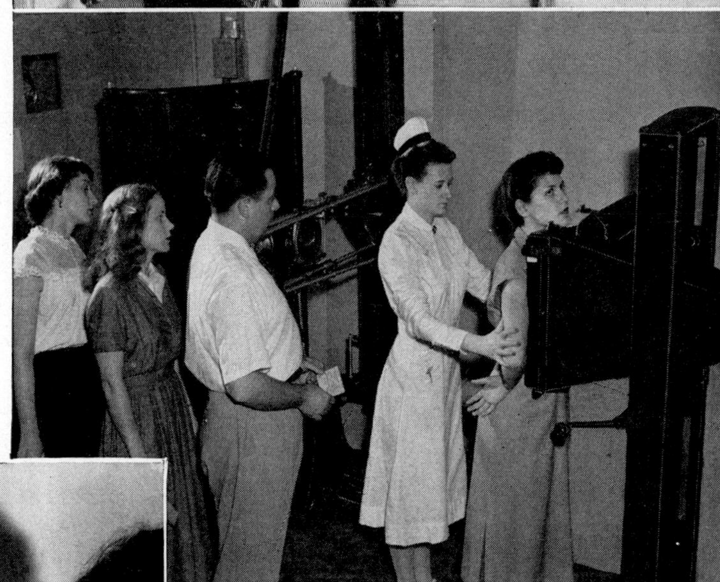

## INJECTING TUBERCULIN

In the Mantoux test for tuberculosis, a small amount of a substance called tuberculin is injected into the skin. If injected area becomes red, hard, and swollen, person has been infected by TB germs at some time.

Top and Bottom Photos,
Emerson Yorke Studio, N. Y.

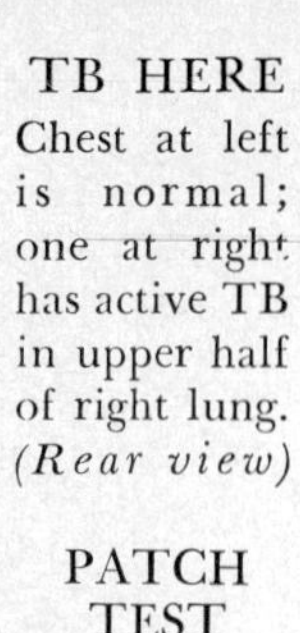

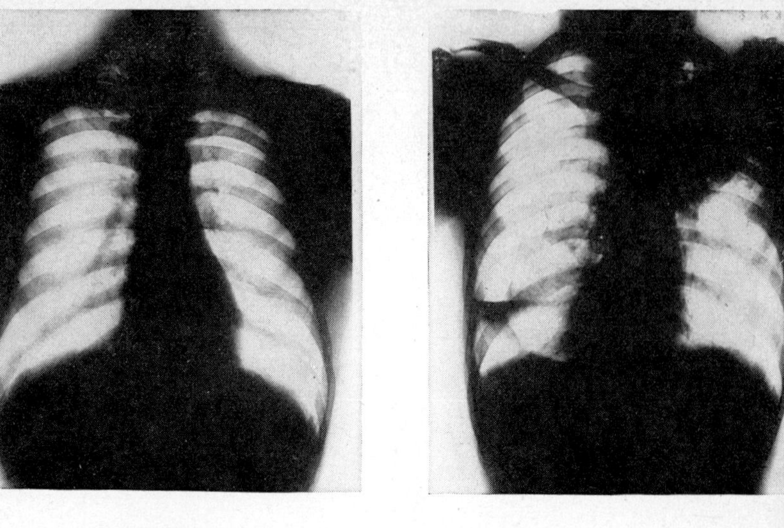

TB HERE

Chest at left is normal; one at right has active TB in upper half of right lung. *(Rear view)*

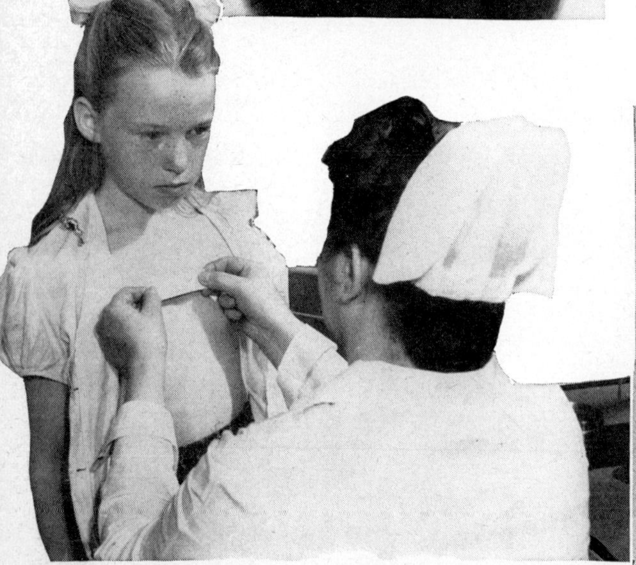

PATCH TEST

Gauze soaked with tuberculin is applied to skin.

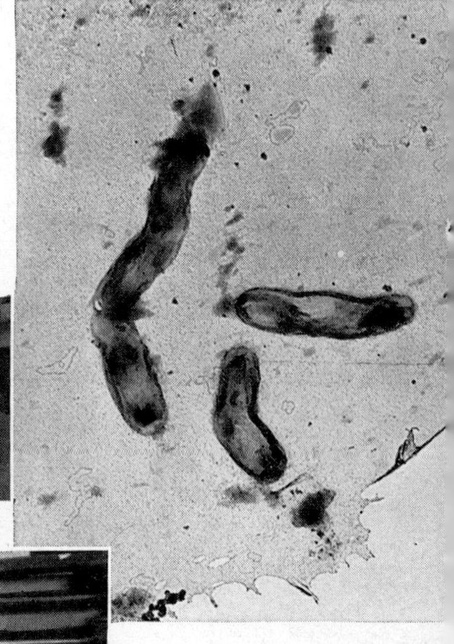

HUMAN TB GERMS

They may attack the spine, bones, glands, eyes, or other tissues, besides lungs. (Enlarged)

LAB TESTS

In the war against TB, laboratory technicians play big role, detecting the presence of germs.

***Warning Signals of Tuberculosis of the Lungs.*** It is urgent that medical opinion as to the possible presence of tuberculosis be sought if the following occur: (1) the spitting of blood; (2) cough persisting over two or three weeks, especially in a young person; (3) repeated chest colds or "flu"; (4) unexplained fever, weight loss or fatigue; (5) wet pleurisy or ill health in persons who have had a wet pleurisy in the past.

A first sign of tuberculous infection may be a pleurisy with fluid collecting between the lung and chest wall. At that time there may be no detectable evidence of disease within the lung itself, but a large number of such patients may develop tuberculosis even after a period of years. Inflammation of the lung cover (pleurisy) is the only common cause of chest pain in tubercular infection. It does not occur with involvement of lung tissue by itself.

***Diagnosis of Tuberculosis.*** With any of the above warning signals present, an X-ray of the chest showing lung changes in the portions of the lungs above the second rib is very suggestive of tuberculosis. Chronic tuberculosis of the lungs almost always starts in the top part of the lungs. The diagnosis is confirmed by the finding of tubercle bacilli in the sputum. Some persons do not have sputum and, in these, washings of the stomach often reveal the germs. Sputum is present but it is swallowed.

When the bacilli are so few that they cannot be found, sputum may be innoculated into a guinea pig and later the bacilli are demonstrated in the test animal after time is allowed for their growth. Artificial culture media (mixtures of agar with materials needed by the bacilli to grow) are now frequently used to grow the tubercle bacilli for diagnostic purposes. In wet pleurisy the fluid obtained from the chest is examined for the germs.

***Tuberculin Tests and What They Show.*** Tuberculin is the bacillus-free product of the growth of tubercle bacilli in culture media. To the individual who has never been infected by the germ, tuberculin is non-injurious to the skin. After infection the skin alters in its response to tuberculin. Now a minute amount of tuberculin solution injected in the skin causes a local redness and swelling in twenty-four to seventy-two hours. This is a positive tuberculin reaction. It signifies that such a person has at one time been infected with tubercle bacilli. This may have occurred years ago in a mild childhood type of infection and the disease for years may have been arrested.

***Meaning of a Positive Reaction.*** A positive reaction is of no value in telling whether active disease is present or not. However, if a negative reaction is present it may be of help in ruling out tuberculosis. Furthermore, the development of a positive reaction may point out that a child is exposed whereas the X-ray may be of little help in diagnosing a mild infection. An immediate search among adults to which the child is exposed may then disclose the source of infection.

Formerly at least 80 to 90 per cent of adults showed positive tuberculin reactions. Now in some localities the adult positive reactors may be as low as 50 per cent and in some communities a rate of only 10 per cent may be found in adolescents.

***Tuberculin Patch Test.*** A tuberculin patch test is now used frequently in young children. Gauze or paper saturated with tuberculin is applied to the skin and held on by adhesive. In this way injection by a needle is avoided but the test is not as reliable as the ordinary tuberculin test.

***Mass X-Ray Surveys and Symptomless Tuberculosis.*** It is important to realize that tuberculosis in its earliest stages shows no symptoms whatsoever. Also at this time, unfortunately, ordinary physical examination of the chest by the physician does not disclose its presence. For this reason X-ray surveys of large groups of persons or even whole communities have been advocated. A new method of photographing the fluoroscopic image of the chest on a small film has greatly reduced the cost of such a survey. Suspicious cases are then re-X-rayed by the ordinary film technique. Such X-ray surveys have greatly increased the finding of cases of symptomless tuberculosis. Many physicians have a routine X-ray of the chest made as a part of their yearly check-ups on their patients.

***Treatment of Tuberculosis.*** The most important treatment in tuberculosis is rest. With most patients it is best that care be at least started in a sanatorium. Absolute bed rest may be prescribed by the physician, and patients with active symptoms may have to be fed. Such bed confinement should be carried on for months before slight graduated physical activity is permitted. If healing fails to ensue or if a cavity is present, further rest of the lung may have to be produced by artificial means. The simplest of these is artificial pneumothorax, or collapsing the lung.

***Collapsing the Lung.*** In this treatment, air is injected into the pleural cavity producing a partial collapse of the diseased lung. In this way the diseased tissue is put at rest which favors healing, and the walls of a cavity are brought closer together, which helps in the obliteration of a cavity. Such a collapse is maintained by refills of air (the air gradually becomes absorbed) every few days to several months, as the case may require. Pneumothorax may be continued for a period of eighteen months to three or four years.

***Use of Surgery.*** In more advanced diseases or where extensive adhesions of the pleura prevent adequate pneumothorax, thoracoplasty may be necessary. This is a surgical procedure in which portions of the ribs overlying the diseased lung are removed so that the chest wall collapses and thereby brings about a maximum collapse of the diseased area.

***Drug Treatment for Tuberculosis.*** In just the last several years specific drug treatment for tuberculosis has been discovered. The most important advance as far as chemical treatment goes is streptomycin. This is an antibiotic (like penicillin) which must be given by injection. It has two outstanding drawbacks: (1) After a period of time the bacilli grow resistant to its action; (2) the auditory nerve may be affected so that permanent dizziness results or, more rarely, deafness occurs as a result of toxic action of the drug. About two-thirds of the cases of miliary tuberculosis without a complicating tuberculous meningitis have recovered on treatment with streptomycin. Formerly it was fatal.

Streptomycin is also highly useful in tubercular lobar and bronchopneumonia. It is not nearly so helpful and is only used as an adjunct in the treatment of the average case of chronic tuberculosis of the lungs. It may be used to check an acute spread in a chronic process or in flare-ups in the opposite lung after thoracoplasty. In "hard" lesions its use is greatly restricted.

Recently a modification of streptomycin called dihydrostreptomycin has been thought by some to be less toxic and just as useful as the original drug. With it and altered dose schedules vertigo now occurs less frequently than with the older treatment. Still another chemical aid is para-aminosalicylic acid. This drug has some direct effect on tubercle bacilli but its most important effect is that it hinders the development of streptomycin resistance by the bacilli. For this reason the combination of dihydrostreptomycin treatment with para-aminosalicylic acid is becoming increasingly popular.

***Climate and Diet.*** Special climates are not stressed for tuberculosis as was the fashion in the past. With proper care the patient may get well in any climate. The diet should be ample in quantity and quality. Above all, a calm, optimistic, cheerful attitude should be developed in the patient. As activity increases, occupational therapy is important.

***The Sickroom.*** Both at home and in the hospital, proper disposal of sputum is essential to prevent spread of infection to others. It should be collected in cardboard containers and burnt. All utensils used by the patient in eating and drinking should be isolated from the rest of the household and sterilized by boiling. Similar attention should be given to bedclothes and towels. Upholstered furniture should be removed from the bedroom and the remaining furniture should be such that it is easily cleaned.

***Contact with Arrested Tuberculosis Cases.*** A word should be said about the irrational fear of some persons of contact with individuals who have arrested tuberculosis. Such an individual has full knowledge whether or not his sputum contains tubercle bacilli. If it is negative, he cannot transmit infection. Moreover, because of his education in the disease, the person with arrested tuberculosis is much more careful of conveying any kind of germs by cough than the average person. The danger is from exposure to an infected person with undiagnosed and unsuspected tuberculosis.

## ASTHMA

Asthma or bronchial asthma is a recurrent condition consisting of attacks of shortness of breath with a peculiar noisy respiration called wheezing. About 1 per cent of the population have asthma. It may begin at any time from infancy to old age although the majority of cases begin before the age of forty.

***Associated Conditions and Heredity.*** Asthma is frequently associated with other disorders due to allergy, such as allergic eczema, both in the infant and later in life, seasonal and perennial hay fever, recurrent hives, stomach and intestinal upsets due to particular foods and others. Extrinsic asthma (asthma provoked by contact with substances in the environment) has a strong hereditary pattern. The individual inherits the tendency to become sensitive. Most often there will be found a history of asthma or other allergies in his parents, brothers or sisters, grandparents or other relatives. Intrinsic asthma (asthma without apparent external cause) begins later in life and an allergic heredity frequently is not to be found. Infection is thought by many to be the common incitant.

***Causes of Asthma.*** The most frequent causes of extrinsic asthma are substances breathed in from our environment. Foremost are the *air-borne* pollens of trees (elm, oak, beech, birch, poplar, hickory, pecan, ash), grasses (Timothy, June grass, redtop, sweet vernal,

orchard, and Bermuda) and weeds (especially r
ragweed and grass pollen are by far the most importa

Probably the most important inhalant is house dust
pillows, mattresses, upholstered furniture, draperies, and rug
home. Animal danders are outstanding, such as those from feat
cats, dogs, and horses. Certain molds may give rise to microscopic
particles called spores, from which new plants are produced. In some, these may act like pollen as a cause of respiratory allergies.

***Foods As Causes of Asthma.*** Foods have been overrated as causes of asthma. In children under two they may be of prominence, but after ten they are of only occasional significance. Even in young children after infancy the inhalants supersede foods as provocative agents. Any food may be a cause in a particular case; frequently listed as important are eggs, fish, milk, wheat, chocolate, tomato, and orange.

Drugs taken into the body, such as aspirin and the sulfa drugs are rare sources of trouble. Infection in the teeth, tonsils and adenoids, sinuses and bronchial tubes may be of importance in the type of asthma known as intrinsic.

***The Way Asthma Develops.*** Fortunately only about 5 per cent of persons inherit the tendency to develop sensitivities to common substances in our environment. Of these, only one-fifth acquire the special allergic disorder known as asthma. In such a predisposed individual, exposure, for instance, to ragweed pollen or house dust may cause the appearance within his body of new chemical substances called antibodies, which are capable of reacting to the specific allergen (incitant of allergy) such as ragweed pollen or house dust. These antibodies anchor to cells in the lining of the bronchial tubes. When the offending substance, such as house dust (or whatever particular substance the patient is sensitive to), is breathed in, the house dust unites with its special antibody located in the bronchial lining.

As a result of this union, there is released from the tissues a chemical known as H-substance (histamine or a histamine-like substance). This substance causes swelling of the lining of the fine bronchial tubes, spasm of the involuntary muscles surrounding the tubes and the outpouring of mucus by the mucous glands of the bronchial lining. The swelling, spasm, and mucus all contribute to obstruction of the fine bronchial tubes. This obstruction causes the attack of asthma.

***Other Predisposing Causes.*** Fatigue, nervousness, emotional upset, menstrual disorders, climatic changes may favor the development of an asthmatic attack. These are secondary influences and cannot of themselves initiate asthma. Irritating fumes of frying meat, DDT, noke, and others may aggravate the asthmatic but are not rgens.

*ptoms of Asthma.* Frequently an attack may begin by some zing and itching of the nose. Soon a tightness of the chest and rhaps a dry cough begins. Shortness of breath is then experienced. It is hard to breathe and especially hard to breathe out. Respiration is noisy and, especially with the long expiration, wheezing, whistle-like sounds are heard. The victim must sit up to breathe better. The attack may last only a few minutes, several hours or even days. The termination of the attack is frequently associated with the coughing up of a thick sticky grayish mucus.

Attacks are especially likely to come on during the early morning hours. This cannot be fully explained, although in many cases it is due to sensitivity to substances in the bedroom. Attacks may be widely spaced and between attacks the person may be entirely free of cough and shortness of breath.

***Severe Asthma Symptoms.*** In severe cases the spells become more and more frequent. Sometimes some wheezing may be present continuously. With chronic distention of the lungs present, changes in the chest and disruption of the tiny air sacs of the lungs may take place (emphysema). The chest becomes barrel-shaped and the breathing capacity of the lungs is greatly reduced. Shortness of breath is now present even in the free period between attacks. This is frequently complicated by chronic bronchitis with constant cough and purulent sputum.

***Symptoms in Children.*** In children especially, but also in adults, a common cold may precipitate asthma even though the primary cause is a sensitivity to the substances noted above. In young children asthma frequently manifests itself by what appears to be recurrent chest colds or bronchitis but is really of allergic cause. It may be several years before the typical asthmatic attacks develop.

***Seasonal Symptoms Become Permanent.*** Often in persons with asthma there is a history of only seasonal hay fever at first. After several years wheezing may occur at the end of the season. If untreated, many of such patients are victimized eventually by frequent nasal symptoms and wheezing during the entire year.

***Diagnosis of Causes of Asthma.*** It is well to remember that the asthmatic patient does not have one single outstanding sensitivity, but usually several. Skin testing is an important diagnostic help, but its value is overestimated by the public. The patient's own account of his case is the primary cause-finding tool of the physician. In many cases the personal history alone will disclose the offending substances. Skin tests are done by two main methods. Scratch tests consist of making shallow scratches in the skin, which do not draw blood, and then rubbing a bit of the powder or solution of the suspected substances in the scratch. Other tests are made by injecting minute amounts of sterile solutions of the test substances into the superficial layers of the skin. In both methods a positive test results in a small hive or swelling which usually itches at the site of the test. The reactions appear within five to twenty minutes. The procedures are not painful and give rise to only a small amount of temporary discomfort.

Diets eliminating certain foods or the prescription of only a certain number of foods for a limited time may be used in diagnosing food allergies. Environmental change, such as removal of the patient to another house for a visit or for a stay in a hospital may give valuable clues.

***Treatment of Asthma.*** *For the acute attack,* epinephrine (one of the trade names is Adrenalin) by hypodermic injection is the most important measure. It usually gives relief in a few minutes. The patient or one of his family may be taught by the physician to give the injections. Epinephrine is useless when swallowed. However, it may be used in solution in a fine mist nebulizer with a hand bulb. The spray is inhaled as the bulb of the apparatus is squeezed. This is useful in mild attacks, but overuse is frequent and harmful.

Ephedrine has an epinephrine-like effect and may be taken in tablet form. Aminophyllin is frequently given by the physician by intravenous injection when epinephrine fails to relieve an attack. It is also frequently prescribed in tablets and as rectal suppositories. Iodides are commonly given to liquefy tenacious bronchial secretions. They form the basis of many patent medicines for asthma. Asthma powder and cigarettes (containing stramonium and nitrates) are not usually as helpful as the standard remedies. Unfortunately, the new antihistaminic drugs relieve attacks of asthma in only an occasional patient. For most patients they are worthless and may be harmful as they tend to promote thickening of the mucus in the bronchial tubes. In prolonged attacks of asthma hospital treatment is often necessary.

***Removing the Offending Substance.*** To control the occurrence of asthma, treatment must be directed to its causes. When these have been found, the ideal course, if possible, is avoidance of the offending substances. A dog may be removed from the home; feather pillows may be replaced by rubber foam pillows or covered by impervious casings; egg may be eliminated from the diet. However, most inhalants cannot be avoided. House dust exposure may be reduced by covering with special cases the pillows and mattress in the bedroom and eliminating non-washable rugs, draperies, upholstered furniture, and dust-collecting objects from the bedroom.

***Desensitizing the Patient.*** Few persons can afford to go to ragweed-free resorts for six weeks each year during the fall ragweed season. For these and other inhalant allergies where avoidance cannot be accomplished, desensitization treatment is necessary. This is carried out by the frequent hypodermic injection of solutions of the offending substances in gradually increasing amounts, working up to the desired top dose. A relative immunity or tolerance is thus produced to exposure to the substances to which the patient is sensitive.

The physician prefers to speak of control rather than cure of asthma. In most instances desensitization treatment has to be maintained indefinitely. Asthma frequently returns some time after treatment is discontinued even though control was good during its course. No other means of treatment besides avoidance, however, offers as much to the asthmatic patient.

***Treatment of Sources of Infection.*** If infection is a cause, sources such as infected tonsils, adenoids, and sinuses should be treated. Surgical measures are usually necessary. If an acute bronchitis is a precipitating cause, sulfa drugs and the antibiotics may be of great help.

***Value of Climate Change.*** Climate change, although frequently recommended by one's friends, is rarely of aid. In persons with a complicating chronic bronchitis or intractable sinusitis, a warm, dry climate may be valuable. Many cures of asthma attributed to change in climate are really due to the removal of an offending substance from one's household environment.

***Prevention of Asthma.*** Some measures should be adopted by allergic parents to prevent the occurrence of asthma in their children. Dust precautions should be instituted in the bedroom, paying especial attention to the covering of the mattress and pillows with dust-proof covers. Pets such as dogs and cats, if permitted, should be kept strictly outside the house to minimize contact with animal dander. Respiratory infections should have prompt and efficient treatment. Chronically diseased tonsils and adenoids should be removed as soon as the physician advises the procedure.

A great number of persons afflicted with hay fever develop asthma and many persons date the chronic asthma from attacks starting first during their hay fever season. Asthma may also be preceded by the symptoms of perennial nasal allergy. For this reason all hay fever and nasal allergy of any severity, especially if the warning signals of cough or slight wheezing occur, should have desensitization treatment. The antihistaminic drugs, very useful for symptoms of hay fever and chronic nasal allergy, do not prevent the development of asthma.

## EMPHYSEMA

Emphysema of the lungs is a condition in which the lungs are continuously overdistended as a result of loss in elasticity of the lung tissue. The change may be illustrated by comparison of an old lax rubber band to a new and fresh one. The walls of the air sacs are broken down in many portions of the lungs. The chest becomes barrel-shaped—remaining more or less fixed in the breathing-in position.

Most often the condition is secondary to chronic bronchitis, with its constant cough or to severe chronic bronchial asthma. Occasionally it arises from other infections of the lungs. Sometimes it begins later in life without apparent cause. In this instance, perhaps, there is a constitutional weakness of the lung tissue with premature and accelerated aging in that tissue.

***Symptoms of Emphysema.*** Shortness of breath on exertion is the outstanding complaint. If chronic bronchitis is present or supervenes, cough and sputum are prominent. Wheezing occurs in the asthmatic cases.

***Treatment of Emphysema.*** If bronchial spasm is present, antiasthmatic remedies are of value. With bronchial infection, expectorant drugs, such as iodides, may be helpful. Respiratory infections aggravate the condition greatly and acute ones are usually treated with sulfa drugs or the antibiotics. Professionally prescribed breathing exercises may accomplish much in improving breathlessness. Smoking had best be prohibited. In suitable cases an abdominal binder which elevates the diaphragm is of aid. Oxygen is sometimes used in the treatment both at home and in the hospital.

## PLEURISY

Pleurisy is an inflammation of the pleura, the delicate membrane lining the thorax and covering the lungs. There are two types: dry (fibrinous) pleurisy, in which the membrane develops a rough thick discharge on its surface; wet pleurisy (pleurisy with effusion) in which fluid develops in the space between the chest wall and the lung.

***Causes of Pleurisy.*** In lobar pneumonia there is almost always a fibrinous pleurisy. Occasionally fluid develops. Other kinds of pneumonia may give rise to pleurisy but it is infrequent with virus types. Tuberculosis may give rise to a wet pleurisy and this may be an initial manifestation of the disease. Malignant disease may spread to the pleura and give rise to fluid in the pleural cavity. Fluid may arise as a complication of the pneumothorax treatment of tuberculosis. Sometimes a fibrous pleurisy arises without apparent cause.

***Symptoms of Pleurisy.*** With a dry pleurisy the outstanding feature is a severe knife-like pain, usually on one side of the chest, made worse by cough and deep breathing. Sometimes the pain is referred to the abdomen. If the pleura over the upper surface of the diaphragm is involved, pain may be felt in the shoulder and side of the neck. An irritating cough is frequently present. If fluid develops, the pain disappears. If the fluid is large in amount, shortness of breath may occur.

***Treatment of Pleurisy.*** Analgesic drugs are given to relieve the pain. Frequently the chest is bound or strapped by the physician. Specific treatment is directed to the cause if it is one of bacterial origin. In wet pleurisy without obvious cause, special investigations are made to determine whether tuberculosis is present. For bacteriological study and for the removal of fluid when it embarrasses breaththing, the chest is frequently tapped.

## EMPYEMA

***Causes of Empyema.*** Pus rather than simpler fluid may collect in the pleural cavity as a complication of infection of the lung. This is called empyema. Common causes are pneumococcal, streptococcal, and staphylococcal pneumonias. Viruses do not cause empyema. In advanced tuberculosis of the lungs a tuberculous empyema may develop. Rarely, an empyema complicates pneumothorax treatment (collapsing the diseased lung). Antibiotic treatment both by injection, and instillation in the chest cavity by injection of solutions through the chest wall after tapping is used in the treatment of those cases arising from the pneumonias.

***Symptoms of Empyema.*** Fever, chills, and chest pain occur early. Later, when the abscess drains in a large bronchial tube, foul sputum is produced.

***Treatment of Empyema.*** In the early stages penicillin and perhaps some of the other antibiotics may clear up the disease. If the abscess becomes chronic, surgical treatment is necessary.

## FOREIGN BODIES IN THE BRONCHI

The breathing of foreign bodies into the windpipe or the bronchial tubes occurs most frequently in children. They naturally gravitate downwards and usually pass through the windpipe to a lower bronchial tube, most often on the right since the right bronchus is straighter than the left. All sorts of things may be inhaled, such as pins, tacks, screws, buttons, false teeth, food particles, nuts, seeds, etc.

***Symptoms.*** If the material stops at the larynx there is wheezing, cough, and loss of voice. But in a large majority of cases these symptoms are not extreme. When it lodges in the trachea, violent coughing is produced. Often in young children with bronchial aspiration there are few or no symptoms for a while. Later however cough, sputum, and then fever and chills begin. X-ray is of great help in the diagnosis.

***Treatment.*** The foreign body is removed through a special instrument called the bronchoscope.

## INFLUENZA

***Causes of Influenza.*** Influenza is an acute, often highly contagious disease caused by a filterable virus. It has occurred in world-wide epidemics, periodically. The last one of severity was that of 1918. It occurs sporadically during the winter months in minor forms.

***Symptoms of Influenza.*** The incubation period is about two days. The disease begins suddenly. A chill or a sense of chilliness is experienced. Fever rises usually to 101 or 102°F. Prostration is marked. There is aching, sometimes severe, of the muscles, especially in the back and legs. In about twenty-four hours, sneezing and irritation of the eyes and throat develop. Later there are hoarseness and some cough and sputum. As a rule, fever and symptoms subside in four or five days. Weakness and fatigue may be present for a week or more.

In the severe type which occurred in the great epidemics such as in 1918 death was frequent, due to a peculiar type of bronchopneumonia.

***Treatment of Influenza.*** Treatment is only to relieve the symptoms. The sulfa drugs and the antibiotics such as penicillin and aureomycin are ineffective in this disease. Bedrest and abundant liquids are important. Aspirin and codeine are used most frequently for the aching. Whether the new drugs would be effective in the complicating bronchopneumonia remains undetermined since the severe epidemic form has not occurred since their discovery.

***Prevention of Influenza.*** Temporary immunity may be produced by the injection of influenzal virus A and B. There are probably other types not isolated, so that complete protection is not afforded. It must be repeated yearly.

## BRONCHIECTASIS

***Causes of Bronchiectasis.*** Bronchiectasis is a chronic condition in which there is abnormal widening and inflammation of the bronchial walls with destruction of their lining due to infection. It may affect the bronchial tubes of all lobes of the lungs but usually it is less widespread and may be confined to only one lobe. In many patients there is probably a congenital weakness of the walls. Some cases seem to date from an attack of pneumonia, whooping cough, measles, or severe influenza. Chronic bronchitis at times may be a factor.

***Symptoms of Bronchiectasis.*** The history is one of many years' duration. Cough is outstanding, with the production of large amounts of purulent sputum, sometimes foul and blood-tinged. Bouts of pneumonia are frequent. Often the ends of the fingers enlarge ("clubbing") and this is helpful in diagnosis.

***Diagnosis of Bronchiectasis.*** X-rays often reveal little despite the severe distressing symptoms. The diagnosis is confirmed by placing an X-ray-opaque oil in the bronchial tubes, and then the widened places in them can be seen on an X-ray film.

***Treatment of Bronchiectasis.*** Treatment has greatly advanced in recent years due to improvement in surgical measures. One or two lobes of the lung are often removed with cure of the condition if it is not widespread. Penicillin is helpful in acute spread of infection in the surrounding lung but does little for the chronic basic condition.

## PNEUMOCONIOSIS

***Causes of Pneumoconiosis.*** Pneumoconiosis is a condition of thickening of lung tissue due to inhalation of inorganic dust. Many particular types are recognized but the only important and serious ones are those resulting from the inhalation of silica dust and asbestos, which is a silica compound. Quartz miners, stone cutters, and sand blasters are particularly exposed. It is an occupational disease.

***Symptoms of Pneumoconiosis.*** Chief symptoms are chronic cough and shortness of breath. Persons with silicosis have a great tendency to develop tuberculosis so that frequently the two diseases exist together.

***Preventive Measures.*** Prevention lies in reducing exposure to silica dust. Respirator masks which filter the air may be used. Water jets and steam sprays to prevent dissemination of dust and exhaust ventilation in closed areas are some of the measures used in industries where silicosis is an occupational hazard.

## PULMONARY EMBOLISM

This is a condition in which a blood clot lodges in one of the branches of the large artery supplying the lungs. The clot usually arises from a vein in the legs or pelvis where clotting (thrombosis) occurred. This most commonly arises as a complication after surgical operations in the abdomen. Much stress is now placed by surgeons on the recognition of thrombosis of leg veins after operation.

Anticoagulants such as dicumarol and the tying off of the large superficial vein of the thigh are sometimes used to prevent pulmonary embolism from clots which arise in the leg veins after surgery.

CHAPTER 4

# THE HEART, BLOOD, AND CIRCULATION

**The Circulatory System and How It Works . . . How Disease Affects the Heart . . . Congenital Heart Disease . . . Heart Palpitation . . . Pericarditis . . . Endocarditis . . . Myocarditis . . . Congestive Heart Failure . . . Heart Strain . . . Coronary Disease . . . Acute Coronary Thrombosis . . . Heart Block . . . Angina Pectoris . . . High Blood Pressure . . . Low Blood Pressure . . . Pernicious Anemia . . . Hardening of the Arteries . . . Hodgkin's Disease. . . Leukemia . . . Hemophilia . . . RH Babies . . . Varicose Veins . . . Varicose Ulcer . . . Varicocele . . . Piles . . . Hygiene of the Heart, etc.**

THE tissues of the human body, like all living tissues, must receive food in order to perform their work. The circulatory system, consisting chiefly of the heart, blood vessels and blood, is the mechanism for carrying the necessary food materials to the various parts of the body as well as for carrying away waste materials from those parts.

The blood is the fluid in which these materials are carried. By means of the blood, the tissues receive oxygen from the lungs, nutritive material from the intestines, hormones from the glands, and substances to counteract germs or poisons. The blood also conveys heat from the part of the body where it is generated to all other parts of the body. Waste materials thrown off by the tissues are carried by the blood to the kidneys and skin, and carbon dioxide is brought to the lungs, from which it is exhaled.

Circulation of the blood is achieved, actually, by two systems: the pulmonary circulation, which conveys the blood through the tissues of the lungs, where it is purified; and the systemic circulation, which carries the blood throughout the rest of the body.

***The Heart and Its Work.*** The organ that drives the blood through both the pulmonary and the systemic circulations is the heart. It lies between the lungs in the front part of the chest cavity. It is a hollow organ composed of muscle, weighs not more than half a pound, and is as large as the fist of an adult.

The heart is divided into right and left halves, the left half sending the blood through the systemic circulation and the right half sending it through the pulmonary circulation. Each of these halves consists of two chambers, the upper ones called the auricles and the lower ones called the ventricles.

The heart expands and contracts continuously. During expansion, or diastole, the blood from the veins enters the auricles. The contraction, or systole, of the auricles force the blood into the ventricles which in turn contract and drive the blood into the arteries. Heartbeats are the sounds made by the muscular contraction of these chambers. The chambers of the heart and the openings of the great blood vessels are equipped with valves which prevent the blood from flowing backward when the contractions cease.

The heart, when the body is at rest, does work which can be compared to lifting sixteen pounds of weight three feet every minute. The daily work of the heart is equivalent to lifting about eighteen thousand pounds a height of about forty inches.

## THE BLOOD VESSELS AND WHAT THEY DO

There are three kinds of blood vessels in the body: the arteries, veins and capillaries.

***The Arteries.*** The arteries are the vessels through which the blood purified in the lungs is carried from the heart toward the body tissues. The aorta is the great artery which arises from the left ventricle. It is the main trunk from which the network of systemic arteries arises.

***The Veins.*** The veins are the vessels through which the impure blood travels away from the body tissues and back to the heart. The veins, like the arteries, are made up of a network of branches which unite with one another until they form the great veins entering the right auricle.

***The Capillaries.*** The smallest branchings of the arteries and veins connect with, and are connected to, each other by the capillaries—a network of very tiny blood vessels in the tissues. The walls of the capillaries are so thin that they permit an exchange of substances between the blood and the tissues.

## THE SYSTEMIC CIRCULATION

The blood of the systemic circulation, in other words, flows from the heart into the arteries, from the arteries and arterioles (subdivisions of arteries) into the capillaries of the various organs of the body; from the capillaries into the veins and thus back to the heart. Entering the right auricle the blood passes into the right ventricle, from which it is sent into the pulmonary artery.

## THE PULMONARY CIRCULATION

The pulmonary artery takes the blood into the lungs, where it flows through arterial subdivisions to the pulmonary capillaries. Here the blood gives off carbon dioxide and takes up oxygen from the air we breathe. From the pulmonary capillaries the blood flows into the pulmonary veins, two of which carry it from the lungs to the left auricle of the heart. This process constitutes the pulmonary circulation. From the left auricle the blood passes to the left ventricle, from there it goes into the aorta, thence into the systemic circulation and so on—flowing in an endless circulatory motion.

***How the Arteries Work.*** The arteries, like the heart, propel the blood by means of a series of contractions which can be felt at various points such as the pulse. A pulse is also felt in some of the large veins, such as the jugular vein in the neck. This pulse wave is transmitted through the blood itself from changes in pressure when the right auricle contracts. The tension in the walls of the blood vessels is known as blood pressure.

***The Nervous Mechanism of Blood Circulation.*** The action of the heart is controlled primarily by the heart centers. These are groups of nerve cells in the part of the brain called the medulla oblongata (the seat of control of the body's automatic activities). Heart action is controlled also by the sympathetic nerves and by the vagus nerves.

Nerve fibers carry impulses from all parts of the body to the part of the brain called the cardio-inhibitory center. From there the impulses travel to the heart by way of the vagus nerves, which branch out into the heart tissues. Thus sensations from all parts of the body affect the heart. The vagus nerves are stimulated by depressing sensations such as fear or sorrow, which cause the heart to seem to stand still. The sympathetic nerves, on the contrary, are stimulated by mental excitement, which causes the heart to beat more rapidly. Both the vagus and sympathetic nerves arise in the medulla and pass downward in the neck and into the thorax.

Within the heart there is a bundle of nerve fibers through which the impulses causing contraction of the heart muscle are transmitted from the auricles to the ventricles.

Other influences which can control the activity of the heart are such chemicals as adrenalin, inorganic salts, and hormones; and the mechanical effects of the blood on the muscle fibers of the heart.

The arteries, too, are controlled by nerves which excite and inhibit, in their turn, the muscle walls, resulting in contraction and relaxation of the blood vessels.

All of these nerves are a part of the autonomic nervous system, the system which regulates those automatic bodily functions over which, as the term denotes, no voluntary control is exercised.

## THE BLOOD

Earlier in this chapter, we pointed out the important roles played by the blood in supplying oxygen and food to the tissues of the body and removing waste matter. The blood consists of a fluid called plasma, in which are carried three vital kinds of cells, called corpuscles: red cells, white cells, and platelets. The red corpuscles (erythrocytes) carry hemoglobin, which combines with oxygen; they also carry various chemicals and fats. The white corpuscles (leucocytes) include a number of different kinds of cells, whose main task is to surround and destroy harmful cells, germs and the like. The chief known purpose of the platelets (thrombocytes) is to enable the blood to clot when necessary, so that too much blood is not lost when a blood vessel near the surface of the body is injured. The plasma serves not only to carry the corpuscles through the blood vessels, but in itself contains various substances important in nourishing the tissues, in protecting them against disease, and in clotting.

## OTHER ORGANS AND THE BLOOD

***What the Spleen Does.*** In order to maintain the necessary amount of blood in the body, the spleen acts as a storage place for red blood cells. It also breaks them down and stores the iron it extracts from them. When hemorrhage occurs, the spleen forms new blood cells, and contracts, sending these new cells into circulation to replace the blood that has been lost.

***The Liver as Part of the Circulatory System.*** Properly an organ of the digestive system, the liver plays a part also in the circulation of the blood. It is in the liver that various properties of blood are manufactured and liberated into the blood stream—fibrinogen, for example, which is important in blood clotting.

***The Kidneys as Part of the Circulatory System.*** While the spleen and liver help to readjust the volume of blood temporarily, the kidneys, which are properly organs of the excretory system, play a fundamental and final role in regulating the volume of blood. When the amount of plasma in the body changes, the urine is found to contain a proportionate amount of the properties of plasma. Thus, by secreting more urine when there is an increase in blood plasma, and less urine when there is a decrease in blood plasma, the kidneys restore to normal the amount of plasma in the body.

## THE LYMPHATIC SYSTEM

There is another circulatory system closely related to that of the blood—the lymphatic system. This system consists of lymphatic vessels, many in number and ranging from the size of veins to capillaries. Working much like capillaries and veins, they carry a fluid called lymph from the tissues of the body to a large vein in the chest into which the lymph is emptied. Lymph is carried only in this direction. The main function of the lymphatic system is the removal of protein from the fluids manufactured in the tissues. The lymph nodes are masses of tissue at various points along the system. They filter certain solid substances, preventing them from entering the blood stream. They also intercept various poisons, such as those resulting from infected wounds. The lymphatics also carry to the blood stream some of the cells of which the blood is composed—the lymphocytes, which are produced in the lymph glands through which the lymphatics pass.

## HOW DISEASE AFFECTS THE HEART

The term "heart disease" covers a variety of different diseases. Common kinds of heart disease are congenital malformation of the heart, syphilitic heart disease, rheumatic heart disease, coronary heart disease, and heart disease resulting from high blood pressure, and others which we shall discuss later in this chapter.

In heart disease the heart muscle is either altered in structure through the influence of poisons—most of which are produced by the germs causing the acute diseases—or the valves of the heart become defective. In other words, the valves do not close properly and are leaky, or else they become obstructed. Such defects constitute what is called valvular disease, which is the most common form of chronic disease of the heart. The effect of such a condition is that the heart does not pump sufficient blood into the arteries, because the blood leaks backward, or is retarded in its flow into the arteries. However, there is a common provision of nature which frequently prevents such a disturbance. This adjustment is called compensation.

### Compensation

This consists in enlargement of the heart and increase in its muscular power sufficient to overcome the defect in the valve. When compensation takes place, there may be so little disturbance produced by the disease of the valves that the patient may be entirely ignorant of its existence. The compensation may be more or less perfect, and may last a longer or shorter time. Occasionally a person may live to a good old age with a valvular disorder of the heart which has been prevented from giving any trouble by the compensating enlargement. When the enlargement is insufficient, or when, after a time, the increase in muscular power caused by the enlarged heart ceases, then disturbances in the circulation appear and are shown by symptoms.

### Causes of Heart Disease

Among all the acute diseases, rheumatic fever is most frequently the one from which heart disease arises. Scarlet fever, tonsillitis, diphtheria, pneumonia, smallpox, erysipelas, blood poisoning, and some others are often responsible for disease of the heart which may either be evident at the time of the infection or occur at a later period.

While children may be born with heart defects, rarely is the tendency to heart disease inherited. Syphilis and gout render the person more liable to its occurrence. Repeated mental stress or physical overstrain also open the way for the development of some forms of heart disease.

Heart disease attacks all ages and both sexes. Valvular disease begins more frequently between the ages of eighteen and forty, and is a little more frequent in women. The changes in the blood vessels which make the vessels more brittle lead to disease of the heart in old age.

### Symptoms of Heart Disease

It may well be asked, "When is a heart normal?" and "At what point does natural aging end and disease begin?" There are, of course, normal standards. But there is no sharp dividing line between the absolutely normal and the beginning of the abnormal.

In general, it may be said that diseased hearts give one or more of the following warning signs and symptoms: rapid, pounding heart; tiring easily; early limitation of effort; shortness of breath or labored breathing on slight or moderate exertion. There may be palpitation, intermittent heartbeats, chest oppression or soreness, and chest pain. Other signs include "gas" pressing on the heart, a sense of congestion in the head, mental sluggishness, dizziness, fainting. Or there may be cardiac asthma, chronic cough, swollen ankles (edema), blueness of the lips or face, or dropsy. The person may need to sit up to breathe; there may be engorged and swollen veins. Vomiting and progressive changes in weight are some of the late signs and symptoms.

## EXAMINATION AND TREATMENT

A careful physical examination of the heart and entire body, made by a physician, is essential whenever heart disease is suspected. It is impossible to form any correct opinion concerning its existence from the symptoms alone. Pains about the joints in children, with or without fever, should always lead parents to secure medical advice because of a possibility of rheumatism and its common result in leading to damage of the heart. What are improperly called "growing pains" are gouty or rheumatic danger signals.

It is impossible to outline any form of treatment, for the treatment must vary according to the kind of heart disease and the specific needs. Above all, however, it is important that patients remain in bed for a sufficient length of time to save the heart and that they be kept in a peaceful frame of mind. Their nutrition should be watched. A diet that will build resistance to infection of all kinds is of great help.

## PAIN IN THE AREA OF THE HEART

Pain in this area cannot always be attributed to heart conditions. Chest pain may, in fact, be in the chest wall. It may be caused by neuralgia between and along the ribs, herpes zoster (shingles), inflammation of the breast, and pain in the breast. Pain in the chest may also be caused by indigestion, pleurisy, pneumonia, and cancer of the lung.

Pain induced by heart conditions may be caused by valve disease, pericarditis, inflammation of the aorta, and other disorders discussed in this chapter. The most serious and severe pain in the heart is occasioned by coronary artery involvement. It is almost always first noted at the end or in the center of the breast bone. Sometimes pain is referred to a distant area, such as the arm, neck or jaw, the point of the shoulder or the elbow.

## CONGENITAL HEART DISEASE

***Symptoms of Congenital Heart Disease.*** This is the condition in which the heart pumps eight to ten quarts of blood a minute instead of a normal three to four. In time, the heart enlarges. As a consequence there is retarded physical development and a tendency to fatal bacterial involvement of the inner lining of the heart. Few patients live out their normal life span if they are not treated surgically.

***Treatment of Congenital Heart Disease.*** For centuries physicians and midwives have been familiar with congenital heart disease as it shows itself in "blue babies." Many of the infants were dead on birth, but a large number survived as invalids. The condition is now capable of being surgically corrected. The surgical procedure is simple in theory, though it is difficult in practice. By it, the blood is diverted back to its proper channel and the structural deformity is corrected.

Important advances in the study of congenital heart disease, especially in young children, have been made. By the use of modern methods, samples of blood can be obtained from the heart for the determination of their content (especially of oxygen). Also, recording of pressures within the heart chambers is possible.

## PALPITATION OF THE HEART

***Causes of Heart Palpitation.*** Palpitation is usually caused by nervous weakness. It occurs more frequently in nervous and anemic women. While in some instances the action of the heart is often rapid and violent, in other examples it beats naturally and quietly even when the patient imagines it is beating tumultuously. This shows that the condition arises often from unnatural sensitiveness of the patient to the action of the heart; for in true organic disease of the heart muscle, even when the action is unusually strong or rapid, the patient is, in most instances, completely unconscious of it.

Palpitation is generally not a symptom of serious heart disease. It is, however, commonly significant of nervous weakness.

Palpitation is complained of more often by women at puberty, during menstrual periods, or during the "change of life," when the nervous system is more sensitive. Fright, excitement, grief, and anxiety—emotional instability in general—may occasion it. Excess in alcohol, coffee, tea, and tobacco are frequently responsible for palpitation. Indigestion with wind or flatulence is a common cause. Overwork, nervous exhaustion, hysteria, and sexual excitement may open the way for its occurrence. Palpitation is more apt to appear when the body assumes certain postures, as for example, lying on the left side. During an attack the increased action of the heart may be seen or felt with the hand on the chest, the face may be red, and the pulse rapid. In other instances no change can be detected.

***Symptoms of Heart Palpitation.*** A test of the normal condition of most of our organs is our unconsciousness of their existence. In palpitation of the heart the movements of the heart become uncomfortably noticeable, and there is an indescribable discomfort or distress over the heart. More commonly there is a beating, throbbing, fluttering, or jumping of the heart. At the same time there may be a sensation of "goneness" and weakness in the pit of the stomach, or nausea and pains about the heart.

Palpitation is not continuous. There are intervals of freedom from distress. The attacks may last for a few minutes or even for an hour or more.

***Treatment of Heart Palpitation.*** Physical causes should be avoided. If coffee, tea, alcohol, or tobacco bring on palpitations, the patient should stop indulging in them. Proper exercise sometimes relieves the condition. When the patient is having the attack, he should get complete rest, however. Since the disease is often psychological in origin, and founded on worry, the patient should seek to cultivate a relaxed frame of mind. Psychotherapy may be of help in achieving this aim.

## PERICARDITIS

***Causes of Pericarditis.*** Pericarditis is an inflammation involving the heart sac. The disease may be limited to the sac; but more frequently there is at the same time inflammation of the heart muscle. Inflammation of the heart sac may occur in the following conditions: acute rheumatism and chorea, acute specific fevers, pneumonia, scarlet fever, and general tuberculosis. It also occurs in septic conditions and as the result of chronic disease of the kidneys, diabetes, and conditions that weaken the body. It may occur as an extension from nearby organs—from pleurisy and pneumonia, for example.

After an attack of pericarditis, the two layers of the sac adhere to each other. This in itself causes no ill effects. Sometimes, however, the outer layer of the sac adheres to the chest wall. This, known as adherent pericarditis, is a serious condition. It occurs in about 20 per cent of persons suffering from rheumatic fever.

***Symptoms of Pericarditis.*** In most of the infectious forms of acute pericarditis, the patient may be seriously ill before he is fully aware of his condition, because the symptoms may be few and not obvious. They are of great variety, owing to the very many forms there are of this disease, and are often masked by the associated diseases.

The main symptoms of pericarditis are pain, labored breathing, fever, weakness, and oppression in the area of the heart. There may also be cough, shortness of breath, hoarseness, an enlarged and tender liver, altered heart sounds, and altered pulse pressure rate.

The dry form of acute pericarditis, as a rule, occurs during an attack of rheumatic fever. There is an increased rise of temperature, and increased frequency of the pulse and of breathing. There is also pain over the heart area.

The main signs and symptoms of pericarditis with effusion, in which fluid collects within the heart sac, are extremely variable. They depend on the amount of fluid and on associated conditions. When there is much fluid, the heart is compressed. The effects of this compression show themselves as increasing rapidity of heart action, shortness of breath, blueness of the face and lips, upper abdominal pain and vomiting.

***Treatment of Pericarditis.*** Rest in bed is of vital importance. Since the causes of the condition are many, the exact one must be found before the condition can be treated. The introduction of the sulfonamides and of penicillin and specific antiserums have materially lowered mortality in cases of pericarditis produced by germs. Sulfadiazine and specific serum—for example, anti-meningococcus or anti-pneumococcus—are often effective. In acute rheumatic pericarditis salicylate drugs are of undoubted value.

## ENDOCARDITIS

Endocarditis is an inflammation of the lining membrane of the heart and its valves. It is usually associated with rheumatic fever and occasionally with other severe diseases. The condition is one of the most common which afflict the human heart. Three well-known forms of the disease are simple acute endocarditis, acute bacterial endocarditis, and subacute bacterial endocarditis.

***Causes of Simple Acute Endocarditis.*** Simple acute endocarditis, except when occurring during fetal life, is almost always confined to the left side of the heart. It is a disease mainly of early life—a first attack is rare after thirty years of age. In children it may be the single sign of rheumatism. Probably 90 per cent of the persons afflicted with it suffer from rheumatic fever. Endocarditis begins early in the course of the disease, and each succeeding attack of rheumatic fever increases the possibility that it will occur. Other infections may also be contributing causes.

***Symptoms of Simple Acute Endocarditis.*** There are no characteristic symptoms which indicate simple acute endocarditis. If a child in the course of rheumatic fever complains of palpitation and distress in the region of the heart, and it is discovered that the heart action is rapid, without increase in joint involvement, the possibility of endocarditis should be kept in mind.

The signs may be few, irregular fever being the most constant. The patient may be pale, and feel weak and uncomfortable.

***Causes of Acute Bacterial Endocarditis.*** Bacterial infection of the inner lining of the heart, particularly of a valve or valves, is an extremely serious disease. Often a valve is destroyed by such infection, and its function seriously impaired.

Acute bacterial endocarditis is caused by blood-destroying streptococci arising from blood poisoning following childbirth, septic sore throat or other serious body infections.

***Symptoms of Acute Bacterial Endocarditis.*** The symptoms are extremely variable. The primary disease usually foreshadows the signs and symptoms of the complicating endocarditis. There is fever, usually high and notably irregular, associated with repeated chills. Profuse sweats follow. The prostration is extreme and progressive. The pulse rate is high. Sometimes there are symptoms in and around the joints. At times blood clots are sent into the circulation, plugging arteries of various organs, especially those of the heart, kidneys, eyes or brain.

Pain is sometimes severe in the area of the heart.

There is shortness of breath, diarrhea, and sometimes sudden blindness.

Of the signs, one of the most significant which a physician discovers on physical examination is the presence of a heart murmur, especially a diastolic one. This and the irregular fever, chills and sweats make the diagnosis practically certain. A great increase in the number of white cells in the blood is also found.

The outlook in this disease is extremely grave. Prompt treatment with streptomycin has recently affected many cures.

***Causes of Subacute Bacterial Endocarditis.*** This is a slowly progressive infectious disease of the valves of the heart or muscle lining of the heart. It is usually caused by a germ called streptococcus viridans and sometimes by those germs which induce influenza and gonorrhea.

***Symptoms of Subacute Bacterial Endocarditis.*** The patient complains of feeling ill and has symptoms which resemble many other diseases. As a rule there is a low-grade fever, weakness, and aching in the joints and muscles, lasting for months. The first symptoms are sometimes caused by a blood clot in some artery—in the brain, spleen, kidneys, eyes or lungs. This is sometimes followed by a resulting paralysis, bloody urine, disturbed vision and even bleeding from the lungs. There is agonizing pain over the area of the plugged vessel. There are also irregular fever, chills and sweats.

Clubbing (short, stubby formation) of the fingers and toes is a significant sign.

***Treatment of Endocarditis.*** Sulfadiazine and penicillin are used. If the germ (discovered in the blood) is one that is susceptible to the effects of streptomycin, treatment is given with this drug.

## MYOCARDITIS

Myocarditis is an inflammation of the muscular walls of the heart. There are degenerative changes in the heart muscle, in most instances owing to lack of oxygen or the inability of the muscle cells to use oxygen adequately.

The condition, acute or chronic, is one of the most common afflictions of man.

***Causes of Myocarditis.*** True inflammation of heart muscle is caused by direct invasion of the heart by an infecting agent, by toxic substances released by this agent, or by infecting agents which are taken into the stomach. Specific causes include pneumonia, influenza, typhoid, scarlet fever, diphtheria, tonsillitis, septic sore throat, etc. There are also some examples of unknown cause.

***Symptoms of Myocarditis.*** In acute myocarditis which is secondary to other diseases, the symptoms, in the main, are those of the primary disease, with the addition of the heart disturbances. Depending on the cause, there may be signs of rheumatic fever, septic states, subacute bacterial endocarditis and sometimes of tuberculosis and of syphilis.

The symptoms may also be indefinite. There may be acute cardiac failure. The pulse may be feeble and easily accelerated. The apex beat and heart sounds are feeble; there may be a systolic murmur.

***Treatment of Myocarditis.*** Bed rest is necessary, and treatment must be given for the disease responsible for inflammation of the heart muscle. A good diet should be maintained to build resistance to further infection.

## CONGESTIVE HEART FAILURE

***Causes of Congestive Heart Failure.*** This is a state of the heart in which the heart muscle is no longer able to handle the circulatory load. Congestive heart failure is the common end-stage of a number of diseases involving the heart. It may be a consequence of rheumatic heart disease, long-standing high blood pressure, syphilitic disease, or occlusion of the main artery of the heart or its smaller branches. It may also occur without any apparent cause.

***Symptoms of Congestive Heart Failure.*** The symptoms include weakness, easy fatigue, shortness of breath on exertion. Cough and sometimes blood-tinged expectoration are also noted. These are usually signs of failing power of the left ventricle of the heart. In primary failure of the right ventricle, the patient is aware of swelling of the ankles at the end of the day, decreased urination, increased body weight and pain under the ribs on the right side. Dull pain over the heart and down the left arm and up the left side of the neck is often a striking manifestation.

As the heart failure progresses, less and less physical effort can be borne without inducing shortness of breath.

***Treatment of Congestive Heart Failure.*** Digitalis still remains supreme among the drugs used in the treatment of heart disease, especially in patiënts with irregularity of the heart—in fact, in heart failure from any cause. In general the drug is used for the treatment of actual or threatened congestive heart failure when there is low heart output. In heart failure of severe degree, large doses are usually required. It may be given (not without a physician's orders) either in the form of a tincture or tablets.

## HEART STRAIN

This is a condition which produces damage to the heart muscle as a result of some unusual effort.

In the acute form the symptoms come on during or immediately after some strenuous work. There is pain over the area of the heart or below the breast bone, weakness, shortness of breath, palpitation, disability, heart failure. Sometimes where there is a previous heart disease, death occurs. The treatment includes rest, and avoidance of strenuous effort.

## CORONARY DISEASE

As a rule the first complaint may not be pain around the heart but a sense of indigestion, with vague discomfort lower down, or fullness at the end of the breast bone, especially from exertion after a heavy meal. Like all forms of heart disease, it requires a physician's attention. It is frequently relieved to some extent by rest, belching, or taking of nitroglycerin on prescription.

## ACUTE CORONARY THROMBOSIS

Thrombosis denotes the clotting of blood in any part of the circulatory system—heart, arteries, capillaries, or veins. The clot is called a thrombus. When a thrombus blocks the coronary arteries—the blood vessels that supply the heart with blood—the condition is called coronary thrombosis.

***Causes of Acute Coronary Thrombosis.*** Previous arterial disease is always present. Hence predisposing causes are high blood pressure, arteriosclerosis, atheroma (nodules of the blood vessels), chronic nephritis, and syphilis. Worries often precede attack. Excess of food and alcohol are possible factors.

***Symptoms of Acute Coronary Thrombosis.*** The disease process may be present without giving definite symptoms, especially in a person with great feebleness of the blood circulation. In others, symptoms of angina pectoris occur.

There may be sudden pain or distress, under the breast bone, in the area of the heart or over the stomach. This pain is prolonged, and may occur either during rest or exertion. Nausea, vomiting, and the signs of circulatory failure in the body may occur at the beginning. There is an increase of leucocytes in the blood. Premature beats, heart flutter, and sometimes heart block are noted. Shock and fever may be present.

The pulse is rapid and of low volume, the heart sounds are faint, and the blood pressure falls. Breathing may be labored. Acute edema of the lungs is common.

A second coronary thrombosis is usually fatal. There is further risk of an embolus or blood-vessel obstruction for at least four weeks after an attack.

***Diagnosis of Acute Coronary Thrombosis.*** The condition is kept in mind when a person who has shown symptoms of cardiac weakness, without labored breathing or pain, suffers a sudden anginal attack, breathes heavily, and shows signs of gradually increasing cardiac weakness.

Electrocardiographic changes are not constant, but usually aid in the diagnosis. Indications are also found by taking the pulse and blood pressure.

***Treatment of Acute Coronary Thrombosis.*** Most patients with blockage of the coronary artery recover or die, regardless of what the physician does. For occasional patients, treatment may be life-saving. At the beginning of the attack, adrenalin is administered. It may be necessary to bleed the patient. He is confined to bed for four to six weeks. The fluid intake is reduced. The diet should consist of about eight hundred calories. Morphine is of great benefit. If labored breathing is severe, oxygen and hypertonic glucose afford relief. A drug called dicumarol has been found to prolong blood-clot formation.

Though it has been the practice to treat patients with coronary occlusions in bed for six weeks and away from work for three to six months, many can be allowed out of bed in three weeks and most should go back to work, at least part-time, much sooner than has hitherto been the practice.

## HEART BLOCK

Any interference with the conduction of stimuli through the heart is termed heart block. The regular contractions of the auricle (upper chamber) are maintained, but those of the ventricle (lower chamber) do not follow in proper sequence.

***Symptoms of Heart Block.*** The symptoms, as a rule, depend on the condition of the heart muscle. In some examples, however, the ventricles either fail to beat for a considerable period or contract at very low rates. As a result, fainting attacks ensue, sometimes associated with convulsions.

***Treatment of Heart Block.*** The outlook in a patient suffering from heart block depends on the extent of heart-muscle disease. In the chronic form it is always serious. Rest is absolutely necessary. There is no special treatment beyond that of treating the condition that causes the trouble. Ephedrine occasionally prevents recurrences. Digitalis is *not* given, as it may increase the heart block.

## ANGINA PECTORIS

***Causes of Angina Pectoris.*** Angina pectoris is a condition characterized by paroxysmal chest pain. An attack may be brought on by exertion, emotion, or change in temperature.

Angina pectoris is not a disease in itself. It appears to be a spasm of the artery to the heart-muscle which causes inadequate blood flow into the muscle itself. The predisposing factors are: hardening of the coronary arteries, syphilis, and arteriosclerosis. The condition may have associated with it inflammation of the fibrous tissue of the heart muscle, insufficiency of the aorta, and syphilitic disease of the aorta.

Angina pectoris is a disorder of later life. It occurs more often in men. It is uncommon in women. Frequently the afflicted person belongs to the professional classes.

Anginas are sometimes divided into two classes, the angina of rest and the angina of effort. The distinguishing feature of the latter is that it occurs in association with physical exertion or mental excitement. Both, however, may occur under a great many circumstances, and usually precede or follow plugging of an artery in a bundle of heart muscles.

***Symptoms of Angina Pectoris.*** Angina of rest is spontaneous, paroxysmal, not always intense, usually located behind the breast bone, in the area of the heart or upper part of the abdomen. It often radiates to the arm but is sometimes experienced in the shoulders, elbow, jaw or wrist. The pain is influenced by movement of the joints of the extremity affected.

Angina of effort is more readily recognized, but the location of pain is variable. Primary pain may be in the jaw, wrist, elbow, neck, upper part of the abdomen rather than below the breast bone. Pain in the chest or upper abdomen, which is clearly started by effort, is usually owing to insufficiency of the arteries supplying the heart with blood. When the pain increases in severity and is brought on by less and less effort, plugging of an artery by a blood clot in the heart muscle is probably near.

In the beginning there may be no more than a mild uneasiness or an indefinite sense of discomfort in the area below the breast bone. No matter what the causal agent is, the symptoms are similar. The pain, although it does not last long, is agonizing, and associated with a sense of constriction as if the heart is compressed in a vise. There is great anxiety, with fear of death.

Angina attacks are ordinarily brought on by effort or some form of emotional excitement when the volume of blood expelled by the heart in a minute is increased but the blood supply to the heart muscle is inadequate for the extra work demanded of it. The increased burden on the heart during digestion also, in all likelihood, accounts for the common occurrence of angina following a heavy meal. The pain is evidently directly related to the lessened blood supply to the heart muscle.

Any form of heart disease that produces acute paroxysmal shortness of breath and angina-like pain may be associated with periods of unconsciousness.

The occurrence of pain over the heart, shortness of breath and collapse strongly suggest the possibility of coronary artery disease.

Where there is no evidence of heart-muscle damage, the attack is described simply as angina. The term "false angina" is no longer used. A person either has angina pectoris or he has not. The pain is anything but false.

***The Outlook for Angina Patients.*** Many people have suffered from anginal pain, and yet have lived to old age. There is a natural tendency to recovery over a period of months, following the development of a collateral (secondary) circulation in the heart muscle fibers. On the other hand, sometimes sudden death occurs. The outlook is determined to a large extent by the general condition of the system of blood vessels, the size of the heart, and how frequent and severe the attacks are. The outlook is obviously poor in those patients with advanced changes in the system of blood vessels, and the gravity of the situation is still further increased by the frequent occurrence of severe attacks.

***Treatment of Angina Pectoris.*** The medical treatment of angina pectoris is based on the following measures: rest, physical and mental, for a period of weeks or months and avoidance of exertion in the cold air or wind; reduction in weight; avoidance of tobacco and alcohol to a *large extent;* and use of certain drugs which seem to have a beneficial effect. Morphine and oxygen are of great value, especially for persons with congestive heart disease. A light, mixed diet is part of the treatment.

Nitroglycerin, when prescribed by the physician, is given in the form of tablets. They should be carried by the patient on his person, and at the beginning of an attack one tablet should be placed under the tongue and permitted to dissolve there.

## BLOOD PRESSURE

In children up to ten years of age, there is little if any difference in blood pressure in the two sexes. From the tenth to the thirteenth year girls tend to have a slightly higher pressure than boys, but in the later teens and throughout adult life men usually have higher blood pressure than women. As old age is approached, there is a slight fall in blood pressure.

It is important to remember that perfectly normal people may show wide variations from the average in blood pressure. But it can be observed that blood pressure in some people is persistently and abnormally high. A persistent elevated blood pressure should be considered as a physical sign that reflects disordered function of the blood-vessel system.

## HIGH BLOOD PRESSURE

***Causes of High Blood Pressure.*** High blood pressure is not only a disease of the heart, kidneys and brain, but also involves the entire body, damaging any tissue to a greater or lesser degree, as the tissues and blood vessels suffer changes. The kidneys have always been considered as playing a major part in the production of high blood pressure.

Blood pressure is influenced by a number of conditions, such as age, sex, muscular exercise, digestion and posture. Excitement and emotion tend to raise the blood pressure, but only temporarily.

An increase in blood pressure may or may not be accompanied by changes in the walls of the blood vessels. When there are no changes, the increased pressure is merely functional. When there is hardening of the walls of the arteries, the condition is called arterio-sclerosis.

The functional or benign increase may be caused by one of several factors, the most important of which is obesity. Second in frequency and importance are emotional influences such as excitement, fear and worry. On the other hand, true hypertension or the malignant type is caused by changes in the walls of the arteries. The modern theory generally accepted and proven by animal experimentation is that the disease is caused by the deposit of a substance called cholesterol on the lining of the arteries. This substance is a special kind of fat and is believed to originate from an excessively rich diet over a period of years. These deposits gradually form scar tissue which in turn causes inelasticity of the arteries.

The actual causes of hypertension are unknown. Although many people believe that alcohol and smoking cause increased pressure, neither is in any way a factor.

In general, hardening of the arteries is considered as an accompaniment of advancing years. This does not mean that every aged man or woman has inelastic arteries, nor does it mean that it does not often exist in both men and women who are not of advanced age.

***Symptoms of High Blood Pressure.*** These include headaches, quick fatigue, dizziness, awareness of the heart, pain in the area of the heart, and ringing in the ears. Any one of these signs alone may not be meaningful, but if several are present and persist, the condition calls for a prompt examination.

***Treatment of High Blood Pressure.*** Persons suffering from high blood pressure should be under a physician's care. In regard to active medical treatment, habits of living and diet must be changed. If the pressure is not very high, only slight restrictions in living habits have to be imposed. In extreme examples, complete rest is necessary. In general, it is best to arrange a program of leisure or frequent rests. Psychotherapy also has its use.

Tobacco and alcohol should be excluded if they disagree with the patient.

There is no adequate drug treatment of high blood pressure. However, sedatives—small doses of phenobarbital, for example—are helpful for the control of nervousness, apprehension, insomnia, awareness of the heart, and discomfort in the area of the heart, of which many patients complain.

In regard to diet, regulation of weight in the overweight patient is of first importance, because decreasing the body weight decreases the strain on the heart and thus prevents heart failure.

Diets that have been found useful in the treatment of arterial high blood pressure include, besides the low-calorie diet—frequently a successful form of treatment—the low salt diet, rice diet, and low cholesterol diet. Sodium in the diet is restricted.

# Disease and the Emotions

Based on the film produced by The National Film Board of Canada

High blood pressure, allergies, other ailments often have emotional causes, rooted in patients' childhood. Take the case of Margaret, who is 23 years old. She does not enjoy mixing with people, has few friends. She suffers with sick headaches, stomach upsets, fatigue. Doctors can find no cause. Only a psychiatrist, probing Margaret's past, is able to discover source of her troubles — too much protection in childhood, discouragement of efforts to assert herself. This has led to crippling fear of failure, leaving girl insecure and inarticulate. Hidden conflict between desires and fears has made her ill.

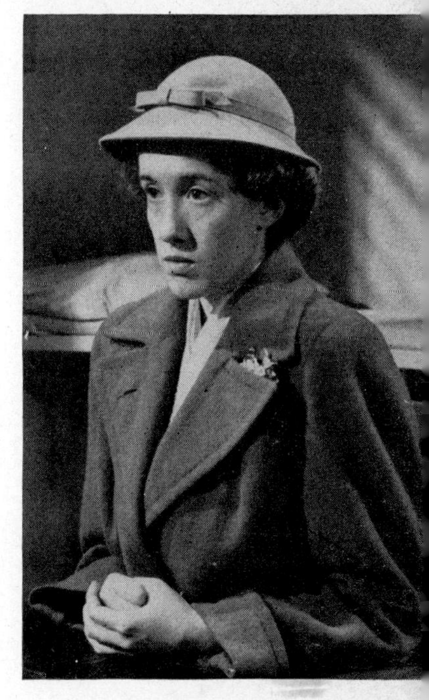

*(Right)* Driven by overwhelming sense of despair, Margaret comes to psychiatrist for help. She looks older than her 23 years, is really sick. He draws out story of her life. Incident by incident, pattern emerges, revealing feelings of rejection from childhood on. She had never realized cause of trouble.

*(Left)* When Margaret was little, parents showed preference for younger sister, played with her but did not invite Margaret to join in. She felt that she was unwanted.

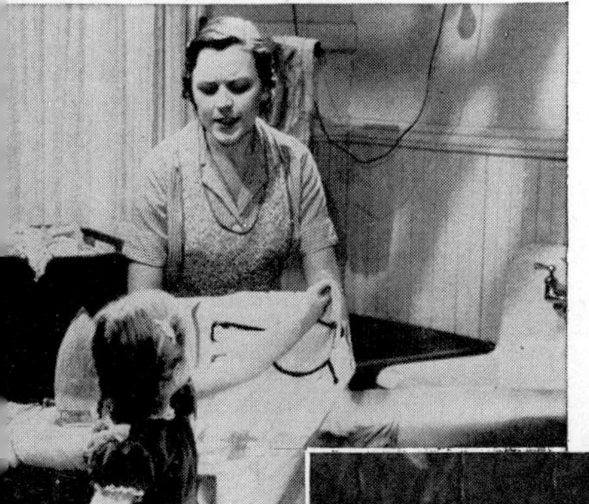

*(Left)* Margaret, proud of finger painting she made, brings it to mother for approval. Busy ironing, mother chases child away. Many times Margaret finds her "too busy to be bothered."

*(Bottom left)* Ironically, when mother does pay attention to child, she is too careful with her. Margaret is kept in own yard, not allowed to play with friends. She feels left out of things.

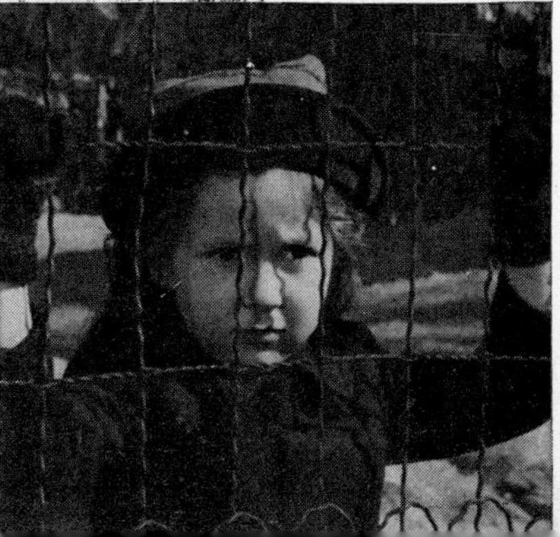

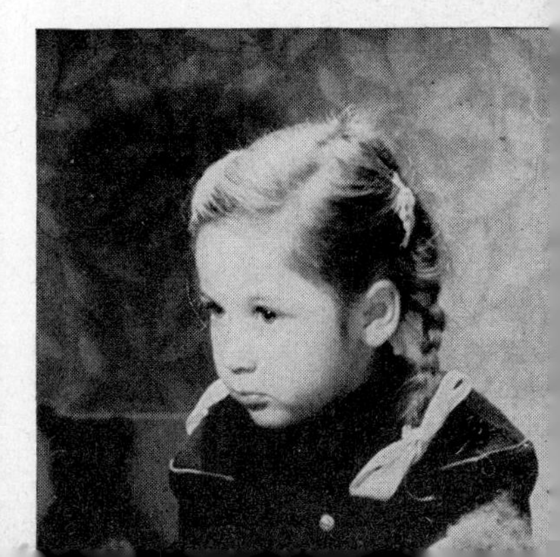

*Far right)* Discourged from more acive play by parents, Margaret sits quietly n corner with her dolls. This way, she inds father and nother like her beter. But child's spirit ias been shattered.

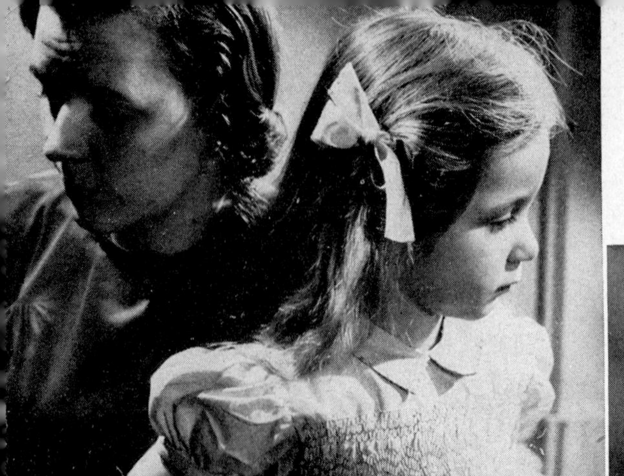

*(Left)* Gradually Margaret becomes "model child" in mother's eyes. She is afraid to play with other youngsters or leave mother's side. Phrase "Mommy doesn't like little girls who do that!" gains fearful meaning.

*(Right)* In school, Margaret is unable to voice opinions. She wants to take part, but, because of home training, fears to say anything that might offend.

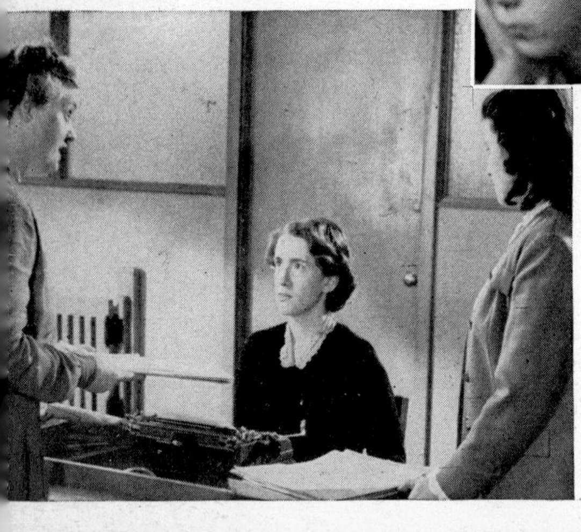

*(Left)* Grown up, Margaret gets job as stenographer. At office, she consents to work overtime, although she does not want to. Her dissatisfaction results in familiar headache, feeling of weakness.

*(Bottom left)* At home, Margaret's younger sister refuses to do her share of housework when it interferes with her entertainment plans. Margaret, unable to stand up for herself, does sister's work.

*(Below)* With psychiatrist's help, Margaret breaks away from habit of blind obedience rooted in fear of losing love. New, free life opens up.

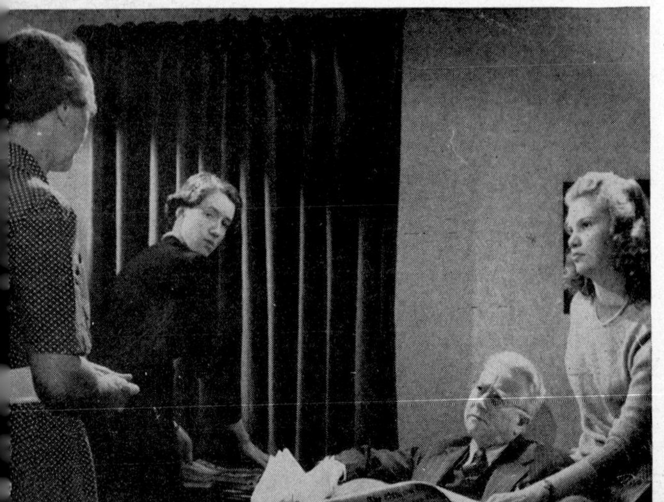

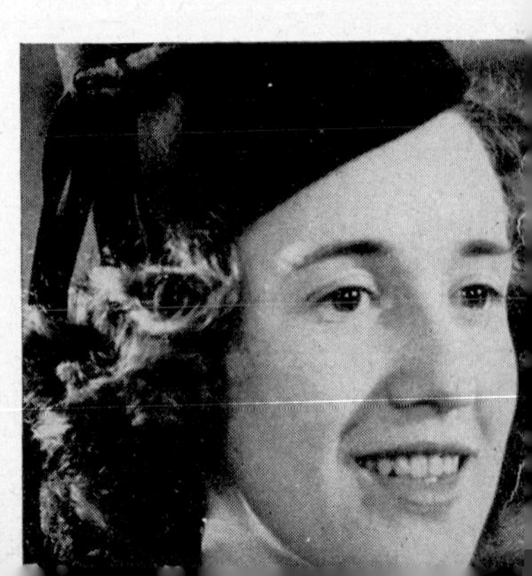

***Rice Diet for High Blood Pressure.*** This diet may be given for five weeks or for almost three years, depending on the condition. The diet is low in salt, low in proteins and low in fats. It includes sugar as well as fruits. There is a daily ration of two thousand calories.

A patient takes an average of nine to twelve ounces of rice (dry weight) daily. Any kind of rice may be used, provided that no sodium chloride, milk, etc., has been added during its processing.

The rice is boiled, or stewed in plain water, or fruit juice, *without* salt, milk or fat. If the sodium concentration of the ordinary water available is high, distilled water should be used.

All fruit juices and fruits are allowed, with the exception of nuts, dates, avocados and any dried or canned fruit or fruit derivatives to which substances other than white sugar have been added. Not more than one banana a day should be taken. White sugar and dextrose may be used without restriction. Tomato and vegetable juices are not allowed. Usually no water is given and the fluid intake is limited to a maximum of a quart of fruit juice a day. Supplementary vitamins are added. No other medication is given unless it is specifically indicated.

***Surgery for High Blood Pressure.*** In extremely high blood pressure of long standing, when all else fails, resort is sometimes had to surgery. The operation is called a sympathectomy, and involves the cutting of certain nerves that connect with blood vessels.

## LOW BLOOD PRESSURE

***Causes of Low Blood Pressure.*** Low blood pressure is a symptom rather than a disease. It may be caused by one or more of a variety of conditions. Sometimes it follows an acute infectious disease, like influenza. It is often associated with worry, and occasionally with anemia, tuberculosis, and diseases of the heart and adrenal glands.

***Symptoms of Low Blood Pressure.*** The patient feels weak, irritable, exhausted. He is subject to fits of depression that he cannot seem to shake off. He may perspire freely when not engaged in any effort.

***Treatment of Low Blood Pressure.*** First of all, the condition that is keeping the blood pressure down—anemia, for example—requires treatment. Sensible living habits must be followed faithfully, and the patient should get plenty of rest as well as exercise in the open air. A wholesome diet, with adequate amounts of milk, eggs, fresh fruits and vegetables, meat, and fish, is important.

## HOW KINDS OF BLOOD PRESSURE AND HEART LESIONS ARE DIAGNOSED

***The Blood Pressure Machine.*** This is an apparatus with a column of mercury in a measuring tube. A flat, hollow rubber tube is fastened around the arm above the elbow. This tube connects with the machine and is filled with air from a bulb. A stethoscope is placed over the artery nearest the surface just below the band, and the doctor listens to the two types of heart sounds—those of the systolic phase, when the blood is forced out of the heart, and the sounds of the diastolic phase, when the heart dilates to receive the blood from the veins. The average systolic pressure in young male adults is 120 and the diastolic is 80. In females of the same age, the normal is slightly higher.

Few physiologic processes have been more accurately and critically studied than the mechanical and electrical events that accompany the contraction of the heart. To the experienced ear, the heart sounds can yield much valuable information, particularly with regard to the condition of the heart valves. In addition, they may indicate the vigor of the contraction of the ventricles.

***The Electrocardiograph.*** This records the electrical differences that develop in the heart during contraction. These are the most easily and accurately recorded of the manifestations of heart activity. The electrocardiograph gives accurate information regarding the spread of activity through the heart and may indicate muscular damage. However, it yields no information about the mechanical events of heart contraction except by inference, and supplementary tests must be used for accurate diagnosis.

## AVERAGE ARTERIAL BLOOD PRESSURE IN HEALTHY PERSONS

| | *Male* | | *Female* | |
|---|---|---|---|---|
| *Age in Years* | *Systolic* | *Diastolic* | *Systolic* | *Diastolic* |
| Birth | 20-60 | .. | 20-60 | .. |
| 1-5 | 75-90 | 50-60 | 75-90 | 50-60 |
| 7-8 | 85-95 | 50-65 | 85-95 | 50-65 |
| 10-12 | 95-105 | 50-70 | 95-105 | 50-70 |
| 14-15 | 97-120 | 60-72 | 95-115 | 57-72 |

| Age in Years | Male Systolic | Male Diastolic | Female Systolic | Female Diastolic |
|---|---|---|---|---|
| 17-18 | 106-122 | 60-70 | 93-110 | 57-73 |
| 20-24 | 108-132 | 65-77 | 100-120 | 55-70 |
| 25-29 | 110-130 | 65-80 | 100-120 | 55-75 |
| 30-34 | 110-130 | 65-80 | 100-120 | 60-75 |
| 35-39 | 110-130 | 65-80 | 105-125 | 60-80 |
| 40-44 | 110-140 | 65-85 | 110-130 | 60-80 |
| 45-49 | 110-140 | 65-90 | 110-140 | 65-85 |
| 50-59 | 115-142 | 65-90 | 110-145 | 65-90 |
| 60-69 | 115-145 | 65-90 | 115-155 | 70-90 |
| 70-79 | 120-160 | 65-90 | 115-165 | 70-90 |
| 80 Up | 120-155 | 65-90 | 115-160 | 70-90 |

## PERNICIOUS ANEMIA

This is a severe, progressive anemia, marked by a persistent and swift decrease in the number of red blood corpuscles. The precise cause is unknown. The course of the disease is often interrupted by periods when the symptoms appear to be absent, and the patient feels considerably better.

*Signs and Symptoms of Pernicious Anemia.* The disease begins gradually, with increasing languor, weakness, pallor, and fainting attacks. Finally, there is extreme weakness and exhaustion. The skin acquires a lemon tint. The heart is dilated and heart palpitations are common. Gastro-intestinal symptoms are frequent, and there is sore tongue, loss of appetite, nausea, and indigestion. There are also numbness and tingling of the feet and hands, and the sense of touch is impaired.

*Diagnosis of Pernicious Anemia.* The blood examination shows distinctive characteristics. The red blood cell count may be as low as half a million, although it is usually between four and a half and six million. The hemoglobin is relatively high. Another diagnostic means is a careful study of the patient's bone marrow. This is obtained by puncture of the breast bone.

*Treatment of Pernicious Anemia.* Treatment by a physician is necessary. Bed rest is of great importance. One-half pound of lightly cooked liver is eaten daily, and it is advisable to prepare this in as many ways as possible—soups, pastries, sandwiches, etc. If it causes a stomach upset, liver extract may be given as a powder or injected in the muscles. A maintenance diet of liver may be required for the rest of the patient's life.

A uniform maintenance dose of purified liver extract may be given weekly. All persons with red blood cell counts below one and a half million should be hospitalized before starting liver therapy, for after the first two or three days of this therapy, there is sometimes a drop in the red blood cells, which may cause collapse. A transfusion is urgent when there are signs of collapse, or transfusions may be indicated as routine at stated intervals.

## HARDENING OF THE ARTERIES (ARTERIOSCLEROSIS)

In hardening of the arteries, the elasticity of the arteries decreases. How many arteries are affected, it is never possible to determine. When a vessel is involved, there is a change in the lumen or passageway, which in turn increases the difficulty of forcing the blood through this vessel, and consequently makes the heart pump harder. Thus the blood pressure is increased.

***Causes of Arteriosclerosis.*** It is not definitely known exactly what causes this condition. Many theories have been advanced. The most logical is the chemical theory. The advocates of this theory claim that the condition begins many years before there are any symptoms and is due to indiscretions in diet. They say there are too many proteins taken into the system, which form a fatty substance called "cholesterol." This is deposited on the surface of the arterial lining. Cholesterol later forms a sort of fibrous tissue which, in turn, causes a contraction of the blood vessel and consequently a narrowing of the passageway.

The only definitely known cause is syphilis. This does not mean that all cases of syphilis have arteriosclerosis, but the vast majority of incorrectly treated and neglected *early* cases will later in life develop hardening of the arteries. Alcoholics were once thought to be candidates for this disease, but it is now definitely settled that alcohol does not cause these hardening changes. Tobacco likewise is not a cause.

***Symptoms of Arteriosclerosis.*** The disease may be present for years before any symptoms manifest themselves. This is because the disease is so slow in developing. Headaches, dizzy spells, sleeplessness, nervous irritability, pounding of the heart, and shortness of the breath are all prominent symptoms when the disease has fully developed. The blood pressure is always raised, sometimes as high as 200 to 250. When this happens, there is great danger of a rupture of a small blood vessel in the brain, causing what is called an apoplectic stroke, with more or less paralysis following.

***Treatment of Arteriosclerosis.*** As we grow older, there is generally some deposit of calcium in the blood vessel walls. A certain rise in blood pressure is as much an accompaniment of old age as white hair and diminished muscular activity. Consequently too much must not be made out of this fact. Many persons with considerable rise in pressure live to be old, provided they live a life in keeping with their age. There is no drug that will change the condition in the arterial walls. If the pressure produces many symptoms, then a few days' complete rest in bed will bring down the pressure.

Again, one must be guarded in putting an aged person to bed for any period of time. There is always the danger of hypostatic pneumonia. Quieting drugs or sleeping pills may be prescribed by the doctor. They should never be taken without professional advice. They may do more harm than good. If there is history of syphilis and the Wassermann test is positive, then anti-syphilitic treatment should be started without delay. Many such cases get remarkably better under this treatment.

## HODGKIN'S DISEASE

***Causes of Hodgkin's Disease.*** This is a variety of anemia marked by enlargement of the lymphatic glands and of the spleen. The cause is unknown.

***Symptoms of Hodgkin's Disease.*** The disease may be local, confined to one group of lymph nodes, or it may become generalized. Lymph nodes of the neck are usually involved first. Gradually the other lymph nodes become enlarged.

The disease begins slowly, with weakness, loss of appetite, and loss of weight. The enlarged lymph nodes are not tender. An irregular fever, mild or severe, is usually present. The liver, gastro-intestinal tract, bone marrow, thymus, lungs, skin, and the central nervous system may be involved by direct extension through the blood or lymph.

There is an anemia, and the red cells and hemoglobin are diminished. The white cells are not much altered but there may be a moderate increase, especially of the lymphocytes. The blood changes are neither constant nor distinctive.

***Diagnosis of Hodgkin's Disease.*** The disease is discovered through a microscopic examination of one of the lymph nodes removed surgically.

***Treatment of Hodgkin's Disease.*** X-ray treatments may relieve the patient temporarily. The disease proves fatal after a number of years.

## LEUKEMIA

Leukemia is a disease of blood-forming tissues characterized by a great increase in the leucocytes, or white blood cells. The normal number of 7500 white blood cells per cubic millimeter of blood is multiplied many times over. There is a severe anemia.

There are a number of different varieties of leukemia. They include acute leukemia, chronic myelogenous leukemia, and chronic lymphatic leukemia. The cause of leukemia is unknown.

***Acute Leukemia.*** This is a disease occurring in children and young adults, characterized by multiple hemorrhages, rapid anemia, fever, enlargement of the spleen, and general glandular enlargement.

***Chronic Myelogenous Leukemia.*** The spleen is often enormously enlarged. The blood is greenish-yellow and clotted like pus. There is progressive weakness, swelling of the legs and nasal bleeding. The anemia may not be extreme. The white blood cells are from one million to two million per cubic millimeter.

***Chronic Lymphatic Leukemia.*** There is enlargement of the spleen and glands throughout the body. White blood cells are present from fifty thousand to one million per cubic millimeter.

***Treatment of Leukemia.*** Blood transfusions and X-ray treatment of the spleen and bone marrow are helpful in prolonging life. Eventually the patient dies from fatigue, severe anemia, and other complications.

## HEMOPHILIA

***Cause of Hemophilia.*** This is a hereditary disease in which the clotting of the blood is retarded, so that the patient may bleed to death from a minor wound. It is transmitted to the male members of the family by a mother who is herself not a bleeder, but who is the daughter of one. The tendency for bleeding usually appears within the first two years. The cause of the disease is unknown.

***Symptoms of Hemophilia.*** External bleeding occurs either spontaneously or from slight wounds. There are many hemorrhages in and around the joints. The larger joints, especially the knee, are usually most affected.

***Treatment of Hemophilia.*** Blood transfusions are given. Local treatment is usually ineffective, but certain special extracts will help clot the blood. For example, an extract of snake venom may be applied locally. It is effective in all examples of hemophiliac bleeding and in other continuous bleeding—after tooth extractions, for example, nose bleeds and wounds about the body. Horse serum and fresh human blood are sometimes injected to aid clotting.

## RH BABIES

There is a certain blood element, known as the Rh factor, which is present in the blood cells of approximately 85 per cent of all white people. The blood of these people is therefore called Rh positive. The remaining 15 per cent are called Rh negative, since they lack this factor. Almost all Negroes are found to be Rh positive. We must know whether this factor is present before giving a blood transfusion, since it is dangerous to give Rh positive blood to a person whose blood is in the Rh negative group. Serious anemia may develop.

When a father is Rh positive and a mother is Rh negative, the consequences for their offspring must be considered. The infant may suffer from congenital edema, which is fatal. There may be jaundice, developing within twenty-four hours after birth and often fatal, and congenital anemia.

These diseases usually develop only after one or several successful pregnancies with live and healthy children. The diseases are due to the growth of substances called antibodies, which form in the mother's blood as a reaction to the Rh factor transmitted through the fetus from the father; these antibodies pass through the afterbirth (placenta) and destroy the red blood cells of the fetus.

***Features That Suggest the Rh Factor.*** The mother may have had one or more normal children followed by stillbirth, or a child that developed jaundice within twenty-four hours of birth. In previous pregnancies, there may also have been excessive water in the bag of waters at birth.

The mothers of infants with blood-destroying disease are likely to have labor complications.

***Signs of the Rh Factor in the Newborn.*** There may be jaundice of the skin and in the jelly surrounding the umbilical cord; generalized swelling, the child being above average weight at birth; afterbirth large, thick, pale and easily crumbled; small hemorrhages; enlarged liver and spleen; and increasing pallor during the first few weeks of life.

***Treatment of Rh Factor.*** The child receives intravenous transfusions of Rh negative blood (the same as the mother's), the object being to give him red blood cells which will remain unaffected by the antibodies of the mother, produced while the Rh-positive child was in the womb. However, the mother's own blood is never given.

Oxygen is also administered, and the body heat of the infant is maintained.

The child should *never* be breast-fed.

## VARICOSE VEINS

Varicose veins are permanently enlarged veins which commonly occur on the legs; they are, however, also seen in other parts of the body. They stand out from the skin as bluish, knotty, winding cords which flatten out when pressure is made upon them, and in most cases shrink in size when the patient lies down. Sometimes bluish, small, soft, rounded lumps or a fine, branching network of veins may be seen.

***Causes of Varicose Veins.*** Varicose veins are more frequent in women, especially in those who stand for long periods of time. Any obstruction to the return flow of the blood from the veins toward the heart, such as a tight garter about the leg, will produce varicose veins; as will also the pressure upon the veins by the large womb in pregnancy, or of tumors in the same region. Heart and lung diseases also predispose to the formation of varicose veins. Heredity is a factor.

***Symptoms of Varicose Veins.*** Often varicose veins, if not extensive, may go on for years without either increasing in size or causing any trouble whatsoever. When they are of long duration, the legs may become swollen and hard, and there is often an associated eczema, with itching. This leads to scratching and sores. The sores may enlarge and become what are called varicose ulcers. These are difficult to heal. Occasionally an old varicose vein may break open and give rise to profuse bleeding. Some patients suffer little or no discomfort, but seek treatment because of the unsightliness. Most patients complain of a heavy, tired feeling in the legs, particularly after standing or walking. Others complain of pain in the affected part of the vein, frequently worse at night.

***Treatment of Varicose Veins.*** These enlarged veins are exceedingly common. If they are not extensive and produce no discomfort, they may be ignored. Otherwise, it is well to have an elastic stocking made which will come at least to the knee. The patient should lie down while putting on and removing the stocking. Cold bathing, outdoor exercise, everything which will improve the general health and tone are desirable. Avoidance of constipation is also of importance. Bleeding from a broken vein is stopped by pressure of a bandage, and by having the patient lie on the back with the foot raised on a pillow. In very aggravated conditions surgical operation will effect a cure.

The injection treatment is extremely successful in less severe cases. The vein is obliterated by the injection of chemical solutions. However, a darkish discoloration of the skin often remains. In an extremely extensive condition it is sometimes advisable to tie the main vein (saphenous trunk) in the upper part of the thigh, and to inject the veins in the leg. The veins should not be tied and injected, however, if the patient is of advanced age, or in pregnancy; nor in the case of debilitating disease, severe damage to the arterial supply of the affected part, previous or present inflammation of veins, tumors in the pelvis, or any other mechanical obstruction to the flow of blood through the veins.

## VARICOSE ULCER

***Causes and Symptoms of Varicose Ulcer.*** This type of ulcer is caused, as the term implies, by varicose veins. The skin around the vein may become infected, and the sore develops. Sunburn or any trivial injury of the leg may start the ulceration. The ulcer varies in size from that of a pin head to that of a hand. It has a deep reddish appearance, is usually moist, and may discharge a yellowish fluid or yellow-green pus. The edges are firm. Ulcers are usually formed near the ankle, but may be located on other parts of the leg or foot.

***Treatment of Varicose Ulcer.*** Almost all varicose ulcers can be healed by putting the patient to bed for a long time, with the leg elevated, and by using warm, wet boric acid dressings.

For patients who are not put to bed, a frequently effective treatment consists of application of the following (obtained at any drug store): zinc oxide, 100 grams; gelatin, 200 grams; water, 300 cubic centimeters; glycerin, 400 cubic centimeters. This material in sheet form is cut in slices, heated in a double boiler and applied.

The ulcer is sometimes treated by compression bandages (made of elastic and gauze to exert pressure) applied to the veins, or the veins are injected with some obliterating solution each time the bandage is removed. Sulfathiazole ointment or powder is applied to the ulcer to induce healing. If the ulcer is infected, which is usually the case, and if the germs are sensitive to penicillin, this drug is used. After the infection has been wiped out, healing is sometimes hastened by skin grafting.

Once a patient has had an ulcer, there is always a tendency that the ulcer will re-form following an injury.

## VARICOCELE

***Cause of Varicocele.*** Varicocele occurs usually in young, unmarried men. It often disappears of itself in later life. It is a form of varicose veins. It consists of enlargement of the veins in the scrotum above the testicle, usually on the left side. Constipation helps produce it.

***Symptoms of Varicocele.*** The large veins of the scrotum feel more like a bunch of earthworms than anything else. If they cause no discomfort, they are not of the slightest consequence, and may be entirely ignored. Even when they produce trouble, it is usually largely imaginary, since these veins are a universal source of worry in young men in case of any irregularities in the sexual functions. Advantage is taken of this fact by quacks, who find it profitable to advertise all sorts of horrible (and impossible) results of the condition.

The testicle on the diseased side may become smaller than its fellow, but in few cases does any serious consequence result from varicocele. Pain in the hollow of the back may be its only symptom, where there are any symptoms at all. However, there may be dragging pain in the groin, pain in the testicles, and around the rectum, and in the bladder, which may cause justifiable complaints.

***Treatment of Varicocele.*** When treatment is necessary, the application of a snugly fitting suspensory bandage—which can be procured at any drug store–and bathing the testicles night and morning in cold water, with avoidance of constipation, will be sufficient to relieve any discomfort arising from varicocele. The enlargement of the veins will not, of course, be altered by this treatment. Absolute cure can be effected only by a surgical removal of the veins. This is not a serious undertaking, but is rarely necessary.

## PILES (HEMORRHOIDS)

***Causes of Piles.*** Piles are varicose veins in the wall of the rectum. They are caused by constipation, by pregnancy, or by tumors in the pelvis which interfere with the circulation of the blood in the rectum. If they protrude beyond the sphincter—the muscle which controls the lower opening of the alimentary canal—they are called external piles; if they do not, they are termed internal piles.

It is never safe to assume that bleeding from the rectum is caused by piles. Cancer or some other disorder may be responsible. A physician must always be consulted to make the diagnosis.

### External Piles

***Symptoms of External Piles.*** These piles appear as bluish swellings or little lumps which project from the rectum and anus, interfering with walking and with the bathing of the parts. They are sometimes exquisitely tender and painful when inflamed. They may bleed when the bowels are moved. In the course of time, piles become mere projections or fringes of flesh, and cause no trouble unless they become irritated through uncleanliness or other reasons.

***Treatment of External Piles.*** The treatment of external piles may be summed up in great cleanliness—washing the parts thoroughly after each movement of the bowels. In addition, rest in bed, if the soreness is great; application of cold water or powdered ice in a rubber bag, or of hot poultices, and of various drugs are part of the treatment. Among the drugs are witch hazel, with which the parts may be frequently bathed; an ointment of nutgall and opium; or extract of equal parts of belladonna and glycerin. Sitting in a tub of cold water, night and morning, also proves serviceable.

The more rapid and effectual method of cure consists in the opening of the recent pile by a surgeon, who clips off the fleshy projections.

The bowels should always be kept regular in any variety of piles by small doses of milk of magnesia taken in ¼ glass of water on going to bed. If this is ineffectual, extract of cascara or compound licorice powder may be taken at night.

### Internal Piles

***Symptoms of Internal Piles.*** In the beginning, patients with internal piles feel as if the bowels were not wholly emptied after a passage. Sometimes there is difficulty in urinating, and there are also pains in the hollow of the back and in the thighs. There is often pain during movement of the bowels, and blood follows the passage. Later, blood may be lost at other times, and the loss may be so great as to cause pronounced paleness and weakness. Itching at the anus is a frequent occurrence. Mucus and pus (matter such as comes from an abscess) may also be discharged. Loss of sexual desire and power is frequently experienced. There may be associated external protrusions.

If the pain is very severe during and also after a passage, it is probable that there is present a fissure or a crack in the flesh, or an ulcer at the exit of the bowel which needs surgical attention. It often happens that piles come out during the bowel movement; in this case, they should be thoroughly washed, greased, and pushed back. Sometimes this is impossible, although after the patient lies down for a while, applying an ice bag or cold water, the mass may shrink so as to admit of its return. When a large mass is thus protruded and cannot be returned, and becomes nipped by the anus muscles, it becomes inflamed and is very painful.

***Treatment of Internal Piles.*** The hot sitz bath in the morning is useful. Ointments may be introduced into the bowel with the finger, or suppositories may be used. Injection treatment given by a physician is the best and quickest cure.

***Operation for Piles.*** There are only two reasons for carrying out an operation for the removal of piles; profuse and recurring bleeding, and uncontrollable protrusion. Slight and occasional bleeding is not of great importance, but when a person loses great quantities of blood at every action of the bowels, his health soon begins to suffer. He becomes anemic, and the anemia gets steadily worse. Under these conditions, the sooner an operation is performed, the better. As long as the protrusion can be reduced, and does not recur until the next clearing of the bowels, it is only a nuisance and can be tolerated for the time being.

## HYGIENE OF THE CIRCULATORY SYSTEM

Among the measures which can help maintain the normal functioning of heart and circulation are: good nutrition, especially in childhood; avoidance of obesity in adult life; and avoidance, if possible, of other strains on the heart, such as excessive nervous tension or over-strenuous activity. Other measures include regular, selective exercise; good posture; and the general health measures which help prevent the diseases that have harmful effects on the heart, blood and blood vessels.

***Heart Disease and Air Travel.*** Questions sometimes arise in judging the physical fitness of passengers for air travel when they have disorders of the heart or circulation.

Various factors that create a tendency to travel sickness may be nullified by simple precautions. Proper rest, a light meal about an hour before taking off, and evacuation of the bowels before flight are advisable. Food taken during the trip should be light and easily digestible. Persons prone to air sickness should dress warmly and protect the ears against aircraft noise by cotton plugs.

Since all air-passenger planes are now "pressurized" (that is, built to withstand any increased or diminished air pressure when flying at great heights), there is no hazard to anyone having or having had a heart lesion. However, if there has been a coronary thrombosis as recent as *six months,* it is inadvisable to fly higher than five thousand feet. Transcontinental flights may necessitate flying as high as fifteen to twenty thousand feet, but in the modern plane there is no discomfort felt by the passenger.

CHAPTER 5

# THE DIGESTIVE SYSTEM



## HOW THE DIGESTIVE SYSTEM WORKS

Most of the foods we eat must be specially prepared within the body for use by its cells. This process is termed digestion. A few foods, such as water and certain salts, can pass without change directly into the blood or lymph, but all others must be digested. Starch must be broken down to sugar, oil to soaps, and protein to amino acids, before any of them can pass through the cell walls. Digestion must change the molecules of the food into molecules the body can use.

The system of tubes through which the food passes from the time it enters the mouth to the final stage of the excretion of the indigestible part at the anus, is called the alimentary canal.

***What Happens to Food in the Mouth.*** When food enters the mouth there is an immediate flow of saliva from the salivary glands. The main constituent of saliva is an enzyme called ptyalin. Ptyalin acts only on the starchy parts of the food, changing them into sugar. Food in the mouth is thus subjected to chemical changes which prepare it for digestion. It is also subjected to the physical action of chewing. As a result of this, the food is cut up into small masses. Thorough chewing of food is of great importance to digestion. When chewing is insufficient, either through loss of teeth or the habit of gulping one's food, extra work is thrown on the stomach. Faulty chewing is a frequent cause of indigestion.

Food remains in the mouth only a short time, and salivary digestion is not completed there. The ptyalin continues its work after the food leaves the mouth.

***How We Swallow.*** Swallowing is a somewhat complicated process, but its main features may be easily understood. The tongue, first of all, gathers together the particles of food in the mouth, where they have been mixed with mucus, and shapes them into a bolus or mass. Then, tilting this mass backwards, the tongue forces it into the pharynx. In the pharynx, the food mass is grasped by the muscles of the pharynx. Here are the posterior openings of the nose. They are closed by the raising of the soft palate, so that the food can now pass into either the esophagus or gullet (the path to the stomach) or into the windpipe (the path to the lungs). If it were to pass into the windpipe, choking would, of course, result. This accident is prevented by the raising of the voice box and also by the action of the epiglottis or lid of the windpipe, which falls over, covering the entrance to the lungs.

The food propelled by the muscles of the upper pharynx now has only one way to go, into the gullet. When it has passed into the upper part of this tube, it is seized by the gullet muscles and propelled downward into the stomach.

The gullet or esophagus extends downward from the pharynx and through the diaphragm to the stomach. This tube is lubricated by its lining membrane. The muscular contractions of the tube push the food into the stomach. No change occurs in the food in passing through the esophagus.

***What Happens to Food in the Stomach.*** The food next passes through a round muscle, or sphincter, which controls the entrance into the stomach. The stomach is shaped like a pear. It lies in the upper part of the abdomen, just below the diaphragm, which separates the abdomen from the chest. The stomach is elastic. It is capable of changing its shape and size to accommodate its contents.

When the food arrives in the stomach, that organ receives an additional blood supply for the stomach glands to help them produce their juice. The stomach juice is poured out upon the food from the stomach's glands in drops. Since millions of these glands are present in the walls of the stomach, in the course of a single day a large amount of this juice is produced. Gastric juice contains hydrochloric acid and is acid in character. Two other essential constituents of the gastric juice are pepsin and rennin. The stomach secretion also contains a large amount of water and a variety of minerals.

When food enters the stomach, the muscular walls of the stomach churn the food to mix it thoroughly with the gastric juice. The hydrochloric acid formed by the stomach spreads throughout the food and brings salivary digestion to an end. Rennin coagulates milk, changing the milk protein into casein, a soft curd. Casein, however, is insoluble. It cannot leave the stomach quickly in solution. Therefore, it remains in the stomach to be acted upon by pepsin. Pepsin attacks the proteins of the food, including the casein, and splits them up into smaller substances.

A fat-splitting enzyme called lipase is also produced in the stomach.

***The Small Intestine.*** Small amounts of churned food—now called chyme—are pushed from the stomach into the small intestine, which is twenty-three feet long. The major part of digestion occurs in the small intestine. Secretions from the liver and pancreas insure the splitting of the foods into substances which can be absorbed into the blood. Tiny glands distributed over the inner surface of the intestine also give off intestinal juices which are necessary for the completion of digestion.

***How Food is Absorbed.*** The end products of digestion—simple sugars, amino acids, fatty acids and glycerol—plus other elements of food, such as vitamins, salts and water, are of no use until they are absorbed into the blood and carried to the cells of the body.

Most absorption takes place in the small intestine. The exceptions to this are the absorption of alcohol by the stomach, and the absorption of water, some inorganic salts, and sometimes glucose by the large intestine.

Finger-like extensions of the lining of the small intestine project into its hollow part. These extensions are called villi. They expose an enormous surface along which absorption can take place. Movements of the villi, from side to side and up and down, are brought about by smooth muscles in their walls. In helping to churn the contents of the intestines, these movements aid in the digestion and absorption of substances. Each villus contains a blood capillary loop and a small lymph vessel. Sugars and amino acids pass through the cells of the villi and diffuse into the capillaries. They are then taken off by the blood. Most of the fat passes into the lymph vessels. Some water and salts are also absorbed into the blood here. The digested foods are now carried to the cells of the body. These foods are used for energy, heat, and the growth and repair of tissues.

***The Large Intestine.*** The large intestine, in comparison with the small intestine's twenty-three feet, is only about five feet long. It goes up on the right side of the lower abdomen, crosses the abdomen about midway on the trunk, and goes down on the left side. Then it extends backward and downward to form the rectum. The indigestible part of our food is passed through the large intestine and out of the body.

## ACUTE GASTRITIS ("ACUTE INDIGESTION")

***Causes of Acute Gastritis.*** Gastritis is an inflammation of the stomach. The common causes are food poisoning (mainly bacterial), too much alcohol, overeating, certain kinds of indigestible food (for example, unripe fruit), and chemical poisons.

***Symptoms of Acute Gastritis.*** In mild conditions there is abdominal discomfort, loss of appetite, furred tongue, nausea and vomiting. There may be fever and diarrhea.

In severe conditions the attack begins suddenly, with or without a chill. There are the symptoms mentioned above, but they are more intense. The vomiting is at first of food and then of bile. There are acid belchings and nausea.

***Treatment of Acute Gastritis.*** This consists in eliminating the irritating food or substance from the diet. Solid food should not be taken for twenty-four hours. Warmth to the extremities gives relief, and an electric pad may be applied to the upper abdomen. An enema is of help. If there is no vomiting, it should be brought on with an emetic. Diluted milk, farinaceous foods, tea, and boiled fish may be served. Avoid fatty foods. Where there is poisoning, the treatment requires the attention of a physician.

## CHRONIC GASTRITIS ("DYSPEPSIA")

***Causes of Chronic Gastritis.*** The causes are many and varied. Chronic gastritis may be produced by faulty dietary habits, hurried meals, insufficient chewing, excessive use of alcohol or coffee. Poorly cooked food may bring it on. Vitamin $B_2$ deficiency and mental and physical exhaustion are sometimes responsible.

***Symptoms of Chronic Gastritis.*** Symptoms are heartburn, discomfort in the area of the stomach after eating, and flatulence after meals. Loss of appetite, especially in the morning, but improving during the day, is a frequent complaint. At times there are nausea and vomiting, mainly of saliva and mucus. Little food is vomited. Chronic belching is a prominent symptom.

***Treatment of Chronic Gastritis.*** If the disturbing food or drink is identifiable, it should of course be eliminated and a bland diet substituted. One-half to one teaspoonful of bicarbonate of soda or bismuth subcarbonate in water is helpful, as are vitamins A, B-complex, and C. Medication should be prescribed by a physician.

***Diet in Chronic Gastritis.*** The patient's preferences should be considered. The digestible articles of food include: chicken, mutton, game, boiled fish, especially whiting and sole; spinach, asparagus, toast; meat cut up very fine and lightly cooked. The indigestible foods include: pork, beef, and any twice-cooked or overcooked meat; condiments, any fried food, cabbage, freshly baked bread, brown bread, pies, and pastries. Fats should be taken in strict moderation; sugar is restricted. Farinaceous foods may be taken at breakfast. At least 2½ pints of fluid should be taken daily between meals. A strict milk diet is rarely indicated.

## STOMACH AND INTESTINAL ULCER

In this condition there is loss of tissue in the mucous membrane and deeper coats of the stomach. The ulcer may be acute or chronic.

***Causes of Ulcer.*** Some of the principal causes are: excessive production of hydrochloric acid, centers of infection, emotional upsets, inflammation of the lining of the stomach or of the upper part of the small intestine, with consequent lowered vitality of the cells and digestion of the tissue itself by the gastric juice.

The most recent thought about ulcers of the stomach or intestine is that they may be produced by nervous strain or emotional upset.

***Symptoms of Ulcer.*** There is usually a history of stomach discomfort, with ups and downs—a tendency to remissions and worsening. The distress occurs periodically, almost always when the stomach is empty. The pain bears a definite relation to the taking in of food. It is usually relieved for one-half to two and one-half hours after meals. It is a gnawing, burning sensation, often felt at the end of the breast bone; it may also be felt in the back. In some instances a variable amount of blood is found in the stools. There is always tenderness on pressure over the pit of the stomach.

A characteristic feature of the pain is that it can be relieved by eating or drinking anything bland or by the taking of alkalis, antacids, milk, or sodium bicarbonate.

Vomiting may occur, with blood in the vomitus. There may be collapse if there is a severe hemorrhage.

Some patients complain only of heartburn, belching and a sense of fullness after eating.

In duodenal ulcer (of the small intestine), the pain—of a boring character— is usually not as severe as in stomach ulcer and is felt in the upper part of the abdomen. The pain comes on late after meals—later than in stomach ulcer. It begins, as a rule, about three hours or more after eating, and sometimes awakens the patient from sleep. Vomiting is rare.

***Diagnosis of Ulcer.*** The diagnosis is made by the characteristic symptoms: pain, felt locally in the stomach region after eating, and eased by alkalis and vomiting; deep, localized tenderness and muscular rigidity in the area of the stomach; and blood in the vomit and in the stools. The condition is confirmed or disproved by X-ray examination.

Ulcer of the small intestine occurs about ten times as often as ulcer of the stomach.

***Treatment of Ulcer.*** If the patient is suffering from shock because of excessive bleeding, a surgeon must be summoned immediately. Before his arrival, the arms and legs should be snugly bandaged so as to collapse the superficial veins. Elevate the foot of the bed in order to send the blood to the head. Do not allow the patient to drink anything.

When there is no emergency, the following facts regarding the diet must be kept in mind: No foods which irritate the stomach—chemically or otherwise—should be given. The diet should be supplemented by vitamins. The diet should be bland.

In ulcer, mental and physical rest are essential. If there is bleeding, the treatment should be placed in the hands of a physician promptly. The patient is put to bed, kept warm and quiet. The physician usually gives a hypodermic injection of morphine if there is excessive bleeding. For one or two days nothing is given by mouth. Mouth hygiene receives attention. The bowels should not be opened for four to seven days; then an enema is given. Rectal saline injections of six to eight ounces with dextrose (2 per cent) are given every four hours. If the hemoglobin falls to 40 per cent, it is an indication that a blood transfusion should be given.

When the bleeding has stopped, half-strength normal saline should be given by mouth every four hours for a period of twelve hours.

Milk feedings may now be begun, using the Sippy method.

***Sippy Diet.*** First three weeks: about three ounces of equal parts of whole milk and 20 per cent cream every hour from 7 A.M. to 7 P.M. Take other foods, adding something each day to the previous day's menu, as follows: first day, no addition; second day, soft eggs at breakfast; third day, cooked cereal at 4 P.M.; fourth day, soft egg at 6 P.M.; fifth day, cooked cereal at 8 A.M.; sixth day, soft egg at 2 P.M.; seventh day, cereal, custard, or soup at noon; eighth day and thereafter, toast or crackers with jelly or grated cheese. By now the patient gets six small meals a day, in addition to his hourly milk and cream. Fourth week and thereafter: three or more small meals on the light diet may be taken, if all has gone well, and the milk and cream may be partly or completely discontinued.

For ulcers not complicated by hemorrhage, a modified Sippy diet is now used. The object of the Sippy diet is to protect the ulcer from the natural hydrochloric acid in the stomach. This is accomplished by giving large doses of alkali after the feedings, and of atropine before the feedings, and by using milk and cream as the basis of the diet.

In the modification of the Sippy diet, feedings are given at 2- and 2½-hour intervals; an alkaline powder or neutralizing substance is taken one hour after, and olive oil and atropine are taken before the feedings. A good neutralizing powder consists of sodium bicarbonate, heavy magnesia, and bismuth carbonate, which can be had at drug stores.

Milk is the best neutralizing food substance and the addition of sodium citrates, on the physician's prescription, not only prevents the formation of curds but also increases the neutralizing effect.

Powdered skimmed milk has been substituted for the milk and cream in the Sippy diet and the alkalis are given *with* the milk rather than between feedings. The alkali may be heavy magnesium oxide, bismuth subcarbonate, or calcium carbonate, which can be had at any drugstore. A one-teaspoonful mixture of bismuth subcarbonate, sodium bicarbonate, magnesium oxide, and lactose should be taken after each meal.

## PAIN IN THE STOMACH (GASTRALGIA)

***Causes of Stomach Pain.*** All varieties of stomach discomfort occur in persons with nervous temperaments. The condition is especially common among worrying women at the change-of-life period. In the paroxysmal variety there is severe pain in the upper part of the abdomen which radiates to the back. The pain has no relation to the intake of food.

***Treatment of Stomach Pain.*** The cause should be found and removed if possible. The application of dry heat and the taking of sodium bicarbonate in water—one tablespoonful—are comforting. However, taking bicarbonate should not become a habit.

## VOMITING AND INDIGESTION

***Causes of Vomiting.*** Vomiting may be caused by disorders of digestive organs. Among these are acute indigestion, especially in children; chronic indigestion, ulcer of the stomach, cancer of the stomach, poisons, alcohol, etc., in the stomach.

Irritation of other abdominal organs may also be the cause of vomiting. Such irritation includes: inflammation of the bowels, appendicitis, and irritation produced by pregnancy; intestinal obstruction, which may cause obstinate and complete constipation; colic from gallstones, kidney stones, or bladder stones; menstruation, worms, and diseases of the liver and pancreas.

Still other irritations may be the cause. Among them are irritation of the throat, with cough, such as is experienced in consumption, whooping cough, or severe cough of any kind, or irritation of the brain, such as tumors.

There are a number of miscellaneous causes, such as car, train and airplane sickness; hysteria; severe pain; ether, chloroform, etc.; diseases of the ear, diabetes, kidney disease, and sick headache (migraine).

In the course of the following diseases, especially during the first stages, there is often vomiting: influenza, malaria (particularly in babies), scarlet fever, smallpox, and yellow fever.

***Vomiting in Indigestion.*** Vomiting from indigestion is the most common and the least serious type. Sometimes the vomiting is only the symptom of indigestion, but usually it is caused by some indiscretion in the diet. One or more of these symptoms are usually present: coated tongue, bad taste in the mouth, pain or discomfort in the stomach or bowels, headache, drowsiness and listlessness, and diarrhea. Diarrhea is a condition accompanying acute indigestion of babies.

***Vomiting and Disease.*** Disease of the other abdominal organs, of which vomiting is a symptom, is usually associated with severe pain in the region where the trouble is located, as in appendicitis, inflammation of the bowels, distention of the abdomen, and colic from the passage of gallstones or kidney stone.

In disease of the brain, the vomiting is usually accompanied by one or more of the following symptoms: severe and constant headache, stupor or unconsciousness, convulsions or paralysis.

***Treatment of Vomiting.*** Swallowing large quantities of hot water results in a washing out of the stomach. Injections of warm soapsuds should be made into the rectum until the bowels move satisfactorily. Do not give cathartics of any kind; they only exaggerate the condition. The patient should rest quietly in bed, and an electric pad should be placed over the stomach.

No food should be taken for twelve to twenty-four hours, or until nausea and vomiting cease. A teaspoonful of cracked ice and water, or hot water (if more agreeable), may be sipped as often as necessary to relieve thirst. When vomiting ceases, the patient may take milk mixed with one-third its bulk of limewater. Clam juice, beef juice squeezed from a slightly broiled, rare steak, or albumin water (see p. 413) are also helpful. Any one of these can be given in teaspoonful doses every two hours at first, and the amount increased if the patient retains the food satisfactorily.

Among drugs, two tasteless white powders are perhaps the most successful in relieving vomiting of indigestion: subcarbonate of bismuth in doses of a third of a teaspoonful, and cerium oxalate in doses of five grains. They should be used only on advice of a physician. The diet may be supplemented with milk toast, cooked cereals, etc., as improvement takes place.

***Vomiting After Drinking.*** Nausea and vomiting following excessive drinking may be relieved by washing the stomach and bowels, as previously recommended, and by giving drop doses of tincture of nux vomica on a physician's prescription. As soon as easily digested nourishment can be retained, such as soft-boiled or dropped eggs on toast, hot milk, etc., improvement is generally rapid.

## CHRONIC INTESTINAL INDIGESTION

***Causes of Chronic Intestinal Indigestion.*** In this form of indigestion, the food, after leaving the stomach two or three hours after the last meal, does not properly digest in the intestines. Instead, it begins to ferment and form gas. This distends the intestines and causes distress by pressing on the nerves of neighboring parts.

***Symptoms of Chronic Intestinal Indigestion.*** This condition varies from feeling of a slight amount of fullness and discomfort to intense pain in the pit of the stomach or elsewhere in the abdomen. It is relieved only by belching up wind from the stomach or passing it from the bowels. Palpitation and pain about the heart are also common symptoms. The pain is owing to pressure of the distended stomach, which interferes with the action of the heart.

The skin is not clear and ruddy, but dull and muddy in color;

eruptions are common. The whites of the eyes and inner surface of the eyelids are apt to present a yellowish appearance, and the tongue is soft and flabby, often has a brownish coating, and is marked on the edges by imprints of the teeth.

Constipation is rather the rule, although diarrhea with slime or mucus is also common; these conditions often alternate. The poisons, generated by the decomposing food in the bowels, escape from the system in the urine, and in so doing irritate the urinary organs. Frequent passage of urine often occurs. In their effect upon the nervous system, these poisons cause insomnia or sleepiness, depression of spirits, and the symptoms seen in nervous prostration.

***Complications.*** Physicians believe that chronic intestinal indigestion, with constant absorption of poisons from the decomposing contents of the bowels, leads to such irritation of the heart, kidneys, and other organs that chronic diseases may result. Many "chronic invalids" or hypochondriacs are such by reason of this disorder.

***Intestinal and Stomach Indigestion.*** Intestinal indigestion is to be distinguished from stomach indigestion by the fact that although pain may occur in the region of the stomach, it does not come on until some time after eating, and there are no stomach symptoms, such as nausea or vomiting. The general distention of the abdominal wall, passage of gas from the bowels, and slight yellowness of the eyes, are also characteristic of intestinal indigestion.

***Treatment of Chronic Intestinal Indigestion.*** This consists chiefly of limiting the amount and variety of food. Rest, fresh air, warm clothing, moderate exercise, freedom from care are the first requisites. For a few days, or during the first week of treatment, the diet may be restricted to warm milk containing a third part of barley gruel, lime water (a glass every 2 hours), and sometimes buttermilk—one or all of these, depending on the condition. When milk does not agree with the patient, broths, porridge, and eggs may be substituted; starches must be avoided.

***Diet When Symptoms Subside.*** After this preliminary treatment, and when the symptoms have begun to subside, the following diet should be followed for an indefinite period, not using any vegetables at first: eggs, poached, scrambled, or soft boiled; rare beef, lamb, roasted or broiled; poultry; veal occasionally; but no corned beef, ham, or pork in any form, except crisp bacon; fish of all kinds, except salt fish; oysters, clams, but no lobsters and crabs; rye or graham bread a day old and toasted, with a liberal supply of butter; plenty of water, especially between meals, to the amount of six to eight glasses daily;

green vegetables, such as lettuce (but no mayonnaise dressing); green peas, puréed; string beans, asparagus—only one variety at a meal.

Avoid *all* the following: baked beans, beets, cabbage, carrots, cauliflower, celery, coffee, corn, egg plant, onions, oyster plant, parsnips, potatoes, tomatoes, cereals, candies and sweets of all kinds, pies and pastries, nuts, rich gravies, and thick soups. The simple puddings, ice cream and cooked fruits, such as baked apple, stewed peaches and pears, may be allowed, but no berries.

The bowels must be kept regular every day by some mild cathartic, such as aromatic fluid extract of cascara sagrada, fifteen to sixty drops in water at night, or milk of magnesia, one to two tablespoonfuls. The patient should eat rather sparingly. All excesses should be avoided, and alcohol should be used with the greatest moderation. An occasional glass of light wine is stimulating.

## SEASICKNESS

The vomiting of seasickness may be prevented in some cases by the taking of preliminary precautions. It is a great help if persons about to undertake a sea voyage refrain from unnecessary fatigue. Iced, dry champagne will sometimes relieve the vomiting, if given in tablespoonful doses at half-hour intervals. A hot-water bottle at the feet, and a warm or hot electric pad over the stomach are also helpful in severe attacks.

A drug called dramamine has been found to be extremely effective in the treatment of seasickness. One tablet is taken one hour before boarding the ship. Then, one tablet before or with each meal and before retiring. The most common reaction felt upon taking dramamine is drowsiness.

## ACUTE DIARRHEA

***Causes of Acute Diarrhea.*** Diarrhea is brought on by various causes, among which are the following: stomach disorders which prevent the completion of gastric digestion; extension of inflammation nearby, as in peritonitis; or extensive burns. It may be brought on by acute infections, such as typhoid fever; overeating and drinking; changes in temperature, which lower vitality, particularly in children; exposure of the abdomen to cold, wet, and draughts.

Certain articles of food—indigestible or excessive food, especially unripe fruit—may be the cause. Also, chemical or toxic poisons, such as those generated in milk which has been kept too long and improperly handled, or has become contaminated with dirt and germs, are often responsible for diarrhea.

Acute diarrhea is also attributable to cream-puff poisoning, poisons swallowed by accident or intent, and germs existing in decomposing animal and vegetable foods, as in food improperly home-canned, overripe fruit, or impure drinking water.

Sometimes diarrhea is produced by purely nervous causes, as by fright and anxiety. For example, it often attacks students before examinations and surgeons before difficult operations.

***Symptoms of Acute Diarrhea.*** Diarrhea consists of frequent and soft or watery discharges from the bowels, varying in number from two or three to a dozen or more daily. It is commonly caused by catarrhal inflammation of the mucous membrane lining the inside of the intestines. This, or another cause, increases the nervous irritability and the movements and secretions of the bowels, so that their contents are expelled more rapidly than usual and in a more liquid state.

The passages are commonly light yellow, but they may be greenish from excess of bile, slimy from mucus, or colorless and watery. Diarrhea is often accompanied by pain, either continuous or occurring with the movements of the bowels, and sometimes by fever (temperature 101° to 102° F.), nausea, loss of appetite, and vomiting. Rarely there are also cold sores on the lips and pains in the muscles and joints.

***Treatment of Acute Diarrhea.*** Children and adults with severe attacks should remain in bed. No solid food should be taken. A mild cathartic is advisable at the beginning of the attack. If, however, the diarrhea has been present severely for several days before beginning treatment, the cathartic may be omitted.

Milk porridge, made by boiling flour in milk, boiled rice, or milk toast constitutes the best diet for diarrhea. If nausea or vomiting are present, a teaspoonful of cracked ice with a few drops of brandy may be taken at frequent intervals. Water is permissible in all instances, but in small quantities at a time, and often enough to relieve thirst. Cracked ice is preferable.

Pain in the abdomen is treated by applications of hot towels, a mustard poultice, a flannel wrung out in turpentine and afterward in hot water. To avoid irritation, use one half teaspoonful of turpentine to a basin of hot water. This is a very valuable remedy. An electric pad at the required temperature may be applied to the painful area.

The best remedies to stop the diarrhea are bismuth subnitrate, a quarter teaspoonful every three hours, or chalk mixture, one tablespoonful every two hours as long as the attack lasts. Both of these drugs may be a factor in causing severe constipation following the diarrhea. They should be used on doctor's prescription only.

## CHRONIC DIARRHEA

***Causes of Chronic Diarrhea.*** This is a chronic inflammation of the mucous membrane lining the intestines. It results in the formation of ulcers and in the destruction of tissue. Ulcers are suggested by the appearance of blood and pus in the bowel passages. Chronic diarrhea follows acute diarrhea, dysentery, and sometimes typhoid fever. It is apt to occur among persons crowded together, as in camps and prisons, when bowel discharges and urine are not properly disposed of or disinfected. Diseases of the nervous system may also cause chronic diarrhea.

***Symptoms of Chronic Diarrhea.*** Diarrhea often alternates with constipation. The number of daily passages varies from one to eight. The discharges from the bowels are loose. They often contain mucus or slime, sometimes in the form of sagolike grains, or in white, opaque masses. Pus, blood, and shreds of tissue are usually signs of ulceration, or raw, sore spots which eat into the lining membrane of the bowel. The discharges are of various colors: yellow, brownish yellow, green, black, slate, or white. Pain in the belly, rumbling noises in the bowels, and distention of the abdominal wall are common conditions. Loss of appetite, coated tongue, a bad taste in the mouth, depression of spirits, general weakness, emaciation, and pallor usually follow in time.

***Treatment of Chronic Diarrhea.*** The outlook in this disease is especially unfavorable for children and elderly persons, and in those weakened by other disorders. Months and years may be required for recovery, and during this time there may be many reverses. The longer it has lasted, the more difficult is it to cure. Since this condition is a symptom, the cause must be removed. There is no home remedy that can be safely prescribed, since the wrong judgment may be used. Sometimes it is better to leave the bowel to itself until it gets rid of the offending cause. For pain, hot turpentine stupes are very valuable. A stupe is made by putting turpentine in hot water (one teaspoonful to one quart), then dipping into it a piece of flannel cloth wrapped in a towel. Wring out thoroughly, and place on the patient's abdomen. Watch your stupes carefully so that the patient's skin does not blister. Rest in bed is essential and a bland diet—no meat, no fried food, and no vegetables that are not easily digested. Paregoric and bismuth are the two drugs most often used, but should be taken only on doctor's prescription.

## ULCERATIVE COLITIS (MUCOUS COLITIS)

***Causes of Ulcerative Colitis.*** A form of chronic diarrhea, common to nervous women between the ages of twenty and forty-five, ulcerative colitis is not caused by actual inflammation of the mucous membrane, but probably by constant irritation of the bowels, produced by chronic constipation combined with a highly nervous disposition. Most of the patients are emotional, overworked, or in a condition of chronic worry, or have so-called "nervous prostration," hysteria, or some other form of nervous weakness. This disease is also called mucous colitis.

***Symptoms of Ulcerative Colitis.*** Chronic constipation and a history of indigestion lasting for a long period are forerunners of this disease. There are numerous painful passages of mucus, either alone or mixed with the ordinary bowel discharges, as well as rumbling noises in the bowel. This is because the mucus sticks closely to the walls of the bowel, and great effort is required to detach and expel it. The mucus appears as a transparent jelly-like substance, as slime, or in the form of white strings, and occasionally as a piece of tubular membrane.

An attack, characterized by pain and numerous passages of mucus alone or mixed with bowel discharges, lasts several hours or days. During freedom from the trouble there is usually constipation. Worry or emotion tends to bring on the disorder.

***Treatment of Ulcerative Colitis.*** The essentials in the treatment are rest, warmth and a sufficient non-residue diet with extra vitamins. Usually a considerable amount of plain food can be digested in small quantities at intervals of 2½ hours. Bread and toast, biscuits, butter, eggs, non-fatty fish, meat extracts and meat jellies can be given freely. Orange juice and puréed vegetables (spinach, potato) are allowable.

Excess use of fats, except butter, should be avoided. Also to be avoided are raw milk, cream, fruits, green vegetables, corn, salt meat, candy, sweets and concentrated sugars.

The nervous manifestations must be treated and brought under control.

## CONSTIPATION

***Meaning of Constipation.*** Constipation refers to delay in the bowel evacuations or movements. The term is also applied to a drier or harder movement than natural. The normal person usually has one movement in twenty-four hours, but some persons have naturally two or three passages daily, while others have habitually but one movement every two or three days, and suffer no inconvenience.

***Causes of Constipation.*** Constipation is brought about in various ways. If, on one hand, the food is too coarse, there is too much residue left in the bowel. On the other hand, if the food is not coarse enough—and this is much more common—there is not enough undigested residue remaining in the bowels to stimulate the normal intestinal movements. Lack of regularity in attending to the bowels, persistent use and abuse of cathartics, lack of exercise, and overeating are common causes of constipation.

Many diseases provide conditions in which constipation develops. These are anemia, "nervous prostration," disorders of the spinal cord, liver, stomach, tumors pressing upon the bowels, or narrowing of the bowels from disease or spasm. Weakness of the walls of the abdomen, as in fat persons and in women who have borne many children, is a common source of constipation. Elderly people are very prone to it, due to loss of muscular tone.

***Common Form of Constipation.*** The more common form of constipation is that brought about by sedentary habits, deficient exercise, irregularity in going to the toilet, and improper diet. In most of these instances there is merely a sluggishness of the bowels, caused by deficient tone in the nerves or muscles which control the movements of the bowels.

More rarely the bowel is contracted in some part by irritation, so that the passages are ribbon-like or occur in small, hard balls. This latter trouble happens more often in persons suffering from nervous disorders. Worry and anxiety are frequent causes of constipation by enfeebling the nervous mechanism which regulates the bowels.

***Constipation and Disease.*** In dealing with the treatment of constipation, this book does not discuss the constipation which is caused by special diseases of the various organs mentioned, nor the constipation caused by mechanical obstruction, by tumors, etc. In such examples, there are usually other symptoms suggesting the presence of these diseases. Their greater importance will lead the patient to seek professional advice.

***Symptoms of Constipation.*** In many persons, constipation present for a week produces no disturbance, while in others, absence of one daily movement occasions unpleasant symptoms. Headache, dullness, a bad taste, a coated tongue, with a feeling of fullness or colicky pains in the abdomen, nausea, and belching of wind are among the more common effects of constipation. Mental depression and dizziness are not uncommon. Long continued constipation often produces piles.

***Treatment of Constipation.*** Outdoor exercise is most valuable. When this is impossible, exercise of the abdominal walls is useful. Rubbing and kneading the belly on the right side for five or ten minutes each morning should be practiced. A helpful exercise consists in repeatedly bending the body at the waist, with the arms held above the head, till the finger tips touch the floor. If the abdominal walls are weak, a tight-fitting abdominal support or elastic belt will be helpful.

***Habit As an Aid in Constipation.*** Every individual should go to the toilet at some regular hour each day and attempt to move the bowels, whether there is a desire to do so or not. If the body is bent forward, so that the back is as nearly as possible on a line with the floor, the muscles will have more effect in causing an evacuation. This is very important.

Violent straining is not desirable. After attempting to move the bowels for three to five minutes unsuccessfully, it is best to give up the trial till the same time the following day. It is unwise to attach much importance to failure to secure a movement of the bowels, as the trouble usually corrects itself within a few days. Never rely on cathartics; use only mild laxatives. Preferably rely on correct diet.

***Diet As an Aid in Constipation.*** Abundance of water is an important aid in having an easy movement of the bowels. Six to eight glasses of water should be taken during each twenty-four hours, preferably between meals. One glass of hot or cold water should be taken before breakfast. (See page 402.)

***Drugs and Enemas in Constipation.*** These should be used only as a last resort. Enemas are more desirable where other means fail. The patient should lie flat on the back, and take the enema slowly from a fountain syringe, which should be at head level. Half a pint of warm water or soapsuds may be taken each night, and retained with the aim of having a movement in the morning. A pint of warmed olive or cotton-seed oil may be injected each night for a week or more, and retained until the next morning.

A glycerin suppository introduced into the bowel in the morning is often effective.

Among drugs for chronic constipation, the following are most appropriate: compound licorice powder, one teaspoonful at night; aromatic fluid extract of cascara sagrada, fifteen to twenty-five drops night and morning. These can be bought at any drugstore. Mineral waters, such as Hunyadi Janos, Apenta water, etc., or the Saratoga Springs laxative waters should never be used. After a time they do harm by irritating the colon lining.

When the constipation is caused by anemia, take iron in some form—a Blaud's pill, for instance, three times a day for ten days. These, too, can be had at the drugstore. It is better to let your doctor decide on any drugs taken.

## APPENDICITIS

***Causes of Appendicitis.*** The frequency with which this disease attacks man gives it much importance. It is more common between the ages of ten and thirty than at other ages.

The appendix is poorly supplied with blood, and can but poorly resist the inroads of germs, which enter the appendix from the intestines. The germs which cause appendicitis very often are also the cause of the diarrheal diseases of childhood, and start the infection in the appendix at that time.

There is no way in which the adult can avoid appendicitis. The old theories that grape seeds, etc., are the cause of the disease are not founded on fact. Constipation is one of the most frequent causes.

***Symptoms of Appendicitis.*** Pain is usually the first symptom. This often begins about the navel, shifting after a while to the right lower part of the abdomen. The pain begins suddenly in most instances, and is usually continuous and often agonizing. Nausea and vomiting accompany the pain and may last, at more or less frequent intervals, throughout the attack. The patient lies with legs drawn up toward the abdomen so as to relax the muscles of the abdominal wall.

The most important point in distinguishing this disease from others causing pain in the same area is the fact that there is tenderness over the inflamed appendix. The point of tenderness is in the lower part of the abdomen on the right side, usually midway between the navel and the bony prominence of the hip. Even when the pain is situated in the middle of the abdomen, it will be found that there is more tenderness on pressure of the hand in the right lower part of the area than at any other point. An extremely important sign is the greater pain brought on when the fingers are withdrawn (rebound tenderness) from the area after making downward pressure. The pulse may be 80 to 120 or more, and the temperature from 100° to 102° F., or even higher. When there is the suspicion of formation of an abscess or gangrene, a blood count will give a fairly reliable index as to whether the diagnosis of appendicitis is correct or not.

Appendicitis, then, differs from ordinary intestinal colic caused by indigestion in the following particulars. The pain is continuous rather than intermittent. There is local tenderness on pressure, whereas in colic the pain is not increased, but often diminished, by pressure and lying on the abdomen. The pulse and temperature are usually increased in appendicitis.

***Outcome of Appendicitis Attack.*** Appendicitis may last a few hours, days, or weeks. In its outcome, there are a number of different possibilities: The patient may entirely recover and never have another attack. He may suffer more or less pain constantly, not sufficient to require him to stay in bed, but enough to make him very uncomfortable, and he is likely to have another acute attack at any time. He may apparently recover completely and yet have another attack at any time—this is the more common result. The attacks may begin as has been described and the patient may die in twenty-four hours or may continue in pain. After some days a lump may form in the lower right side of the abdomen, and this may soften down into an abscess. This may subside in a few weeks or may break internally and cause death, or its contents may escape through the bowels. Many other complications may occur.

The appearance, in the course of the disease, of chills, rapid feeble pulse, general swelling and drumlike condition of the abdomen, with anxious pinched countenance, cold sweats, and coldness and blueness of the hands and feet, are grave signs.

***Treatment of Appendicitis.*** The most successful treatment consists in the surgical removal of the appendix within the first twelve hours after the beginning of the attack. The best results are obtained if the appendix is removed after the acute attack is over and the patient is apparently well. The most important point is quickly to get an expert opinion by calling your doctor.

In patients ill with appendicitis, in whom a severe spreading peritonitis is present, streptomycin is used.

## PERITONITIS

***Causes of Peritonitis.*** Acute general peritonitis is an infection of the peritoneum, the membrane which lines the abdomen and covers most of its organs. This disease is caused by extension of inflammation, for example, from the intestines, stomach, appendix, or gallbladder. It may follow an external perforating wound.

***Symptoms of Peritonitis.*** The disease begins fairly suddenly, with a chill and severe pain in the abdomen. There is fever and vomiting. The abdomen soon becomes distended and rigid, and the tongue dried and cracked. There is severe constipation from paralysis of the bowel. The pulse becomes quick and feeble. The patient lies with legs drawn up. The expression is anxious and the face has a sharp, pinched appearance. Death may occur in three or four days.

***Treatment of Peritonitis.*** There should be no delay or attempt at treatment with household remedies or drugs of any kind. A surgeon should be summoned *at once* when there are symptoms that suggest peritonitis. He makes the decision regarding treatment, which may involve surgical operation and administration of penicillin. Bed rest and regulation of diet are important helps in relieving or curing this condition.

## GALLSTONE COLIC

***Causes of Gallstone Colic.*** This disorder is more frequent in women over forty years of age. The gall bladder is situated immediately under the lowest rib, about 1½ inches to the right of the navel. The pain usually accompanies the escape of gallstones from the gall bladder, where they have been formed, into the passage which conveys the bile from the gall bladder to the bowels. Infection of the gall bladder is a common cause of the stones.

***Symptoms of Gallstone Colic.*** The pain begins suddenly. It is often agonizing and of an aching, tearing character. Sometimes it is not continuous, but occurs in violent attacks with comparative ease between them. The pain is felt in the region of the stomach, but more in the right lower chest and right shoulder blade. This pain in the right shoulder blade is characteristic, and differentiates this disorder from kidney and appendix colics. Pressure below the ribs on the right side may at first give relief, but tenderness in this region soon appears. It is the most distinguishing feature of this form of colic.

The patient commonly suffers intensely. He is pale, covered with

## SELF-OPERATION

*(Right)* Photograph shows doctor removing his own appendix; assistant and nurse helped him to hold instruments. He did this to "get patient's attitude."

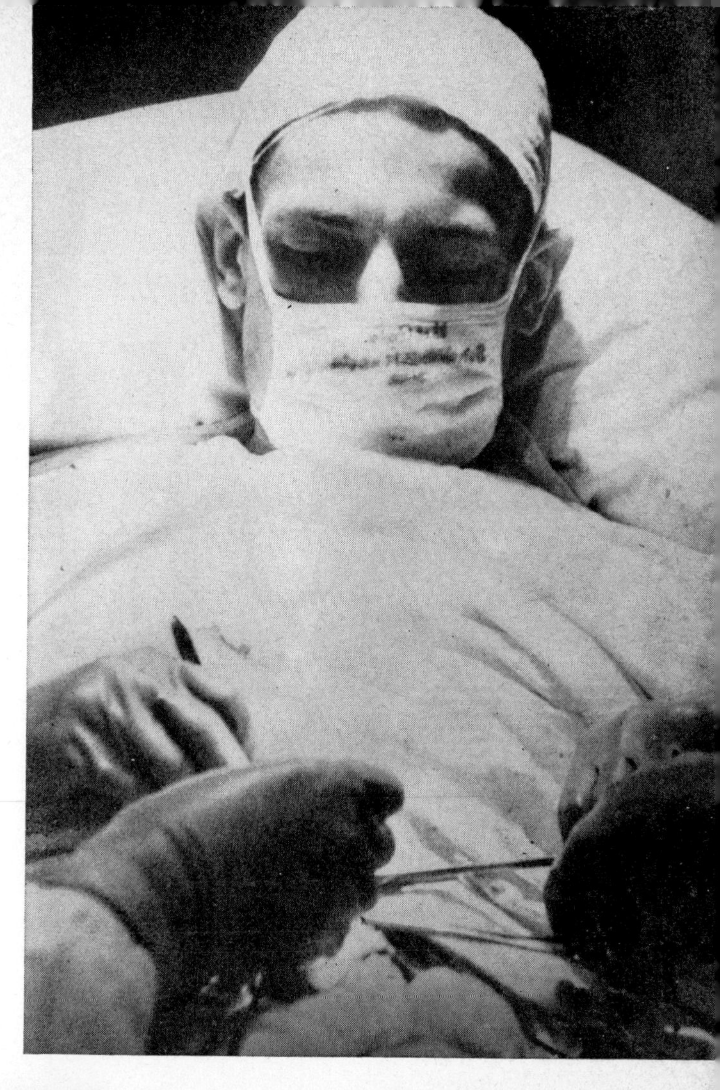

## A MIRACLE OF MODERN SCIENCE

Press Association

*(Bottom left)* Nail swallowed by four-year-old boy was successfully withdrawn from his duodenum when doctors induced him to gulp chocolate malted milk containing magnet attached to thread. X-ray shows magnet in contact with nail, which appears as curved line beneath it.

## BLIND, BUT SHE CAN WORK

*(Bottom right)* Blind people, like girl above, can do many jobs efficiently. Handicap is minimized with help of Seeing Eye dog.

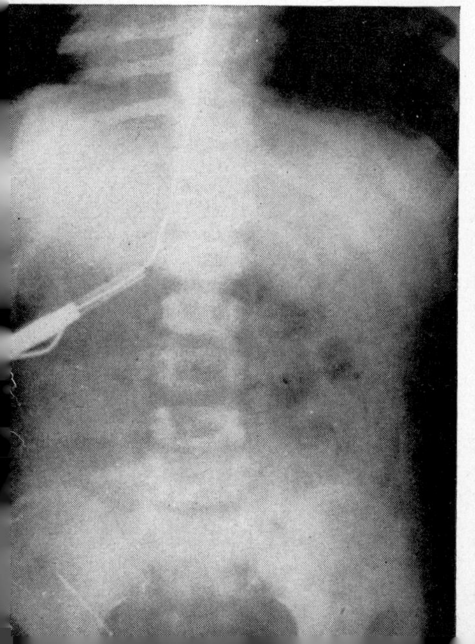

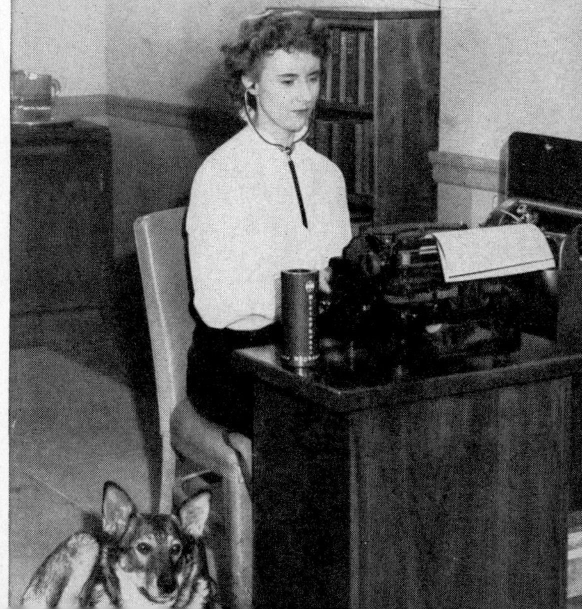

# Stomach Cancer

## CANCER NEVER RESTS

Cancer cells do not limit their damage to the area where they first start. If unchecked, some of them break off and make their way through the lymph and blood vessels to other parts of the body. Illustration shows stomach cancer and its closeness to the lymph nodes.

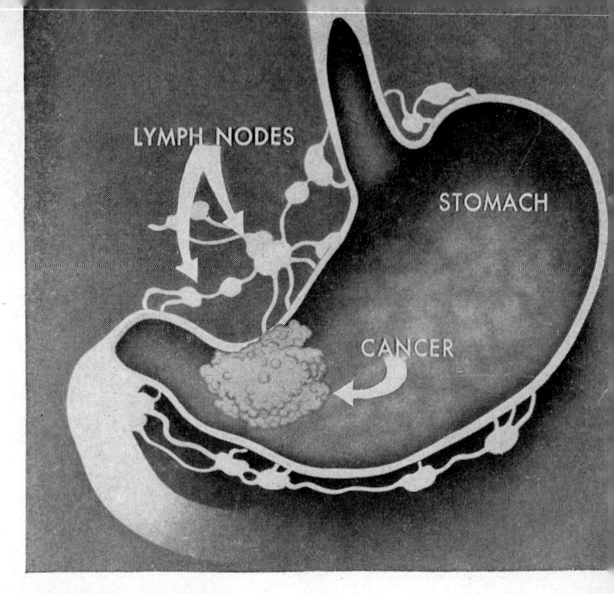


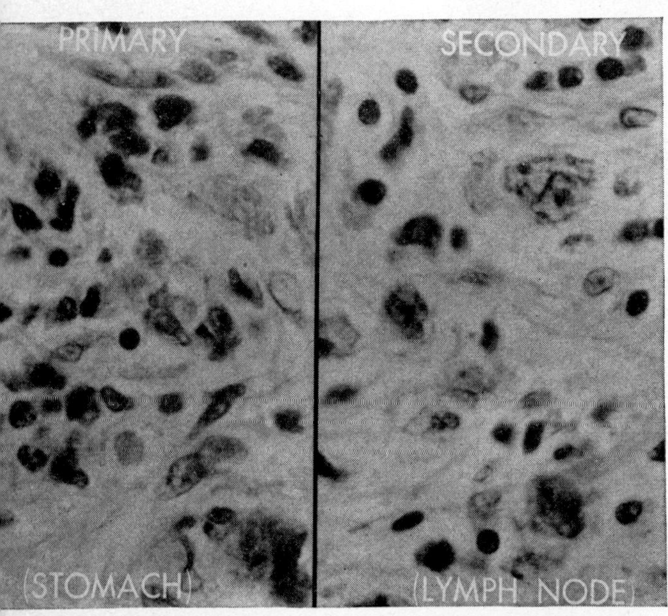


## SECONDARY CANCER

Cancer cells, carried to a secondary site, as from the stomach to the lymph nodes, have the character of those found in the first site. Photomicrographic study of cells in stomach and lymph nodes shows similarity.

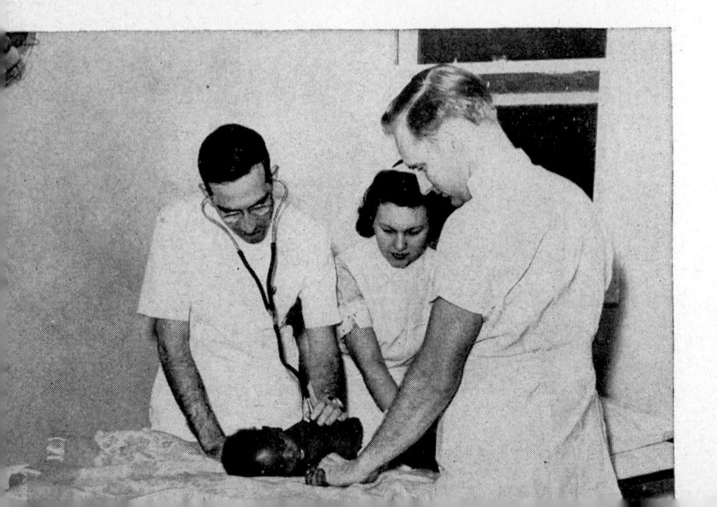

## CHILDREN ARE NOT SPARED

Cancer respects no age, race, or class. In the United States, about 1400 children under fifteen years of age may die of cancer in one year. It is important that children be examined regularly.

cold sweat, and vomits frequently, while the pulse is feeble. There is often chilliness at the beginning of the attack, and this is followed by fever with a temperature of 102° to 103° F.

The pain may last a few hours or, with intermissions, for days or weeks. It is occasionally continuous and dragging instead of occurring in sharp attacks. Jaundice coming on either with or after an attack of pain, such as described, is another characteristic symptom. Taken together with violent pain and tenderness over the gall bladder, it points to a diagnosis of the presence of gallstones. Jaundice is shown by yellowness of the eyes, tongue, skin, and urine, with whiteness of the bowel discharges. However, jaundice is not always present.

***Treatment of Gallstone Colic.*** During an attack, the patient should be put to bed and an electric pad applied to the upper right area of the abdomen. The physician will give a hypodermic injection of morphine. Diet should be restricted to fluids for at least forty-eight hours. (See Diet, Gallstones.)

A surgical operation may be required and sometimes becomes urgent.

## JAUNDICE

This is otherwise known as icterus. It is a symptom characterized by an increase in the blood of bile pigment. This pigment is distributed in the skin and mucous membranes, with resulting yellow appearance of the patient.

***Causes of Jaundice.*** These are rather numerous. In general, the trouble is some interference with the normal flow of the bile in the gall bladder. As a result, the bile is absorbed by the blood vessels. Any infection of the ducts of the bile tract; any disturbance of the liver function; any mechanical pressure of the bile ducts such as tumors of the neighboring organs, especially tumors of the stomach or pancreas; any destructive disease of the blood itself, such as the anemias or such as occurs in the late stages of a malignant tumor in any part of the body—all these will cause jaundice.

Jaundice is more often than not present with such diseases as malaria, yellow fever, and other tropical diseases that cause a destruction of the red blood corpuscles. There is also marked bronze discoloration of the skin associated with Addison's disease, which is a disease of the pituitary gland.

***Jaundice in the Newborn.*** There is one other type of jaundice, known as physiological jaundice, which is found very frequently in the newborn. This is due to the delayed establishment of the normal bile flow. It lasts only a few days, when the yellow appearance of the skin disappears.

***Symptoms of Jaundice.*** This is really a contradiction, since it has been mentioned that the discoloration of the skin is itself a symptom of an underlying disease or condition. However, there is one characteristic that is nearly always present—severe itching of the entire skin. This may be greatly disturbing and yields only to the removal of the cause.

***Treatment of Jaundice.*** The discoloration of the skin and mucous membranes will disappear if the patient is treated properly for the underlying disease.

## OBSTRUCTION OF THE BOWELS

***Causes of Bowel Obstruction.*** This condition in adults is caused by compression of the bowel at some point, as in the opening through which a "rupture" occurs; or by compression from a band of tissue resulting from former attacks of inflammation. These are called adhesions. The obstruction may result from operations or from unnatural conditions arising in the development of the patient before birth. A frequent cause of obstruction of the bowels in children is a slipping of one portion of the bowels into a neighboring part, the way one joint of a telescope slips into another. Twisting of the bowel on itself is still another source of obstruction, and even an almost knotted condition may at times occur. The existence of an accumulation of hardened feces in the bowels may give rise to complete obstruction.

***Symptoms of Bowel Obstruction.*** The pain is usually in the neighborhood of the navel. It begins suddenly, is at first intermittent, but later becomes continuous. It varies in intensity from moderate to excruciating pain. Vomiting is also a prominent symptom. First, the contents of the stomach are expelled; then greenish, bilious matter; and, finally, after a day or two, a brownish-black substance having an unmistakable odor of feces.

Constipation is the third symptom of importance; often it is complete, but, particularly in the obstruction common to children, there escapes from the bowels, with much straining, slimy and bloody material. The temperature may rise to 102°F., or higher. The abdomen is often much distended with gas, and although not tender to the touch at first, it rapidly becomes so. A lump may be felt in the abdomen, especially in children.

The effect of obstruction of the bowels on the general condition is profound. There are great prostration, feeble pulse, cold hands and feet, and anxious, sunken features and cold sweats. If the obstruction is not relieved, the patient will not live more than three to six days.

***Obstruction and Other Diseases.*** Absolute constipation with constant vomiting and tenderness and distention of the abdomen often occurs in other conditions than obstruction of the bowels, as in appendicitis and peritonitis. The appearance of vomitus having the odor of feces is characteristic of obstruction of the bowels and nothing else.

***Treatment of Bowel Obstruction.*** This condition requires urgent surgery.

## RUPTURE (HERNIA)

***Causes of Rupture.*** Hernia or rupture consists of a protrusion of a part of the bowel, or its covering (or both), through the abdominal wall. The common danger points for rupture are at the navel and in the groin. Rupture at the navel is called "umbilical hernia"; that in the groin either "inguinal" or "femoral," according to slight differences in location. Umbilical hernia is frequent in babies, but occurs as a rule in only 5 per cent of all ruptures; rupture in the groin accounts for some 94 per cent of all ruptures. There is still another variety of hernia which occurs in the scars of wounds in the abdomen, after injuries or surgical operations. This type may arise in almost any area of the abdominal wall.

Rupture is sometimes present at birth. In other cases, it results from various causes, natural weakness of the part involved being chief among them. Rupture is three times more frequent in men than in women, and conditions favorable for it are provided by severe muscular work, obesity, chronic coughing, constipation, diarrhea, sudden strain, or blows on the abdomen.

***Early Symptoms of Rupture.*** An external rupture first appears as a fullness or swelling on some part of the abdominal wall, more noticeable when standing, lifting, coughing, or straining. It may disappear entirely on lying down, or on pressure with the fingers. In the beginning there may be discomfort after standing or walking for any length of time; later the patient often complains of a dragging pain or uneasiness, or a sensation of weakness or griping at the seat of the rupture. When the protruding section of the bowel cannot be returned, the rupture has reached a more serious stage, called "irreducible," or "strangulated."

***Dangers from Strangulation.*** The great danger of hernias is the likelihood of their being strangulated. When this occurs, there is a constriction of the hernial wall in such a way that the blood supply is first interfered with and finally stopped. As a rule, the passage of feces (intestinal waste) is stopped. Strangulation may be present on the first appearance of a hernia, usually in children, but it more often results from additional contents being forced into a long-standing rupture.

***Later Symptoms of Rupture.*** There is sudden and complete constipation. During some unusual effort, such as coughing or straining, the patient is seized with acute pain localized at one of the hernial areas, with a variable degree of shock during the early stages. He feels faint, cold, and clammy. His pulse is slow and weak, his temperature subnormal. Vomiting soon follows—of stomach contents at first, then bile, and finally yellowish or brown and offensive (so-called "fecal") vomiting. Pain meanwhile increases and spreads to the whole abdomen, which becomes tender, distended and full of gas.

Gangrene of the bowel sometimes occurs, accompanied by a fall in temperature and cessation of pain, but the pulse gradually becomes weaker, and extremely rapid. The patient, if not promptly treated surgically, dies of blood poisoning or general peritonitis.

In some conditions, where the obstruction is not complete, the symptoms are comparatively milder, consisting of occasional vomiting, with slight pain, and incomplete constipation.

***Treatment of Rupture.*** If the patient cannot return the protrusion speedily, a surgeon should be summoned at once—the patient meanwhile lying in bed with an ice-bag or cold cloths over the rupture. When the patient is hospitalized, the surgeon replaces the protruding part by "reducing" it, under ether, or by operation.

Strangulation of any rupture may occur, but of course it is less likely to happen when a well-fitting truss (supporting appliance) is worn. However, strangulation is always a dangerous possibility, and this fact, added to the likelihood that the rupture may increase in size, makes a surgical operation for complete cure advisable in persons for whom surgery is safe.

***Preventive Treatment.*** Preventive treatment should be started early in life. The new-born infant must be repeatedly examined by the attending physician to discover any possible rupture at the usual sites. Later, attention should be directed to digestive disturbances and to coughs and crying spells. A truss may be used in incipient, incomplete, or complete but reducible hernias of infancy, in the navel and inguinal varieties where a cure may often be expected, especially during the first year of life. The great majority of spontaneous cures are in infants under one year of age, and the earlier the use of the apparatus the greater the prospect of a permanent cure.

***What to Do about Umbilical Rupture in Babies.*** Umbilical rupture in babies is very common after the cord has dropped off. There is a protrusion at the navel which increases in size on coughing, straining or crying. If the rupture is pushed in and the flesh is brought together from both sides in two folds over the navel, so as to bury the navel out of sight, and held in this position by a strip of adhesive plaster reaching across the front of the belly, complete recovery will usually take place within a few months. It is well to cover the plaster with a compact flannel band around the body. The plaster should be replaced as need be, and should be applied, in all cases, by a physician. Authorities in the surgery of hernia hold that all such conditions in infants should be operated on as soon as they are diagnosed.

***Operation for Rupture.*** Operations for complete cure of hernia in the groin are successful in ninety-five cases out of a hundred. The sooner the operation, the better the results.

## DIABETES

There are two forms of diabetes, one entirely different from the other. The more serious is diabetes mellitus or "sugar diabetes." This is not a disease of the kidneys but of the pancreas. The internal secretion of the pancreas, insulin, which regulates the amount of sugar in the intestinal tract, fails in this condition, and the body does not utilize the sugar properly. The other form is called "diabetes insipidus." This is a disease of the pituitary gland and has nothing to do with sugar excretion.

***Causes of Diabetes Mellitus.*** There is no definite knowledge as to the cause of this disease. That it is a disease of the pancreas is definitely established and exactly what structures in the pancreas are involved is also known. But why the natural insulin fails is still a mystery.

***Symptoms of Diabetes Mellitus.*** There are four cardinal and typical symptoms: (1) insatiable thirst for water, (2) enormous appetite, (3) the passage of excessive amounts of urine that contains sugar, and (4) progressive loss in body weight. If not recognized in time, there are associated changes in the circulatory system which will end in gangrene of the toes and foot or even the leg. Later the liver is involved, which leads to a state of what is called acidosis and then coma and death.

***Causes of Diabetes Insipidus.*** The only thing that is definitely known is that the disease often follows head injuries and may be associated with tumor of the pituitary.

***Symptoms of Diabetes Insipidus.*** This disorder more often attacks the young. Although the thirst is excessive and very large quantities of urine are passed there is no sugar in the urine. There may be increase in appetite and loss of weight with emaciation. If the cause is an injury, the patient may recover without any treatment. Extract of pituitary is helpful in many cases.

***Treatment of Diabetes Mellitus.*** There is no hard and fast rule for general treatment. Every case is different. It is almost a "must" that as soon as a diagnosis is made the patient should go to a well-regulated hospital for a few days. In the hospital many difficult tests are done. The blood sugar and urine sugar are estimated, at different times of the day and under the influence of different diets. The conclusions drawn from these tests will determine the further treatment that the patient can carry out in his home. For example, he is taught exactly what to eat and how to give himself insulin, which is given by injections. He must learn how to sterilize the hypodermic syringe with which he injects the insulin. He will learn when to take it and how much to take. Regulation of diet is an important feature of treatment in controlling the sugar taken into the body. Often proper diet makes the taking of insulin unnecessary.

It is rare that diabetes is completely cured, but under careful professional guidance the patient can live into old age.

### How to Give an Insulin Injection

To give a hypodermic injection of insulin, you require: absorbent cotton; 70 per cent grain alcohol; an official insulin syringe; insulin; and at least two rustless needles, one-half to five-eighths inches long, 25 gauge. Keep the insulin in its box in a cool place, and always have an extra syringe and extra needles on hand.

Wash hands thoroughly, and place the syringe (with plunger withdrawn) and needle in a large strainer. Lower the strainer into a pan of water so that the syringe and needle are completely submerged. Boil for five minutes. (If you have no strainer, you can boil the syringe in a pan of water.) Take strainer out of the boiling water and dispose of the water. (If you are traveling, and there are no facilities for boiling the syringe and needle, you can rinse them thoroughly in pure alcohol.) Fit the tip of the syringe to the needle and turn the needle hub to the left until you feel that it is affixed securely. Avoid touching anything with the needle or syringe; place the syringe with the inserted needle on top of a box so that the needle does not come in contact with anything.

Take a piece of sterile absorbent cotton, soak it in alcohol, and with it wipe the rubber cap of the insulin bottle. If protamine zinc is the variety suggested by your physician, merely *roll* the bottle between your hands—do not shake it forcibly—before cleaning the cap.

Push the needle through the rubber cap on the bottle, and push out all air from the syringe into the bottle. Turn the bottle upside down so that the needle is in the insulin, and pull the plunger back to the mark of the designated dose, and draw the needle out of the bottle. Slowly push the plunger until air bubbles are out of the syringe. You will accomplish this by holding the syringe vertically. (Be sure the full dose is in the syringe before you take the needle out of bottle.) Put the syringe back on the box top, again being careful not to touch any object with the needle.

Change the place for the injection often. The insulin may be placed under the skin of the upper arm (deltoid muscles), in the upper part of the abdominal wall, or along the side of the thigh. With a piece of sterile absorbent cotton soaked in alcohol, wipe the skin where you are going to make the injection. Stretch the skin tight, or pinch it with fingers spread at least a few inches apart. Insert the needle quickly at an angle under the skin. Draw the plunger back a little to make certain that you have not entered a blood vessel. If you see blood, withdraw the needle and inject in another spot. If no blood shows, press plunger down slowly as far as it will go. Withdraw the needle and wipe the area of injection with sterile absorbent cotton soaked in alcohol.

CHAPTER 6

# THE VITAL ENDOCRINE GLANDS AND THEIR HORMONES

**How the Hormones Work . . . The Pituitary—the "Master Gland" . . . Role of the Thyroid Gland . . . Abnormal Conditions of the Thyroid . . . Goitre . . . The Parathyroid Glands . . . The Pancreas . . . The Adrenal Glands . . . Female and Male Hormones—What They Do . . . The Pineal and Thymus Glands . . . The Basal Metabolism Test . . . Treatment with Hormones, etc.**

AN ENDOCRINE secretion or hormone is a natural drug of the body. Instead of being poured into the body through a duct, as is the case with the secretions of non-endocrine glands, the hormone is absorbed by the blood as the blood passes through the gland. The hormone is then carried by the blood to all parts of the body.

The glands which produce the hormones are called the glands of internal secretion or endocrine glands. Some glands produce both an internal and an external secretion, as for example, the pancreas. The sex glands also have internal and external secretions.

The hormones secreted by the endocrine glands have many varied jobs to perform. They play a role in transmitting nervous stimulation, control of salt and water balance, reproduction, metabolism, growth, production of insulin, and control of blood pressure, and they also influence the digestive processes. The hormones perform their specific tasks far from their "habitats." For this reason they have been called "chemical messengers."

When rapidity of action is essential, the body is organized and controlled through the central nervous system. When there is no harm in the action's being slow or even extremely slow and prolonged, then the body makes use of the chemical, rather than the nervous, means of control. An example of slow coordination in the body is the growth of the bones. Such growth is rarely complete until a person has reached adult age. Therefore, for twenty years the rate of growth of each bone in the body has to keep pace with the rest. This coordination is brought about by minute doses of an internal secretion from the pituitary gland, which is poured into the blood from before birth to old age. The rate of growth of different bones is coordinated by means of a hormone.

The endocrine glands secrete hormones in varying number. The thyroid, parathyroid, and pancreas apparently secrete one hormone each. The adrenals and sex glands secrete at least two each while the anterior pituitary gland secretes eight or more. Each gland has certain characteristic functions, the disturbance of which causes various changes in the appearance and workings of the body.

The endocrine glands are located in different parts of the body. The pituitary is situated at the base of the skull; the thyroid, in the neck; the parathyroid, also in the neck; the pancreas and the two adrenal glands, above the kidneys; the sex glands, which include ovaries and testicles, in the pelvic region; the pineal gland, in the brain; and the thymus, under the breast bone until puberty.

Not many ideas in connection with how the body works are entirely new. The idea of control by hormones, although it dates from the beginning of the twentieth century, is a revival and elaboration of an idea which used to be held widely in the Middle Ages. In ancient times it was believed that the body was controlled by four "humours." Illness was thought to be caused by an upset in their balance. The four cardinal fluids of the body, according to this view, were blood, phlegm, and yellow and black bile, which were correlated with the four alchemical elements—fire, earth, air and water.

"The body of man," wrote Hippocrates, the Father of Medicine, "has in itself blood, phlegm, yellow bile and black bile; these make up the nature of his body, and through these he feels pain or enjoys health. Now he enjoys the most perfect health when these elements [substitute "hormones"] are duly proportioned to one another . . . The flesh of glands is different from that of the rest of the body, being spongy and full of veins; they are found in the moist parts of the body where they receive humidity . . ."

## HOW THE HORMONES WORK

The actions of the various hormones differ widely. Yet their basic chemical structure is similar. These natural drugs of the body are active in extremely small dilutions. They are present in the blood, in the lymph and in the glands in small quantities. We have said they control such extremely vital functions as growth, nutrition and sex. They also influence mentality and personality. They are closely related. They may have stimulating, as well as inhibiting, action on one another.

No single hormone acts entirely by itself. The secretions of two endocrine glands may exert opposite effects upon the same organ or tissue. Thus, for example, insulin increases the quantity of carbohydrate stored in the muscle; while adrenalin causes a decrease in the quantity of carbohydrate. If one gland "falls down on the job" it may exert an influence on other endocrine glands. For example, castration in childhood is followed by excessive growth in the long bones.

## THE PITUITARY GLAND

This gland, which lies at the base of the brain, is about the size of an acorn. It contains three lobes: anterior, intermediary and posterior. The anterior pituitary controls the activities of *all* the endocrine glands. It is indeed the "master gland."

The anterior and posterior lobes of the pituitary have different structures. The posterior lobe secretes two hormones, and the anterior lobe secretes eight or more active principles. Extracts of the posterior pituitary are used, for example, to increase the force of contractions of the womb in labor. These extracts are also used for asthma, abdominal distension and in a variety of diabetes called insipidus.

### The Eight Anterior Pituitary Hormones

At least a dozen or more varieties of effects on the body have been attributed to the anterior lobe. Eight of these have been proved to be caused by the action of distinct hormones: a growth hormone exercising control over the development of the body; a hormone which stimulates the growth and maturation of the ovarian follicles; a hormone which causes the formation of the corpus luteum of the ovarian follicles; a hormone which is essential for normal thyroid development; a hormone which induces the flow of milk in mammals; a hormone which acts to decrease the sugar action of insulin; a hormone which stimulates the outer part of the adrenal glands; a hormone which stimulates the thyroid gland.

Excess secretion of the growth hormone before full development of the ends of the bones results in gigantism (abnormally large size and height).

The milk-producing hormone is secreted when the estrogen in the blood decreases, after the delivery of the "afterbirth." The hormone is administered to increase inadequate milk secretion in women.

The function of the anti-insulin factor is to prevent overaction of insulin.

There is thus to be noted a harmonious relationship in the body between the various endocrine glands. Abnormal function of a specific endocrine gland may cause disturbed function of another gland. The anterior pituitary influences other glands, and other glands influence the anterior pituitary.

### The Anterior Pituitary Lobe

The removal of the anterior pituitary in young animals has a great influence on their growth: the formation of bone tissues is brought to a stop, no more teeth come through, and sexual and mental development ceases. Dwarfism is produced. On the other hand, increased activity of the anterior lobe results, as previously stated, in gigantism. Sometimes the gigantism is local, affecting only the head, hands, and feet. This condition is known as acromegaly.

Anterior lobe deficiency leads to underdevelopment of the reproductive system. It also has a profound influence on the carbohydrate metabolism of the body. The anterior pituitary is regarded as being responsible for a great many functions. It is puzzling to understand how so many secretions can be formed within a gland that is no larger than a large green pea. This has lead to the assumption that the anterior pituitary works as an activator of other glands, producing its effect by indirect action rather than directly.

### Posterior Lobe of the Pituitary

Two different extracts have been derived from the posterior lobe of the pituitary. One causes a contraction of smooth muscles, particularly of the blood vessels and womb. The other has a notable effect in increasing the output of urine. The first of these two active principles is used in labor. When the contractions of the womb are too feeble to be effective, an injection of posterior pituitary is sometimes given in order to increase their strength. Removal of the posterior lobe of the pituitary does not cause any profound disturbance in the body.

The posterior part of the pituitary gland probably plays a part in water regulation of the body.

A connection between the posterior lobe of the pituitary and the stomach has been demonstrated by investigators. When an extract of the posterior lobe of the pituitary gland was injected into rabbits, in twelve hours there was intensive bleeding in the acid-bearing area of the stomach of the rabbits. This seems to prove that there is a relationship between the base of the brain and the stomach.

***Location of Pituitary in the Brain.*** An interesting point about the pituitary is its location. It is the only endocrine gland, except the pineal, which is intimately connected with the brain. It is of great significance that it is connected with that part of the brain, the thalamus, which is assumed to be related to the emotional life. By virtue of its close connection with the thalamus, the pituitary is influenced by the thalamus. The thalamus is also influenced by the pituitary. This area at the base of the brain may be regarded as a meeting place of chemical secretions and of nervous impulses.

## THE THYROID GLAND

The thyroid gland lies on both sides of the trachea or windpipe. It is a double gland. It produces thyroxin, the hormone which influences metabolism and growth. The thyroid gland must have a certain amount of iodine in order to function properly.

***Abnormal Conditions of the Thyroid.*** If the thyroid is overactive, food is burned too quickly in the body. Then the person loses weight, his pulse becomes rapid, and he is nervous and unable to sleep. If the thyroid is underactive, development of the body is also not normal. In an adult with a mildly underactive thyroid, there is great sensitivity to cold. The hands and feet are cold. The patient also finds mental activity difficult.

Some secretion of the thyroid is absolutely necessary for the maintenance of life. Complete absence of the gland produces a condition known as myxedema. This consists in a general swelling of the body; the face becomes puffy, and the skin dry and wrinkled like that of the aged. There is a general decline in the activity of the body and a slowing of the heart, and, finally, death. Arrest of development of the thyroid at an early age results in cretinism. In this condition, growth stops. Stunting of the body is linked with a corresponding backwardness of mental and sexual development. When a cretin is given thyroid extract, his condition improves. Indeed thyroid is sometimes given to children to encourage growth even when they show no signs of cretinism.

### Symptoms of Overactive Thyroid

There is an increased activity of the body metabolism associated with a quickened pulse. The patient becomes overactive, anxious, emotional and tremulous. These symptoms occur in patients who are afflicted with exophthalmic goitre, a disease characterized by a swelling in the area of the thyroid gland. The disease is associated with bulging eyes. That this condition is caused by an excess of thyroid secretion is proved by the fact that it is relieved by the surgical removal of part of the gland. Removal of the *entire* thyroid would produce the reverse condition of myxedema; therefore, sufficient gland must always be left for the normal requirements of the body.

Hyperthyroidism (an excess of thyroid secretion) is especially apt to occur in women during puberty, pregnancy and lactation.

Psychic states, particularly anxiety and excitement, stimulate the action of the thyroid. In many patients suffering from exophthalmic goitre, the condition occurs after a period of excessive emotional disturbance.

***Prevention of Goitre.*** In order to prevent the formation of goitre it is merely necessary to provide iodine where the drinking water is deficient in it. Iodized table salt is used to prevent goitre. The nearer the ocean, the fewer the cases of exophthalmic goitre. Sea water is rich in iodine.

### Treatment of Goitre with Radioactive Iodine

Goitre specialists are among the first practical peace-time users of atomic energy. They are treating and often curing toxic goitre with radioactive iodine. The physician gives the patient a small "tracer" dose of the radioactive atoms to see whether the thyroid takes it up from the blood stream. The overactive gland is always eager to get new iodine atoms for the manufacture of thyroxin. If the glands avidly take up iodine, a Geiger counter held near the patient's throat indicates this fact to the physicians. The counter is an extremely sensitive electric instrument which records each of the invisible "atomized" explosions which constantly occur in all radioactive substances. If the tracer dose of radioactive atoms is not absorbed by the thyroid, it shows that the patient does not have an overactive thyroid. If, however, the tracer atoms show that toxic goitre is the seat of the patient's trouble, then the remedy is fairly simple and inexpensive, with radioactive iodine available.

A carefully measured dose of radioactive iodine is dropped into a glass of orange juice and given to the patient to drink. (Orange juice is used because most people like it, not because the iodine, in such small quantities, is distasteful.)

What the atoms do to cure the toxic goitre, in effect, is to cut down the quantity of thyroxin manufactured by the thyroid.

When radioactive iodine is taken into the gland it destroys the electrical balance of many of the tissue cells. These cells become inactive. This cuts down the number of "workers" in the thyroid factory. It also lowers the quantity of thyroxin released into the blood stream.

The quantity of iodine needed to destroy exactly the right number of thyroid cells is easily calculated.

The drug thiouracil may also be used to treat hyperthyroidism. However, it is slightly toxic and must be taken regularly over a long period of time under the direction of a physician. Formerly, the standard procedure was nearly always surgery.

Radioactive iodine treatments must be carried out with great caution and under the supervision of a highly skilled physician.

Too many radioactive atoms in the thyroid would curtail the production of thyroxin too much. This would result in hypothyroidism instead of hyperthyroidism, and render the patient sluggish and inactive. For this, however, there is a ready antidote: the hormone thyroxin can be given in tablet form to restore the proper action of thyroid cells.

The thyroid is a good example of a gland influencing personality. A cretin, given thyroid medication, may become a normal person. The same is true of an adult with underactivity of the thyroid.

## THE PARATHYROID GLANDS

Removal of these "false thyroids" in animals causes death. They are quadruple glands that lie alongside the windpipe. They are covered by part of the thyroid gland. They seem to exercise two effects, one on the utilization of calcium and phosphorus in the body; the other on the central nervous system.

The normal amount of calcium in the blood is very small—as low as from 8/1000 to 10/1000 of 1 per cent. However if that percentage falls to 6/1000 of 1 per cent or less, there will be trouble in store. There will be headache, a feeling of weakness and radiating pains in the limbs; apprehensiveness and consciousness of "quiverings" throughout the body. Then come cramps, particularly of the muscles of the fingers and palms of the hands. These cramps spread to the wrists, forearms, feet and finally to the trunk muscles. If the condition extends to the muscles that control breathing, there is always a possibility of death by asphyxia (cutting off of oxygen). All these symptoms are the result of depletion of calcium in the blood. The treatment is concerned with raising and bringing back to normal the calcium in the blood by high calcium feeding and injections of calcium salts and use of Vitamin D and allied substances to increase the absorption of calcium from the intestinal tract.

## THE PANCREAS

This gland is not ductless. It provides a digestive juice. In addition, it forms an internal secretion, insulin, a protein hormone, that exercises a powerful influence over the use of carbohydrate in the body. Insulin lowers the blood sugar. When insulin is given in proper dosage to a person suffering from diabetes mellitus, the blood sugar is maintained at a normal level and the urine remains sugar-free. Fat is also burned and, as a result, dangerous symptoms do not appear.

The action which lowers the blood sugar is prolonged when insulin is combined with protamine. It has been found that the addition of a zinc salt to a mixture of protamine and insulin further prolongs the activity. Protamine zinc insulin is therefore the proper remedy for those persons suffering from diabetes mellitus for whom standard insulin is unable to provide adequate control unless it is administered several times daily.

Insulin can be purchased in at least four different concentrations. The insulin is usually injected under the skin about thirty minutes before meal time. The action is established within one hour and lasts from two to four hours.

With the use of insulin mixtures, the control of severe diabetes is successful with but one injection of insulin daily.

## THE ADRENAL GLANDS

Certain hormones such as those secreted by the adrenal cortex are absolutely essential to life.

The adrenal glands (which lie on top of the kidneys) are composed of two parts, a cortical or outer layer and a central or medullary part.

***Adrenalin and Its Uses.*** From the medullary part of the adrenal glands an extract, adrenalin, was long ago obtained which had the effect of constricting blood vessels. It is now used for the purpose of diminishing the blood supply to any specified part of the body. It is often applied to the mucous membrane of the nose in order to reduce bleeding during an operation. When injected into the blood stream, adrenalin produces the general effect of raising the blood pressure. The drug has a reverse effect on many of the muscle layers of the internal organs, causing relaxation.

Any emergency that provokes fear or anger causes the adrenals to throw an excess of secretion into the blood. Thus the adrenals mobilize the body for the activities that may be necessary to meet that emergency, whether the activities are flight or fight. Consequently, the adrenals are referred to as the emergency glands of the body. While the action of these glands serves a useful function and is helpful, it should be realized that in certain circumstances the results of their activities might prove harmful. A state of chronic fear or anxiety leads to a prolonged excess of adrenalin in the blood, causing a prolonged rise in the blood pressure. Excessive blood pressure can be harmful.

***Secretion of the Adrenal Cortex.*** We know less concerning the functions of the outer layer of the gland than about those of the central part. There are, however, reasons for believing that the outer layer produces a substance which neutralizes the poisonous products of nitrogen use in the body. It is also known that increased activity of the outer layer or cortex accentuates masculine sex traits both in young males and in young females. If a girl develops a growth in the adrenal cortex, she loses many of her feminine characteristics and tends to develop those of the male. Her breasts diminish in size, she develops hair on the face, and her voice becomes more like that of the male. A successful surgical removal of the cortical tumor causes the disappearance of these abnormalities.

## THE SEX GLANDS

The sex glands or gonads have internal secretions which have much to do with the secondary sex characteristics. The secretion of the ovaries, for example, is essential to normal feminine appearance. The secretion of the testicles probably gives to the male his masculine characteristics. Their greatest influence must therefore be exerted during adolescence.

***The Ovaries.*** Estrogen (or estrogenic hormones) produced by the ovaries helps produce the changes occurring in the reproductive organs of females. It plays a vital role in menstruation and pregnancy.

The corpus luteum hormone (in the ovary) and its derivatives are called progestins because they are directly concerned with pregnancy and its successful completion.

### What the Estrogenic Hormone Does

The estrogenic hormone plays a most important part not only in the reproductive function but also in the general well-being of woman. In addition to its part in the menstrual cycle it has the following functions:

It maintains the normal size, capacity and functional activity of the womb, Fallopian tubes and vagina. It preserves the normal epithelial (cell) layers of the vagina. It influences normal contraction of the womb by its stimulating effect on the muscular activity of that organ. It acts upon the anterior pituitary so as to control the production of other hormones. It promotes the growth of the duct tissue of the breast. It helps maintain the normal condition of the nasal and oral (mouth) mucous membranes. It is responsible for the womanliness of woman as expressed by the secondary sex characteristics: bodily contour, distribution of fat, distribution and growth of hair, breast development and psychic attitudes. It has definite constitutional effects directly on the physical and mental health of the normal, hormonally-balanced mature woman.

## USES OF SYNTHETIC ESTROGEN

The synthetic estrogenic hormone is used on the basis of a number of its actions on the body. In general, estrogen treatment makes use of the following effects of the hormone: action on the development of the reproductive organs; inhibition of pituitary hormone; and constitutional effects in both younger and older women. Here the estrogenic hormone produces an increase in muscle strength, bodily vigor and mental faculties.

### Hormones for Menopausal Symptoms

These effects are present without exception during the administration of the estrogenic hormone for other purposes, as for example, treatment of menopausal symptoms. The hormone is an important factor in the patient's restoration to full health. Progress in the treatment may be judged by the lessening in number and disappearance of the flushes and sweats, by relief of irritability, of insomnia and fatigue, and by the general improvement in the well-being of the patient. A method of determining the response to treatment by estrogen is through a study of vaginal smears.

It is found that if estrogens are administered to the patient in decreasing amounts over a period of about one year, the symptoms are suppressed during the course of the treatment and do not recur when the treatment is finally discontinued.

There is some evidence that estrogen treatment in humans may have a cancer-producing effect. There is not any chance of such action unless estrogen is administered unrestrictedly. The dosage should be carefully adjusted so that the desired effect is produced with a minimum dose. This should be particularly the case in patients with a history of breast cancer in the family.

Other disturbances which occasionally occur at the menopause respond to treatment with estrogens—for example, menopausal arthritis and menopausal high blood pressure.

Loss of menstrual flow—the result of estrogenic hormone deficiency—is often restored by the use of the hormone. Painful menstruation, or premenstrual tension, too, is frequently benefited by the use of the hormone, as are also breast disorders and bleeding of the womb.

### The Breasts and Estrogen

The mammary glands or breasts are under pituitary and sex hormone control. They are subject to notable changes at puberty, throughout pregnancy, during lactation and after change of life. The influence of the female hormones is seen in the temporary breast swelling and soreness which often occur at each menstrual period.

Abnormally small breasts may occur with other symptoms of inadequate hormone supply, or as an isolated sign. In either case the breasts may be developed by treatment with estrogen, particularly when supplemented by local applications of ointment. It has been shown that estrogens can be absorbed through the skin of the human female into the breast tissue and by this route can produce their characteristic stimulation of normal mammary growth. This is very meagre in its action and is rarely used for this purpose.

## THE MALE HORMONES

Members of this group are known as androgens. They possess masculinizing properties. The principal androgen is the male sex hormone itself, testosterone. It is the primary male sex hormone, actually obtained from the testicle.

The ancients were aware that the loss of the testicles caused profound changes in the development of the penis and other sexual organs, as well as in the general appearance and behavior of the male of any species. It is only if castration is performed early in life that all these changes are produced. Removal of the testicles in adult life has less effect, because the body has already reached its full development.

### The Sex Hormones and Sex Characteristics

The main function of the internal secretion of the testicles and ovaries, then, is the development in the body and mind of the distinctive characteristics belonging to each sex. The secretions of these glands are specific, that is, one makes for maleness and the other for femaleness. However, both may be found in the body of the male, and of the female. This being the case, it is not surprising that various forms of intersexuality are found. It is recognized that in addition to the masculine male and the feminine female there exist effeminate men and masculine women. In certain instances this blending of the two sexes in a single individual is so notable as to be pathologic. There have been persons of whom it is difficult to say whether they are truly male or truly female.

The testicles have two functions. One is the production of spermatozoa. The other is the production of the male sex hormone. These two functions go on more or less constantly during the period of sexual maturity. The spermatozoa are produced within a series of slender canals, imbedded in loose, connective tissue. This tissue contains the cells which secrete the male sex hormone. (See page 192.)

Complete normal development of the sexual organs and the secondary sex characteristics depends on the proper coordination of the gonads (sexual glands) and the pituitary gland.

## THE PINEAL AND THYMUS GLANDS

The pineal gland (in the brain) and the thymus (in the chest) are believed to be endocrine glands. Great precocity—mental and sexual—has sometimes been observed in boys whose pineal gland has been destroyed, as by a tumor. For this reason it has been assumed that it provides a secretion which acts as a hindrance to sexual development.

The thymus is situated behind the upper part of the breast bone.

Little is known about its function. It is assumed that it reaches its full development in childhood and shrinks at puberty.

## THE BASAL METABOLISM RATE

One very important means of diagnosis of glandular imbalance is the "basal metabolism test." This is an ingenious procedure which should be a part of every complete physical examination, especially in those cases in which the symptoms point to some disturbance of the endocrine glands. The basal metabolism rate is the term applied to the heat production of a person who, though awake, is as nearly as possible at complete muscular and mental rest and is in the "post-absorptive" state, which means from twelve to fourteen hours after a light meal, when it is assumed that the digestive processes are quiescent. The patient refrains from any undue muscular exertion or fatiguing effort of any kind for twenty-four hours beforehand. The light meal is taken not later than 7 o'clock the night before the test, which is taken at 9 A.M. For a period of thirty minutes before the test, the patient should be lying down comfortably in a room with subdued lighting.

The instrument which is used for the test consists of a bell-type spirometer. This is a hollow, double-walled cylinder. In the narrow space between the two walls fits a second inverted hollow cylindrical bell. This is counterpoised so that it rides easily up or down in the circular space between the two walls. This space contains water which acts as a seal. At the commencement of the test sufficient oxygen is admitted from an oxygen tank to raise a pointer on the spirometer bell to the zero mark upon a scale. A rubber plug is inserted into the mouth to fit tightly between the lips and teeth. This mouthpiece is connected with the breathing tube of the cylinders. The nose is clamped to keep out any air. The breathing of the patient through the inspiratory and expiratory tubes keeps the air circulating through the system.

As oxygen is consumed, the spirometer falls and from this difference in the levels of the pointer at the beginning and the end of the test, the oxygen usage is calculated and the heat production is determined. The test lasts seven minutes. There is no discomfort connected with the test, but there must be complete relaxation in order to get an accurate reading. The result of the calculation shows whether the metabolic rate is above or below normal. From these and other findings the cause and nature of the disorder are determined.

### Endocrine Treatment Requires Care

The results of the treatment of the endocrine glandular diseases are among the most satisfactory that we have today in our therapy. At times the cures are startling.

The selection of the hormone and amount given must be chosen accurately and by an experienced physician. The routine use of endocrines may prove very harmful. Many of the drugs sold for reduction of body weight contain thyroid, and their continuous use is very dangerous. Since each gland has its individual treatment, the need of experience in handling these cases is paramount.

CHAPTER 7

# THE BRAIN AND NERVOUS SYSTEM

**Functions of the Brain . . . Social Stress and Nervous Disorder . . . Neurasthenia . . . Hiccough . . . Sleeplessness . . . Facial Paralysis . . . Neuralgia . . . Sciatica . . . Shaking Palsy . . . Delirium Tremens . . . Epilepsy . . . Grand Mal . . . Petit Mal . . . Hysteria . . . Dementia Praecox . . . Paranoia.**

THE CENTRAL NERVOUS SYSTEM is the mechanism by which the various activities of the body are coordinated and made to work in harmony. Through this system, too, the body is made aware of changes in its surroundings. Because our central nervous system is highly developed, adjustments to inner and outer changes can be made in an instant.

***The Brain and Spinal Cord.*** The chief structures in the central nervous system are the brain and spinal cord, and the vast number of nerves to which these give rise. The whole of this coordinating system, with its "headquarters" in the brain and cord, may be compared to a great collection of offices which keep in touch with the working of the body by means of an intricate system of telegraph wires. In the main, the brain controls psychic life, with the messages arriving through the special senses. The spinal cord deals with movement and with the other activities of the body.

Actually, the part of the nervous system to which is assigned the all-important work of supervising the vital activities of the body is the junction of the brain and the cord. It is the region of what is known as the bulb or medulla oblongata. This contains the centers which regulate body temperature, blood pressure, respiration, and other essential body functions.

***Central and Sympathetic Nervous Systems.*** The central nervous system, then, consists of the brain and spinal cord. From the spinal cord, protected by the vertebral column and by a fluid, there issue thirty-one pairs of nerves which run to different areas of the body. The brain gives rise to twelve pairs of cranial (head) nerves. These are chiefly concerned with the special senses of sight, hearing, taste and smell.

There is still another system of nerves, the sympathetic system, which is formed as a kind of offshoot from the spinal nerves. It takes its own origin from the spinal nerves at a short distance from the place where they emerge from the spinal cord. While the main central nervous system functions chiefly in receiving sensations and causing movements, the sympathetic system regulates, almost entirely, the purely automatic functions of the body, such as the activity of glands, the contraction and expansion of blood vessels, and the movements of the intestines.

## FUNCTIONS OF THE BRAIN

As an example of the precision with which scientists are mapping out the brain centers to find what work they do, there is the discovery of the speech centers—a tiny area, on the left side of the brain only, which is concerned with speech, and another which controls the faculty of writing. Information has also been gained about how the brain hemispheres work, by seeing what happens when they are removed.

It is probable that the physical bases for the emotional impulses are the gray nuclei which are situated at the base of the brain. From these nuclei, fibers run toward the so-called silent areas in the forebrain, and it is believed that through these fibers an emotional tone is imparted to man's thoughts. In this region two streams of consciousness meet—those of thought or cognition (clearly understanding fact), and emotion. The intermingling of these streams of thought and feeling is necessary for the psychic life; one reacts upon the other.

## SOCIAL STRESS AND NERVOUS DISORDER

Physical disease or change in the brain or nervous system is not the only cause of mental derangement. The tendency of modern times is toward nervous and mental disorder. In the large cities the pace of life is too swift, the strain is too constant, the struggle is too keen. Human beings are witnessing the greatest luxury the world has ever seen and a large proportion of persons in cities are living beyond their means, striving to be rich or to appear rich. It is as if stress and strain are voluntarily invited.

In many cases, persons who are nervous or neurotic from early youth are so placed that unusual demands are made upon them. Adversity brings necessity for overwork, duties are manifold, and responsibilities are heavy. They are ignorant of the fact that they are on dangerous ground, because they have no reserves of psychic health.

Driven by circumstances, they are apt to overwork, cut short their sleep, and conscientiously press on. Such persons may finally lose their mental balance. Neurosis or, in more serious cases, insanity is often the result.

The insane are simply ill; therefore all insane should be cared for sympathetically. To consider the insane as constantly malevolent is a relic of the old-time absurd belief that insane people were "possessed of the devil." It is no disgrace to be insane, and the feeling of chagrin at discovering disease of the brain in a relative is another absurdity. How to keep the mind healthy should be studied with as much devotion as how to avoid tuberculosis.

## NEURASTHENIA

***Causes and Symptoms of Neurasthenia.*** This common nervous disease is a neurosis or functional nervous disorder characterized by a tendency to mental and physical fatigue. It may arise from an "escape into illness"—an attempt to protect oneself from the difficulties encountered in daily life. The quick and prolonged fatigue is often due to absorption and waste of mental energy in repression and conflict. The patient has slight impairment of memory and slight depression, associated with palpitation, trembling, sweating, fainting, and breathlessness on exertion. The symptoms are usually worse in the morning, and tend to improve during the day.

***Diagnosis and Treatment.*** The diagnosis is made by the physician on the appearance of the patient and his history. The main consideration, however, is not to overlook some organic disease which may be present at the same time as the neurasthenia. Treatment consists in regular work, abstention from excesses of all kinds, frequent holidays and frequent rest, and adequate physical exercise. Psychotherapy is of great value.

## HICCOUGH (SINGULTUS)

***Causes and Symptoms of Hiccough.*** Hiccough is a brief spasm of the midriff (diaphragm). The causes are: reflex hiccough, due to stimulation of the sensory nerves of the intestines (particularly the nerves called the vagus and phrenic) by indigestion, alcoholism, distension of the stomach, air swallowing (as in infants), pleurisy or gastric ulcer. Sometimes it is caused by irritation of the phrenic nerve (which supplies the midriff muscle) by tumors or a large gland. Disease of the spinal cord, uremia, and hysteria are other possible causes. In apoplexy and meningitis, peritonitis and intestinal obstruction, hiccough may become a grave symptom.

***Treatment of Hiccough.*** Treatment consists of an attempt to remove the cause. Hot baths and large doses of sedatives often stop the attack. Babies, in their early months, hiccough regularly after taking the bottle. A drink of warm water is then helpful. For adults, inhalations of aromatic spirits of ammonia, or five drops of spirits of camphor, are often effective. An icebag applied to the back of the neck sometimes stops the spasm. Holding the breath or breathing into a bag to rebreathe the exhaled carbon dioxide may prove curative. Drugs and inhalations of oxygen and carbon dioxide give relief in severe cases.

In prevention, avoid heavy meals which may give rise to indigestion.

## SLEEPLESSNESS (INSOMNIA)

***The Meaning of Sleep.*** Man's knowledge is extremely limited as to the actual condition of the brain which induces sleep. It seems probable that the same waste products which accumulate in the blood and produce fatigue after exertion also act as narcotics and induce sleep at night. According to another theory simple tiredness of brain cells may account for the oncoming of sleep. It is known that a tired man, if not overtired, goes to sleep more readily than the man who is not tired.

During the day, then, waste products accumulate in the blood; by the evening the amount is at the maximum, and they send the person to sleep. At night these substances, which are really poisonous, are carried away by the blood; in the morning they have almost all disappeared, and the sleeper awakens refreshed.

The healthy man who works hard, especially at an occupation requiring extreme muscular exertion, sleeps soundly; the indolent man, as a rule, is a poor sleeper. Of all afflictions, want of sleep is one of the most trying to a person, and one which needs most careful management at the hands of a physician.

***Causes and Symptoms of Insomnia.*** Passing insomnia may arise from noises, worry, depression, excitement, changes in working hours to night time, and high blood pressure. It is usually an affliction of light sleepers. Persistent and severe insomnia usually occurs on the basis of numberless disorders which produce pain, headache, cough, nausea, shortness of breath, palpitation, diarrhea, etc. Insomnia is common in various mental disorders, particularly those associated with depressions, anxiety states, excitements, and fears. It may also be common among those addicted to alcohol and coffee.

***Treatment of Insomnia.*** The condition is often cured by removing the cause, if possible. Outward conditions demand attention, and, if the cause is removed, the patient is automatically cured. Sedatives may be supplied by the physician. Sleeping tablets or potions of any sort must be taken strictly as he directs. When insomnia is caused by pain, only a physician is competent to treat the conditions.

## FACIAL PARALYSIS

***Causes and Symptoms of Facial Paralysis.*** This is a common nervous disorder, due frequently to exposure to cold—as, for example, cold air blowing on one side of the face while sleeping near an open window. Disease of the ear is a cause, especially in children; also injuries about the ear.

The paralysis comes on rapidly, usually with little pain, although there may be earache. The patient may first discover the paralysis on looking in the mirror, or on trying to eat, talk, or whistle. The face is smooth and expressionless on the paralyzed side. The eye on that side cannot be closed and weeps; the mouth is drawn over to the well side, and saliva may flow from it. Whistling becomes impossible. Eating is interfered with, and the food collects in the cheek of the paralyzed side. Speech is somewhat difficult.

***Treatment of Facial Paralysis.*** Facial paralysis following exposure to cold usually disappears, with complete recovery in from two to six weeks. Persons have been known to have several attacks. Hot applications should be made about the ear for the first few days. If there is running from the ear, or earache, an ear specialist should be consulted. The most valuable measures aiding recovery are electricity and massage, which must be under the direction of a physician.

## NEURALGIA

***Causes and Symptoms of Neuralgia.*** This is a symptom, not a disease, although in some instances an acute inflammation of a nerve seems to be the cause. It is a convulsive attack of pain in the course and distribution of a sensory nerve or its branches. It is frequently a symptom of disease, such as syphilis in the third stage and herpes zoster (shingles). It may be psychologic in origin, as in hysteria. It may be reflex, from disease of the intestines. Children are rarely affected.

Neuralgia is characterized by sudden stabbing pains, with longer or shorter intervals between paroxysms. In the arm (brachial neuralgia), pain shoots downward. Constitutional diseases and those of the vertebral column and spinal cord are the most frequent causes. If the pain is in the chest—between or along the ribs—it is sometimes caused by herpes zoster (shingles). Sciatica is a special form affecting the nerve of the same name in the thigh. It is the most frequent variety, and men are usually affected.

***Treatment of Neuralgia.*** The basic treatment is the continuous application of dry heat. An electric pad is effective. One tablet of empirin three or four times a day is often very helpful in relieving the pain.

## SCIATICA

The word sciatica, as ordinarily used, has a loose meaning, being applied to a number of painful conditions along the course of the sciatic nerve. It almost always affects one side of the body.

***Causes of Sciatica.*** Sciatic symptoms occur in men, as a rule, in adult life, often during the years past middle age. Sciatica may occur after exposure, overexertion, or in the course of, or following, infectious diseases such as gout, rheumatism, diabetes, or diseases within the pelvis.

***Symptoms of Sciatica.*** The pain of sciatica starts in the middle of the upper, fleshy part of the thigh, at the back, and extends down the middle of the back of the leg, even to the foot. There are tender spots along this course, especially in the upper and middle part of the back of the thigh. The pain is usually intense, burning or boring in character, worse at night and on walking. At the beginning it may be felt only after exercise, or when the leg is held in certain positions. A characteristic sign of the disease is noted when the patient attempts to rise from a chair, using the affected side and holding his back while he bends the painful leg. Walking becomes difficult (or impossible), even if the weight is borne on the toes with the knee bent. The patient is usually compelled to remain in bed, and the disease may last for months, with occasional improvement followed by return of the painful episodes. A thorough examination by a physician is required to find the cause.

***Treatment of Sciatica.*** In preventive treatment, dental hygiene is of importance. The treatment obviously depends on the cause. Rest in bed and fixation of the limb in a splint for several weeks, with applications of heat, may be necessary. Diathermy is sometimes helpful. Aspirin and phenacetin are given by the doctor. The patient should remain in bed until he is free of pain on standing or walking.

## SHAKING PALSY

***Causes of Shaking Palsy.*** This disease of the nervous system is a progressive destruction of the brain and nerve centers of coordination of muscular movements. The cause is not known. Hardening of the arteries (arteriosclerosis) is supposed to play a part in the cause of the disease. The condition rarely appears in persons under fifty years of age.

***Symptoms of Shaking Palsy.*** These begin with slight tremors of the hands, then the legs. The tremors gradually increase in frequency and severity until the patient cannot hold any article firmly and will have to be fed. Walking, too, becomes difficult and unsteady. The disease is long standing, covering years before the patient may become incapacitated. Other than the tremors, there are no symptoms.

***Treatment of Shaking Palsy.*** There is no cure. The patient may reach advanced age and die from an entirely different cause.

## DELIRIUM TREMENS

***Causes of Delirium Tremens.*** Delirium tremens occurs not in those given only to occasional drinking sprees, even if prolonged, but in the habitual, heavy drinker. It is brought on by an unusual excess in drinking, or by some nervous shock, from bodily injury or an acute disease, especially pneumonia.

***Symptoms of Delirium Tremens.*** The attack begins with sleeplessness, depression, and restlessness, for a day or two, and then the patient experiences a mental change. He talks continually in a rambling, disconnected manner, and is in constant motion, determined to go out to attend to this or that matter; and he commonly experiences illusions—objects which he imagines he sees, such as rats, snakes, and monsters, all driving him into such a state of terror that he continually attempts to escape. He may even try to jump out of the window, or attempt suicide in some other way. There is usually some fever, a weak and rapid pulse, muscular weakness, and trembling of the hands and tongue.

Recovery from the first attack is the rule—unless some other condition complicates the delirium tremens, such as pneumonia or surgical accident. After three or four days the patient secures good sleep, which is usually the favorable turning point of the disorder. Rapid improvement then follows, until another attack is provoked by more drinking. In conditions that prove fatal, the ravings, sleeplessness and restlessness persist, while prostration and weakness of the pulse increase until the patient dies of heart failure.

***Treatment of Delirium Tremens.*** The patient must be confined to a room and watched every minute. The attendants must treat him with gentleness and great patience. It may be necessary to restrain him in bed if he is weak. A sheet may be fastened across both the patient's body and the bed, but it is unwise to tie his limbs. Feeding with strong soups, beef tea, milk, and raw eggs every two hours is of chief importance. Alcohol should not be given. If the pulse is weak, administer aromatic spirit of ammonia (twenty drops in a wineglass of water) every hour. To procure sleep, the physician will prescribe sedatives.

A cold bath, or sponging with cold water, may produce a quieting effect, especially if there is fever. Call a physician, particularly to discover and treat any underlying and complicating condition, such as pneumonia, broken rib, or other injury; also to judge whether the patient's general condition warrants the use of such powerful remedies as are sometimes required, and to manage the mental aspect of the disorder. Most alcoholics suffer from malnutrition and vitamin deficiency, and a corrective diet should be established by the physician.

## EPILEPSY

***Causes of Epilepsy.*** Epilepsy is a chronic nervous disease. There are periodic seizures of convulsions with disturbance of consciousness. The actual cause is unknown. Both sexes are equally liable to epilepsy.

***Symptoms of Epilepsy.*** The only apparent difference between epilepsy and accidental or occasional convulsions in children is one of duration. The attacks are similar; it is impossible, on first view, to distinguish between them; but in epilepsy the fits are repeated and the condition is chronic. Two kinds of epilepsy are to be noted: a severe form (grand mal) with insensibility and spasms; and a milder form (petit mal) with transient loss of consciousness, without spasms.

### Severe Form of Epilepsy (Grand Mal)

There are sometimes four stages in the attack. First, a preliminary "warning" or "aura" occurs in cases of most of those afflicted. It consists of a sense of unreality and dizziness, of great fear, with various sensations of taste, hearing, and sight. This aura, as a rule, lasts only a few seconds.

Second, the patient may turn around rapidly, or even run swiftly. More often a terrible cry or low gurgling groan is emitted, and the patient falls to the ground unconscious. In the fall the victim may then, or usually in the next stage, injure himself by biting his tongue. The body is stiff and arched upward, with the head thrown back or to one side, or the body is bent sidewise. The face is pale at first, but quickly becomes dark or bluish, with jaws rigidly set; the legs are outstretched, but the arms are bent at the elbow with the fingers tightly clenched in the palms. This is the rigid stage, and lasts only fifteen to thirty seconds.

***The Convulsive Stage.*** The third is the convulsive stage. The spasms begin; the limbs jerk violently; the face is contorted and working. The eyes are wide open and rolling, the pupils dilated and the whites of the eyes showing. The jaw may be firmly set and the tongue or lips bitten, or the mouth may be open with the lips flapping loosely in breathing, and the mouth covered with froth, which may be bloody. Sometimes urine escapes, and less often the contents of the bowels. The fit lasts several minutes. There is a short period of unconsciousness.

***The Relaxed Stage.*** In the fourth stage, the patient gradually becomes relaxed and quiet, and may recover after a variable time. Sometimes he comes to himself very soon, in a dazed and bewildered state, suffering from a dull headache. At other times he remains unconscious, with red face and noisy breathing, in a stupor, from which he may be aroused after a time, or may not awake for hours.

### Epilepsy Without Spasms (Petit Mal)

In this form of epilepsy there is momentary unconsciousness, but the patient does not have spasms. Sometimes it is a mere interruption in his occupation. He becomes suddenly pale, the eyes are fixed, and he stops whatever he is doing—talking, eating, playing piano or cards—only to continue in a few moments where he left off. He may be walking when the attack comes on, may continue mechanically, and then come to himself, finding that he has been unconscious. Any glass or spoon or other object which may be held at the time usually falls from the hand. There may be some confusion in speaking or dizziness after the attack, or the patient may perform some act unknowingly, such as to begin to undress, or even to do acts of violence.

***Fainting and Epilepsy.*** There are many varieties of this milder kind of epilepsy, but it usually ends in the severer form, with fits, as described previously. Fainting is most likely to be confused with the mild form of epilepsy, but in fainting the patient usually falls and the pulse is feeble or imperceptible, while in this variety of epilepsy the patient does not fall, as a rule, and there is a history of similar attacks. The pulse is not much affected.

### Treatment of Epilepsy

The epileptic should lead as normal a life as possible. If he is employed, he should avoid certain hazards—mental and physical. He should not work near moving machines, nor drive an automobile. He should avoid marriage because he is usually a poor provider and may transmit the disease. If he displays antisocial conduct, owing to mental retardation (which is not infrequent) or deterioration he should be placed in an institution.

***Emergency Measures for Epilepsy.*** Emergency treatment of a patient in a "grand mal" seizure consists of protecting him from injury. Measures to prevent or shorten the attack are useless. The patient should be permitted to remain where he falls. The collar should be loosened, a folded coat or blanket placed under his head, and a soft object inserted between his teeth to prevent biting of the tongue. Artificial teeth should be removed, when possible. If the tongue apparently obstructs breathing, the jaws should be drawn forward and the head turned to one side. The patient should be permitted to sleep until he awakes. Certain drugs give some relief from frequency of attacks and severity of the seizures. They are prescribed by the physician.

## HYSTERIA

***Causes and Symptoms of Hysteria.*** The general conception is that an individual is hysterical when he or she screams, tosses the limbs about, and has fits of weeping, or fainting spells.

Much of this may only be a tantrum, a display of bad temper, as is often seen in children, who will throw themselves upon the floor, kicking and screaming.

In pronounced hysteria, there is usually a history of peculiar, different kinds of symptoms. There are nervous tendencies, headaches, weakness and a general nerve instability.

The mentality of hysterical persons is very susceptible to any kind of suggestion. Any kind of excitement, overwork, or unusual happenings may bring on an attack. Impressions will develop into fixed ideas and obsessions, and nothing can at the time sway the hysteric. Reasoning is largely ineffective in calming the attack. On the contrary, the patient appears subconsciously to use the attack as a means of avoiding the need to face certain aspects of life that are unpleasant to him, highlight his feelings of inadequacy, or injure his ego in some way. We seem to be dealing here, in many cases, with a phase of psychoneurosis.

***Treatment of Hysteria.*** The attacks must be differentiated from epilepsy. When they are mild, they pass away after a while. In serious cases, which recur again and again, only a psychiatrist can accomplish any results. He must be consulted early in the patient's life if the condition appears in youth.

## DEMENTIA PRAECOX (SCHIZOPHRENIA)

This is a form of insanity which includes a large range of mental disorders. These occur in late adolescence as a rule and are marked by melancholia, self absorption, and loss of coherence in thoughts and acts, terminating in a mental weakness of an emotional nature.

The effects of this serious illness could in many instances be minimized if the introverted child were given careful mental training before he reached adolescence. Here is the type of case that at least in its less pronounced phases is usually benefited by psychoanalysis. Treatment should be carried out in a sanitarium. However, the outlook for cure is very uncertain.

## PARANOIA

***Causes of Paranoia.*** This form of mental derangement is a chronic, slowly progressive disease of the mind characterized by the presence of delusions built up in logical form.

It is claimed that heredity is an important factor in its cause. If

# Overdependency

Based on the film produced by The National Film Board of Canada

'arents can hurt a child by giving him too ittle love—or too much. Where to draw the ine is a problem. A child needs sympathy, ut he must learn to overcome small disap- ointments if he is to surmount the big ones f adult life. Innocently, the overprotective nother harms her child. Jimmy—his story is llustrated here—was a "little accident." Moreover, he nearly died at birth. After not wanting him, his mother never overcame fear of losing him. She overprotected and babied him through childhood and even after he grew up. Self-reliance he should have developed was stunted. Often, when confronted by problems, he fell ill. His symptoms were real, but cause was psychological.

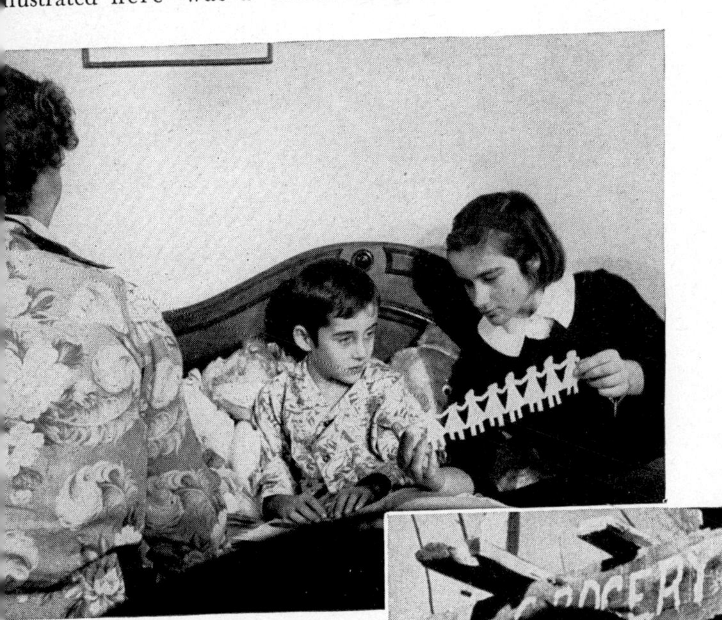

Mother and sister lavish attention on Jimmy, pamper him after tonsil operation — instead of helping him to develop own resources, as child should. Often being sick in early years, Jimmy grows to depend on comforting by female members of family. He will still demand it of wife when he marries.

Playing store with sister and her friends is natural for Jimmy. Girls make fuss over him, cater to his whims. He is not encouraged in normal boy's activities by father and brother.

Jimmy goes fishing with his father—but only in dreams. He would really like to go, but unsympathetic father will not take him. Nor is he allowed to help father in tool shed, although brother is.

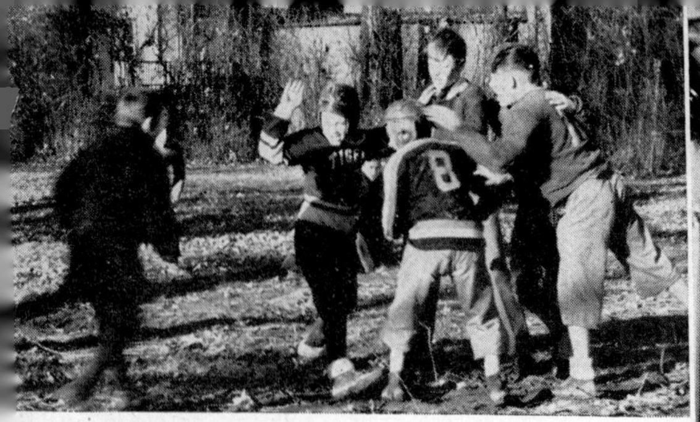

When Jimmy does attempt to play with the boys, they shoo him away as being too "sissified" for rough games. Hurt, he continues depending on females.

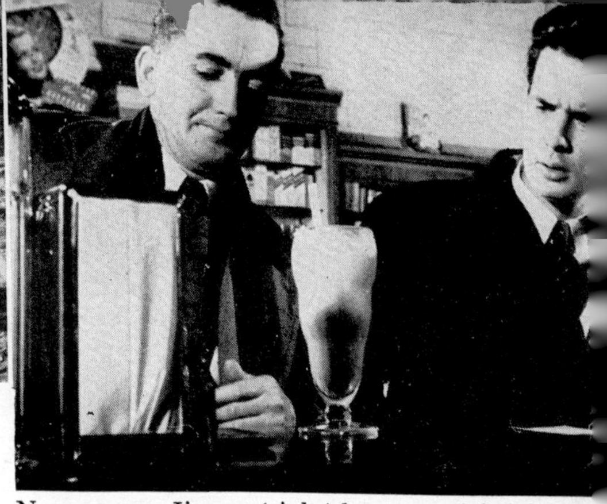

Now a man, Jimmy *(right)* borrows nickel from friend to make a phone call. He also lets friend pay for his soda. It is in such "little" things that people show overdependency, vex others.

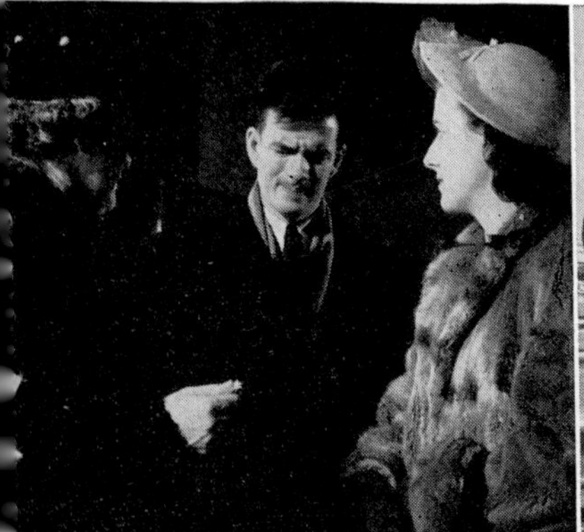

Jimmy has date which may mean better job. Mother invites him to dinner at same time, and he can't decide what he should do.

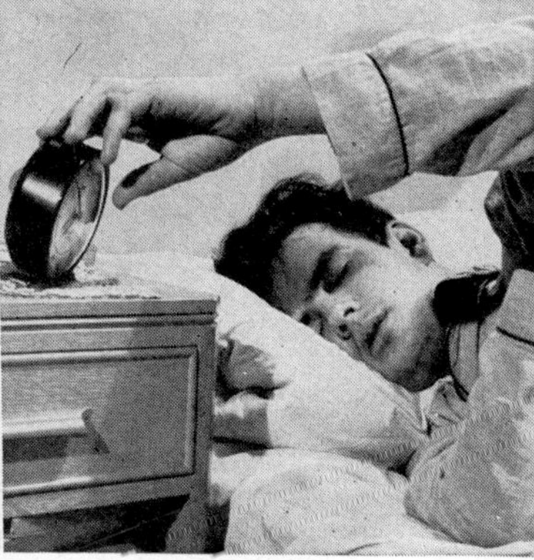

Facing difficult task at the office, Jimmy becomes sick. He turns off alarm, stays in bed. He's done it before.

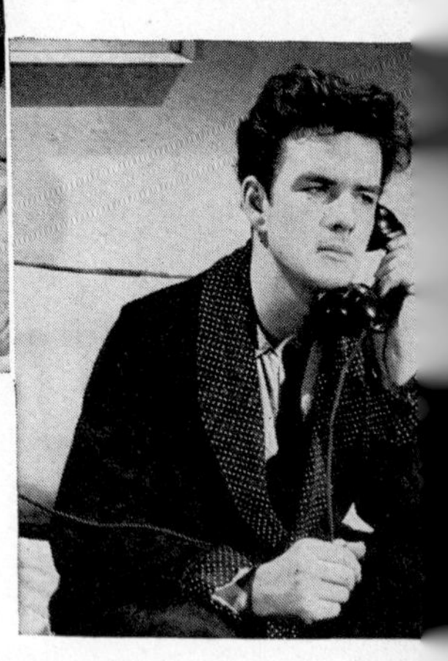

Jimmy phon wife, who has ready gone work, asks her make appoin ment with docto He could do th himself, but used to wife ranging thing

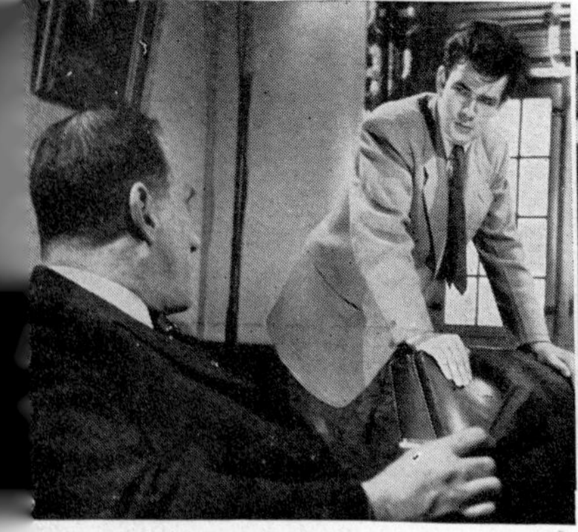

Doctor, finding Jimmy physically sound, concentrates on his emotional background. He suspects psychosomatic disorder—ailment with a psychological cause.

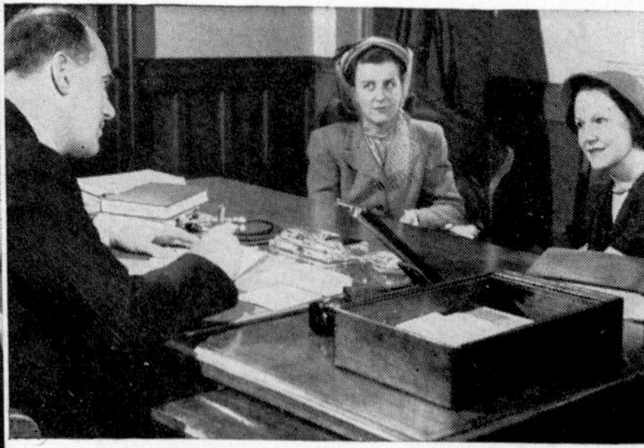

With Jimmy's consent, doctor interviews his family. He tells them how they can help Jimmy stand alone.

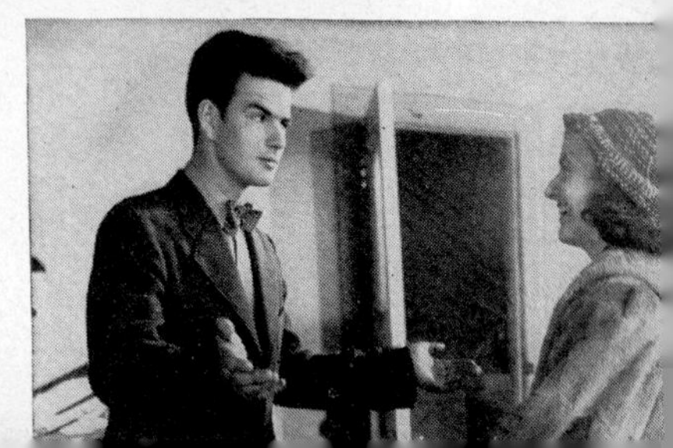

After psychiatric treatment, Jimmy is less dependent, accepts responsibility.

those who suspect they possess a heredity history of paranoia marry, they should not have children before competent medical advice indicates their offspring will be free of the disease.

***Symptoms of Paranoia.*** These frequently manifest themselves in early childhood. In the adult there is a state of worry about health. The patient imagines he is being watched and he does not feel normal. Although in reality no one is speaking, he hears voices. He then reaches a stage of imaginary persecution. He feels he is menaced by some person or organization; the "persecutor" may be some friend or relative, Nazis, Communists, or perhaps even spirits—an infinite variety is possible. This condition sometimes leads to delusions of grandeur in the patient. He pictures himself as a saint, a great patriot, an heir to untold wealth, or a dignitary of some sort.

***Treatment of Paranoia.*** These are cases for the psychiatrist. The eventual outlook is not favorable.

CHAPTER 8

# WOMAN'S REPRODUCTIVE ORGANS, MENSTRUAL DISORDERS, AND CHANGE OF LIFE

**Sexual Organs of the Woman . . . The Pituitary Gland . . . Sex Glands and Our Development . . . Normal Menstruation . . . Precautions During Menstruation . . . The "Safe Period" . . . Signs and Symptoms of Change of Life . . . Treatment of Change of Life . . . Painful Menstruation . . . Absence of Menstruation . . . When Menstruation Stops Suddenly . . . Scanty or Delayed Menstruation . . . Excessive Menstruation . . . Irregular Menstruation . . . Uterine Hemorrhage after the Menopause . . . Severe Hemorrhage from the Womb . . . Discharge from the Vagina, etc.**

WOMAN'S reproductive system is made up of external and internal genital organs. Her external genital organs are known as the vulva. They consist first, of the mons pubis, which is a rounded elevation at the lower part of the abdomen. It lies above the pubic bone, and is covered with hair. Also, the lips or folds at the entrance of the vagina, which is the canal extending from the external sex organs to the uterus or womb; then, the clitoris, which is a small organ corresponding in structure somewhat to the penis in the male. There are also two openings—the opening of the vagina and the opening of the urethra, the tube that carries the urine to the outside. The entrance to the vagina is protected by a membrane called the hymen.

***The Internal Reproductive Organs.*** The internal genital organs consist of the vagina, womb (or uterus), Fallopian tubes, and the ovaries. The vagina is a long canal leading from the outside of the body to the womb. The womb is a hollow, pear-shaped and highly muscular organ. It is suspended within the pelvis with the neck or narrow part downward. At each upper corner it is joined by a Fallopian tube, and it ends below in the neck (cervix) which projects into the upper part of the vagina. The uterus is lined with cells that are particularly rich in glands.

The ovaries are two oval sex glands lying in the lower part of the abdomen, one on each side. They contain thousands of minute cell groups or follicles which have two uses—the production of ova (eggs) and of female hormones. Each month a ripened ovum breaks off from a follicle and is passed into the mouth of one of the two Fallopian tubes. Here the ovum awaits fertilization by a male sperm.

The internal secretions of the ovary periodically, once a month, prepare the womb for pregnancy. If fertilization does not take place, menstruation occurs. The menses (monthly periods) were called by ancient writers "the tears of the uterus"—tears supposedly shed because of the failure to conceive.

Fertilization takes place when one of the sperm deposited by the penis in the vagina succeeds in reaching and combining with the ovum in the Fallopian tube. The fertilized ovum travels from the Fallopian tube to the womb. It becomes implanted in the lining of the womb, where it proceeds to develop into an embryo. This is the beginning of pregnancy.

## THE PITUITARY GLAND

The activities of the ovaries in women (and the testicles in men) are conditioned by hormones from the pituitary gland, which is situated at the base of the brain. The front lobe of this gland produces hormones (gonadotropic) which act on the reproductive organs to stimulate the growth and development of the ovaries. The front lobe hormones from the pituitary gland are ultimately responsible for normal sexual development in both the male and the female.

In youth, the pituitary gland produces growth hormones. After having developed under the influence of these hormones, the body is ready to carry out its reproductive function. To accomplish this, the pituitary takes on a new task, and secretes a hormone to help in the maturing of the sex cells. Excess quantities of these hormones (as with almost all hormones) pass out of the body in the urine.

When the ovum arrives in the womb without having been fertilized, it is expelled in the menstrual flow. On the other hand, when an ovum is fertilized, a chemical messenger is sent to the pituitary gland, which now works to prevent the formation of more ova.

## SEX GLANDS AND OUR DEVELOPMENT

For centuries it has been known that the sex organs influence physical development, and in some way the personality, or psyche. The sex glands remain quiescent as a rule till somewhere around thirteen or fourteen years of age. Then, under the influence of the front lobe of the pituitary, as we have seen, they begin to develop.

With this development they, in their turn, secrete into the blood hormones which start the development of both primary and secondary sexual characters, till they reach adult size and function. In males, sex glands enlarge and begin to produce ripe, motile spermatozoa capable of fertilizing a mature ovum. The penis grows in size. Hair appears in the pubic region, under the armpits, and on the face. Characteristic male contours of the thighs, the chest, and the neck develop, and the voice breaks. The personality also undergoes changes.

Similar changes occur in the girl, but they begin somewhat earlier. The ovaries produce one ripe ovum per month. Since, in civilized communities, these ova are not fertilized, they are incapable of settling in the uterus; and the menstrual periods begin. Their first occurrence marks the ability to conceive, and hence the development from girlhood to womanhood. The age at which this change occurs varies with race, climate, heredity and environment. Meanwhile, the external sex organs (genitalia) enlarge, as do the vagina and womb. Secondary changes appear in the growth of the hair in a characteristic fashion in the pubic region and under the armpits. The breasts enlarge. The pelvis broadens, and by a characteristic disposition of fat under the skin, the body takes on definitely female contours. The voice is more vibrant and rich, but contrary to the case of the boy it does not alter in pitch. These changes, in both male and female, are the result of increased secretion into the blood stream of the sex hormones.

When young women continue undeveloped, this condition may be corrected by treatment with female sex hormones. These will generally bring on the development of the physical and mental characteristics of the adult woman.

## MENSTRUATION

The lining of the womb undergoes a complex cycle of change each month in preparation for a possible pregnancy. This lining, known as the endometrium, is at rest for only a few days in each month. Most of the time it is in a state of great activity. The cycle of change which it undergoes, may be divided into four stages: quiescence, construction, destruction, and repair. During the constructive stage the lining becomes greatly thickened. This change is followed by a destructive stage, during which blood leaves the smallest blood vessels and leaks into the womb tissues. A few days later, the blood finds its way to the surface and together with cast off epithelium (lining tissue) and other debris appears as a discharge. This is the menstrual flow. As soon as it has ceased, the repair of the lining begins again.

The whole of this cycle is controlled by the internal secretions of the ovaries and of the pituitary gland.

***When Menstruation Is Normal.*** Menstruation normally occurs at regular intervals in the woman who is not pregnant or nursing. While the rule is to menstruate only once in twenty-eight days, some women have an interval of as little as twenty-one days; others are unwell at the end of every thirty days. When a woman becomes pregnant, menstruation ceases, and does not return till after the child has been born or the mother has ceased nursing her baby. However, there are sometimes exceptions.

The duration of the discharge is generally four or five days, although the flow may go on for only three days, and sometimes for as many as six or seven. The amount of blood lost averages about one tumblerful.

While menstruation is of regular occurrence in most women, there is irregularity in others. For these, this irregularity may be the normal thing. Menstruation may stop during the course of wasting diseases, such as tuberculosis of the lungs, or for other reasons, which we shall discuss later.

The approach of the menses, or flow, is generally accompanied by discomfort, headache, irritability, a sense of weight and tenderness in the breasts and about the loins, and some restlessness. Mothers should instruct their daughters concerning this experience so that they may not be alarmed when it occurs for the first time. They will then be saved needless worry about a natural condition.

***Precautions During Menstruation.*** Strenuous exercise or overfatigue should be avoided during "the period" chiefly because it may induce excessive bleeding. Otherwise, the normal routine can be followed. Taking a sponge bath or a shower daily is desirable for the sake of cleanliness. Warm water is preferable. Sanitary napkins should be changed regularly.

## THE "SAFE PERIOD"

Ovulation tends to occur at approximately the midphase of the monthly cycle, so that this time is most fertile, while other days in the cycle are relatively less so. Whether a period of *absolute* sterility ("safe period") actually occurs is still unknown. However, where it is desirable to insure the very best conditions for conception, coitus should be carried out during the midphase of the cycle. Where natural contraception (birth control) is the purpose, it is relatively safe if coitus is limited to those days in the cycle which are generally considered "sterile."

When calculating the limits of the "safe period" in a specific instance, various factors should be considered, such as illness, nervous shock, unusual excitement, the use of certain drugs, strenuous exercise, and change of environment and climate. These factors may alter the normal menstrual rhythm, and the time of ovulation.

## CHANGE OF LIFE

This period is usually reached between the ages of forty-five and fifty years, or somewhat later. It is also called the female climacteric. Its diagnosis is usually simple. Apart from the fact that the monthly flow stops, the most characteristic symptom is the hot flush followed by sweating. There may be shortness of breath on exertion. In addition there are frequently emotional and nervous disturbances, such as headache, feelings of faintness, insomnia, and emotional instability. Occasionally more severe symptoms, such as melancholia, high blood pressure (hypertension), diabetes, or overactivity of the thyroid gland make their first appearance at this time. On the other hand, the discomfort may be quite slight. Medical treatment can relieve or cure all of these symptoms.

***Psychic Effects of Change of Life.*** The psychic effects of the "change of life" depend, of course, upon the patient's emotional balance. Various psychological disturbances may make their appearance. It has been considered the "dangerous age" for women—the stress state—during which various aberrations become marked in the person with a predisposition to them. Nervousness, excitability, irritability, impairment of memory, tiring easily, falure of concentration, and depression may be notably in evidence.

***Physical Changes.*** There is a tendency to obesity affecting the whole body, thinning of the muscles, and wrinkling of the skin. The vulva atrophies and shrinks. The vagina, too, shrinks and becomes inelastic. The ovary shrinks to about a third of its normal size and is converted into fibrous tissue.

Physical changes may also involve: the joints, producing various symptoms; also the skin, the texture of which may be altered; as well as changes in the genital tract. Senile inflammation of the vagina, which may occur at this time, is directly attributable to deficiency of estrogen, which leads to thinning of the vaginal lining, thus preparing the ground for infection. Like other symptoms of the menopause, it responds readily to treatment by estrogen.

Ordinarily, women soon recover their poise after the menopause, putting on more flesh, and becoming less sensitive in regard to flushes, sweats, etc., as well as somewhat less active. However, after the flow has finally disappeared, following an irregularity of several months, there may be a mucous discharge which occurs at intervals. If there is a profuse flow at this time, it indicates that some uterine disorder is present which calls for the attention of a surgeon. Women frequently endure nervous disturbance from removable causes for years, erroneously thinking they are still undergoing "change of life." Many suffer silently, often quite unnecessarily. In all such examples, a physician should be consulted.

***Treatment of Change of Life.*** As a rule, when estrogen is administered, the symptoms of change of life are promptly and dramatically relieved. The physician decides what particular product is to be used and the dosage. The manifestations in and around the joints, the high blood pressure, the psychic disturbances, senile changes in the vagina, and other changes are all favorably influenced by the treatment.

## PAINFUL MENSTRUATION (DYSMENORRHEA)

Dysmenorrhea is not a disease but a series of symptoms, in which pain in the lower abdomen is the most prominent.

It is estimated that menstrual pain occurs in over one-half of all menstruating women. The aching recurs more or less in the same form and at the same time each month. It generally persits during the first and occasionally also during the second day; it rarely lasts throughout the period. In the majority of women, menstruation is painless until about the age of seventeen to nineteen, but occasionally "aching pain" may be felt from puberty onward.

***Causes of Painful Menstruation.*** Painful menstruation is frequently experienced in the absence of actual tissue changes. In such purely functional cases, the pain usually begins either shortly before, or at the same time as, the flow, and subsides when it ends. In painful menstruation caused by organic changes, the pain tends to begin at, or shortly after, the onset of the flow, and persists throughout the bleeding period or even after.

Pains during the flow may be due to tumors, displacement of the womb, or inflammation of the mouth of the womb. They may also be caused by diseases of the ovaries or tubes, by chronic appendicitis, or by other conditions.

***Suggestions for Control of Pain in Menstruation.*** For the immediate attack in painful menstruation, a 50-milligram Demerol tablet may be taken and repeated, if necessary. Avoidance of physical and mental exertion is important, and in severe conditions rest in bed is advisable.

Pain is greatly reduced and frequently forgotten in other cases through healthy recreation and pastimes, outdoor life, and sufficient sleep. In the avoidance of pain, it is necessary to treat constipation, for a loaded rectum and colon add greatly to pelvic congestion. Hot stimulating drinks, heat applied locally by means of an electric pad, diathermy to the pelvis, warm enemas or hot sitz baths, all may give temporary relief. The doctor may also prescribe drugs for relief.

With young girls, pain is often psychological in origin. As we have already advised, it is important that the adolescent girl be informed that menstruation is a natural function and a normal condition of healthy life, and not something to be regarded with fear and disgust.

***Corrective Use of Hormones.*** The functional variety of painful menstruation responds to treatment by hormones. In some women the womb is undeveloped, bent and displaced. In such conditions it is necessary to administer follicular hormone for its effects on development. In other cases—where the womb is of normal size—it may be treated with hormone from the back lobe of the pituitary, to lessen the stimulation of the muscles of the womb.

## ABSENCE OF MENSTRUATION (AMENORRHEA)

Amenorrhea means absence of flow—either temporary or permanent. It is considered abnormal when it occurs within the limits of the reproductive period, or when a woman is neither pregnant nor nursing a child. Amenorrhea has been classified as primary and secondary. Primary refers to conditions in which menstruation has never occurred, although the normal time for it has long passed. Secondary amenorrhea refers to a condition where the menses cease at some time after menstrual function is established.

***Causes of Amenorrhea.*** Among the causes are: irregularities in development; injuries; disorders of the ovaries; inactivity of the pituitary and thyroid glands; certain blood conditions (pernicious anemia, leukemia); wasting diseases such as tuberculosis, diabetes, and malnutrition; or toxic agents, such as alcohol, morphia, lead. The cause may also be chill, such as cold sea bathing or exposure just before a period is due.

***Treatment of Amenorrhea.*** First, the underlying cause must be found. In a large proportion of patients, the condition is often transient and self-limited and in no way inconsistent with good health. Amenorrhea that lasts a long time requires the attention of a physician.

Use of estrogens in the treatment of amenorrhea is based on the certainty that adequate doses induce favorable changes in the lining of the womb. These should be given by injection.

## WHEN MENSTRUATION STOPS SUDDENLY

If the monthly flow has begun, and is suddenly checked by fright, exposure to cold, etc., there may be a chill, fever, headache, backache, bearing-down pains in the lower part of the abdomen, as well as pains in the legs, and frequent urination.

The patient should take a hot sitz bath, or full bath, for twenty minutes; she should go to bed and take a teaspoonful of Hayden's Viburnum Compound in a wineglass of water every two or three hours. If the pain continues and a physician is not available, a suppository containing ¼ grain of belladonna extract should be introduced into the rectum.

Following such an attack the regular periods may be suppressed for several months.

## SCANTY OR DELAYED MENSTRUATION

When the monthly flow is scanty, or late in appearing, there are often symptoms such as pain low down in the abdomen, thighs, and legs; backache, pain and fullness in the top and front of the head; also cold hands and feet. All the symptoms which usually indicate that menstruation is coming on are present, and yet there is no flow. This condition may last for days, or even a week or more. At other times the flow may be very scanty and afford but little relief from these symptoms.

***Treatment.*** In such cases it is best for married women to take douches of six quarts of water, as hot as the elbow can bear. The best position is lying flat on the back, with the hips raised on a douche pan, and using a fountain syringe. These douches should be taken night and morning every day between the periods. They should be stopped when flowing occurs. Young girls should not take them. In all cases the general health must be improved in every way possible, and if relief is not speedily obtained recourse should be had to a physician.

***The Pregnant Woman.*** Delayed menstruation in women who are conscious of the possibility of pregnancy should receive no treatment. A physician may afford comfort, and should be consulted if possible. He may be able, early in the situation, to give a probable opinion as to pregnancy based on the Ascheim-Zondek test.

## EXCESSIVE MENSTRUATION (MENORRHAGIA)

***Causes of Excessive Menstruation.*** This is excessive loss of blood during the period, the duration of which may or may not be prolonged. There are a number of possible causes: inflammation of the "tubes" and ovaries; tumors–fibroids, particularly in the wall of the womb; displacement of the internal sexual organs. The cause may be functional (poor blood clotting); or endocrine–thyroid gland inactivity, pituitary gland overactivity; or ovarian–excessive activity of the ovaries, in the absence of corpora lutea and good blood conditions generally.

At the age of puberty the beginning of menstruation may be attended by severe bleeding; more often, however, there are spells of floodings and irregular losses, the bleeding occasionally being so severe as to endanger life. The condition is probably caused by lack of balance in the endocrine glands.

The approach of the menopause (change of life) may also be associated with this variety of menstrual trouble, though here too the losses are liable to be irregular.

***Treatment of Excessive Menstruation.*** It is obvious that in order to relieve or cure the condition, a physician must first find and treat the cause. Complete rest in bed during the period is important, together with restriction of strenuous exercise for a few days before menstruation is expected.

Drugs are used chiefly to promote contraction of the womb. A few have a sedative effect, relieving anxiety and probably diminishing blood pressure; others promote coagulation of the blood. Ergot has long been in use for this purpose. Calcium gluconate promotes blood coagulation. Pituitary gland products are often effective, as well as thyroid preparations.

Vaginal douches—three or four quarts of saline solution—as hot as can be tolerated (115° to 118° F.), two or three times daily, stimulate the contraction of the womb and small arteries.

Surgery is sometimes required to relieve the condition.

## IRREGULAR MENSTRUATION (METRORRHAGIA)

***Causes of Irregular Menstruation.*** This term is used for departures from the normal in rhythm and in amount of flow. The causes are usually local—in the womb or pelvis; they may be related to the glands (endocrine) or general. Of the local causes, fibroids (tumors) are the most common. Next are cancer, and erosion or ulceration along the genital tract. Conditions outside the womb may be found in the tubes (acute or chronic inflammation), or infection of an ovarian cyst. An acute fever, such as influenza, may cause sudden bleeding between periods.

***Treatment of Irregular Menstruation.*** Such bleeding demands full investigation to find out the cause, and must always be regarded as a serious symptom until proved otherwise. Only a physician is competent to plan the treatment.

## UTERINE HEMORRHAGE AFTER THE MENOPAUSE

Bleeding may be said to be "post-menopausal" when it occurs six months after the menstruation has definitely ceased. Probably over 50 per cent of examples of such bleeding are due to non-malignant conditions. The causes, in order of frequency, are: polyps in or at the mouth of the womb; ovarian tumors (malignant); cancer of the mouth of the womb; fibroids; and tuberculosis of the cervix of the womb.

*All women suffering from post-menopausal bleeding (occurring six months after menstruation has ceased) should be examined without delay, and complete investigation should be made.*

## SEVERE HEMORRHAGE FROM THE WOMB

This may be due to many causes, chief of which are tumors (fibroids, especially), cancer, labor, and abortion (during the process or immediately thereafter). Fibroids are not of themselves painful, and may develop to a considerable size without giving any hint of their presence. The symptoms vary according to the presence or absence of complications. Symptoms common, in variable degree, to all fibroids are: hemorrhage, pain, vaginal discharge, and abdominal enlargement. Hemorrhage usually occurs as menorrhagia (excessive menstruation), and occasionally as metrorrhagia (irregular menstruation). Pain is of an aching or "bearing down" character. Pressure on the nerves and veins occurs only when the tumor is anchored in the pelvis. Retention of urine, sudden in its beginning, liable to recur, and caused by pressure on the ureter (duct carrying urine from kidney to bladder), is the most important. Fibroids, when small and not causing symptoms, require no immediate treatment, but the patient should always be kept under observation for early evidence of complications. Treatment is given by the physician, and may include X-ray or surgery. Small fibroids during or after menopause often disappear after X-ray treatment.

## LEUCORRHOEA—DISCHARGE FROM THE VAGINA

Leucorrhoea is not a disease, but rather a sign of disorder of the female sexual organs, or of the whole body. When it occurs for a few days before and after the monthly periods, during the change of life, and accompanying pregnancy, it may be regarded as a natural occurrence, provided it is not associated with any other condition suggestive of disorder of the sexual organs or of the body as a whole. In ordinary conditions of health, however, there should be no perceptible discharge from the vagina in women, and if it occurs, with the exceptions just noted, it should be regarded as a symptom of local or general disorder.

The discharge is not by any means always white, as the common name for it, "whites," would suggest, but yellow, brown, reddish if mixed with blood, or colorless like the white of an egg. Indeed, it varies greatly in color, consistency, and amount.

***Causes of Leucorrhoea.*** Among general disorders causing a discharge from the vagina are: debility (weakness); anemia; malaria; tuberculosis; and acute diseases, such as scarlet fever, measles, diphtheria, and typhoid fever. Exposure to heat, dampness, and emotional excitement may cause leucorrhoea. When the trouble follows a disturbance of the general system, the discharge is usually white or watery, and not thick and yellow.

So-called "whites" is one of the most frequent symptoms of inflammation of any part of the sexual organs—the womb, tubes, ovaries, and neighboring structures; also of tumors and injuries of these organs, such as follow tears occasioned by childbirth. It is also produced by faulty positions of the womb and by irritating injections.

Excessive sexual intercourse is sometimes responsible for a passive congestion of the pelvic organs and the mouth of the womb, with an increased secretion which causes the patient to complain of the "whites." Trichomonas vaginalis is a parasite responsible for many of the leucorrhoeal discharges in women. The diagnosis can always be confirmed by demonstration of the parasite in either a fresh wet drop or a vaginal smear.

***Symptoms of Leucorrhoea.*** In all such conditions of local disease of the sexual organs, other symptoms are usually present, such as pain in the lower part of the abdomen and back, or in the vagina, frequent—and perhaps painful—urination, and a discharge which is more apt to be thick and yellow, like that coming from a boil. Such conditions should never be neglected, since sometimes serious disease may be averted by submitting to treatment by a physician during the early stages of inflammatory disease of the sexual organs.

Leucorrhoea is a common disorder of old age, owing to natural changes in the womb. At such times the discharge is apt to be profuse, watery, and very irritating. In cancer of the womb the discharge is copious, dirty-colored, has a foul odor, and is often accompanied by flowing. As the result of a continuous discharge pouring out on the skin about the entrance to the vagina, much irritation and itching are produced, and often there is chafing and rawness of the parts.

There is sometimes a simple white or watery discharge from the front passage with no other unhealthy local or general disturbance. In this case it is safe for the patient to try the simple and harmless measures recommended farther along. There are other conditions in which there are symptoms of local inflammation in some part of the sexual apparatus, such as pain, disturbances of urination, flowing, and thick discharge like pus. These demand immediate attention of a physician. There is still a third class where the discharge is caused by some disorder of the general health, for which the patient should also consult a doctor. While the discharge itself causes weakness and a drain on the system, it is more often true that the discharge is caused by a general condition of weakness (or local inflammation) than that the general weakness is the result of the discharge.

***Treatment of Leucorrhoea.*** The treatment suggested here is suitable when the discharge is associated neither with general ill-health nor with other symptoms suggestive of disorder of the sexual organs, such as pain, disturbance of urination, flowing, etc. Over the vulva the patient should wear a pad of absorbent cotton, held in place by a napkin worn in the usual manner. Many women have a prejudice against wearing cloths for a discharge of "whites," believing that covering increases the discharge. This is not so, and cleanliness is an important agency in cure. The pad or tampax should, of course, be changed as often as it becomes soiled.

The vagina should be douched with boric acid solution, as hot as the elbow can bear, using a fountain syringe, night and morning. A powder composed of boric acid, 10 per cent; zinc stearate, 20 per cent; lactose, 42.5 per cent; lactic acid and trichomonacide, is curative when repeatedly blown into the vagina with a hand syringe and used with viogorm—a grayish powder.

Douches are commonly used, but though they are helpful they are not curative. After marriage some women continue the habit of douching regularly, either with a view to cleanliness or more frequently with the object of preventing an early conception. After a time they complain of a vaginal discharge. This is due to an infection following the constant chemical irritation set up by the douching—especially when Lysol, vinegar, or mercury is used.

CHAPTER 9

# THE MALE REPRODUCTIVE ORGANS

**The Prostate Gland and What It Does . . . Inflamed Prostate Gland . . . Enlarged Prostate Gland . . . The Testicles, and How Sperm Are Formed . . . Role of the Male Hormone . . . Undescended Testicles . . . Sterility in Men . . . Physical and Psychic Causes of Sterility and Their Correction . . . Decline of Sexual Powers (the Male Change of Life) . . . Its Nervous, Circulatory, Sexual Symptoms, and Treatment with Male Hormones.**

## THE PROSTATE GLAND

THIS important gland, present in the male only, lies at the neck of the urinary bladder and completely surrounds the urinary canal, about one and one-half inches from the bladder entrance. It reaches full development at puberty, when it is the size of a horse chestnut and similar to it in shape. Its nearness to the rectum and bladder is significant—disturbances of the gland are intimately associated with disturbances of both the rectum and bladder.

The prostate is made up of hundreds of minute glands which are held together by a firm fibrous sheath. Each one of these has a little duct or canal. These ducts collect the secretion from the hundreds of minute glands and carry it to larger collecting tubes, which finally empty into the prostatic portion of the urinary canal.

The secretion which the prostate manufactures is necessary to give movement to the spermatozoa, which are the reproductive elements of the semen. Without the addition of healthy prostatic secretion to the semen, the sperm cells do not move. Consequently reproduction cannot take place, and the man is sterile.

Disturbances of the prostate are numerous and frequent. The predominating disturbance is congestion of the prostate, which causes an enlargement. This is only transient and occurs often in young men long before they reach the so-called "prostatic age," which is about the fifth decade of life, when a large number of men have a true enlargement of the gland.

## INFLAMED PROSTATE GLAND (PROSTATITIS)

***Causes of Inflamed Prostate Gland.*** Twenty-five per cent of men between twenty and forty have prostate trouble. That is not generally known.

The predominating disturbance in young men is congestion, which means an enlargement of the gland due to too much blood in its structure; this enlargement with its accompanying symptoms, described below, is only transient, disappearing with simple conservative treatment and removal of the cause. This congestion may be caused by mechanical irritation or, as is the case more frequently, by sexual irregularities.

Any constant force or pressure on what is called the perineum—the area between the legs just above the rectal opening—may cause prostatic congestion. This is seen in men who are in the saddle for long periods daily, such as cattle-men, and in office workers, who are seated for many hours each day.

Prostatic congestion may also be produced by any abnormal disturbance of the sex function, which may be overindulgence or underindulgence and, most important of all, long periods of sexual excitation without completion of the act. In marital life, this latter is the case where offspring are not desired and the unhygienic practice of withdrawal or "coitus interruptus" is indulged in.

***Symptoms of Inflamed Prostate Gland.*** As a rule there is an urgency or frequency of urination. When the desire to urinate is felt, haste is necessary or there is loss of control of the bladder. Discomfort is constant over the bladder region, which is the lower area of the abdomen. In addition, there may be, and often is, a urethral discharge, which resembles an acute gonorrheal infection, but which on microscopic examination shows definitely it is not; associated with this there is often burning or discomfort on urination. Finally, the inability to have satisfactory intercourse will manifest itself. This combination of symptoms, especially when the last mentioned occurs, will cause the man to seek professional counsel.

When there is stagnation in the rectum—constipation—increased fermentation occurs and the bacteria which are normal for the normal lower bowel find their way through the rectal wall into the prostate, thus setting up an inflammation. Prompt removal of the cause or relief of the constipation will get a prompt restoration to normal.

***Treatment of Inflamed Prostate Gland.*** The first consideration is the removal of the cause. Intercourse should not be indulged in until all symptoms disappear. If there is considerable discomfort, a few days' rest in bed will be helpful. A hot sitz bath two or three times a day is necessary. After the acute symptoms have disappeared, gentle prostatic massage is indicated. It is much preferable to employ a specialist for this. It requires experience to massage the prostate correctly.

## ENLARGED PROSTATE GLAND

***Causes of Enlarged Prostate Gland.*** The actual cause of this condition is unknown. It is especially likely to occur in men who had frequent inflammation of the prostate in early life. Enlarged prostate is a true tumor formation, and a certain percentage become cancerous.

***Symptoms of Enlarged Prostate Gland.*** The symptoms that are present due to prostate obstruction are usually very typical. They begin with frequency of urination during the night. At first the patient may have to get out of bed to urinate only once or twice. This simple condition may exist alone for two or three years; then frequency occurs also during the day. Work and pleasure are interfered with. Pain gradually develops which at first is a burning sensation, soon becoming cramplike at the end of urination.

If the urine is examined at this time it will be found to contain some pus and not infrequently blood. If at this time treatment is instituted, usually the severe symptoms will subside, but the frequency will persist, which means that the condition is not cured. If relief is not obtained or not sought, complete retention of urine occurs, the patient cannot void any urine, and, unless relieved by the passing of a catheter, he will suffer intensely and much damage will be done to the kidneys by the urine backing up into them from the overfilled bladder.

So it is quite evident that early treatment is very necessary, and that many men, if treated at the beginning of their urinary difficulty, will be spared any progressive discomfort and certainly any operative procedure.

***Treatment of Enlarged Prostate Gland.*** There are many cases recorded where patients have had rational prostatic care for as long as fifteen years. They had no more annoyance than having to get up once at night to empty their bladders although they had been told many years previously that an operation was necessary.

In the recommended method of treatment, regulation of the bowels is important, and so are hot sitz baths and massage. The patient should have daily bowel movements. Suppositories are used to reduce the inflammation. Ichthyol, 4.00; extract of belladonna, 0.195; and cocoa butter to make twelve suppositories—this prescription will be made up by the druggist. The suppositories should be kept in the refrigerator, and lubricated with cold cream or vaseline before use. One should be inserted immediately before the sitz bath. The sitz bath, lasting fifteen minutes, should be taken before going to bed at night.

The patient should see his doctor once or twice a week for gentle prostatic massage.

Although 25 per cent of men past fifty years of age have prostatic enlargement, only a small percentage of these really need any surgery. The eager and radical surgeon will disagree with this statement, but many years of experience prove that the majority of men who have symptoms of prostatic disturbance causing bladder disturbance can be kept in comparative comfort for an indefinite number of years.

Why the stress on conservatism? Because more than half the cases of true enlargement are associated with inflammation, so that the enlargement producing the obstruction to free urination can be greatly reduced by simple measures and surgery avoided. There is no doubt whatever that too many men are operated on unnecessarily for prostate gland enlargements.

## THE TESTICLES

The testicles have two major jobs to do: They manufacture spermatozoa, just as the ovary manufactures ova, and they form an internal secretion or hormone which is responsible for sex desire and the secondary sex characteristics—deep voice, hair, and muscular strength.

***Sperm Formation.*** The manufacture of the spermatozoa takes place in the tiny tubules of the testicles, which number over a thousand in each gland. The process is called spermatogenesis. The mature sperm has a head, neck, and tail, and under the microscope has form and movement almost identical with the pollywog's.

After the sperm reach full formation, they circulate through the tubules into a collecting duct which finally carries them into two little receptacles situated on either side of the prostate, the seminal vesicles. The seminal vesicles are a store-house for the accumulation of the completely formed sperm. When orgasm takes place, these reservoirs force the sperm through a little canal into the urethra (urinary canal), where they are diluted with prostatic secretion, thus completing the formation of the semen.

When the sperm contacts an ovum, the head enters it and the neck and tail disappear; thus fertilization of the ovum has occurred.

The process of spermatogenesis continues unceasingly throughout the period from puberty to the male climacteric, which may be reached at varying ages from fifty to sixty-five. Active sperm have been found not infrequently in men over eighty. It is estimated that with each ejaculation, which occurs at orgasm, between fifty and two hundred million spermatozoa are present. Each sperm is about one five-hundredth of an inch in length, and it requires but one sperm to effect fertilization.

## THE MALE HORMONE

The other function of the testes is the formation of internal secretion, which is the male sex hormone. The manufacture of this hormone continues during the entire period of sex activity. The secondary sex characteristics and sex potency are dependent upon this secretion. Without it there is no sex power and the physical development and energy output are reduced. This male sex hormone is called testosterone.

The testicles have an intimate relationship with other glands of internal secretion, such as the pituitary gland, which lies at the base of the brain, and the thyroid. Males whose production of the male hormone is deficient are generally undeveloped and undersized. The genital organs of these individuals are not developed and there is retardation of the physical sexual differentiation, such as feminine appearance, high pitched voice and absence of pubic hair.

The psychologic development, too, is delayed. At early age these unfortunates avoid the customary activities of normal boys.

The use of manufactured testosterone has been widespread in the past ten years. It is of inestimable value in many cases but will only influence those physiological changes which are deficient results of the male hormone production.

## UNDESCENDED TESTICLES

In about 10 per cent of males, at birth, the testicles are not in the scrotum; this is called undescended testicles. It is important that these glands should be in their proper position, and the majority of them do eventually go into the scrotum without any interference.

However, there is no medicine, drug, or hormone that will influence the testes to move into their sac. If the glands are allowed to remain either in the groin canal or in the abdominal cavity, there is danger of either the loss of function from pressure or malignancy (cancer) from the continued irritation.

If one or both of the testes do not reach the scrotum by the age of ten, they should be submitted to surgery, but before the age of ten operation is not indicated.

## STERILITY IN MEN

***Meaning of Sterility.*** Physiologic impotence, or sterility, may occur at widely varying ages in different individuals. No average age can be given. A man may be perfectly normal in every respect except that he is unable to produce healthy sperm, or the process may be reduced. This man is said to be sterile. Congenital sterility of the male is uncommon. Sperm production, of course, changes with age (see discussion of the male climacteric below), but here we are concerned only with an abnormal condition.

There must be a clear understanding between the ability to produce children and the ability to have satisfactory intercourse. They are two separate and distinct activities. A man may be capable of having intercourse and yet not have normal semen. The opposite may also be true.

Psychic impotency is a true psychosis. A good psychiatrist will accomplish wonders with this type.

***Treatment of Sterility.*** The first requirement is the examination of a fresh specimen of semen. This should reach the physician not more than an hour after discharged. Chilled sperm soon lose their motility. If there is a reduction in the number of sperm to less than one half, or deformities of the sperm, or inactivity of the sperm, or a total absence, then we have found the source of the sterility.

The next procedure is to have a complete physical examination, paying special attention to the blood examination to see if there is any anemia, and to rule out the possibility of a latent syphilis. There should be an investigation of the other hormone glands by means of a basal metabolism test.

If all other possible conditions are ruled out, the conclusion is that the testicles are at fault. For this condition hormones are given by muscular injections.

## THE MALE CLIMACTERIC

***Decline in Sexual Powers.*** The term "male climacteric," which has come into use only in the past ten years, means a physiological loss of power of production of sperm and internal secretion of the testicles, which, according to the term, should be expected to occur at a fairly regular time of life in all men.

However, such a definite period does not exist. Some cases appear in men before the normally expected shrinking of the sex organs, others in men past middle age.

The production of the secretion of the cells which have to do with sexual potency reaches its highest level between the ages of twenty-two and twenty-five, maintains this level for from five to ten years, then gradually declines. This decline becomes more rapid between the ages of forty and fifty until at sixty, in most instances but by no means all, it approaches that which existed before puberty.

The parallel of this process in the female is the rise and decline of the female productive elements in the ovaries.

***Symptoms of the Climacteric.*** It should be understood that this so-called climacteric in the male is by no means a grouping of sex symptoms and disturbances alone. More often than not professional counsel is sought for the other manifestations characteristic of these symptoms.

The symptoms should be divided into three groups: (1) nervous and mental manifestations, (2) circulatory disturbances, and (3) sexual disturbances.

***Nervous Symptoms.*** Most patients describe a feeling of tension, an inward tremulousness. They are irritable and easily angered. Insomnia is often present. Numbness and tingling of the hands and feet are complained of. But most important are the mental disturbances, the decrease of memory and ability to concentrate, and the presence of a depression which may reach the stage of melancholia.

***Circulatory Symptoms.*** The circulatory symptoms are characterized by a sudden redness of the face and neck that is akin to blushing and is due to the sudden dilation of the superficial blood vessels of the skin. It is an uncomfortable sensation that may last a few seconds or an hour or more. This flushing is usually followed by a profuse perspiration of the face and neck and sometimes the entire body. It may occur once or several times daily.

In addition there may be an increase of the heart beat (tachycardia) and an irregularity of the beat (palpitation).

***Sexual Symptoms.*** The sexual symptoms may be overshadowed by those just described and these symptoms may be elicited only on questioning. However, they are always there and may include a complete loss of desire (libido) or/and loss of sex power (potency). On the other hand the reverse often exists, and consultation is sought for the sex disturbances, the nervous and circulatory symptoms being secondary.

***Treatment of Male Climacteric.*** Within certain age limits, relief is obtained in most cases. Practically all of the mental illness due to reduction or imbalance of the hormones can be relieved or cured.

Early in this century extracts of testes were used with some satisfactory results, but nothing convincing. Then, about ten years ago, came the advent of testosterone, a potent preparation which provided the physician with the weapon to combat these symptoms just described.

A note of warning must be sounded. This drug in the hands of the inexperienced can be productive of much harm. When it is used indiscriminately, without definite indications, or in the presence of definite signs against its use, such as high blood pressure, it may spell disaster.

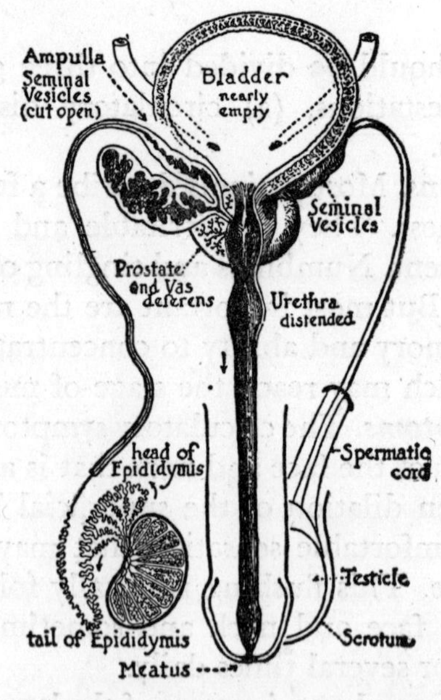


MALE SEXUAL ORGANS

CHAPTER 10

# SEXUAL HYGIENE

**Responsibility of the Parents . . . Six Rules for Teaching Your Child the Facts of Sex . . . The Truth About Masturbation . . . How to Prevent Masturbation in Infancy . . . What Every Young Person Should Know . . . Danger of Venereal Disease . . . Continence and Health . . . Preparation for Marriage . . . Common Sex Difficulties in Married Life—Basic Advice on How to Overcome Them . . . Securing Help to Solve Sex Problems.**

EVERY child should know the names of the sexual organs, and how to care for them, as well as the names of any other parts of the body —provided that the teaching is done by the proper person and at the proper time and place. Such accurate information should be given to children at an early age by parents, guardians, teachers, or physicians. If this is neglected, because of ignorance or false modesty, mistaken ideas of the nature and purpose of the sexual function will surely be supplied at a later period by ignorant and possibly evil-minded persons, with correspondingly bad results. No other responsibility in the whole range of parental duties is so commonly shirked, and with such sad consequences.

In order to help clarify sexual matters for the child, the parent may want to give him explanatory books. It is important that these books, as well as any other sexual information furnished, should be suitable for the child, and should fit into his needs in relation to his own day-to-day experiences. The parents should make every effort to find out what is on the child's mind, and there should be no evasion of any questions.

Sex is the central fact of life and there is urgent need for a clear understanding of this subject that greatly affects every member of society. To be prudish is silly and sentimental. What is called "modesty" must be disregarded when the child's immediate peace of mind and future happiness are at stake.

The particular information that parents give to their children as regards sex is not so important as the attitude which they themselves create towards sex from the child's earliest days. It is not what they say, but how they say it, that is significant. The subject of sex should be removed from the morbid and seductive mystery with which custom has foolishly surrounded it. Otherwise, the first lesson the child will learn about sex is that it is associated with the idea of shame. It should be considered in the same spirit with which the anatomy and hygiene of the digestive or respiratory systems are studied. Then it will be found possible to give instruction about the sexual function in a natural way, without exciting unhealthy and undue curiosity.

### SIX RULES FOR TEACHING SEX

Dr. George E. Gardner, the child guidance expert, gives some valuable advice to parents as teachers of sex. He writes: "Always use the correct scientific words to designate the anatomical areas or parts you are discussing with the child.

"Be as unemotional and matter-of-fact as you can in presenting sex information.

"What you tell your child about sex should be the truth and nothing but the truth.

"Even though the truth and only the truth should be told to children in answer to their questions, you do not have to give the child the whole truth about sex matters at any one time.

"It must not be assumed that the child is going through school . . . without finding some answers to his questions in the conversations of his schoolmates and friends.

"Do not use the sex life of animals and plants as a means of conveying information regarding human anatomy and physiology to the young child."

Evasive replies, with the intent of putting off the explanation dreaded by the parent, do no good; they may result in unexpected harm. By winning the child's confidence at the start, you may not only keep yourself informed of his actions, but also protect him from seeking or even listening to bad counsel. It is perfectly natural that the young should wish to know something of the origin of life, and how human beings come into the world.

### MASTURBATION

Much has been said as to the harm produced by masturbation, or abuse of the sexual function. The injury thus received has been purposely magnified by quacks. These, for their own selfish reasons, work upon the fears of their victims.

Masturbation or abuse of the sexual organs in the young is usually due to the almost criminal neglect or ignorance of the parents. Far from inspiring worry in the child, as many parents do, they should try to help him rid himself of the habit, by kindly instruction and judicious supervision. In this way no serious damage to the child will result.

The opposite teaching is that of the quack who prophesies every imaginable evil, including complete loss of sexual function and insanity. Any real or fancied disorder of the sexual function in itself is extremely apt to lead to much mental anxiety and depression. A cheerful outlook is therefore essential in inspiring an effort to correct bad habits. Such an outlook is actually fully warranted in view of the entire recovery, in most cases, of the young who earlier have abused their sexual organs. It is a sad fact, however, that the practice of masturbation or self-abuse is generally in the young, at least in boys, under the prevailing custom of failure of parents to exercise proper supervision over the sex education of their children.

Self-abuse often leads to temporary physical and mental suffering but it does not commonly result in permanent injury. Children at an early age—three to four years—should be gently taught not to touch, handle, rub, or irritate their sexual organs in any way whatsoever except as far as is necessary, in urination or in the course of daily cleansing. If there seems to be any inclination to do so, it will usually be found that it is caused by some local trouble. A physician's attention should be called to it; it can usually be readily remedied by him.

***How to Prevent Masturbation in Infancy.*** It is always advisable to ask a physician to examine babies for any existing trouble and abnormality of the sexual organs. There may be a tight, adherent, or elongated foreskin in boys, and, rarely, a corresponding condition in girls, which may give rise to much local irritation and nervous disturbances. The presence of worms may lead to irritation in the bowels. This excites masturbation in children. Girl babies should be watched to prevent them from irritating the external parts by rubbing them between the inner surfaces of the thighs.

## WHAT EVERY YOUNG PERSON SHOULD KNOW

***Danger of Venereal Disease.*** At the age of puberty the child should be warned against the moral and physical dangers of sexual intercourse. The physical dangers refer to the great possibility of being infected with one or both of the common venereal diseases—syphilis and gonorrhea—which are acquired by sexual contact with an individual suffering from these diseases. It is usually impossible for a layman to detect the presence of these diseases in others, or rather, to be sure of their absence. The permanent damage which may be done to the sufferer and to others with whom he may have sexual relations is incalculable.

It is widely known that syphilis is a disease to be dreaded. It is perhaps not known that it endangers not only the life and happiness of the patient, but also of future generations of his descendants. Gonorrhea—the much more common disease—while often treated lightly by youth, may lead to long, chronic, local disease; if neglected, may even result fatally. When the time comes for marriage, it may cause infection of the wife, resulting in chronic invalidism which requires surgical removal of her maternal organs. These possibilities often occur long after the patient thinks he is wholly free from the disease. Gonorrhea in women is the most frequent cause of their sterility.

Gonorrhea is so alarmingly prevalent that it is stated, on good authority, that the disease occurs in 80 per cent of all males at some time during their lives. It is not confined to prostitutes, but is found much more commonly than is suspected, in all walks and classes of life and at all ages. Even among boys attending boarding schools and similar institutions the disease is only too frequent.

It is particularly important that the true situation be explained to boys about to leave home to enter college or a business career, for it is at this period of life that their temptations become greatest. Alcohol is the most dangerous foe, next to bad companions, with which they must contend in this matter, for, when they are weakened by its influence and associated with persuasive friends, their will gives way and all the advice and warnings they may have received are forgotten. Idleness is also another indirect but influential factor in causing sexual disease. Hard physical and mental work are powerful correctives of the sexual urge.

***Continence and Health.*** The voluntary exercise of the sexual function is not necessary to health. In this regard, the function differs from that of any other important organ. Even after maturity it is quite possible to maintain perfect health through life, without exercising the sexual function at all.

## OF SPECIAL INTEREST TO THOSE ABOUT TO MARRY

When young adult life has been reached, it is desirable for the parent, or the family physician, to give the young man or woman—especially one about to enter a marriage engagement—certain information. For example, to explain that close and frequent personal contact with the opposite sex, especially when the affections are involved, will necessarily, though involuntarily, excite local stimulation of the sexual organs. For this reason long engagements—when the participants are frequent companions—are peculiarly unfortunate. It is only when the sexual functions are normally exercised in adult life, as in sexual intercourse, that sexual excitement is not harmful.

Young women about to marry should receive instructions from their mothers or family physician with regard to sexual relations which will exist after marriage. Most girls are allowed to grow up ignorant of such matters. In consequence they may be greatly shocked and even disgusted by sexual relations in marriage. They may fancy that there must be something unnatural and wrong about such relations because the subject was never alluded to by those responsible for their enlightenment.

***Common Sex Difficulties.*** At the couple's first coming together, everything may go easily. Oftener, though, some degree of difficulty may be met. The man is apt to be so eager that intercourse is incomplete. He may be temporarily impotent, or unable to have an erection because of nervous excitement. Both he and his wife should realize that the impotence of the new bridegroom is merely evidence of his desire to do especially well. A little later, or the next morning, or at some other time in the next few days, he will perform satisfactorily.

Meanwhile the wife has corresponding problems. Unless her hymen has been gradually stretched in preparation for marriage, either by herself or by a doctor, it may present a more or less serious obstacle. In a small percentage of women the hymen is practically nonexistent, and offers no barrier to intercourse; in a small percentage at the opposite extreme it is so thick and tough and inelastic that it prevents intercourse unless it is first nicked or stretched as a surgical procedure. Of the women in the middle group, some possess hymens that offer only a moderate barrier to entry at the time of intercourse, and others have hymens that are a considerable but not insuperable obstacle.

***Breaking the Hymen.*** The hymen is a perforated drumhead partially shutting off the outer opening of the vagina. It can be stretched sidewise, a little at a time, until it is pushed aside far enough not to be in the way in early intercourse. If that is not done, it can usually be quickly stretched or broken at the time of the first intercourse.

This is not especially painful, in most instances, as the area is not well endowed with nerve endings.

If the hymen is too hard to break, a gynecologist or other doctor can be consulted, even at this late date, as to whether it needs to be cut or stretched by him as an office procedure, requiring a local anesthetic.

***Sex Problems of the New Husband.*** A further fact the wife needs to understand is that the average man is very sensitive about even temporary impotence or premature discharge. The teaching of adolescent girls and young women by society at large is still so unlike the casual sex education picked up by boys and men, and the sex make-up and functioning of women is so different from that of men, it is not strange that the two find it hard to understand each other. Rare is the bride who is not overcome by chagrin or shame because she thinks she is not doing well in the first sex relations of marriage. Equally rare is the man who does not tend to feel ashamed, or at least deeply embarrassed, if his sexual performance seems to him not up to par. Most bridegrooms think they will lose rank in the bride's eyes, as they do in their own, if they cannot immediately consummate the marriage.

***Time Difference in Intercourse.*** The time difference between the man and woman is not confined to the stage of preparation. The intercourse itself tends to run quickly to its climax in the man, with an average duration estimated to be from two to five minutes; while the woman usually has to have several times as long a period, from ten to fifteen minutes or more, to bring her to a climax.

Fortunately, this time difference can often be largely made up by the preliminary love play before intercourse is begun. The man can also learn to delay his climax by inactive periods, deep breathing, forcing his attention to switch to a neutral subject such as the walls or curtains, talking, changing position, and renewing his courting. Resolving the time difference between the two is an important principle of good sex adjustment.

***The Climax.*** It is advisable that the wife not worry over whether she will have an orgasm or not, since that kind of attitude might interfere with her natural tendency to respond in such a way as to lead to her having one. The orgasm, or climax of intercourse, varies greatly in intensity among different women, as it does among different men. In the same individual it is also very different from time to time. The quieter episodes are not necessarily less happy occasions, though of different quality.

***Securing Help to Overcome Discomfort in Intercourse.*** At the same time it must be emphasized that if a woman feels persistent discomfort throughout intercourse, in spite of the husband's exercising great care to woo her adequately at each approach, she should not delay in consulting a careful doctor, if possible a gynecologist, to find out if some pathological condition needs treatment. Even if she was examined before marriage, something requiring attention may have come up since.

CHAPTER 11

# VENEREAL DISEASES

**How Penicillin Helps Prevent Venereal Diseases . . . Congenital Syphilis Comes Under Control . . . How to Avoid Gonorrhea . . . Its Social Danger . . . Gonorrhea in Men . . . Gonorrhea in Women . . . Three Stages of Syphilis . . . Its Complications . . . The Marriage of Syphilitics . . . Difference Between Congenital and Hereditary Syphilis . . . "False Positive" Wassermann Tests . . . Conditions That Produce These Reactions.**

ALTHOUGH no one can give a definite estimate as to the total number of cases of gonorrhea and syphilis infections that have occurred since, let us say, the close of World War II, both diseases have undoubtedly increased in frequency. The cures, however, have been startling, the efficacy of treatment remarkable, and the ultimate results beyond all predictions.

Your question logically is, why the increase in number of infections? Probably one reason is that the efficacy of the treatment is well known to most of the lay public through the wide circulation of information about the "wonder drug" penicillin. As a consequence, men and women have become devil-may-care in their attitudes.

Gonorrhea has increased more than syphilis. Yet this is countered by the fact that ninety-eight per cent of the cases in males can be cured in twenty-four hours by a single injection of penicillin. Because of the promptness with which the infection is brought under control, it is very unusual to see any complication.

How do we know that gonorrhea is cured in twenty-four hours? First, the urethral discharge in the male disappears and the patient is thoroughly examined at the end of one week and then once a month for three consecutive months. He is then dismissed as cured.

It would not be scientifically accurate to make the twenty-four-hour statement about females, since the wider area of possible distribution of the germs makes the conclusions less definite.

During World War II our eight million men in the armed forces were constantly instructed about venereal disease prophylaxis. The frequency of both gonorrhea and syphilis among the men in continental United States dropped in some areas to less than twelve per one thousand soldiers and sailors, but as soon as peace came and penicillin catapulted into prominence, all the teachings about prophylaxis were cast to the winds. Recent clinical experiments with penicillin show definitely that the drug is not only curative but also preventive.

Proof of this is shown by a typical report from an army post. Fifteen hundred soldiers who admitted exposure were given a preventive treatment of penicillin. One case of gonorrhea developed among the fifteen hundred given the test.

## PREVENTIVE MEASURES REDUCE SYPHILIS

Similar preventive results are reported against syphilis. A most striking example is found in a report covering 309 men. All admitted exposure. Half were given the preventive treatment and half did not receive it. Of the half who took the treatment 6 per cent developed syphilis and 62 per cent developed it among the untreated.

When we restate some of the horrors of syphilis of bygone days, the diseased babies, the destruction of any part of the human body, the late manifestations of inadequately treated cases resulting in paresis (softening of the brain) and locomotor ataxia, and compare our present-day results, it is indeed gratifying to the scientists and medical profession who brought all this about. So when the statement is made that venereal diseases are on the increase, it is in frequency alone, for the results of treatment are of far greater import.

For example, from 10,000 cases reported, 859 were selected who had varying manifestations of the primary and secondary stages. Those are the chancre and infectious eruption. All possibility of contagion from these cases disappeared in from four to eight days. This coincides with the results in general, so it is seen that even though we do have more cases, they more rapidly reach the stage of not being contagious. This fact may be a forerunner of the possibility of stamping out *contagious* syphilis in a few years.

## CONTROL OF CONGENITAL SYPHILIS

The greatest single achievement in the treatment of syphilis is the prevention of congenital or hereditary types. Here medical progress stands out as monumental. It is now definitely established that a pregnant syphilitic, if given adequate treatment any time during her pregnancy, will in 98 per cent of instances give birth to a syphilis-free baby. Before penicillin the birth rate of surviving syphilitic babies was 70 per cent, in which over 50 per cent had eye involvement resulting in partial or total blindness.

There still remains a high percentage of still-born babies and spontaneous abortions in the untreated cases. These are of course to be found most often in the lower strata of society.

All women who have taken treatment for syphilis during pregnancy are followed for a period of one year after childbirth. Both baby and mother take blood tests at varying periods during the year and a thorough physical examination is given at the same time.

The last group of cases to be mentioned are the neuro-syphilitics. These are those who suffer from paresis and locomotor ataxia. In the ten thousand cases of syphilis already referred to, there were 1866 of these unfortunates. The infection of all these cases occurred as long ago as twenty years. They were, of course, inadequately treated or recieved no treatment at all.

Under penicillin all these cases improved markedly. Their disease was *arrested,* but no damaged area of the brain or spinal cord could be replaced. If our predictions hold good, the future will show few cases of brain or spinal cord involvement.

One point should be emphasized—syphilis is an evasive disease. Its primary and secondary lesions often go entirely unnoticed and not always does a blood test give evidence of the presence of the disease. Therefore, promiscuity in sexual relationships should have *periodic* blood tests as a safeguard.

One of the greatest pieces of legislation ever to be adopted in this country is the requirement of a blood test for syphilis before a couple can get a license for marriage. This is now law in most of our states. It has helped prevent many a needless tragedy.

## GONORRHEA, A PREVENTABLE DISEASE

***How to Avoid Gonorrhea.*** Aside from continence, chemical as well as mechanical measures on the part of the male have long proved their value. There is no disputing that mechanical prophylaxis, as by means of a condom, assures a certain measure of protection. There is also evidence that sulfathiazole taken by mouth before and after intercourse may prove of practical value to both men and women. The drug is given on prescription by the physician before possible exposure, repeated after the act, and again the following day.

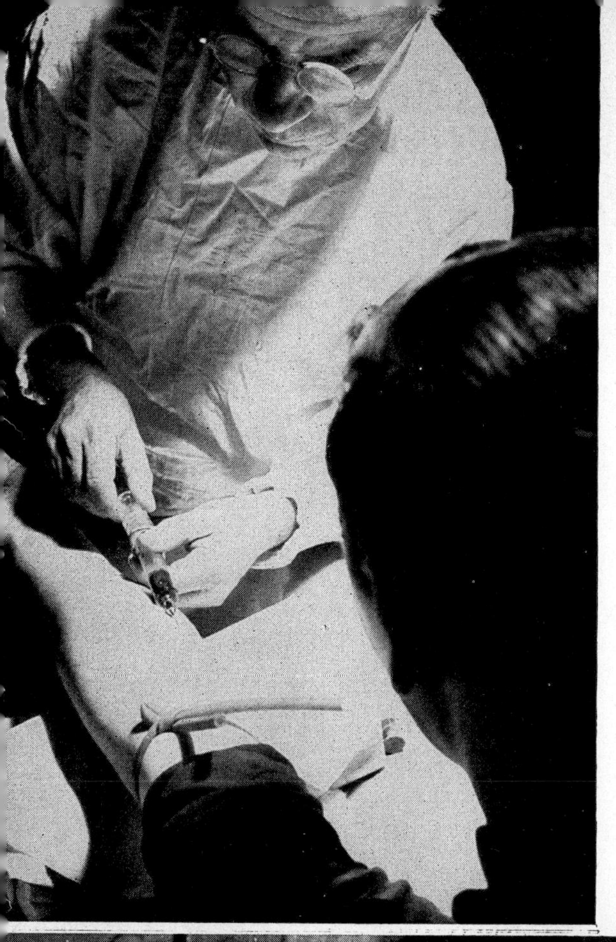

# Detecting Venereal Disease

## WASSERMANN TEST

This test, generally performed on a blood sample, is an excellent means of detecting syphilis early. Disease, highly contagious, is transmitted by close personal contact. Penicillin soon renders syphilis noninfectious, but treatment is needed till blood has been completely cleared of germs.

## HUNTING SPIROCHETES

Laboratory worker examines blood specimen for syphilis-causing spirochetes, under microscope. When he finds them, they appear as pale, spiral-shaped germs. Before development of penicillin, they were responsible for many deaths, particularly of infants, infected through mother.

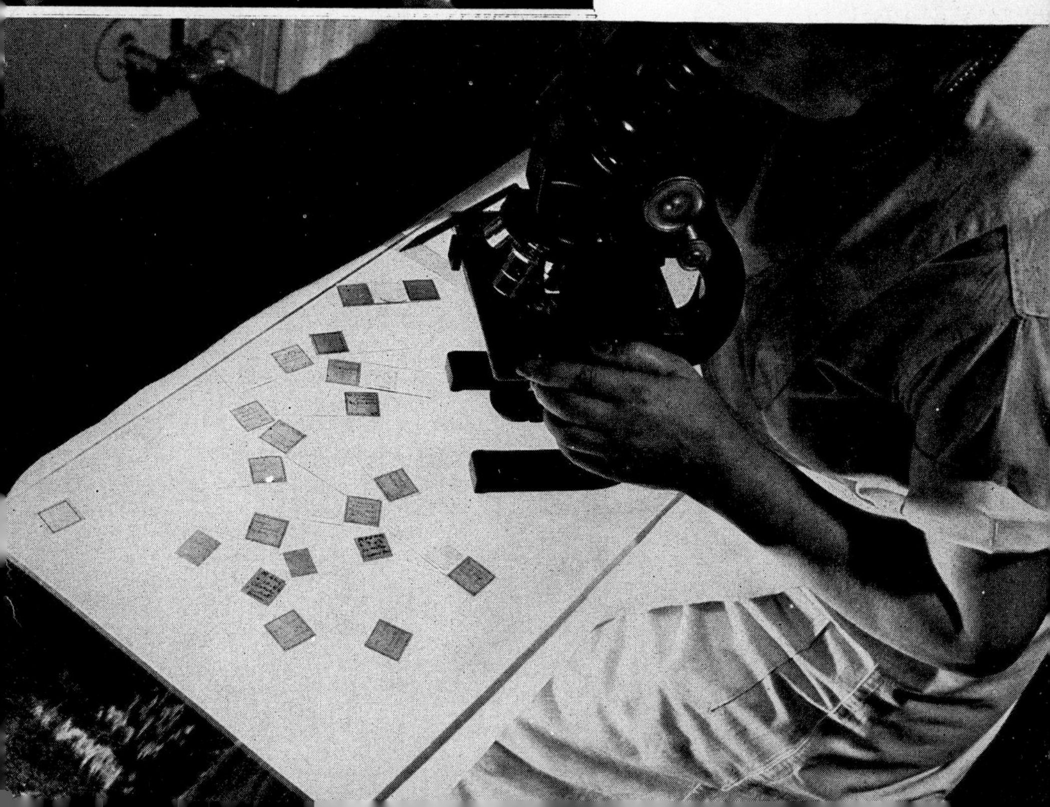

# Sex, Age, and Cancer

## WHERE CANCER STRIKES IN MEN AND WOMEN

Diagram below shows percentages of occurrence of various kinds of cancer in both sexes. Differences in habits and occupations probably account for these variations. Men, more apt to develop cancer of digestive tract and mouth, should cultivate regular eating and bowel habits, practice proper hygiene of teeth and mouth. Women should examine breasts periodically, avoid tight-fitting or chafing clothing.

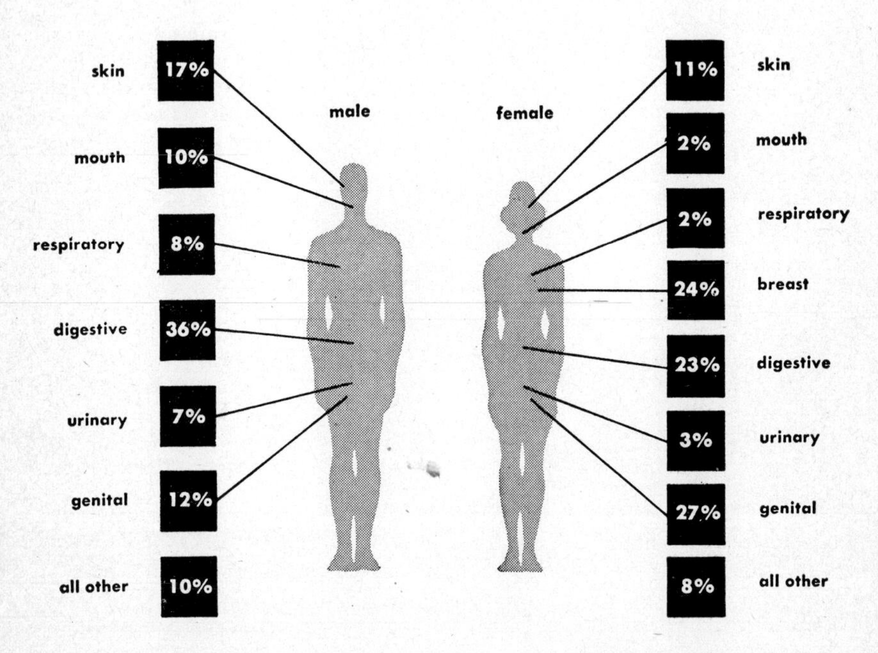


American Cancer Society

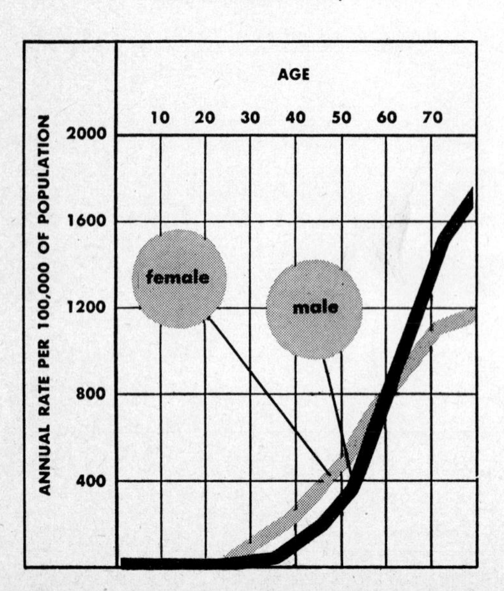


## WHEN CANCER STRIKES

Chances for developing cancer increase rapidly as people grow older. Below age of twenty, fewer than ten people in 100,000 develop cancer in a year. Cancer is Number 1 killer of women between ages thirty and fifty-five. Forty is the age when men become particularly susceptible— increase from then on is steady as they become older. Seven danger signals to watch for are: (1) any sore that does not heal; (2) lump or thickening, in breast or elsewhere; (3) unusual bleeding or discharge; (4) any change in a wart or mole; (5) persistent indigestion or difficulty in swallowing; (6) persistent hoarseness or cough; (7) any change in normal bowel habits.

## GONORRHEA IN MEN

***Signs and Symptoms of Gonorrhea.*** There are indications that several million persons are infected with gonorrhea every year. This contagious inflammation of the urethra, accompanied by a yellowish discharge, is caused by a specific germ, the gonococcus. It is acquired through sexual intercourse with a person suffering from the disease. The mucous membranes of the mouth, of the lower part of the bowel, and of the eyes may also become infected through contamination with the discharge, though this is not common. The disease in males usually begins three to seven days after sexual intercourse with a person suffering from the disease.

There are at first symptoms of burning, smarting, pain on urination, and a watery discharge from the passage. This is soon followed by a yellowish secretion. Swelling of the penis, frequent urination, and painful erections are also common symptoms if treatment is delayed.

***Treatment of Gonorrhea in Men.*** So remarkably prompt is the action of penicillin in gonorrhea that there is a real danger that the disease may come to be considered as trivial. The drug has made all other forms of treatment obsolete. A single course of treatment results in complete cure in 98 per cent of the cases. In long-standing, neglected gonorrhea, more prolonged treatment is necessary. However, there is no longer anything like the old treatment which often had to be carried on for months and even years.

## GONORRHEA IN WOMEN

Gonorrhea in women is a much more frequent and serious disease than was formerly supposed. The general impression among the public has been that gonorrhea in females is limited to the prostitute and those who indulge in licentious relations. This is not the case. There is perhaps more gonorrhea, in the aggregate, among virtuous and respectable wives than among professional prostitutes, and the explanation is simple. A large proportion of women are infected by their sexually promiscuous husbands.

***The Social Danger of Gonorrhea.*** The danger from gonorrhea introduced after marriage is not limited to health risks incurred by the women themselves. When a woman thus infected bears a child, the contagion of the disease, as has been stated, may be conveyed to the child's eyes in the process of birth. Gonorrheal pus is one of the most virulent of all poisons. A single drop transferred to the eye may destroy this organ in from twenty-four to forty-eight hours. It is estimated that from 75 to 80 per cent of all babies blinded at birth have suffered from this cause, while from 20 to 30 per cent of blindness from all causes is attributable to gonorrhea. The horrors of this disease in the newborn have been mitigated by the use of penicillin ointment or silver nitrate solution in the eyes immediately after birth, but it remains one of the most common factors in the causation of blindness.

Another social danger is due to the pus which is conveyed to the genital parts of female children, either at birth or by some object upon which it has been accidentally deposited, such as clothes, sponges, diapers, etc. This state of affairs was formerly common in babies' hospitals and institutions for the care of children. The pus may be passed from child to child by means of an improperly cleaned thermometer, or is the result of sexual exposure to an infected person.

***Symptoms of Gonorrhea in Women.*** In women, gonorrhea is usually not so acute and painful as in men, unless it involves the urethra. It rarely begins with smarting and painful urination, but there is abundant discharge from the front passage. If the infection spreads to involve the Fallopian tubes, there may be severe abdominal pains, with fever and chills. This is rarely seen nowadays. In the majority of cases, if the infection travels upward, it settles in the deeper parts, that is, in the neck or body of the womb. In this location it may not give rise at first to painful symptoms, and the patient often attributes the increased discharge to an aggravation of leucorrhea (discharge from the vagina) from which she may have suffered.

The special danger to women from gonorrhea is that the inflammation is apt to be more severe during the menstrual period, and the germs of the disease may ascend to the cavity of the womb, the tubes and the ovaries.

***Treatment of Gonorrhea in Women.*** The treatment for women is the same as for men, except for certain complications of the disease. Women suffering from inflammation within the abdomen (of the tubes), or with fever, are put to bed and given treatment with penicillin or sulfa drugs.

The most common error in treating gonorrhea is failure to treat the infected partner.

The infection in immature girls is treated with penicillin and estrogen (theelin).

## SYPHILIS

Syphilis is a contagious disease caused by a germ called Treponema pallidum. It affects the entire system. While commonly acquired through sexual intercourse with a person already infected, it may be inherited from the parents—one or both. It is often acquired through accidental contact with sources of contagion.

It is to be noted that syphilis is not always a "venereal" disease, that is, acquired through sexual relations. It may be communicated by kissing, by accidental contact with a sore on a patient's body, by the use of pipes, eating or drinking utensils, or contact with any object upon which the germ, Treponema pallidum, has been deposited. Any part of the surface of the body or mucous membrane may be inoculated with the infecting organism of syphilis. The contagiousness of the disease is supposed to last during the first three years of its presence. There are, however, many authentic examples of contagions occurring after four or five years of syphilis.

***The Primary Stage of Syphilis.*** Acquired syphilis may be divided into three stages. The first stage is characterized by the appearance of a pimple or sore on the surface of the sexual organ, lips, or mouth not usually earlier than two, nor later than five to seven, weeks after sexual intercourse. The first sore or "chancre" is characteristically a single, more or less circumscribed, superficial ulcer which is always painless (unless secondarily infected), and is always accompanied by enlargement of the adjoining glands of the groin. The ulcer presents a moist worm-eaten base, occasionally crusted, with a hardened border which feels like a rubber button when touched with the gloved finger. Rather characteristic is the painlessness of the enlarged glands.

The appearance of this first sore is subject to such variations that it is, on rare occasions, impossible for even a skillful physician to determine positively at first glance the presence of syphilis in any person. A blood examination has first to be made and the report given of a "positive Wassermann" test, or a positive Kahn test. Following the pimple on the surface of the penis, comes a raw sore with hard deposit beneath, as of a coin under the skin. It may be so slight as to pass unnoticed, or it may become a large ulcer, and last from a few weeks to several months, if untreated. There are a number of other kinds of sores which have no connection with syphilis, and yet may resemble the syphilitic sore so closely that it becomes impossible to distinguish between them except by the later symptoms to be described.

***The Second Stage.*** The second stage appears in from six to seven weeks after the initial sore, and is characterized by the occurrence of a copper-colored rash over the body which resembles measles considerably, but appears less often on the face. Sometimes a pimply or scaly eruption is seen following, or in place of, the red rash. At about, or preceding, this period other symptoms may develop, such as fever, headache, nausea, loss of appetite, and sleeplessness, but these may not be prominent. Moist patches may appear on the skin, in the armpits, between the toes, and about the rectum. There is sore throat, with frequently grayish patches on the inside of the cheeks, lips, and tongue. The hair may fall out in patches. Inflammation of the eye is a frequent sign. These signs and symptoms do not always occur at the same time, and some may be absent or less noticeable than others.

***The Third Stage.*** The third stage comes on after months or years; in those subjected to treatment, it may not occur at all. This stage is characterized by sores and ulcerations of the skin and deeper tissues, and disease of different organs of the body, including the muscles, bones, nervous system, and blood vessels. Every internal organ is susceptible to syphilitic change.

In untreated patients many disorders of the internal organs—the heart, lungs, liver, kidneys, brain and spinal cord—are directly caused by syphilis. The central nervous system is peculiarly susceptible to the action of the syphilitic poison, and when affected may show the fact through paralysis, crippling, disabling, and various disfiguring disorders.

Years after a presumed "cure" has followed improper treatment, patients are more liable to certain nervous disorders, such as locomotor ataxia, which attacks only syphilitics; and general paresis, all the cases of which occur in those who have had syphilis.

***Inherited Syphilis.*** Children born with syphilis, of syphilitic parents, may show the disease at birth or usually within one or two months, or not until puberty. They present a gaunt, wasted appearance, suffer continually from snuffles or nasal catarrh, have sores and cracks about the lips, loss of hair, and troublesome skin eruptions. The syphilitic child has been described as a "little old man with a cold in his head." The internal organs are almost invariably diseased. Sixty to eighty per cent of the infants dies. Those who live to grow up are puny and poorly developed, so that at twenty they look not older than twelve, and are always delicate.

***Diagnosis of Syphilis.*** The prompt diagnosis of early syphilis is of extreme importance. It is a matter of record that the earlier treatment is begun after diagnosis, the earlier the condition is arrested and cured.

***The Treatment of Syphilis.*** In the past few years, as we said earlier, the treatment of syphilis in all its forms has undergone a radical change. The latest directives from the United States Department of Public Health discard all forms of mercury, bismuth and arsenic derivatives. In their place, penicillin is now the only drug used, except in special cases where the drug is not well tolerated, such as syphilis of the heart and circulatory system.

For practical purposes the treatment is divided into three classifications:

1. The contagious stages, that is, the primary stage or the chancre; and secondary stage or the eruptive stage, that is, when there is a breaking out of the skin and the mucous membranes.

2. The late stages, when the only finding is the positive blood test (Wassermann reaction).

3. The prevention of hereditary infection. This is the treatment of the pregnant woman who has syphilis, which also may be only determined by the blood reaction.

The treatment for the primary and secondary stages is by the injection into the buttocks of large doses of penicillin for eight consecutive days, then taking a blood test once every month for a year.

The treatment of the late stages is also with the muscular injections of penicillin, but the doses are not so large. Here again, the blood is watched for one year.

To prevent the mother from infecting her baby before it is born, at any time during the pregnancy when the blood shows positive, large doses of penicillin are given. When the baby is born, its blood test is also taken, and the baby as well as the mother is watched for one year.

## THE MARRIAGE OF SYPHILITICS

The eligibility for marriage of a syphilitic should be determined on the basis of liability to transmit infection to the healthy marital partner and the offspring of such a union. Marriage should be strictly forbidden during the early stages of syphilis even if the Wassermann test is negative, because infectious relapse may occur at any time. In adequately treated cases the danger of transmitting the disease after the eruptive or secondary stage decreases with time. A fair rule for both male and female is that five years should elapse after the infection started before marriage is allowed. The Wassermann and spinal fluid tests should remain negative for two years following the completion of treatment.

As has been pointed out, a most serious factor in women is the transmission of the disease to offspring. A woman may continue to transmit syphilis to her child during the whole child-bearing period.

The burden of responsibility must be borne by the family physician. He must warn the patient that marriage may not be entered into, and, if his advice is not taken, then he must know all the facts so that he can watch both mother and children and administer proper treatment.

Unfortunately, the laws enacted to prevent the marriage of venereally infected men and women are evaded. The medical examinations may be made in a cursory manner by physicians of limited experience who may make inconclusive interpretations of the history of the case and the blood examinations.

The question of the infectiousness of syphilis must be decided on the age of infection, the special reactions and responses of the individual patient and the results of persistent and systematic treatment and repeated physical examinations, with special attention to the central nervous system, the *heart and blood vessels.*

We must understand the difference between congenital and hereditary infection. The former means the transmission of disease during birth; in the latter the infection is carried to the child through the circulation of the blood during the period of gestation (pregnancy).

One per cent of all births in the United States are syphilitic! Fortunately, 25 per cent or more of the pregnancies in syphilitic families result in miscarriages or still-births.

Appropriate treatment of a syphilitic pregnant woman, if begun early, will prevent in 98 per cent of all cases the birth of a syphilitic baby.

The question is often asked if syphilis can be transmitted to the third generation. It is safe for a person with hereditary syphilis to marry and have children, provided he or she has had prolonged treatment, has had repeated negative Wassermann and spinal fluid tests, and has no mental defects. Under these conditions, there is no possibility of a man transmitting the disease to his wife or of a mother transmitting the disease to her child.

## "FALSE POSITIVE" WASSERMANN TESTS

There is probably no more dramatic experience for both physician and patient than the sudden discovery of a positive blood reaction to a Wassermann test, when there is no history of a previous syphilitic infection.

What happens then? Immediately more blood is taken and divided into two or more parts and sent to two or more other laboratories. In the absence of any syphilitic taint, of course, the final tests come back negative—except in those instances where there is present one of the many conditions which may cause the so-called "false positive" test.

## OTHER CONDITIONS CAUSE THE REACTIONS

There are many conditions that may exist in the human body that can give this so-called "false positive" blood reaction.

For example, there is one person in every seven hundred who has under quite normal conditions either a temporary or permanent positive Wassermann. If one has been infected with malaria, as so many were in World War II, he is sure to have the positive blood reaction for two to four weeks following, or even longer. It is still a matter of speculation as to how long the malarial parasite remains in the body, but it is well established that one hundred per cent of infected individuals will give a positive blood test for some time following malarial infection. This is a very important point since so many soldiers were stationed in the malarial mosquito-infested areas.

Typhus fever, although rare in our country, did affect many of our overseas soldiers. This disease frequently will give a positive false blood test, which disappears on recovery from the disease. In addition to these, there are fifty odd tropical diseases, many of which were contracted by our soldiers. These also will cause this type of test reaction. It is claimed that as high as eighty per cent of persons so infected have this blood reaction for an unknown period of time.

Although these tropical infections are foreign to our soil, it must be remembered that a great number of our soldiers were exposed during World War II. Despite the great precautions taken in detecting those infected, it is reasonable to suppose that some disease parasites were brought back into the United States.

If you have recently been vaccinated against smallpox, you may have a positive blood reaction. This is not generally known, but it is estimated that between ten per cent and thirty-five per cent of small-pox vaccinations will cause this positive blood test as long as four months after vaccination.

A severe bite by one of the rodent family may cause a fever. This is usually a rat bite and is called rat-bite fever. The same reaction may be produced by the bite of a squirrel or woodchuck. Thirty-five to fifty per cent of persons bitten will give the positive blood test during the course of the fever and possibly for a short time afterwards.

***Laboratory Errors.*** Technical errors in the laboratory, of course, should never occur; yet the human factor must be taken into account since the blood test for syphilis is one of the most delicate performed in the clinical laboratory. Experienced syphilologists constantly warn against the acceptance of the single, the partial, or in some cases even the repeated, positive tests as final evidence of the presence of syphilis.

***Methods Not Always Final.*** It is almost axiomatic in medical science that the existence of so many different methods for detecting the same condition—be the methods clinical, surgical, or of the laboratory—at once registers a doubt as to the accuracy of any. There are no less than a dozen different methods of testing the blood for the presence of syphilis. The father of them all was Wassermann. Then came Kahn, and since, we have had a galaxy of names attached to some insignificant variation. So, despite the fact that "all roads lead to Rome" we find many bypaths that, to date, may carry us into other places.

One of our most prominent specialists states that "The blood test for syphilis has always been recognized as unfit to stand alone." When we add to this the fact that there are a number of conditions in the blood other than syphilis which will give a true positive, the confusion that may arise concerning false positive tests is obvious.

This question of false tests involves another large group of persons besides those about to be married. There are also those requiring blood tests in industry. It is well known and highly commended that every applicant for any position in large or small industries should have a blood test for syphilis as part of his or her physical examination. At the same time it must be emphasized that rigid care in interpretation must ever be maintained in the absence of any real proof of the disease.

It is unfortunate but too true that the industrial examiners are not always acquainted with the dangers of misinterpretation. There are legion records on file where men and women have failed to obtain needed employment or have been discharged from their positions because of the false positive reactions. Another pitfall is the fact that a persistent positive blood test very often exists through life in persons who have had adequate syphilitic treatment.

This must always be evaluated and when there is any doubt there should be expert professional consultation.

There is no desire to give the impression that the blood test in syphilis is of little or no value. On the contrary, it is of the greatest importance in diagnosis and as a guide for type and duration of treatment. But, regardless of the value of the test, we must guard justice for the minority.

CHAPTER 12

# THE PREGNANT WOMAN

**Signs of Pregnancy . . . Tests for Pregnancy . . . Figuring the Date of Baby's Birth . . . The Care of the Expectant Mother . . . Danger Signals . . . Rules for Good Health . . . Some Fallacies Regarding Pregnancy . . . The Increased Demands on Nutrition . . . Recommended Diet . . . What to Take to the Hospital . . . How Labor Begins . . . Preparations for Delivery . . . Convalescence from Childbirth . . . Spontaneous Abortion and Miscarriage . . . Legal Reasons for Interruption of Pregnancy, etc.**

When a woman finds herself pregnant, she should promptly consult her physician. If she cannot afford a private doctor, she should go to a prenatal clinic. These clinics are now to be found in every community of any size. The pregnant woman will receive careful instructions in her care during pregnancy. The "do's and the don'ts" are usually given in printed forms. If there are any doubts in the patient's mind, she should feel free to ask questions. It is most important that the physician in charge should remove any doubts she has and allay the fear which is usually present.

A woman should always remember that her greatest happiness is that of bringing a baby into the world. Giving birth to a baby is the most important function in her whole life.

There are a number of early signs of pregnancy. These include skipping a menstrual period, morning sickness, and changes in the breasts and womb.

***Skipping the Menstrual Period.*** This is the most significant sign of pregnancy. A healthy woman with normal menstruation suddenly misses a period. Her first thought should be of pregnancy.

***Morning Sickness.*** This happens most often during the first pregnancy. Vomiting in the early morning and during the first few weeks of pregnancy is considered normal for a pregnant woman. The condition usually disappears in from five to six weeks, but it may be prevented by taking crackers, dry toast, or orange juice before arising in the morning. It is also usually greatly relieved if the patient eats six small meals a day instead of three large ones.

If the vomiting should persist during the day, and become progressively worse as the weeks go by, it becomes a serious matter. This is usually the case in nervous, high-strung women, and they often require hospital treatment. Psychotherapy may prove of great value, and vitamin $B_6$ has been reported helpful for many patients. Vomiting late in pregnancy is always a danger signal, and is one of the signs of serious toxemia (blood poisoning) heralding convulsions. The bowels must be made to move daily.

***Changes in the Breasts.*** The breasts begin their preparation for milk production soon after conception. The nipples increase in size, pigmentation (coloration) is deeper, and the area around the nipple (areola) also becomes darker. Marks also appear in the skin of the breasts. If the breasts are large and heavy, they need to be supported, but never with a constricting brassiere. The most desirable material for a brassiere is parachute silk, but other strong, light materials, such as batiste, silk, or rayon are also satisfactory.

***Care of the Nipple.*** The nipples require only bathing, until about the seventh month, when they should be kept soft and pliable by oiling them nightly with some bland ointment (olive oil, cocoa butter, etc.), followed by gentle massage (of the nipples, not the breasts). The nipples should never be bathed for the purpose of hardening them, with tannic acid, alcohol, or other means, which tend to make them crack. If the nipples are small and flat, they may be lengthened by gentle pulling with the patient's clean fingers, or with a breast pump. A secretion sometimes forms on the nipples, and dries up, leaving a crust. If cold cream or lanolin is applied at night to soften these crusts, they will usually come off with the morning bath.

***Changes in the Womb.*** About the sixth week after the beginning of the last menstrual period, the physician finds the lower part of the womb softened. By the end of the second month the womb is soft and globular.

In experienced hands, pregnancy can be diagnosed by the end of the second month, with great probability, on the basis of physical examination.

## BIOLOGIC TESTS FOR PREGNANCY

***Aschheim-Zondek Test.*** This test makes use of immature white mice. The concentrate of morning urine or, preferably, a quantity of blood serum from a woman who has stopped menstruating, is injected under the skin of five mice over a period of two days. The mice are killed four or five days after the first injection, and their ovaries are examined. If bloody follicles, or corpora lutea, are found in the ovaries of the animals, the woman's pregnancy is considered certain. The urine used should be fresh, and, if possible, a morning specimen.

The errors with this test are less than one in one hundred.

***Friedman Test.*** This is a modification of the Aschheim-Zondek test. It uses mature virgin female rabbits which have been isolated for a period of four weeks. The concentrate of morning urine from the woman is injected into a vein of the rabbit, and sixteen to twenty-four hours later the rabbit is killed and its ovaries are examined. Ruptured, bloody follicles indicate a positive test of pregnancy.

The only advantage this has over the Aschheim-Zondek test is that a report can be had more promptly. However, in both these tests false positive results may be obtained in certain conditions, such as the menopause, in cases of ovarian deficiency in younger women, disorders of the pituitary gland, tumors above the kidneys, and inactivity and overactivity of the thyroid.

## LATER SIGNS OF PREGNANCY

***The First Feeling of Life.*** This is called "quickening" and is due to the movement of the child in the womb. It appears about the sixteenth week. In later pregnancies this movement is noticed about two weeks earlier than with the first baby.

***Later Movements of the Baby.*** These are when the womb has grown larger and the baby has more room to move; his movements may cause considerable discomfort to the mother. Should they become less noticeable or cease, the doctor should be consulted at once.

***Increase in the Size of the Abdomen.*** At the end of the fourth month, by placing the hand upon the abdomen, one can feel the enlarged womb as a big round ball. This is felt just above the pelvic bones. At the sixth month the uterus has reached the level of the navel. By the eighth month the uterus has reached half way between the navel and the breast bone.

***Settling of the Baby.*** This is called "lightening." It means the descent of the baby into the basin of the pelvis. This is usually more noticeable with the first baby. It brings great relief to the mother. It gives her more room in which to breathe. Associated with this settling there is often an increase in the frequency of urination. This is due to the pressure upon the bladder.

# CHART FOR FIGURING THE PROBABLE DATE OF THE BABY'S BIRTH

## *Directions for Using the Chart*

*In the column of light type and figures, find the date of the first day of the last menstrual period.*

**The probable date of the baby's birth will be found in the next column to the right—in heavy type and figures.**

| *Jan* | **Oct** | *Feb* | **Nov** | *Mar* | **Dec** | *Apr* | **Jan** | *May* | **Feb** | *Jun* | **Mar** | *July* | **Apr** | *Aug* | **May** | *Sept* | **Jun** | *Oct* | **July** | *Nov* | **Aug** | *Dec* | **Sept** |
|---|---|---|---|---|---|---|---|---|---|---|---|---|---|---|---|---|---|---|---|---|---|---|---|
| 1 | 8 | 1 | 8 | 1 | 6 | 1 | 6 | 1 | 5 | 1 | 8 | 1 | 7 | 1 | 8 | 1 | 8 | 1 | 8 | 1 | 8 | 1 | 7 |
| 2 | 9 | 2 | 9 | 2 | 7 | 2 | 7 | 2 | 6 | 2 | 9 | 2 | 8 | 2 | 9 | 2 | 9 | 2 | 9 | 2 | 9 | 2 | 8 |
| 3 | 10 | 3 | 10 | 3 | 8 | 3 | 8 | 3 | 7 | 3 | 10 | 3 | 9 | 3 | 10 | 3 | 10 | 3 | 10 | 3 | 10 | 3 | 9 |
| 4 | 11 | 4 | 11 | 4 | 9 | 4 | 9 | 4 | 8 | 4 | 11 | 4 | 10 | 4 | 11 | 4 | 11 | 4 | 11 | 4 | 11 | 4 | 10 |
| 5 | 12 | 5 | 12 | 5 | 10 | 5 | 10 | 5 | 9 | 5 | 12 | 5 | 11 | 5 | 12 | 5 | 12 | 5 | 12 | 5 | 12 | 5 | 11 |
| 6 | 13 | 6 | 13 | 6 | 11 | 6 | 11 | 6 | 10 | 6 | 13 | 6 | 12 | 6 | 13 | 6 | 13 | 6 | 13 | 6 | 13 | 6 | 12 |
| 7 | 14 | 7 | 14 | 7 | 12 | 7 | 12 | 7 | 11 | 7 | 14 | 7 | 13 | 7 | 14 | 7 | 14 | 7 | 14 | 7 | 14 | 7 | 13 |
| 8 | 15 | 8 | 15 | 8 | 13 | 8 | 13 | 8 | 12 | 8 | 15 | 8 | 14 | 8 | 15 | 8 | 15 | 8 | 15 | 8 | 15 | 8 | 14 |
| 9 | 16 | 9 | 16 | 9 | 14 | 9 | 14 | 9 | 13 | 9 | 16 | 9 | 15 | 9 | 16 | 9 | 16 | 9 | 16 | 9 | 16 | 9 | 15 |
| 10 | 17 | 10 | 17 | 10 | 15 | 10 | 15 | 10 | 14 | 10 | 17 | 10 | 16 | 10 | 17 | 10 | 17 | 10 | 17 | 10 | 17 | 10 | 16 |
| 11 | 18 | 11 | 18 | 11 | 16 | 11 | 16 | 11 | 15 | 11 | 18 | 11 | 17 | 11 | 18 | 11 | 18 | 11 | 18 | 11 | 18 | 11 | 17 |
| 12 | 19 | 12 | 19 | 12 | 17 | 12 | 17 | 12 | 16 | 12 | 19 | 12 | 18 | 12 | 19 | 12 | 19 | 12 | 19 | 12 | 19 | 12 | 18 |
| 13 | 20 | 13 | 20 | 13 | 18 | 13 | 18 | 13 | 17 | 13 | 20 | 13 | 19 | 13 | 20 | 13 | 20 | 13 | 20 | 13 | 20 | 13 | 19 |
| 14 | 21 | 14 | 21 | 14 | 19 | 14 | 19 | 14 | 18 | 14 | 21 | 14 | 20 | 14 | 21 | 14 | 21 | 14 | 21 | 14 | 21 | 14 | 20 |
| 15 | 22 | 15 | 22 | 15 | 20 | 15 | 20 | 15 | 19 | 15 | 22 | 15 | 21 | 15 | 22 | 15 | 22 | 15 | 22 | 15 | 22 | 15 | 21 |
| 16 | 23 | 16 | 23 | 16 | 21 | 16 | 21 | 16 | 20 | 16 | 23 | 16 | 22 | 16 | 23 | 16 | 23 | 16 | 23 | 16 | 23 | 16 | 22 |
| 17 | 24 | 17 | 24 | 17 | 22 | 17 | 22 | 17 | 21 | 17 | 24 | 17 | 23 | 17 | 24 | 17 | 24 | 17 | 24 | 17 | 24 | 17 | 23 |
| 18 | 25 | 18 | 25 | 18 | 23 | 18 | 23 | 18 | 22 | 18 | 25 | 18 | 24 | 18 | 25 | 18 | 25 | 18 | 25 | 18 | 25 | 18 | 24 |
| 19 | 26 | 19 | 26 | 19 | 24 | 19 | 24 | 19 | 23 | 19 | 26 | 19 | 25 | 19 | 26 | 19 | 26 | 19 | 26 | 19 | 26 | 19 | 25 |
| 20 | 27 | 20 | 27 | 20 | 25 | 20 | 25 | 20 | 24 | 20 | 27 | 20 | 26 | 20 | 27 | 20 | 27 | 20 | 27 | 20 | 27 | 20 | 26 |
| 21 | 28 | 21 | 28 | 21 | 26 | 21 | 26 | 21 | 25 | 21 | 28 | 21 | 27 | 21 | 28 | 21 | 28 | 21 | 28 | 21 | 28 | 21 | 27 |
| 22 | 29 | 22 | 29 | 22 | 27 | 22 | 27 | 22 | 26 | 22 | 29 | 22 | 28 | 22 | 29 | 22 | 29 | 22 | 29 | 22 | 29 | 22 | 28 |
| 23 | 30 | 23 | 30 | 23 | 28 | 23 | 28 | 23 | 27 | 23 | 30 | 23 | 29 | 23 | 30 | 23 | 30 | 23 | 30 | 23 | 30 | 23 | 29 |
| 24 | 31 | ——Dec. | | 24 | 29 | 24 | 29 | 24 | 28 | 24 | 31 | 24 | 30 | 24 | 31 | ——July | | 24 | 31 | 24 | 31 | 24 | 30 |
| ——Nov. | | 24 | 1 | 25 | 30 | 25 | 30 | ——Mar. | | ——Apr. | | ——May | | ——June | | 24 | 1 | ——Aug. | | ——Sept. | | ——Oct. | |
| 25 | 1 | 25 | 2 | 26 | 31 | 26 | 31 | 25 | 1 | 25 | 1 | 25 | 1 | 25 | 1 | 25 | 2 | 25 | 1 | 25 | 1 | 25 | 1 |
| 26 | 2 | 26 | 3 | ——Jan. | | ——Feb. | | 26 | 2 | 26 | 2 | 26 | 2 | 26 | 2 | 26 | 3 | 26 | 2 | 26 | 2 | 26 | 2 |
| 27 | 3 | 27 | 4 | 27 | 1 | 27 | 1 | 27 | 3 | 27 | 3 | 27 | 3 | 27 | 3 | 27 | 4 | 27 | 3 | 27 | 3 | 27 | 3 |
| 28 | 4 | 28 | 5 | 28 | 2 | 28 | 2 | 28 | 4 | 28 | 4 | 28 | 4 | 28 | 4 | 28 | 5 | 28 | 4 | 28 | 4 | 28 | 4 |
| 29 | 5 | 29 | 6 | 29 | 3 | 29 | 3 | 29 | 5 | 29 | 5 | 29 | 5 | 29 | 5 | 29 | 6 | 29 | 5 | 29 | 5 | 29 | 5 |
| 30 | 6 | | | 30 | 4 | 30 | 4 | 30 | 6 | 30 | 6 | 30 | 6 | 30 | 6 | 30 | 7 | 30 | 6 | 30 | 6 | 30 | 6 |
| 31 | 7 | | | 31 | 5 | | | 31 | 7 | | | 31 | 7 | 31 | 7 | | | 31 | 7 | | | 31 | 7 |

This chart was compiled by Dr. Herman N. Bundesen, President, Chicago Board of Health.

## THE CARE OF THE PREGNANT WOMAN

***Visiting Your Doctor.*** This is of the utmost importance. The proper care of the prospective mother during the whole of her pregnancy is as important as is her care during labor and delivery. The physician she selects to care for her during her pregnancy may be a general practitioner or an obstetrician. In either case, the expectant mother should visit the physician at least once a month for the first five or six months, every two weeks for the next two months, and once a week the last month. She brings her urine specimen along at every visit, for examination. Through these regular visits, the physician can keep a careful watch over the development of the pregnancy, and give indispensable care and advice for its success.

## DANGER SIGNALS DURING PREGNANCY

If any of the following symptoms arise at any time during pregnancy, do not lose any time in notifying your doctor.

1. Increase in frequency of nausea and vomiting.
2. Severe headaches associated with dizziness.
3. Specks floating before the eyes.
4. Puffiness of the face, especially around the eyelids.
5. Swelling of the feet, ankles, or hands.
6. Increase in desire to urinate, with the passing of only small amounts.
7. Twitching of the muscles of the face.
8. Sudden appearance of fever.
9. Shortness of breath when not exercising especially.
10. Sudden failure to feel the baby's movements after they have once been felt.

These symptoms, either singly or with one or more present, may or may not mean anything, but it is wise to stay on the safe side by reporting what you note to your doctor.

Avoidance of infection, which is always important, becomes even more so during pregnancy. If infection occurs, the welfare and often the life of both mother and child may be endangered. In a pregnant woman, the course of most infections becomes more severe. Even minor infections, if occurring near the time of confinement, may cause blood poisoning. A single condition—rheumatoid arthritis—considered infectious, is an exception to the rule in that it temporarily is benefited by pregnancy. There is no clear explanation for this.

Colds and sore throat are a menace to the pregnant woman. They always carry the threat of pneumonia, which is particularly dangerous during pregnancy. It is therefore best for the pregnant woman not to mingle in large crowds, especially during the winter months. It is also important to avoid fatigue and emotional strain. If, in spite of precautions, an infection does take place, she should make every effort to shorten its duration by remaining in bed. The physician can provide treatment that will also help.

## RULES FOR GOOD HEALTH

***Sexual Intercourse during Pregnancy.*** This should be completely avoided during the last six weeks. If intercourse is engaged in up to the beginning of labor, infection may follow. Between the third and fifth months there is no medical objection to intercourse in moderation, provided the wife is agreeable.

***Avoidance of Indigestion.*** Indigestion is caused by poor eating habits, too many sweets, heavy fried food, poor teeth, fatigue, constipation, and worry. The best treatment is to find the cause and correct it.

***Attitude of Mind.*** A happy prenatal period, free from worry and following a normal routine, is of importance. The mental state of the pregnant woman is often subject to change; that is one of the symptoms of her condition. Her character may seem altered, and she may become irritable and somewhat suspicious. A cheerful habit of mind should be cultivated, and the cares incident to business, social or educational matters should be avoided as much as possible. Unnatural mental states more often appear in the middle period of pregnancy. They call for the attention of a physician.

***What Exercise to Take.*** Moderate exercise is necessary. Walking is the best and safest. Vigorous exercise (swimming, bicycling, or playing tennis) should be avoided or modified according to the patient's physical condition and state of pregnancy.

***Need for Adequate Rest.*** The pregnant woman requires adequate rest to build up a reserve of energy, and to combat nervous and physical strain. A fifteen- or twenty-minute rest period during the day is advisable.

***Baths During Pregnancy.*** Skin cleanliness is very important. The pregnant woman may take warm sponge baths or tub baths, but she should be particularly careful about getting in or out of the tub. (Tub baths are usually given up during the last two weeks.)

***Need for Dental Care.*** The dentist should be visited in the prenatal period and the necessary measures carried out. There is no reason for delaying the extraction of a tooth if it is endangering the patient's health.

***Suggestions as to Clothes.*** Clothes should be comfortable, light, loose, and suspended from the shoulders. Constricting bands around the waist, or circular garters, must not be worn. Maternity clothes, attractive and adjustable, are now the rule. The patient may wear her usual girdle for the first three or four months if it can be adjusted to avoid pressure on the abdomen.

***Need for Suitable Shoes.*** These should be well fitted and comfortable, with low heels. High heels are apt to cause back strain, and there is the added danger of tripping and falling.

## SOME FALLACIES REGARDING PREGNANCY

There are many popular fallacies or mistaken beliefs regarding pregnancy. For example, it is still widely held that all pregnant women crave strange foods, and that a seven-month baby is more likely to live than an eight-month baby. Both of these beliefs are false. As for the second of them, the fact is that the nearer the term of delivery, the better the chance of survival for the fetus.

It is equally untrue that the wearing of high-heeled shoes during pregnancy may cause the child to be cross-eyed, or that three Caesarian babies is the limit any woman can have. Contrary to popular opinion, too, a woman can become pregnant while she is nursing her first child.

Many people believe that maternal impression—looking at an ugly person, or a mouse, for example—will leave its birthmark on the offspring. This contradicts the medical facts. What a woman thinks or sees cannot imprint itself physically on the child she is bearing.

## THE INCREASED DEMANDS ON NUTRITION IN THE PREGNANT WOMAN

There is sufficient evidence available to prove that poor nutrition kills more babies than does congenital syphilis!

The complex mechanisms behind the formation of the eggs in ovaries and fertilization with the sperm undoubtedly require a nicety of adjustment. The accurate timing of these momentous details are particularly dependent upon the environment in which they occur. Many investigators in the role of nutrition in pregnancy have stressed the importance of nutritional balance when trying to become pregnant, as well as in pregnancy. In rats, for example, congenital malformations can be induced by nutritional deficiency. One group of investigators were able to show, by X-ray, bony changes in the hand and foot in the development of the embryo in relationship to the calcium and protein intake of the mother. Various other workers have shown that the deciduous teeth development is dependent upon the prenatal diet of the mother. It is obvious that a patient's tissues on borderline of adequacy will become deficient when she becomes pregnant if her eating habits remain unchanged.

***Mortality among the Newborn.*** The main causes of the frequency of mortality among the newborn are prematurity and congenital debility, or weakness at birth. A baby born to a mother who is in a run-down condition will start life without reserves. The diets of many of our American women have too frequently deteriorated to coffee and a sweet roll for breakfast and a cup of soup and a sandwich for lunch. The National Research Council, analyzing the diets of a large group of women, found that only 10 per cent met all requirements and could be termed good, 40 per cent were fair, and 50 per cent were poor.

It is logical to suppose that large reserves might protect the embryo during the first and most critical periods of its development when the mother's reserves may be depleted by the loss of appetite and vomiting. Many patients during this period have difficulty in taking food or even retaining it. This too may happen to the supplemental vitamins prescribed for them.

## Underfeeding and Overweight

The pregnant woman's meals must be carefully planned, then, so that all essentials of a balanced diet are retained. It is too often taken for granted that an overweight patient must of necessity be well nourished. This, of course, is far from true. Life insurance and medical statistics show that overweight persons may be more poorly nourished on account of their unbalanced diet and that their overloaded machine breaks down, years before it needs to, with "burned-out bearings" of heart and kidney disease.

The amount of weight a patient should gain during pregnancy

will depend on the degree of nausea during the first three months and the weight level when pregnancy began. The average patient loses from twenty to twenty-five pounds in the six weeks following delivery.

***Psychiatry and Pregnancy.*** It is now claimed by some physicians that psychiatry may be helpful in controlling some of these difficult problems. A psychiatrist may be helpful in coping with some of the appetites of pregnancy or distaste for food. A combination of methods may be necessary just as it is in the control of overindulgence of alcohol. The psychiatric approach may find its place just as it is now doing in the care of children. After all, many of the problems are just grown-up feeding problems of childhood.

## DIET IN PREGNANCY

We see, then, that not only is the well-being of the mother preserved and improved by good nutrition, but the child's chances of survival and health are greatly increased. The diet should be simple, nourishing and easily digestible.

Studies of the diets of nursing mothers have indicated that when the diet of the mother falls below a certain minimum, her milk will be inadequate in quality and especially in quantity. Yet a word of caution is necessary with regard to the not uncommon practice of overfeeding patients in an effort to stimulate milk production. Many examples of obesity in women during pregnancy are attributable to such ill-advised attempts at overfeeding.

### The Balanced Diet

A balanced diet is extremely important, as ever. The pregnant woman should have a full quota of proteins, fats, carbohydrates and minerals. The heightened bodily processes of the pregnant woman and the demands of the growing fetus render her dietary requirements different from, and on the whole greater than, those of other adults. The diet must be rich in fruits and vegetables, but even this does not insure a proper intake of vitamins and minerals, since during pregnancy the requirements for protein, minerals, and vitamins may be increased 100 per cent or more.

The fetus acquires two-thirds of its total birth weight in the last three months of pregnancy, two-thirds of its calcium, four-fifths of its iron, three-fourths of its protein, and over ninety per cent of its fat. It is during this period that the serious effects of malnutrition are most likely to appear in the mother if she does not eat properly.

***Mineral Requirements.*** To be healthy, the mature human body must be richer in calcium than in any other mineral element; yet every child is born calcium-poor and iron-rich. The calcium poverty facilitates birth in that the bones are then soft. On the other hand, pregnancy usually results in a depletion of the mother's body calcium.

Pregnancy, then, considerably increases the requirement of calcium. Enough must be supplied to meet both normal adult needs and the demand of the growing fetus. If the dietary supply is inadequate, the skeleton of the fetus will develop at the expense of the mineral content of the mother's bones and teeth. Deficiency may lead to mild or latent tetany in the mother. The main reliance should be placed on green vegetables and milk. Plenty of sunlight or vitamin D (or both) is necessary to insure the greatest possible use of calcium in the diet.

Phosphorus is as essential a dietary element as calcium, but the danger of deficiency is less. A normal intake of meat, fish, eggs and dairy products should insure a good supply. The iodine needs are also higher, and can be met by the use of iodized salt. This is particularly important in areas where the soil lacks iodine, even in the small amount that is necessary for man. Iron is an essential constituent of the human body, and should be available in sufficient quantity in a good diet. The salt and fluid intake should be watched in pregnancy. Extreme salt restriction is ordinarily unnecessary, but sodium intake should be only moderate, since excess leads to fluid retention and swelling.

***Over-all Vitamin Requirements.*** The requirements for all the known vitamins and particularly those of the B complex are increased during pregnancy.

***Vitamin A.*** Vitamin A is essential for normal reproduction and milk production, as well as for resistance to infection. The required amounts may be obtained by the daily consumption of a quart of milk, one egg, one ounce of cheese, one or two servings of green leafy vegetables, and a teaspoonful of cod-liver oil. Carrots and butter are other good sources. In women deficient in vitamin A, maternal deaths have been found to be more than four times as great as in those on a vitamin-A-rich diet.

***Vitamin B Complex.*** The members of the B family of vitamins are all-important in the proper functioning of the human body. The need for the B complex as a whole is much increased in pregnancy.

Its importance in this condition is shown by the scientific evidence that animals completely deprived of it during the first half of pregnancy invariably have abortions.

***Thiamine.*** Thiamine, found in almost all plants, is essential for metabolism and growth. Pork and dried brewer's yeast are good sources. To be sure of an adequate supply of thiamine, include whole-grain breads and cereals, milk, dried beans and peas in the daily diet. Symptoms frequently noted in pregnancy which may indicate a relative lack of vitamins are fatigue, poor appetite, indigestion, nausea or vomiting, disturbed bowel function, palpitation, frequency of urination, shortness of breath, headache, or backache. Proper diet will improve these conditions if they are nutritional in origin.

***Folic Acid.*** The average diet is unlikely to be lacking in folic acid if salads and raw fruits are included. This member of the B complex is best known for its curative effects in certain anemias. It has a maturing effect on the cells of the bone marrow, and plays an essential role in body activity.

***Vitamin C.*** The need for vitamin C is considerably increased during pregnancy, the fetus acting, so to say, as a parasite in this regard. An adequate amount of vitamin C can be supplied by five ounces of unstrained orange juice, or by generous amounts of foods rich in this vitamin (tomatoes, grapefruit, raw cabbage, leafy green vegetables, and potatoes cooked in their skins).

***Vitamin D.*** The need for vitamin D is greater in pregnancy and milk production (lactation) than in any other period after the first year of life. An adequate intake of this vitamin is necessary for the proper absorption of calcium and phosphorus, and for their proper utilization by the bones and other tissues. Because vitamin D is contained in only a few of the foods in the average diet, and only in small quantities, the requisite daily allowance must be provided by some form of vitamin supplement.

***Vitamin E.*** There is a great deal of scientific evidence that a vitamin E deficiency may be one factor in recurrent abortion.

***Vitamin K.*** A vitamin which assumes great importance as pregnancy draws to its close is vitamin K, the anti-hemorrhagic vitamin. Its value is less to the mother (whose diet will usually be high enough in K for her own needs, due to its extensive distribution in natural foods) than to the child, which possesses virtually no vitamin K during the first weeks of life. Hemorrhagic disease of the newborn is associated with this vitamin lack, and it is now common practice to guard against it by administering vitamin K (about 2 milligrams daily) during the last weeks of pregnancy, or just before or during delivery.

***Protein Requirements.*** Protein of high biologic value, in adequate amounts, is essential for the health of a pregnant woman. Milk and lean meat are good sources. The fetal mortality is significantly lowered when the mother's diet has been high in protein throughout pregnancy.

## RECOMMENDED DIET FOR PREGNANCY

*Fruits.* Orange, grapefruit, or tomato juice, one glass (six ounces) daily. Fresh fruit in season, one serving daily. Stewed prunes, apricots, peaches, applesauce or prune juice, once daily, in addition to the aforementioned.

*Vegetables.* Two cupfuls of cooked vegetables daily. Fresh green leafy vegetables and other highly colored vegetables in the form of salads: one cup in amount, using any dressing desired—once daily.

*Fats.* Butter, three squares daily, or not more than two tablespoonfuls of oil.

*Cereals.* Any of the whole-grain cereals, either hot or cold, at least two servings daily. One piece of whole-wheat bread may be substituted for one serving of cereal.

*Eggs.* At least two or three daily—more if desired.

*Meats.* At least nine ounces daily of lean meat, fish, chicken, turkey, and particularly liver and other organ meats.

*Cheese.* At least one and one-half ounces daily (no cream cheese).

*Milk.* Three glasses daily are sufficient.

*Bread.* Whole-wheat; no more than three slices daily.

*Desserts.* Jello, junket, custards, fruits and fruit-whips.

*Starches.* Including potatoes, noodles, rice, spaghetti, corn, macaroni, lima beans, dry beans. One of these may be taken once daily, but not more than one and one-half tablespoonfuls.

*Heavy Desserts.* Heavy desserts, including pastries, nuts, candy, ice cream, fried foods, are not to be eaten.

*Liquids.* Do not drink more than eight glasses in twenty-four hours. (This is to include all milk, water, fruit juices, soup, coffee, tea, cocoa or any other liquid.)

The caloric value of this diet depends upon the manner of preparation and the degree of adherence to the exact amounts indicated.

It is very important in later months of pregnancy that six small meals be eaten rather than two or three large ones.

## SAMPLE MENU FOR PREGNANCY DIET

*Breakfast.* Fruit, two eggs, one-half piece toast, beverage.

*Mid-morning.* One-half cup oatmeal, one-half glass milk, prunes.

*Lunch.* Three ounces cooked meat, fish, poultry; one cup of two vegetables; one-half cup of salad greens; one-half glass milk.

*Mid-afternoon.* Two ounces cheese—cottage or cheddar variety; one-half piece bread, one-half glass milk.

*Dinner.* Three ounces cooked meat, one cup of two vegetables, one-half cup salad greens, simple dessert, one glass milk.

*Before Bedtime.* One egg, one glass milk, one-half slice bread.

Remember, there is as great danger in overweight as there is in underweight.

## READY FOR THE HOSPITAL

The bag containing all the necessary articles for both the prospective mother and the baby should be packed at least ten days before the date of the expected arrival of the baby. It should contain

***For the Mother***

2 bed jackets
3 nightgowns
1 kimono
1 pair comfortable slippers
1 sanitary belt
1 box Kleenex
toilet articles

***For the Baby***

2 diapers (the new kind with snappers)
1 shirt
1 abdominal binder
2 blankets
1 bunting
1 gown or kimono
stockings

## LABOR

The woman whose first baby is coming into the world entertains many misconceptions about labor pains, the use and effects of anesthesia, and other proceedings that may or may not occur during the entire process of labor. She should realize, first of all, that childbirth is a normal process. If she has been under a physician's care during her pregnancy, has followed his advice faithfully, and her pregnancy has run a normal course, she has nothing to fear.

At the beginning of labor, the location of the pains is usually vague and more or less resembles a mild intestinal colic, or gas in the bowel. If it is the calculated time for delivery, before calling the doctor, she should watch the clock in order to get the exact frequency of the pains. If the pains gradually extend toward the back and resemble a real backache, they are more likely to be from the womb than from any intestinal cause. At first the true labor pains occur about every half-hour, gradually increasing in frequency.

If the abdomen is not too fat, a good test for true womb contractions is to place the palm of the hand over the most dependent part of the abdomen and wait for a pain to come. The uterine contractions can then be felt as a sort of hardening of the muscles. This may be misleading, as a bowel contraction may give a similar sensation, but it is worth noting before calling the doctor. If you now call your doctor he will probably tell you to go to the hospital when the pains occur every five to ten minutes.

### Entering the Hospital

So you now go to the hospital promptly. You are shown to your room. Here is what follows in a well-regulated hospital. You are put to bed, your temperature is taken, a specimen of urine is sent to the laboratory and you are shaved. It is curious that this procedure should disturb most women. Maybe it is the extensive paraphernalia, brought in on a large tray, that you might mistake for a sign of some emergency that is being kept from you. But, for aseptic precautions, all the hair of the external sexual organs must be removed. Next you get an enema, which is also necessary.

### The Examination

You are now taken to the examining room. You may walk if you prefer, but do not become frightened if a cart is brought to roll you in. If your own doctor has not yet arrived, you may be examined by the resident obstetrician. You are first prepared by thorough cleansing of the genitals with soap and water, then some mild antiseptic solution. The examiner wears sterile rubber gloves. The examination is for the purpose of learning just how far labor has progressed. This is determined by the extent of the dilation of the mouth of the womb, also by whether or not the "bag of water" has ruptured, which you may or may not have noted.

After this examination there is seldom another. Depending upon the degree of dilation, and the frequency and severity of the pains, you may be taken back to your bed or taken into the delivery room. If the latter, then you are further prepared locally and sterile leggings are put on.

### Relaxing for Delivery

As the pains increase in severity you are told to put into use the relaxation procedures in which you should have been instructed. If you have had no such instruction, then you are given enough anesthetic to take off the edge of the pain. If you have become proficient in relaxing, then you will need little or no anesthetic, but in any case you are not allowed to suffer unduly. Remember that muscular tension has an undesirable effect on the accomplishment of natural spontaneous childbirth.

When the bearing-down stage is reached, you are told when and when not to bring into play the voluntary muscles. Again, you will probably be given a light anesthesia, just enough to relieve the pain, but rarely enough to produce unconsciousness. Above all, have confidence in your physician and in all those around you.

Your cooperation with your obstetrician will make deep anesthesia unnecessary and you will then be able to get that glorious thrill of your baby's first cry. You will be kept upon the delivery table until the afterbirth (placenta) is delivered. This usually takes place in about twenty minutes. Do not worry about this as it is quite painless.

## CONVALESCENCE FROM CHILDBIRTH

Nowadays the mother is gotten out of bed on the third day after childbirth and sent home from the hospital on the fifth day. However, she should not immediately take up her household duties again, but should get plenty of rest at home.

To suddenly put a strain on her overstretched organs may cause a descent of the uterus. Therefore it is most desirable to be conservative and go back to one's routine gradually. In this period of adjustment, the mother should have someone to assist her in the care of the new baby and the home.

## SPONTANEOUS ABORTION AND MISCARRIAGE

Abortion and miscarriage are often confused. Here we use these terms in their medical sense, which applies when these conditions occur spontaneously or accidentally, and are not brought on intentionally. We ought also to explain, before going further, that the unborn child, up through the third month, is called an embryo; after the third month it is called a fetus. In an abortion, the embryo is expelled. In a miscarriage, the fetus and the afterbirth are expelled.

Bleeding and pain are the outstanding symptoms of these conditions, and vary according to the stage of pregnancy. In the early stages, pain is intense and bleeding is usually not excessive. In late miscarriage, there is usually less bleeding and more pain, since there is a fetus to be expelled, and there is a complete afterbirth which tends to remain attached until after the birth of the fetus.

The varieties of abortion and miscarriage are as follows:

***Threatened.*** Often the pains and bleeding subside and the pregnancy continues to full time. However, when membranes rupture and the water which surrounds the fetus escapes, abortion is inevitable. Hemorrhage is likely to be profuse, pains continue, and the mouth of the womb spreads.

***Complete.*** When the embryo is expelled entirely.

***Incomplete.*** When the fetus is expelled, but the afterbirth and membranes which cover the fetus, in part or wholly so, remain.

***Treatment of Abortion.*** At the first evidence of warning signs, such as bleeding, no matter how slight, dragging backache, sense of weight in the pelvis, and cramplike pains, the patient should go to bed. A physician should be summoned at once. He will administer hypodermic injections and decide whether or not the abortion is inevitable.

## REASONS FOR INTERRUPTING PREGNANCY

There is no justifiable cause for interrupting pregnancy save when its existence threatens the mother's life. This may occur in certain circumstances. Even then a consultation of reputable physicians is advisable to determine upon such a grave and important step. The only course open to a woman who fears pregnancy is to wait. If she is not pregnant, time will prove it, and no harm will have been done by waiting. If she is pregnant, that also will become evident, and no harm will have been done. There is no reason for hasty action in such an event, and every reason for waiting for time to reveal the true condition.

***Criminal Abortion.*** There is no drug or other means known to the medical profession by which it is possible for a woman to bring on a miscarriage without greatly endangering her life. This is entirely apart from the ethical and legal aspects. Even if the patient is but a week pregnant, there is the same difficulty in causing a harmless abortion, the same danger to the patient's life, and the same degree of crime. Persons who perform abortions are usually as incompetent as they are criminal. All too frequently blood poisoning and death of the patient result. The very secrecy required is, of itself, sufficient to prevent the abortionist from giving the patient proper care, even if he were competent to give it.

## CHAPTER 13

# STERILITY AND HOW IT IS TREATED

**Meaning of Sterility and Infertility . . . Conditions Required for Conception to Take Place . . . The Fertile Period . . . Causes of Sterility . . . Physical Defects That Prevent Conception . . . Treatment of Sterility . . . The Male Must Be Examined . . . Help Afforded by Hormones and Surgery . . . The Role of Vitamin E in Preventing Abortion . . . Psychiatric Treatment Aids Some Cases . . . Two Types of Endocrine Treatment, etc.**

STERILITY means that one is unable to produce a living child. Some women never conceive; others conceive, but are unable to carry the child to an age where life after birth may be expected. Still others who have given birth to a child cease to be fruitful. Sterility is considered primary when the woman has never been pregnant. It is considered secondary when she has borne a child and then becomes sterile. Temporary sterility generally occurs during the milk-producing period, and as a result of serious illnesses. The term infertility is often used to denote the inability on the part of a woman to give birth to a child capable of living outside the womb.

***Fertility.*** Fertility is dependent on the deposit of healthy spermatozoa in a normal vagina. The mouth of the womb and the womb itself must be in a state favorable for the transmission of spermatozoa, and the lining of the womb must be in a suitable condition for embedding the ovum or egg. The ovaries must produce ova and function normally, and the Fallopian tubes must offer no obstruction to the passage of healthy ova. There must also be normal secretions in both the man and the woman, with biochemical reactions which are not incompatible. The ovaries must, of course, produce healthy ova. A failing in any of these factors may result in sterility, and in an effort to solve the question, they must all be tested methodically.

The period of fertility is commonly measured by the length of menstrual life, but there are exceptions on record where women long past the menopause have borne children. Menstruation is not absolutely essential to conception, for many women conceive while suckling a child, even though menstruation has not begun again since its birth.

## CAUSES OF STERILITY

It has been estimated that some 12 per cent of marriages are involuntarily childless. The causes of sterility include physical defects, prolonged use of contraceptives, venereal diseases, and the various psychological stresses of modern life.

Formerly, the investigation and treatment of sterility centered almost solely on the wife. Lately, it has become increasingly obvious that in one-third to one-half of barren unions the husband is responsible for the state of affairs. The woman usually accepts the suggestion that she is at fault and is willing to submit to everything to remove the stigma, if stigma it is. Frequently the man refuses to listen to the suggestion that the responsibility may possibly be his. Often he refuses to submit himself for examination.

A great proportion of women who are sterile have defects in development. These are total or partial absence of genital organs; imperfect development of the ovaries; arrested development of the tubes or womb, or both; bent or displaced womb; and closure of the mouth of the womb. Acquired defects which prevent conception are usually the result of inflammation in the pelvis, which may close or distort the tubes. There are in addition many other causes, some of which have already been suggested.

Another little-known cause of sterility in women is increased acidity of the vaginal secretion. Spermatozoa are quickly killed in an acid medium. Therefore the chemical reaction of the vaginal secretion must be determined. The treatment for this is douching with lime water before coitus.

## TREATMENT OF STERILITY

A careful consideration of all the conditions that contribute to sterility should make the diagnosis definite. The diagnosis obtained in the examination of sterile couples will suggest the method or methods of treatment. Treatment should always begin by an examination of the male member of the marriage, to discover possible abnormal genital conditions, and to test for the presence or absence of live spermatozoa. After a thorough physical examination, especially a pelvic one in the woman, other special tests are made. One consists of determining whether the tubes are open. This is done by blowing oxygen or carbon dioxide gas through them under low pressure.

***Other Helpful Treatment for the Woman.*** Another effective measure is treatment of the mouth of the womb, if there is an abnormality there, and, when necessary, reconstructive surgery. In addition, if necessary, the patient should try treatment with estrogens, gonadotropins, thyroid and iodine; general medical treatment, where that is indicated; administration, before the menstrual period, of large

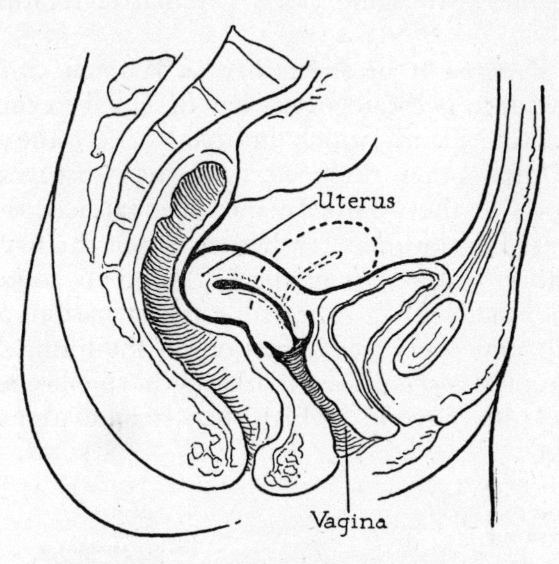


DISPLACED UTERUS

This cross section of the female sex organs shows, with broken lines, the normal position of the uterus or womb. The uterus that is labeled in the diagram is displaced or tilted backward toward the rectum—a condition often responsible for sterility—instead of forward toward the bladder. The small passage to the right of the vagina is the urethra.

doses of progestin, and removal of tumors; also, use of dietary supplements.

The absence, inadequacy, or faulty utilization of vitamin E may be a factor in repeated abortions. A temporary lack of vitamin E may produce a single abortion which does not occur again. The administration of wheat germ oil gives good results with a large number of women.

Another vitamin of great importance, toward the end of pregnancy, is vitamin K—the anti-bleeding vitamin. It is of greater importance to the child than the mother. During the first weeks of life the child possesses almost no vitamin K, and bleeding disease of the newborn is associated with this condition. It has become common practice to guard against this tendency by giving vitamin K during the last weeks of pregnancy or just before or during delivery.

Sometimes, when no physical cause of sterility can be found, the trouble is a psychological one. Rest and avoidance of tension are then recommended. In some cases, psychiatric treatment may be helpful.

***Endocrine Treatment of Infertility in Women.*** Such treatment may be divided into two categories: one designed to correct disturbances of endocrine glands which indirectly affect the reproductive processes, and the other designed to correct disturbances wholly within the ovary or the womb. In specific treatment the first factor which the physician considers is whether or not the maturing of the follicle, ovulation (formation of the egg), and its consequences are taking place normally. Data concerning menstruation, together with those obtained from special examinations of the lining of the womb, vaginal smears, and tests of the circulating hormones, all help in arriving at a definite diagnosis, which then suggests the specific treatment required.

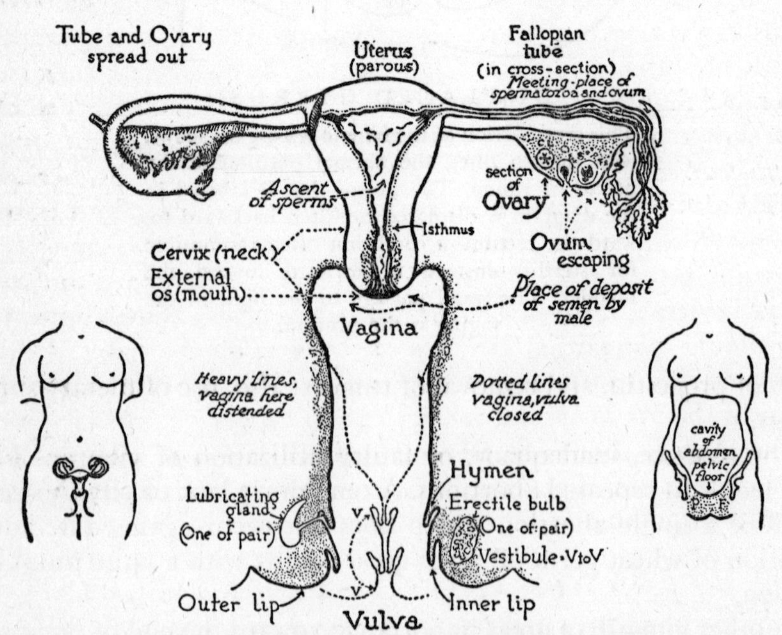


FEMALE REPRODUCTIVE SYSTEM

For conception, a spermatozoön or sperm cell must fuse with an egg; this takes place in one of the two Fallopian tubes, and is called fertilization.

CHAPTER 14

# CARE OF THE INFANT AND CHILD

**The Nursery . . . Clothes to Prepare for Baby . . . How to Diaper a Baby . . . Techniques of Breast and Bottle Feeding . . . Facts About Formulas . . . Preparing the Day's Feeding . . . Solid Foods . . . Diet Up to Third Year . . . Feeding the Sick Baby . . . Important Facts in Food Preparation . . . Teething and Care of the Teeth . . . When Children Cry . . . Bathing and Cleanliness . . . Toilet Training . . . The Baby's Sleep . . . Taking the Baby Outside . . . When to Immunize Your Child . . . Booster Doses and Reimmunization . . . Baby's and Child's Weight and Rate of Growth.**

## THE NURSERY

EVERY CHILD ought, if possible, to have his own room. The nursery should be well screened. The crib should be in a corner protected from drafts. In winter, it is wise to keep a pan of water on the radiator to prevent the air in the room from becoming too dry.

Two great mistakes in city homes are these: using excessive clothing for infants and having the room too warm. These often predispose to skin irritation and rashes. Indeed, overheating the room is just as harmful as underheating. It is best to keep the temperature of the nursery about 70° F.; if the baby is weak, 78° or even 80° is better. At night, during the first few weeks, the temperature of the room should not be below 65° F. After one month the night temperature may go as low as 55° F. and after six months to 50° or even 45° F.

*Fresh Air.* Parents are often fanatical in their ideas about fresh air. Some overdo it; some underdo it. Just remember one thing: Fresh air is not necessarily cold air. The air in the baby's room should always be fresh. This is accomplished by correct ventilation. At no time should a stream of air blow directly upon the baby. A simple glass ventilator can be had very cheaply. The use of this makes regulation of the air in the room very easy.

The nursery should be aired at least twice a day, after the infant is one month old. This should be carried out completely, while the infant is in another room.

## CLOTHES AND OTHER ARTICLES TO PREPARE FOR BABY

The mother should prepare the following clothes and articles for the baby:

2 dozen diapers of soft cotton material
6 shirts, preferably of a cotton and wool mixture. If the weather is hot, pure cotton shirts are preferable.
6 cotton or cotton and wool nightgowns
4 to 6 dresses and slips
2 light and 2 heavier blankets
6 cotton pads for the bed
6 crib sheets
2 rubber sheets
6 bathing towels
6 soft face cloths
1 dozen safety pins
Bathing articles (soap, oil, powder, absorbent cotton, boric acid)
Crib
Bathinette

The best material for diapers is bird's eye cotton cloth. It is absorbent and non-irritating. Disposable paper diapers are a great convenience. There are now available diapers that have snappers, thus completely doing away with safety pins.

## HOW TO DIAPER A BABY

There are at least two ways of diapering an infant. In the first method, the diaper is folded triangularly. The infant is placed on this, the base of the triangle being at his waist-line and the apex pointing downward between the legs. The three points of the triangle are then brought together and pinned flat to the front of the baby's undershirt.

A second method is to fold the diaper so that it forms an oblong, placing the infant's waist over the short end, the length of the diaper being between the legs. This long part is then brought up between the legs and the corners of the diaper are flat to the sides of the infant's undershirt. The oblong diaper is particularly suitable for older infants because it permits freer movements of the legs.

## BREAST AND BOTTLE FEEDING

Unless there is some valid reason to the contrary, approved by a physician, all infants should be breast-fed for the first six months. Mother's milk is superior to formulas, good though they may be. Nor need a nursing mother, in general, restrict her diet.

# Exercise at Six Months

## EXERCISES FOR FUN AND HEALTH

Even at six months, a baby enjoys exercise. Try this as a starter. Have him lie on back, legs outstretched. Let him grasp one of your fingers in each hand. Raise him gently to sitting position, lower him. Repeat.

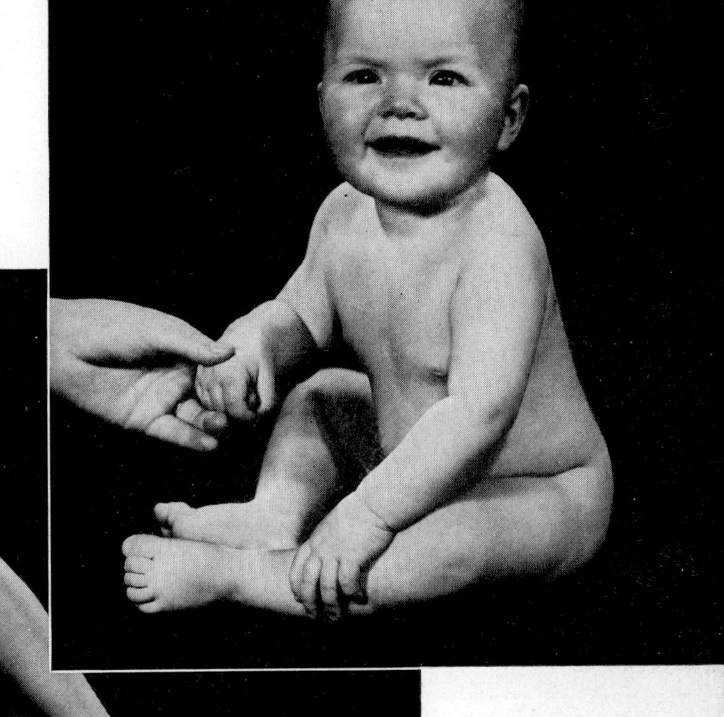

## KNEES UP

With baby lying flat on back, grasp leg below knee, bend knee gently, bringing it up toward abdomen. Straighten leg, repeat with other leg.

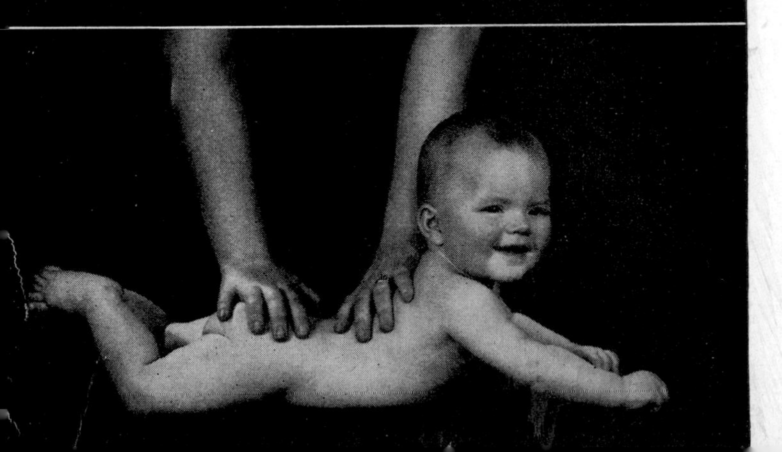

## ROLLING

Rolling baby around in bed is a simple exercise he and you will enjoy. Do exercises with baby in a spirit of playfulness, with frequent pauses.

# Exercise at One Year

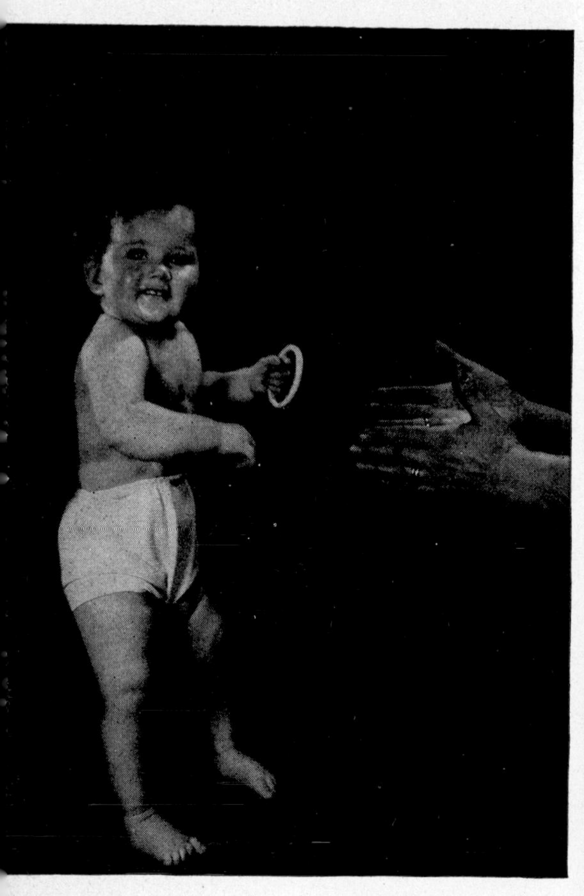

## BABY'S FIRST STEPS

*(Left)* At about twelve months, baby takes his first steps. It is a good game to have him go back and forth between parents. Reassuring hands should be extended to catch him. Equal fun can be had if baby is still in crawling stage. Pause often.

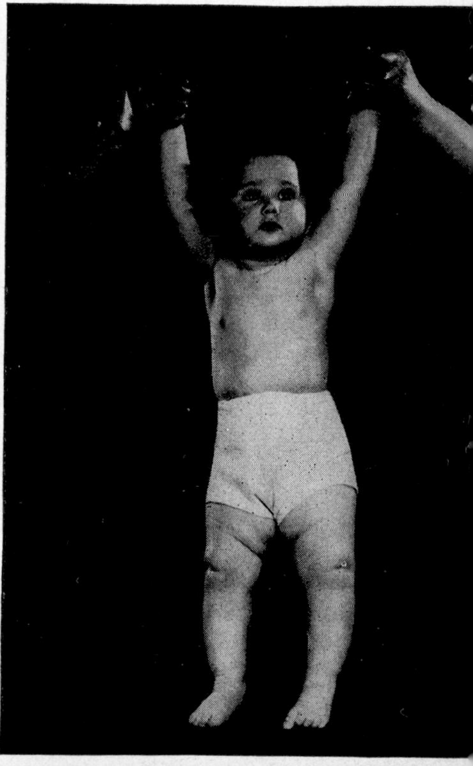

## ARMS UP – ARMS DOWN

With baby standing on table, leaning against your chest, raise his arms up, out, down. Lift him a little. Don't swing him by his hands.

## KNEE BENDING

This is similar to knee-bending exercise on preceding page, only both knees are bent at same time. With one hand on baby's chest, grasp both knees with other, press gently upward, then bring down again.

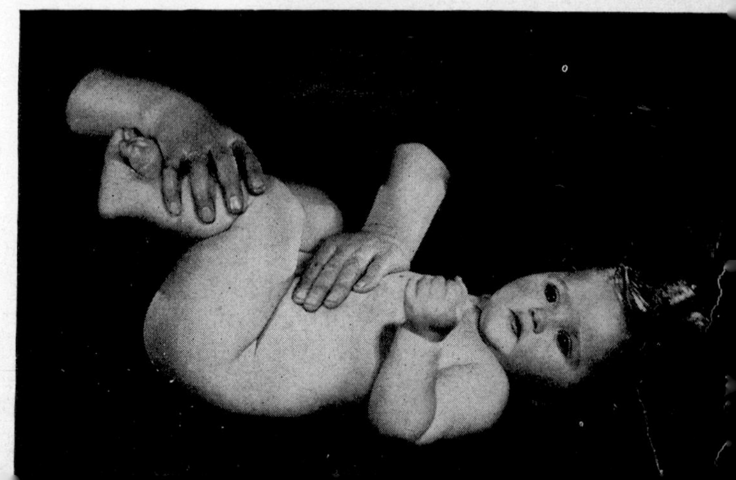

Of course, sometimes breast feeding is just not possible. The need for bottle feeding may be indicated by several conditions: if, after three or four days' trial, the mother has no milk; if, after one week or two of trial, the amount of breast milk diminishes instead of increasing; if, after one month's trial, the breast milk gives out. But an effort should be made to feed the infant by breast. If the breast milk at first appears inadequate, he should receive a bottle, which can later be discarded when the breast supply increases.

## EARLY FEEDING

The newborn baby should be put to the breast from six to ten hours after he is born, and four times during the first twenty-four hours at intervals of six hours.

Afterward, the young infant is usually fed every three hours during the day and every four hours at night, either by breast or bottle. The four-hour interval may be substituted as soon as the capacity of the infant's stomach permits. In case of bottle feeding, it is advisable to determine how much is needed daily, and then to divide it by the number of feedings adapted to the age of the child.

The usual four-hour schedule is as follows: the infant is fed at 6, 10, 2, 6, 10, and 2 o'clock, while the standard three-hour schedule calls for 6, 9, 12, 3, 6, 9, 12 and 3 o'clock as the feeding hours. The important difference between these two schedules, however, is the number of hours which elapse between feedings, and not the specific feeding hours.

It is important to follow a regular schedule in feeding. However, in many instances a "self-selection" schedule has been found to be quite workable. Under this system, the infant is fed whenever he is hungry.

## THE TECHNIQUE OF BREAST FEEDING

Before each nursing period the mother should wash her hands thoroughly with soap and water. She should then wash the breast and nipple using a clean cloth, soap and water. For the final thorough wiping, a sterile cotton pad dipped in boiled water should be used. The mother should not wash with antiseptic solutions as the baby may be affected by traces of the solution which may settle in the creases of the skin surrounding the nipple. After each nursing the breast should again be washed and covered with a clean fold of cloth held in place by a brassiere, not too tightly worn. The cloth absorbs any milk which may leak out.

If the mother has a cold, she should wear a mask while nursing the infant.

The mother should be propped up in bed or seated in a comfortable chair so that her infant rests in a semi-sitting position. This minimizes the amount of air he swallows while sucking.

If the mother has plenty of milk the baby may be offered only one breast at each feeding, alternating each time. The usual nursing period is fifteen minutes. If the supply is scanty, he may be given both breasts at each period, doubling the period and allowing him ample time to empty the first breast before giving him the second.

***Making the Baby "Burp."*** Whether a baby is breast-fed or bottle-fed, and however correctly his feedings are given, he will at some time swallow a little air. Therefore, at intervals of about four or five minutes during his feedings, as well as at the end of every feeding, the mother should lift the baby and hold him against her shoulder, his head leaning over it, and pat him gently on the back with her free hand until he belches or "burps." The mother should lay a clean cloth over her shoulder at these times, for a little of the feeding may come up with the air.

## WEANING

***When Weaning Is Necessary.*** Temporary weaning (accustoming the infant to do without the mother's milk) must be prescribed sometimes in an acute illness of the mother. Menstruation is not a warning against breast-feeding. However, a new pregnancy is a signal to wean the infant, but in this case it must be carried out gradually. Frequent emotional crisis, or any chronic disease, such as disease of heart, kidneys, rheumatism, as well as anemia or serious mental disease, is an indication to stop nursing. The syphilitic infant can safely be nursed by his mother but not by a wet nurse. In an abscess or inflammation of the breast it is usually necessary to stop nursing.

***How to Wean.*** Whenever possible, the baby should be weaned under the supervision of a physician. Sudden weaning should be avoided but, as has been indicated, it is sometimes necessary on account of a serious disease in the mother.

Weaning should be begun by substituting one feeding a day for a nursing; later two feedings are substituted, and thus gradually the child is completely weaned.

Ideally, a mother will nurse her baby as long as the infant requires it, either emotionally or from the viewpoint of nutrition. This period varies in length from three or four months to fourteen or even sixteen months. On the average, a baby is ready to be weaned somewhere between the sixth and ninth months, by which time he is enjoying solid foods and has gotten used to drinking from a bottle or perhaps even from a cup.

Doctors do not agree on whether it is wise to wean a child during the summer months. The step is determined largely by whether or not a safe milk supply can be procured. Today, owing to the protection afforded fresh milk, to the use of evaporated or dried milk, and to advanced knowledge on how to make and prepare digestible formulas, many physicians entirely disregard the weather. They advise weaning whenever the baby is ready for it.

## TECHNIQUE OF BOTTLE FEEDING

Under the heading "Breast and Bottle Feeding," we have already discussed how often the infant should be fed. The amount he takes is limited by the capacity of his stomach. The newborn infant should receive about one ounce at a feeding, at first. However, this amount may be rapidly increased to from two to four ounces in a week or ten days.

***Whole Sweet-Milk Formula.*** A simple method of preparing the formula is by diluting Grade A pasteurized milk and adding carbohydrate (sugar) in sufficient amount to meet the infant's energy requirements. The formula must be changed from time to time as these requirements vary. Your physician will supply new formulas as you need them.

An easy way of calculating the milk formula for an average healthy infant is to start with the amount of cow's milk which will furnish an adequate quantity of protein. This will be from 1½ to two ounces of milk for each pound of the infant's body weight. To this must be added enough boiled water to give a total, with the milk, of three fluid ounces per pound of body weight. For example, a well-nourished infant two months old, weighing ten pounds, will require not less than fifteen ounces of milk and fifteen ounces of water.

The daily calory requirements have been calculated at a minimum of forty-five calories per pound of the infant's weight. Each fluid ounce of milk supplies 20 calories. Each ounce of carbohydrates supplies 120 calories. The amount of carbohydrate added to the total day's feeding ranges from one ounce during the first few weeks of life to two ounces during the latter part of the first year.

The carbohydrates commonly used as additions to cow's milk are table sugar, Karo syrup, lactose (milk sugar), sucrose (cane or beet sugar) and maltose-dextrin mixtures. Dextri-maltose consists of dextrin and maltose. Two level tablespoons of table sugar or Karo syrup, three of lactose and four of dextri-maltose equal one ounce.

Schedule for Healthy Infants—First Half Year

| *Approx. Age (Months)* | *Quantity (oz.) for 24 Hours* | *Quantity (oz.) for one Feeding* | *Feedings in 24 Hours* | *Calories for 24 Hours* |
|---|---|---|---|---|
| 1 | 15-25 | 2½-4 | 6 | 300-500 |
| 2 | 20-29 | 3½-5 | 6 | 400-580 |
| 3 | 24-32 | 4½-6½ | 5 | 480-650 |
| 4 | 28-35 | 5½-7 | 5 | 560-700 |
| 5 | 31-37 | 6 -7½ | 5 | 630-750 |
| 6 | 32-40 | 7 -8 | 5 | 690-800 |

After six months of age, very little water need be added to the cow's milk. As soon as the infant takes carbohydrates in the form of thin cereals, bread, or crackers, the sugar in the milk should be reduced. At eight or nine months of age, if the sugar is added to the cereals, fruits, puddings, etc., this carbohydrate can be omitted from the milk.

Sample Formulas

*2-weeks-old-infant—weight 7½ pounds*

| | |
|---|---|
| Whole grade "A" milk | 14 ounces |
| Boiled water | 7 ounces |
| Lactose | 3 level tablespoons |

7 bottles of 3 ounces each

*1-month-old infant—weight 8½ pounds*

| | |
|---|---|
| Whole milk | 17 ounces |
| Boiled water | 9 ounces |
| Lactose | 3 level tablespoons |

7 bottles of 3¾ ounces each

*2-months-old infant—weight 10 pounds*

| | |
|---|---|
| Whole milk | 20 ounces |
| Boiled water | 10 ounces |
| Lactose | 4 tablespoons |

6 bottles of 5 ounces each

*3-months-old infant—weight 11½ pounds*

| | |
|---|---|
| Whole milk | 23 ounces |
| Boiled water | 10 ounces |
| Lactose | 4 tablespoons |

5 bottles of 6½ ounces each

*4-months-old infant—weight 13½ pounds*

| | |
|---|---|
| Whole milk | 26 ounces |
| Boiled water | 9 ounces |
| Lactose | 4½ tablespoons |

5 bottles of 7 ounces each

*5-months-old infant—weight 15 pounds*

| | |
|---|---|
| Whole milk | 27 ounces |
| Boiled water | 5 ounces |
| Lactose | 4½ tablespoons |

4 bottles of 8 ounces each

*6-months-old infant—weight 16 pounds*

| | |
|---|---|
| Whole milk | 30 ounces |
| Boiled water | 2 ounces |
| Lactose | 4 tablespoons |

4 bottles of 8 ounces each

*7-months-old infant—weight 17 pounds*

| | |
|---|---|
| Whole milk | 32 ounces |
| No water | |
| Lactose | 3 tablespoons |

4 bottles of 8 ounces each

*8-months-old infant—weight 18 pounds*

| | |
|---|---|
| Whole milk | 32 ounces |
| Lactose | 2 tablespoons |

4 bottles of 8 ounces each

*9-months-old infant—weight 19 pounds*

| | |
|---|---|
| Whole milk | 24 ounces |
| Lactose | 1 tablespoon |

3 bottles of 8 ounces each

*10-months-old infant—weight 20 pounds*

| | |
|---|---|
| Whole milk | 24 ounces |

3 bottles of 8 ounces each

***Milk Used in Formulas.*** Besides whole milk, evaporated milk is often used in making formulas. Evaporated milk is whole milk evaporated to one-half or less of its original volume. It is more than twice as concentrated as fresh milk, so that if you mix one part evaporated milk with one part water, you get approximately the concentration of fresh milk. To this mixture, you still have to add the water your formula calls for.

Condensed milk is similar to evaporated milk, but it contains added cane sugar. It has too much carbohydrate to be suitable for feeding infants.

On the other hand, powdered milk is occasionally made the basis of a baby's formula. Four level teaspoons of powdered milk mixed with eight ounces of water are equal to eight ounces of whole milk.

## PREPARING THE DAY'S FEEDING

***Equipment.*** The necessary equipment for the preparation and feeding of the baby generally includes the following: a deep, covered kettle for boiling bottles and other articles; twelve 8-ounce heat-proof nursing bottles; twelve anticolic, ball-top nipples; twelve caps for bottles; covered glass jar to hold nipples. Also, two bottle brushes; a tablespoon; a teaspoon, a small spatula to level off measurements; an eight-ounce measuring glass, marked off in ounces; rack to hold bottles; two-quart aluminum saucepan; a strainer; an aluminum funnel; kitchen tongs for removing bottles, nipples, etc. from the boiling water.

***How to Proceed.*** Strict cleanliness is absolutely essential in the preparation for the feeding of the infant. The preliminary step in preparing feedings is to sterilize everything that will come in contact with the food. Boil the feeding equipment for twenty minutes, throwing in the nipples in the last minute or two. Then keep the nipples in a sterile jar with a lid.

In preparing the milk formula, the feedings for an entire day are made up at one time. The sugar is measured by level tablespoonfuls and dissolved in water; the milk is measured and mixed. The whole mixture is then sterilized by boiling in a saucepan one to two minutes. The milk, while still hot, is strained and then poured into sterile nursing bottles, one for each feeding. The bottles are then tightly capped, cooled by immersion in water and placed in a bottle rack in the refrigerator until needed. At feeding time, the nipple is substituted for the cap and the bottle is warmed. It is important at this time not to touch the part of the nipple that will go into the baby's mouth.

***Holding the Bottle Properly.*** When giving the baby his bottle-feeding, the mother should keep the bottle tipped so that there is always milk in the nipple and neck of the bottle while the baby is sucking; this will decrease the amount of air he swallows. (See p. 240 for the correct way to "burp" a baby.)

## CARE OF MILK IN THE HOME

If pasteurized milk cannot be obtained, the milk used in the home should be heated according to the following directions, which will destroy any disease-producing organisms that may be present.

Fill the lower part of a double boiler with water. Place the milk in the upper part, cover and set over the fire. Heat until the water begins to boil. Allow it to boil for three minutes. Remove from the fire and cool immediately by placing the upper part, containing the milk, in a large pan of cold water. Change the water every few minutes at least five times or until the milk is almost as cold as the water. If the milk in the closed container can be placed in running water, it can be cooked more quickly.

Milk can become infected because of improper care in the home. This usually consists of failing to keep the milk cold, in allowing it to freeze, in failing to clean the top of the bottle, in pouring the milk into unclean or unsterilized utensils and in exposing it unnecessarily in uncovered dishes to dust, flies and other contaminants. Milk cannot be properly kept without ice or mechanical refrigeration, except in cold weather.

Milk should be kept in the original bottle until ready to be used, covered with its cap or a clean inverted glass. It should not be poured into a pail or pitcher for storage. It should not be poured back into the bottle after it has been exposed in another vessel.

## OTHER ESSENTIALS IN THE DIET

***Water.*** The infant requires more water, relatively, than the adult. Milk goes far toward supplying this need, but water which has been boiled and cooled should be offered the baby between feedings, especially in hot weather. It must not, in combination with the feeding, exceed the fluid requirement of three ounces for each pound of body weight. Too much water is harmful because it interferes with digestion and requires an increased elimination by the skin, lungs and kidneys.

***Vitamins.*** Whether the baby is breast-fed or bottle-fed, he needs more vitamins, and foods that contain them must be added to his diet. By the second or third week, he should be receiving one teaspoonful of cod-liver oil daily. This should be continued until he is at least six years old. Orange juice may be given beginning with the third or fourth week.

***Solid Foods.*** Solid foods should be introduced early to assure the baby of a properly balanced diet. Milk and sugar do not furnish all the elements required for growth and development of bones, teeth, muscular and other tissues.

Although authorities disagree as to the exact month at which solid feeding should begin, the consensus is that the third month is not too early to introduce cereal, and the fifth or sixth month not too early to introduce stewed fruits and strained vegetables into the diet of the infant.

The following foods should be added to the baby's diet at the ages given, and the meals should follow the schedules that are indicated:

*One to Three Months.* Orange juice—start with two teaspoonfuls per day, diluted in one ounce of water; increase to two ounces a day by three months. Tomato juice may be substituted, but the amount is twice that of orange juice. Cod-liver oil—give ten to fifteen drops once or twice daily, increasing dose up to 1½ teaspoonfuls a day at three months, and to three teaspoonfuls at six months.

*Three to Five Months.* Cereals, such as Cream of Wheat, Farina, and oatmeal may be given at 10 a.m. in very small amounts to start.

*Four to Five Months.* The diet may be as follows:

6 a.m. Milk formula, six ounces or breast.

Between 9 and 10 a.m. Orange juice, two ounces; cooked cereal, three or four tablespoonfuls; milk formula, six ounces or breast; cod-liver oil, one teaspoonful.

2 p.m. Egg yolk; milk formula, six ounces or breast.

6 p.m. Same as at 9 a.m.

10 p.m. Milk formula, six ounces or breast. (Most properly fed infants sleep from 6 p.m. to 6 a.m. at three or four months of age and do not require a 10 p.m. feeding.)

*Average Diet at Six Months*

6 a.m. Whole boiled milk, sweetened with syrup, six ounces.

10 a.m. Orange or tomato juice, two ounces; cereal with milk, one ounce; milk, six ounces.

2 p.m. Vegetable soup or cooked vegetables; juice, two ounces; milk, six ounces.

6 p.m. Cereal with milk, two ounces; milk, six ounces.

*Six to Eight Months.* Raw egg yolk may be mixed into the formula. (Some infants do not tolerate this very well.) Begin feeding bacon at eight months, the equivalent of one-half teaspoonful, broken up in small pieces. You may increase the amount by one-half teaspoonful or one teaspoonful every two or three days until you are giving a whole slice.

*Seven to Nine Months.* Add fruits: put tomato, apple, prunes, bananas, or apricots through a sieve; zwieback and cookies.

*Eight to Ten Months.* Add puddings, such as junket.

*Ten to Twelve Months.* Add meat, cut up very fine.

## AVERAGE DIET AT TWELFTH MONTH

***Breakfast.*** Orange juice, one cupful, or tomato juice, one tumblerful; cod-liver oil, one teaspoonful; milk, pasteurized, one tumblerful; cereal, four tablespoonfuls, serve with pasteurized milk and small amount of sugar; bread, fresh or toasted, lightly buttered, one slice.

***Lunch.*** Soup, vegetable or cream, one-half cupful; coddled egg, liver, beef, lamb, chicken, or fish, three tablespoonfuls; buttered toast or zwieback, one or two slices; vegetables and potato, three tablespoonfuls each; milk, pasteurized, one tumblerful if cream soup or milk dessert is not included; puddings, mashed or finely cut stewed fruit, or banana, four tablespoonfuls.

***Mid-afternoon.*** (Only if it does not interfere with the appetite at dinner.) Milk, pasteurized, eight fluid ounces; buttered toast, or slice of bread with jam.

***Dinner.*** Cereal, baked or mashed potato, or cottage cheese, three to four tablespoonfuls; buttered toast, zwieback or bread, one or two slices; milk, pasteurized, two cupfuls; baked apple, applesauce or other stewed fruit, or scraped raw fruit, three to four tablespoonfuls.

By the end of the first year the average child is getting baked potatoes, cream soups, cereals, egg, beef juice or meats; fruits, such as prunes, baked apple, or applesauce; and vegetables, such as spinach, carrots, early squash, peas, asparagus, and celery. A diet of approximately 1,000 calories is regarded as safe by most authorities.

## AVERAGE DIET AT EIGHTEEN MONTHS

***Breakfast.*** Fruit, cereal; egg or crisp bacon; bread; milk—six ounces.

***Lunch.*** Soup or broth; scraped meat; liver at least twice a week; potatoes and one green vegetable; bread and butter; cooked fruit; milk—1½ cup.

***Dinner.*** Small portion of potato and vegetable; pudding or rice or bread and milk; bread and butter; milk—1½ cup.

Some stewed fruit may be given between these meals—prunes, apricots or apples.

(As a rule coffee, tea, and cocoa are not allowed during childhood. The child requires no stimulants, and cocoa is apt to spoil the taste for other foods.)

## FEEDING THE CHILD OF ABOUT TWO

***Breakfast.*** (Between 7 and 8 o'clock.) Citrus fruit or tomato juice; cereal; egg or bacon; breadstuff, with butter.

***Lunch.*** (Between 11:30 and 12:30 o'clock.) Meat, potato, one leafy vegetable, one green or yellow vegetable; breadstuff, with butter; dessert; milk.

***Dinner.*** (Between 5 and 6 o'clock.) Cereal, soup; potato or macaroni, vegetable; breadstuff, with butter; cooked fruit, milk.

Water should be given frequently during the day. Cod-liver oil may be given in one or two doses before meals or whenever convenient. Citrus fruit or tomato juice may be given between meals rather than at breakfast. One additional fruit may be given between meals if the child wants a lunch in mid-morning or mid-afternoon.

Continue to give milk at every meal, the total day's amount varying from a pint to a quart. Other dairy products, such as cottage cheese, may be given freely, and cream cheese occasionally.

Orange or other citrus fruit juice or tomato juice should be given daily, one to two cupfuls being desirable. Cereal should be eaten twice daily. A whole egg may be given from three to four times a week, provided the baby has learned to eat the white and tolerates it well. Vegetables should be given in increasing variety, two or three servings being offered daily. Raw vegetables may be introduced at about eighteen months. Potato is given every day, usually at noon, although it may be fed occasionally at supper in place of cereal. Breadstuffs which require chewing may be given from one to three times daily. Fruits, in addition to citrus, may be added once or twice a day if at least one serving is cooked.

Meat, fish and poultry should be included in the daily diet now. Desserts may be given once or twice a day, if all the other foods are being well taken. Soups as carriers for cereals and vegetables may be useful to vary the evening meal. Fat, preferably butter, may be used in small quantities, not more than one tablespoonful daily. Salt should be held to a minimum, except during hot weather, when the child is perspiring freely.

## FEEDING THE CHILD OF THREE

***Breakfast.*** Orange juice, three tablespoonfuls; dark farina, three-quarters of a cup; milk, 1 glass (for cereal and to drink); toast, whole wheat, one slice; butter, one-half teaspoonful.

***Lunch.*** One medium potato, mashed; carrots, steamed and chopped, five tablespoonfuls; toast, whole wheat, one slice; butter, one teaspoonful; banana, one-half in small cubes with one-half teaspoonful of sugar and one tablespoonful of orange juice; milk, 1½ cups; cod-liver oil, one teaspoonful.

***Midafternoon.*** Milk, one glass; 2 whole-wheat crackers.

***Dinner.*** Baked or boiled potato with plenty of butter; any steamed vegetable; one small lamb chop broiled, or small portion of roast beef; pudding of jello or rice or custard; one to two cups of milk.

## FEEDING UNDERNOURISHED INFANTS

Infants who are undernourished as a result of disease or improper feeding need almost as much total food as normal infants of the same age. Unfortunately such undernourished infants are not always able to digest the amount of food required. To supply their need for a concentrated and digestible food, mixtures of acidified milk and sugar are preferable to formulas of diluted whole milk.

## FEEDING PREMATURE INFANTS

For premature infants (an infant born before the thirty-eighth week of pregnancy or one whose birth weight is under 5½ pounds is a premature infant), breast milk is the best food. Feeding must begin a few hours after birth. The infant must be fed at first with a dropper; later a bottle with a small nipple is used. At the beginning the quantity of food must be small. On the first day it is best to begin with one-twentieth of the infant's body weight of human milk. This is divided into twelve parts, and the infant is fed every two hours. The quantity at each feeding is increased daily until the infant receives one-fifth of its own body weight per day.

If human milk is unavailable, artificial food must be given. Evaporated milk (one part with two parts of water) is used, acidulated with lactic acid, and 5 per cent of pure milk sugar is added. (Buttermilk and powdered milk can also be used.)

## FEEDING THE SICK BABY

***Some General Points to Keep in Mind.*** Infants who cannot suck (for example, those with cleft palate, harelip or both) have to be spoon-fed or dropper-fed. Tube feeding is sometimes used.

When predigested food is needed, use peptonized milk, fermented milk or acidified evaporated milk. See that fat content is decreased and that at times other fats are substituted.

In acute vomiting, give no food at all for a while. Sweetened cereal decoctions (boiled until they are very soft) or barley water may be given in place of milk. If the vomiting occurs soon after nursing, the infant has usually taken too much milk. If the vomiting occurs some time after nursing, it is often because the milk is too rich. Be careful not to overfeed the infant.

In mild diarrhea, cereal decoctions, salted and sweetened, may be used. In persistent diarrheas omit all sugar and starches from the diet and give instead buttermilk, or protein milk. Banana powder or apple powder may be added to the milk.

For constipation increase sugar content of the milk—for example, malted wheat germ extract, or honey, or sorghum molasses.

In fevers, give extra amounts of water.

## SOME IMPORTANT FACTS IN FOOD PREPARATION FOR INFANTS

***Cereals.*** Only well-cooked cereals should be given. For preparing the cereals use: one tablespoonful cereal; one-half cup water; one-half cup milk; pinch of salt.

Combine water and milk, heat to boiling, stir in cereal, add salt and cook for one hour in a double boiler. Or, it may be cooked for five minutes over a direct flame, with constant stirring, followed by thirty minutes in a double boiler. Cook oatmeal and whole barley for two hours in a double boiler.

A number of excellent precooked cereals, such as pablum, pabena, or cerevim, can also be employed.

***Spinach.*** To a half pound of cleaned spinach add one pint of water; bring to boil and keep boiling over a medium flame for twenty to thirty minutes until the spinach is soft and most of the water has boiled away. Press the spinach through a fine sieve. If the sieved spinach is too watery, boil away extra water by careful heating. A little butter and a pinch of salt may be added.

***Potatoes, Boiled.*** Boil several washed potatoes in just enough water until they are thoroughly cooked. Remove the skins, mash, and add to the cooking water. Boil the mixture in a double boiler to a thick mush. Potatoes boiled in the ordinary way for the family meal may be used, but by that method some nutritive values are lost.

***Potatoes, Baked.*** Bake in a slow oven for forty-five minutes to one hour; remove skin and mash thoroughly. A pinch of salt and butter may be added. Do not puncture the skin with fork or knife in testing.

***Carrots and Beets.*** Boil several washed carrots or beets in water until thoroughly cooked; peel, slice, mash, and add to the cooking water. If necessary, boil mixture in a double boiler to a thick mush. A little butter and a pinch of salt may be added.

***Cauliflower.*** Discard leaves and stalk, separate into parts, wash carefully and soak in salt water for twenty to thirty minutes. Then drop into boiling water and boil uncovered for similar period of time. Drain, mash with a fork or rub through a coarse sieve. A little butter and a pinch of salt may be added.

***Asparagus.*** Cook one-half bunch of washed asparagus in about a pint of water. When tender, remove from the water, place on a warm plate and scrape out the pulp with a fork, scraping lightly toward the tip. Use only the pulp. Make a sauce, using one-quarter cup of asparagus cooking water, one-quarter cup milk, and one teaspoonful flour. Mix sauce with two to three tablespoonfuls asparagus pulp, reheat, and place on toast.

***Green Peas.*** Cook a cupful of green peas in boiling water, drain and retain cooking water. Rub through a coarse sieve. Make a sauce of two tablespoonfuls of bread crumbs with the cooking water. Mix with the sieved peas.

***Cream Soup.*** Cream soups may be made from vegetable pulp, using one tablespoonful cooked pulped potatoes, peas, asparagus, carrots, spinach, or celery to each one-half teaspoonful flour. Add milk for consistency desired. Cook for two or three minutes; strain if necessary.

***Coddled Egg.*** Bring water to a boil in saucepan, remove from stove, put egg (in the shell) in the water and allow to stand for eight minutes.

***Soft-Boiled Egg.*** Cook egg in boiling water for two minutes.

***Orange Juice.*** Wash an orange, cut it in half, squeeze out juice, strain, and use as directed by physician. If too sour, add small amount of sugar. (Orange juice should be prepared immediately before use as the vitamin C content is gradually destroyed on standing.)

***Prune Juice.*** Wash thoroughly one-half pound dried prunes, cover with cold water and soak over night. In the morning place on stove in same water; cook until tender, add one teaspoonful sugar and strain.

***Applesauce.*** Peel and core six apples, cut into slices, place in an enameled dish, sprinkle with one tablespoonful granulated sugar, add one cup cold water, put on stove and boil to a mush (about thirty minutes).

***Bread.*** Use enriched white bread that is several days old, or whole wheat bread, rye or enriched white bread that has been dried in the oven. Enriched bread contains added vitamins and minerals.

***Zwieback.*** Zwieback is obtainable in all grocery stores. Babies like it.

***Meats.*** Beef steak, lamb chops, and liver are the best meats for the baby. They should be broiled, rather than fried, to make them more easily digestible. Soup meat or chicken meat, well cooked, may also be given, as well as codfish or whitefish. All meats should be finely cut before feeding.

***Scraped Beef.*** Scrape a piece of raw or seared beef with a knife. The tender pulp is then collected and made into a patty which is broiled on both sides.

## TEETHING

Teething is a natural process. The belief that it is the cause of many an infant's illness is mistaken. Moreover, it is rarely, almost never, necessary to cut the gums in order to aid the appearance of a tooth or teeth.

In healthy children there is often fretfulness during teething, and poor sleep. There may also be drooling and loss of appetite. However, there generally are no serious symptoms, such as fever.

The condition of the first teeth depends almost entirely on the mother's diet before the baby is born.

Teething begins with the sixth month, the "milk teeth" appearing as follows:

*Upper*

| | |
|---|---|
| Central incisors | 6 to 8 months |
| Lateral incisors | 9 to 10 months |
| Cuspid (eye tooth) | 18 to 20 months |
| First molar | 14 to 16 months |
| Second molar | about 2 years |

*Lower*

| | |
|---|---|
| Central incisor | 6 to 8 months |
| Lateral incisor | 12 to 14 months |
| Cuspid | 18 to 20 months |
| First molar | 14 to 16 months |
| Second molar | about 2 years |

There are 20 teeth in the first set. At one year a child usually has six teeth.

The permanent teeth appear as follows:

*Upper*

| | |
|---|---|
| Central incisor | 7 to 8 years |
| Lateral incisor | 8 to 9 years |
| Cuspid (eye tooth) | 12 to 14 years |
| First bicuspid | 10 to 11 years |
| Second bicuspid | 11 to 12 years |
| Six year molar | first permanent tooth |
| Second molar | 12 to 15 years |
| Third molar (wisdom tooth) | 16 to 20 years |

*Lower*

| | |
|---|---|
| Central incisor | 6 to 7 years |
| Lateral incisor | about 8 years |
| Cuspid | 9 to 14 years |
| First bicuspid | 10 to 11 years |
| Second bicuspid | 11 to 12 years |
| Six year molar | first permanent tooth |
| Second molar | 12 to 15 years |
| Third molar (wisdom tooth) | 16 to 20 years |

### Care of the Teeth

Proper care of the teeth—which should be made a habit—is essential to the child's health, happiness, and comeliness. To maintain the teeth in good condition, dental hygiene is of the first importance—that is, cleanliness. Brushing the teeth, using tooth paste, should be introduced at twelve to eighteen months of age. Calcium and phosphorus are all-important and must be adequately supplied in orange juice, cod-liver oil or appropriate substitutes.

If small cavities develop in the "milk teeth" they should be filled; if the cavities are large, the teeth should be extracted. When crooked teeth appear, or when teeth are out of place, a dentist should also be consulted.

### When Children Cry

Teething children frequently cry a great deal. The mother should make certain that the cutting of teeth is actually the cause, for there may be one or more different reasons for the crying, as for example:

1. Desire for exercise, or hunger, or thirst.
2. A wet or soiled diaper.
3. A pin sticking the child.
4. Feeling too hot or too cold.
5. Clothing that is wrinkled under him, clothing that is twisted so that it pulls, or clothing that is too tight.
6. Wrinkled bedding, or unsuitable bed or bedding.
7. Itching or chafing from irritation caused by clothing, soap, heat or lack of cleanliness.
8. Pain, colic, or earache.
9. Fear of falling or of a sudden loud noise.
10. Desire for change of position.
11. Discomfort from sunlight or other bright light shining directly in the eyes.
12. Discomfort from gas in the stomach.

## BATHING AND CLEANLINESS

A baby should be bathed daily; in the hot weather, an additional sponge is advisable. During the cold season, it is best to bathe the baby at 5 or 5:30 p.m., before the 6 p.m. feeding. Unless the baby is small and premature or the skin is dry, oiling is inadvisable. After the bath, talcum or cornstarch powder is dusted over the body. The eyes are washed with warm boric acid solution, using one-half teaspoon to eight ounces of boiled water. This can be discontinued by the third month, when the ability to produce tears is fully developed. The nose and ears are gently cleaned with a pledget (wad) of absorbent cotton dipped in oil; toothpicks with cotton or any stiff holders that might injure the mucosa are best avoided. The mouth of an infant should never be cleaned, as more harm than good can result. When at least sixteen teeth are cut, cleaning the teeth with a soft brush and nongritty tooth powder is practiced daily. The scalp may be oiled after the bath and the hair brushed back with a soft baby brush. After the bath, the foreskin is retracted and a little oil or vaseline applied; the labia of the vagina are separated and powdered, and debris and mucus are wiped away gently with absorbent cotton and oil.

## TOILET TRAINING

Bowel and bladder training should begin early. At five months the infant is placed on the "toidy" seat after a feeding and its back supported. If this is carried out regularly, it is surprising how quickly bowel training is accomplished. By the end of the first year, bladder training may be begun by taking the child to the toilet at regularly specified periods. When a certain amount of control has been attained, the diapers are dispensed with during the day. If the child is not given to consuming too much fluid at bedtime, is made to empty the bladder before retiring, and, particularly, is not overstimulated and excited at bedtime, he may soon begin having dry nights; as these become frequent, the diaper is also removed at bedtime.

***Bed-wetting.*** When a child is past three years of age and continues to wet, it is often as much the fault of the parent as of the child. Inadequate training at an early, but not too early, age, an overanxious and emotional parent unwittingly transferring her emotional instability to the child, too much excitement at bedtime, scolding or humiliating the child because of the bed-wetting, are all factors in perpetuating the infantile habit of urinating in bed. A sympathetic attitude on the part of the parent, coupled with intelligent guidance by a physician, will, provided there is no organic basis for the faulty control (which, if present, should of course be eliminated) ultimately lead to successful results.

## THE BABY'S SLEEP

Prolonged and restful sleep has a great influence upon the health and growth of the baby. For the first two months he should average eighteen to twenty hours of sleep. Some doctors claim that it is better not to interrupt the night sleep for the feeding. This of course depends to a great extent on the general robustness and weight of the baby. After the first month many babies will go through the night without waking for food. When about a year of age, the child's sleeping periods average about twelve hours with a nap both in the morning and in the afternoon.

***The Bedtime Hour.*** In the early months this should be established with regularity. If the time set is six or seven, then it should remain at that hour. There should be no excitement before the time to go to sleep. Remember that nervous reaction to the happenings around the baby register almost at birth. So, quiet, before the bedtime hour, is the watchword.

***Position During Sleep.*** Particularly during the winter months it is better to have the baby lie face downwards. This position assures more belly warmth and helps reduce colic to a minimum. You need have no fear that the baby will smother while sleeping on the stomach; this cannot happen.

***Your Baby and Noise.*** From birth, the baby must be made to get accustomed to the ordinary noises that are necessary in a household. Tiptoeing and "shushing" are all wrong. Of course, undue noises should be guarded against. Even the radio should not be shut off, though it should not blare.

***What Causes Poor Sleeping?*** If the baby does not sleep well, there must be something wrong. Maybe he has had either too much or too little to eat. Maybe his clothing is too tight or rumpled. Maybe it is the temperature of the room—too hot or too cold. Watch that. Finally, it may be a wet diaper. Who likes to sleep in wet clothes?

***Preventing Bad Habits.*** Some of the don'ts are: Do not put the baby to sleep with the bottle in his mouth; do not use a pacifier. If he cries, do not run to the medicine chest—maybe all that he needs is a good "burp." Above all things, do not interrupt his sleep to show him off to visitors.

## TAKING THE BABY OUTSIDE

***In Cool Weather.*** After two months it is all right to take the baby outside if the sun is out and there is no wind blowing. Wind does

## WHEN TO IMMUNIZE YOUR CHILD

*(Suggested Schedule)*

| *Age* | *Disease* | *Dosage by Physician* |
|---|---|---|
| 3 months | Whooping Cough | Dosage administered by injection at intervals of one month. First injection in left arm or buttock. |
| 4 months | Whooping Cough | Second injection in right arm or buttock. |
| 5 months | Whooping Cough | Third injection in left arm or buttock. |
| 6 months | Diphtheria and Tetanus | Total dosage administered deeply under the skin or in the muscles in two injections, one month apart. First injection in right arm or buttock. |
| 6 months | Smallpox | Contents of one capillary tube of smallpox vaccine applied by multiple skin puncture. |
| 7 months | Diphtheria and Tetanus | Second injection in left arm or buttock. |
| 8 months | None | None |
| 12-24 months | Scarlet Fever | At intervals of one week, five injections of skin test doses are administered under the skin. |

## BOOSTER DOSES AND REIMMUNIZATION

| *Age* | *Disease* | *Dosage by Physician* |
|---|---|---|
| 12-18 months | Whooping Cough, Tetanus, and Diphtheria | A booster dose administered deep under the skin or in the muscles. |
| 5 years; or when starting school or kindergarten | Whooping Cough, Tetanus, and Diphtheria | A booster dose administered deep under the skin or in the muscles. |
| 5 years; or when starting school or kindergarten | Smallpox | For reimmunization, using contents of one capillary tube by multiple skin puncture. |

If a child lives on a farm or is going to spend the summer in the country, he should be immunized against typhoid fever.

more harm than is usually thought. It stirs up the dust which is laden with all sorts of bacteria. Remember that the baby's resistance in the early months has not been built up.

***In Cold Weather.*** Under two months of age, it is better not to take the baby out of doors. After two months, always use the middle of the day to take the baby out. If it is very cold, then do not keep the baby out for more than fifteen minutes at a time. In bad weather you can give the baby plenty of fresh air by opening the window in his room and either using the ventilator or putting a screen in front of the open window.

***Sunshine.*** Sunshine contains the valuable vitamin D. Also, it contains the ultra-violet rays, which are so helpful in changing some of the mineral elements of the body into bone formation, which is vital to the child's welfare. To get the maximum benefit of these rays, the sun must shine directly upon the skin. Window glass and clothes filter out most of the ultra-violet rays.

***Season of the Year.*** Naturally only in warm weather can the baby be exposed unclothed out of doors. This also depends upon your geographical location. Always protect from the wind. In very hot weather, great caution must be used not to burn the baby. His delicate skin cannot take too much sunshine at one time. In the hot summer months do not go out in the extreme heat of the day; do not expose the baby longer than five minutes on each side of the body. In the shade there is no reason to limit the time that much. It is the direct rays of the sun that are the active ones.

## AVOIDING RESPIRATORY INFECTIONS

Respiratory infections are exceedingly dangerous to the newborn. The source is the nurse, mother or some visitor. The mother's fingers must never be put in the baby's mouth, and the baby should not be kissed on the mouth.

## THE BABY'S WEIGHT

***Average Weights at Various Ages.*** For a child of average weight at birth (7½ pounds), at three months the weight should be twelve to thirteen pounds; at six months, sixteen to seventeen pounds; at nine months, eighteen to nineteen pounds. At five months an average healthy child has doubled its birth weight, and at twelve months he has nearly trebled it.

Healthy infants, as a rule, gain steadily in weight every week during the first year. With most infants there are times during the year when there is no gain in weight, especially from the seventh to the tenth month, and frequently on account of teething. It must be kept in mind that not every infant who gains rapidly in weight is getting along normally. He may merely be getting too much carbohydrate.

At the end of the first year infants usually weigh twenty to twenty-three pounds.

The average baby gains about two pounds a month (seven or eight ounces a week) during the first three months. By six months the average gain is down to a pound a month (four ounces a week). In the last three months of the year the average gain is about two-thirds of a pound a month. Thus, as the infant grows older, his weight gains are slower.

A healthy baby therefore gains fairly steadily in weight. But parents should not be alarmed if the infant's weight does not follow the average course we have indicated. If the infant's appetite is good, if his bowel movements are regular and of normal consistency and color, if he is sleeping quietly and not vomiting, and gains only two or three ounces in weight during the week instead of the seven or eight ounces you expect, don't worry, just so long as he is gaining.

## RATE OF GROWTH

A baby should be examined by a physician every month, until he is a year old. During the second year, examinations may be reduced to one in every three months.

Nothing else reveals so strikingly that a child is making normal progress as his rate of gain in height and weight. In infancy, progress is noted by weeks; in later childhood, by months. A progressive gain in weight and height in an older child is also a sign of health.

Growth in height is rapid during the first year—about nine inches; during the second year about four inches are added. The annual increase during early and late childhood varies from two to three inches a year. There is little difference in the sexes in this increase until the eleventh year when girls begin to grow more rapidly and often surpass the boys, who, however, again pass the girls at about the fourteenth year.

AVERAGE ANNUAL GAIN IN WEIGHT AND HEIGHT

| Age (years) | Boys Weight (pounds) | Boys Height (inches) | Girls Weight (pounds) | Girls Height (inches) |
|---|---|---|---|---|
| 5 to 6 | 4 | 2 | 4 | 2 |
| 6 to 7 | 4.5 | 2 | 4.5 | 2 |
| 7 to 8 | 4.5 | 2 | 5 | 2 |
| 8 to 9 | 5 | 2 | 6 | 2.2 |
| 9 to 10 | 6 | 2 | 6 | 2.2 |
| 10 to 11 | 5 | 1.7 | 7 | 2 |
| 11 to 12 | 6.5 | 1.8 | 9.5 | 2.5 |
| 12 to 13 | 8 | 2 | 11.5 | 2 |
| 13 to 14 | 10.5 | 2.5 | 10 | 2 |
| 14 to 15 | 12.5 | 2.7 | 6 | 1.2 |
| 15 to 16 | 12.5 | 2.7 | 5 | 0.75 |
| 16 to 17 | 6.5 | 1.2 | 2 | 0.50 |
| 17 to 18 | 5 | 0.5 | 1 | 0.20 |

Actually there is no standard weight for children at the different ages. Healthy children of the same age vary a great deal as to height and weight, which are modified by race and family inheritance.

There is a standard weight for children of the same height—approximately; this varies so little in children of different families that it may be taken as a general guide to the child's nutrition. A table showing the *standard* weight for height is given here. The *normal* includes a wider range.

STANDARD WEIGHTS FOR GIVEN HEIGHTS

| Height (inches) | Weight (pounds) Boys | Weight (pounds) Girls |
|---|---|---|
| 42 | 40.5 | 39.5 |
| 43 | 42.5 | 41.5 |
| 44 | 44.5 | 43.5 |
| 45 | 46.5 | 45.5 |
| 46 | 48.5 | 48 |
| 47 | 51 | 50.5 |
| 48 | 53.5 | 53 |
| 49 | 56 | 55.5 |
| 50 | 58.5 | 58 |
| 51 | 61.5 | 61.5 |
| 52 | 64.5 | 64.5 |
| 53 | 67.5 | 67.5 |
| 54 | 71 | 71 |
| 55 | 74.5 | 74.5 |
| 56 | 78 | 78.5 |

Age, however, is a factor which cannot be ignored. An older child should weigh more than a younger one of the same height.

(Weights are taken in the usual indoor clothes without shoes; boys with coats and sweaters removed; heights are without shoes.)

AVERAGE HEIGHTS AND WEIGHTS OF CHILDREN

| | *Boys* | | *Girls* | |
|---|---|---|---|---|
| *Age (years)* | *Height* | *Weight (pounds)* | *Height* | *Weight (pounds)* |
| At birth | 20.5″ | 7.5 | 20.5″ | 7.5 |
| 1 | 29.5″ | 21.5 | 29.0″ | 20.0 |
| 2 | 33.5″ | 26.5 | 33.0″ | 25.0 |
| 3 | 36.5″ | 31.0 | 36.0″ | 29.5 |
| 4 | 3′ 3″ | 34 | 3′ 3″ | 33 |
| 5 | 3′ 6″ | 39 | 3′ 5″ | 38 |
| 6 | 3′ 9″ | 45 | 3′ 9″ | 43 |
| 7 | 3′ 11″ | 52 | 3′ 11″ | 50 |
| 8 | 4′ 2″ | 58 | 4′ 2″ | 58 |
| 9 | 4′ 4″ | 64 | 4′ 4″ | 64 |
| 10 | 4′ 6″ | 71 | 4′ 6″ | 71 |
| 11 | 4′ 8″ | 78 | 4′ 8″ | 79 |
| 12 | 4′ 10″ | 85 | 4′ 10″ | 89 |
| 13 | 5′ 0″ | 94 | 5′ 0″ | 101 |
| 14 | 5′ 3″ | 111 | 5′ 2″ | 110 |

CHAPTER 15

# COMMON DISEASES OF CHILDHOOD



## INFLAMMATION OF THE BREASTS IN THE NEWBORN

***Symptoms of Breast Inflammation.*** This condition is not uncommon. The breasts of either girl or boy babies become swollen and tender, and a few drops of thin milk may exude from them. Ordinarily, the child's temperature is not above normal, nor is the appetite disturbed, and the condition subsides without causing any trouble.

***Treatment of Breast Inflammation.*** The breasts should be gently, yet thoroughly, washed with soap and warm water, and then covered with a few layers of cheesecloth, which has been wet in a warm solution of boric acid (a teaspoonful in half a pint of water). Then cover with oil silk and a flannel band about the chest, with shoulder straps to keep it in place. A fresh, wet application should be applied each day.

***Abscess of the Breast.*** Rarely, abscess of the breast results, with increasing inflammation and redness, formation of "matter" (pus) and fever, loss of appetite, and general disturbance. Such a case, of course, must be referred to the surgeon at the earliest moment for incision.

## RETENTION AND PAINFUL PASSAGE OF URINE

***When the Child Does Not Pass Urine.*** The baby may pass no urine for twenty-four hours after it is born, and yet there may be no cause for worry. If no urine is passed in the first twelve hours, it is well to put the baby in a warm bath. If this does not lead to a passage of urine a physician should be consulted, as there may be some deformity or obstruction.

After a bad attack of colic in some instances, no urine is passed for many hours, but this condition may be relieved by the warm bath.

***Painful Urination.*** Pain during the passage of urine may be observed when the urine is too concentrated and stains the diaper with a reddish or yellowish substance. Giving the baby an abundance of water to drink will relieve this condition.

***Bowel Deformity.*** Very rarely there is no opening for escape of excrement from the bowels. A surgeon must be summoned at once to remedy this condition.

## SMALL OPENING IN THE FORESKIN

***Symptoms of Small Opening in the Foreskin.*** This is seen in the newborn boy baby as a natural condition. The opening is not only small as a pinhole, but the foreskin cannot be drawn back so as to expose the head of the penis.

This state changes naturally as the child grows. However, if it does not, and if the foreskin remains attached to the parts beneath so that it cannot be moved freely over the penis, and if the opening for the passage of urine is very small, several complications are apt to follow.

***Complications.*** The end of the penis is likely to become sore, red, and swollen, and the passage of urine painful. Some discharge may occur. The irritation leads to rubbing of the parts, and the bad habit of masturbation often begins in this way. Bed-wetting is a common consequence of the irritation. Prolapse (falling down) of the bowel, or rupture may be caused by straining to pass water. Various nervous disorders may owe their beginning to a tight foreskin.

***Treatment of Small Opening in the Foreskin.*** This consists of circumcision. The operation is done by a surgeon. Parents should consult a physician when there is any suggestion of trouble such as has been described.

## BLEEDING OF THE CORD AND SORENESS OF THE NAVEL IN THE NEWBORN

***Treatment of Bleeding.*** Bleeding of the cord occurring soon after birth must be stopped immediately by tying a soft string tightly about it as far from the belly as the string will hold without slipping off. Slight oozing after the cord has dropped off is usually of no consequence. Sometimes the cord becomes soft and offensive, and when it comes away leaves a large sore behind it. There may be a little pea-shaped swelling in the sore which discharges "matter."

***Treatment of Sore.*** In the absence of a physician, the sore should be washed three times daily with boric-acid solution (one teaspoonful to half a pint of warm water) and clean absorbent cotton. Then dust it with dry boric acid or aristol powder, and cover it with clean gauze or soft cotton. With such treatment it usually heals.

## PROLAPSE (FALLING DOWN) OF THE BOWEL

***Causes of Prolapse of the Bowel.*** This condition is brought about by great or constant straining caused by diarrhea, constipation, a narrow foreskin with difficult urination, worms, whooping cough, overeating that results in too frequent large movements of the bowels, etc.

***Symptoms of Prolapse of the Bowel.*** There is to be seen a protrusion of the bowel, from one-half inch to several inches long. Ordinarily it presents the appearance of a dark-red or purplish, puckered ring at the point of opening of the bowel. It goes back or can be pushed back into place. It reappears, however, whenever there is much straining, as during a passage from the bowels.

There is usually little pain associated with the prolapse, unless it is large, when—if it remains out for a considerable time—it becomes very painful and inflamed, and may ultimately cause the death of the patient.

***Treatment of Prolapse of the Bowel.*** Treatment consists in removing the causes, if possible. Keeping the feces soft, prevention of constipation, avoidance of straining, and discouraging the spending of too much time on the toilet are the best curative measures.

***Emergency Treatment.*** The first thing to do is to place the child flat on his face, cleanse the protrusion with warm water, grease it with vaseline, and gently push it back. The injection of a little ice water into the bowel (a cupful three times daily) will have a most beneficial effect.

To prevent a return of the trouble, the child should be required to have a movement while lying on its back on a diaper. A baby must not be allowed to sit on a vessel more than five minutes at a time; there is no more pernicious habit for causing prolapse of the bowels than long sessions of this kind. An operation is necessary to cure chronic or large protrusions of the bowel.

## WASTING (MARASMUS)

***Causes of Marasmus.*** Wasting is an extreme state of malnutrition. It may arise from incomplete starvation, protracted malnutrition, persistent intestinal indigestion, and repeated attacks of inflammation of the bowel.

***Symptoms of Marasmus.*** The body is extremely wasted, and the infant appears aged. The face shows wrinkles, the features are drawn, eyes sunken, temples hollow, and cheeks flat. The skin is dry and inelastic, and hangs in wrinkles and folds over the bones. The joints are prominent. The abdomen may be flat or distended. The temperature is subnormal, and the cry and activity of the infant are extremely weak.

***Treatment of Marasmus.*** Human milk should be secured and given in increased quantities. The processed milks (fermented milk, powdered half-skimmed milk, evaporated milk) should be used when human milk cannot be obtained. Vitamins A and B are helpful.

## FEVER

***Some General Facts.*** Fever is only a symptom of many diseases, but until the cause is known the same general treatment may be pursued in all instances. The first thing to do is to take the temperature with a thermometer. This is the only way to be sure of either the presence or degree of fever; no other signs are certain. For an infant, a temperature of less than 101°F. might be called a slight fever; between that point and 103°, a moderate fever; over 103°, a considerable fever; and over 104°, high fever. High fevers are much more common in children, and are not of as serious import as in adults, unless they are continued. A temperature of 100° or over always means some sort of a physical disorder; no single test is as reliable in determining whether a child is sick or not as taking the temperature.

Fevers lasting for a few days are not as harmful as commonly believed, unless the temperature is high. Fever is nature's method of combatting the cause, in most conditions, and moderate fever, unless it continues for many days, need not cause anxiety, as far as the increased temperature itself is concerned. High fever—especially in children—should be reduced, since headache, delirium, and, in infants, convulsions are common. A child with fever should be immediately isolated in a room by himself, and other children should be kept away until it is known that the disease is not contagious. The eruptive diseases of childhood, tonsillitis, grippe, and diphtheria are often first brought to attention through fever.

***Treatment of Fever.*** When fever is high, cold applications should be kept on the head. This is best done by applying a rubber cap containing cracked ice. If this cannot be obtained, a single thickness of soft cotton wrung out of ice water should be placed on the forehead and frequently moistened with ice water as it evaporates. The cloth or ice cap ought to be applied as long as the fever remains high. In addition, the entire surface of the body may be sponged with tepid water.

It is not necessary to reduce the temperature below 102°, in most instances. The application of a cold pack, under your physician's direction, when there is fever with restlessness and sleeplessness, is frequently useful in place of sponging. A rapid way of reducing an excessively high temperature is the administration of a cold water enema.

***Diet and General Care.*** In most fevers the diet must be liquid. Infants on milk should have the mixture diluted a third to a half with water. Milk, broths, albumin water, and thin cereals generally make up the best diet. An abundance of cool water may be allowed in fevers, but the rule is to give a little at a time, and frequently. Rest in bed is imperative. Moving the bowels is also good practice; milk of magnesia or a cleansing enema is often advisable. If vomiting is present, avoid giving any food for twelve to twenty-four hours. Never give a laxative without consulting a physician if there is vomiting and/or the child complains of abdominal pain.

## INFLAMMATION OF THE GLANDS

***Causes of Inflammation.*** Glands are a natural part of the structure of the body. They are, however, not usually noticeable unless they become enlarged through inflammation. This inflammation is simply an extension of an infection from other parts of the body, since glands are a part of a system of vessels (lymphatic system) which drain the tissues all over the body, and empty finally into the general blood stream. The glands may be regarded as acting like traps in a drainage system, to catch the germs, or poisons which the germs produce, and so protect the whole body from invasion, although the glands may themselves become invaded. Germs gain entrance to glands through wounds, sores, abrasions, and inflammation in various parts of the body.

Enlarged glands are commoner in the neck than elsewhere, because inflammation about the throat and mouth is so frequent. Enlarged glands are seen and felt as movable lumps under the skin. They may be more or less tender. In the neck they may be found below or behind the jaw, along the sides, and below the scalp at the back of the neck. Enlarged glands in the armpits arise from extension of inflammation in the hands, arms, or chest; enlarged glands in the groins, where the upper and inner part of the thighs join the body, occur from inflammation in any part of the foot or leg or external sexual organs.

In the neck, enlarged glands at the angle of the jaw and upper part of the sides of the neck are caused by inflammation of the tonsils, by sore mouth and tongue (enlarged glands beneath the jaw), by abscess of the ear (enlarged glands below and behind the ear), or by eczema or lice of the scalp (enlarged glands at the back of the neck). Sore throat from any cause, particularly tonsillitis and the type common to many of the germ diseases, including measles, German measles, scarlatina, diphtheria; adenoids; decayed and loose teeth; cracked lips; and sore tongue and mouth—these are frequent origins of enlarged glands of the neck.

The enlargement of these glands is brought down by treating the underlying cause.

### Tuberculous Glands

***Causes of Tuberculous Glands.*** Enlarged glands of the neck are more often seen in children under ten, and the most serious and important form is that caused by the entrance of the germ of consumption or tuberculosis. This germ may enter the healthy gland. More often it attacks the gland already enlarged and inflamed from the causes enumerated. The gland attacked by the germ of tuberculosis is called a tuberculous or scrofulous gland, or the disease is spoken of as scrofula—an antiquated term.

***Symptoms of Tuberculous Glands.*** Tuberculous glands develop very slowly; one or more lumps appear in the neck; they are not very tender, but persist and tend to increase gradually in size and number. Finally, after weeks or months, they often become red and sore, soften, and form abscesses. The enlarged glands which are not tuberculous usually vanish spontaneously after a time. These are exceedingly common in children, and differ from the tuberculous glands in that they arise suddenly—usually after a sore throat—and although they may be quite tender at first they rarely go on to abscess, but slowly disappear. If they do form abscesses, they do so in a short time after their appearance. But tuberculous glands, after persisting for a long time, may likewise disappear without further trouble.

*Treatment of Tuberculous Glands.* As in other forms of tuberculosis, dietetic and hygienic measures should receive first consideration. Enforced rest is necessary during the most severe period of the infection. Ultra-violet rays, applied generally and locally, are extremely effective. During the summer, sunlight treatment can be used. Certain drugs, like streptomycin, given under the directions of a physician, are valuable curative agents.

## RICKETS

*Causes of Rickets.* Rickets is a nutritional disorder of infancy marked by insufficient amounts of calcium phosphate in the bones. The disease causes softening of the bones, which consequently bend easily and produce deformities of the head, neck, chest, and legs. The abdomen is enlarged. The milk teeth are late in coming through the gums.

Rickets is a preventable disease. It is common especially among the poor. It usually occurs in infants from three months to three years old. Almost invariably it begins during the winter and early spring months. Premature infants are more liable to have rickets than full-term infants. If unchecked, the disease results in severe anemia.

*Symptoms and Signs of Rickets.* The disease begins with restlessness at night on the part of the child, profuse sweating of the head and neck, and increased skin pallor. The muscles become flabby. Soft spots appear in the bones of the skull. There is also swelling of the joints, beading of the ribs, enlargement of certain finger joints and evidence of acquired deformity. (Beading consists of a row of nodules, or knoblike structures, which are found at the junctions of the ribs with their cartilages.) Constipation is common.

*Prevention of Rickets.* Inadequate diet is the chief factor in the production of rickets. The essential dietary factor is vitamin D. This vitamin occurs in milk, cream, butter, egg yolk, and some animal fats. In the strongest concentration, it is found in the oil extracted from the liver of certain fishes (cod-liver oil, halibut-liver oil, salmon-liver oil, etc.). Vitamin D is also manufactured, and in that form is known as viosterol. Cod-liver oil or viosterol, or a combination of these, should be given from the time the infant is two weeks old, and continued for at least two years.

Sunlight is a protection against rickets. (Ordinary window glass interferes with the passage of ultra-violet rays. The child must therefore be placed out-of-doors to obtain the beneficial effects of the sun's rays.)

***Treatment of Rickets.*** Cure and prevention are alike in many respects. The diet should include ample amounts of vitamin-D-enriched milk, egg yolk, butter, and cream. It should be rich in anti-rachitic foods (that is, foods valuable in fighting rickets), which should contain an abundance of calcium phosphate—as is to be found in cheese, nuts, cabbage, and milk—in addition to vitamin D. Dicalcium phosphate may also be given, and daily sun baths are suggested. The various bone deformities should be treated by an orthopedist. Under treatment, most children recover.

## SPASM OF THE LARYNX ("HOLDING THE BREATH")

***Causes of Spasm of the Larynx.*** This nervous disorder occurs especially in children of six months to three years, with rickets. The cause is usually fright, temper, or pain. The attacks are more apt to come on if the child is scolded or stopped from doing something; also after swallowing, or exposure to draughts. The condition is caused by a sudden spasm of the muscles of the throat, so that the air passage is temporarily closed.

***Symptoms of Spasm of the Larynx.*** When an attack comes on, the child suddenly stops breathing, struggles to regain its breath, turns blue, and sometimes almost loses consciousness. Just when suffocation seems imminent, the breath is drawn in—with a crowing sound in many instances—and the attack is over, with the passing of the spasm in the throat. Similar attacks may even occur many times during the day.

***Treatment of Spasm of the Larynx.*** There is no danger. Recovery always takes place. During an attack, you can dash cold water in the child's face, though this is seldom necessary. Daily cold sponging of the body, part by part, drying each part in turn, may be of benefit, unless it increases the spasm through fright.

The spells are apparently related to inadequacies of diet in some cases.

## CHOREA (ST. VITUS'S DANCE)

***Causes of St. Vitus's Dance.*** This disorder is a nervous manifestation of rheumatism. The disease occurs most frequently in later childhood and puberty. It is rare before the age of five. Females are much more susceptible than males. Like rheumatism, it often follows some acute respiratory infection, such as tonsillitis and pharyngitis. The psychic factor is sometimes evident–sudden fright, great grief, or other emotional causes, such as a bad relationship between the parents.

***Symptoms of St. Vitus's Dance.*** As a rule the beginning is gradual. In the mild conditions there may be nothing more than restlessness and inability to sit still. Some slight twitchings of the face and a tendency to involuntary facial grimacing are noted. The irregular movements are exaggerated when the child tries to carry out some normal act, such as handling objects or feeding himself. Sometimes the unexplained dropping of a plate or spoon first draws the attention of the parents to the child's condition.

In moderate conditions, the child shows emotional disturbance—cries over nothing and indulges in queer laughing spells. The characteristic jerking movements are most obvious in the neck and upper extremities. As a rule the movements cease during sleep.

In severe forms of the disease, the movements are greatly exaggerated, so that the child can neither feed or dress himself. In such conditions, the irregular movements are constantly present. The speech also is affected.

***Treatment of St. Vitus's Dance.*** A physician's care is important. The child must be kept quiet and must avoid excitement. In severe conditions, absolute rest in bed is essential, and the child should receive three or four doses daily of aspirin. A high caloric diet is necessary.

Fever treatment seems to be helpful, and is carried out in most hospitals. Fever brought on by the hypodermic injection of typhoid-paratyphoid bacillus often shortens the course of the disease to a marked degree. This is a drastic procedure, which should be resorted to only after careful consideration.

The heart is often affected, and should also be treated by a physician.

After recovery, great care must be taken of a child's general nutrition and health in order to prevent relapses. If the child's tonsils are infected, they must be removed. It is important for the child to be in a happy home atmosphere.

## CONVULSIONS IN CHILDREN

***Causes of Convulsions.*** A convulsion (fit) in a child is not a disease, but a symptom. It may be a sign of some digestive disturbance or of epilepsy. It is sometimes occasioned by incorrect feeding, or by food to which the child reacts abnormally.

***Symptoms of Convulsions.*** Convulsions may begin with squinting of the eyes, restlessness, starting or crying out in sleep, grinding the teeth, bending the thumbs, or slight twitching of the muscles of the face or limbs. Such signs should serve as a warning, particularly if the child is feverish. The patient should be bathed immediately with cool water as described further along.

The fit may begin with a choking sound. The body stiffens and is arched forward, while the head and neck are bent rigidly backward; the eyes are fixed, staring, squinting, and rolling, but sightless; the child neither sees, feels, nor hears, but is wholly unconscious. The face becomes blue, the hands are clenched, and then the body and limbs begin to jerk and twitch, the arms and legs being alternately bent and straightened. The breathing is rapid and noisy; there is grinding of the teeth, and frothing at the mouth; sometimes the tongue is bitten.

The whole attack may last but a moment, and there may be no more; on the other hand, the attack may last for several minutes. Rarely, it may last for hours, or there may be frequently repeated attacks.

If the immediate cause, fever, for example, can be removed at once, there is little probability of a return of the fits. The child, after the convulsions, acts bewildered, begins to cry, and returns to consciousness; or it may fall asleep, or into a stupor.

***Treatment of Convulsions.*** Call the physician. Undress the child and give him an alcohol rub. If this is not effective, place him in a hot bath at once, keeping a cold cloth to his head. The temperature of the water should be 100° to 103° F. One-half cupful of powdered mustard may be dissolved in each gallon of water. Be careful later to rinse all mustard from the folds of the infant's skin.

A better procedure is to use a hot pack made by wrapping the naked child in a blanket or in heavy towels wrung out of water at the same temperature used for the bath. Use either the bath or the pack up to thirty minutes, if necessary.

## POTT'S DISEASE (ANGULAR CURVATURE OF THE SPINE)

***Causes of Pott's Disease.*** This disease is caused by softening and destruction of a part of the vertebrae (bones of the spine) by the germs of tuberculosis. It is a tuberculosis of bone. It begins usually in children between the ages of three and five, although at other periods as well. If it goes on without early treatment, it eventually causes death in about one-fifth of all patients, or leads to deformity of the spine or humpback, and many other conditions, such as abscesses in the groins and back, paralysis, etc. If, on the other hand, treatment is begun early, before there is any, or but slight, deformity, the disease is frequently cured completely. It is of the greatest importance, then, for parents to recognize spinal disease at the earliest moment.

The seat of the disease is more often in the upper two-thirds of the back. The exciting cause in many instances is a blow or fall received a long time before the spinal disease became evident.

***Symptoms of Pott's Disease.*** The disease begins slowly. Before any definite symptoms present themselves, the child appears fretful, lies on the floor, is loath to stand or play, and often has a cough or pain in the abdomen.

The chief symptoms are pain, stiffness of the back, awkwardness in moving, weakness, and deformity. Pain is not usually felt in the back except when jarred, although at night the child often cries out in his sleep, owing to his unconscious movements, which cause pain. Neither is tenderness on pressing the spine common, but pain is felt more often in the belly, as stomach ache and colic.

Stiffness of the back is a very important sign. The child does not bend his back freely, but carries himself stiffly, and, when he stoops to pick up anything, squats down by bending the legs at the knees and hips. Weakness is shown by the child's dislike of standing or walking. He tries to hold on to something for support, totters about on his toes, and falls frequently.

Deformity is usually the first sign which calls attention to the real nature of the disease, unless the parents are alert to the possibility of the disease and consult a physician before the disease is advanced.

The deformity is seen as a knuckle-like projection in some part of the back, and is made much more noticeable by bending the back. Occasionally there is a curvature of the back caused by rickets. In this case the spine is bent outward through a great part of its length, and there are other signs of rickets, such as enlargement of the wrists and beadlike swellings on the ribs. If the spine in the neck is diseased, the shoulders are apt to be held high and there is often a chronic stiff neck. If the disease is in the lower part of the back, the child is apt to lean forward with the hands resting on the thighs.

The temperature in Pott's disease or tuberculosis of the spine is apt to range about 99.5 to 100° F.

The diagnosis is made certain if there is spasm of the spinal muscles and a consequent rigidity of the spine in testing its mobility by passive and active motion. The tuberculin test is positive, and X-ray examination shows more or less destruction of one or more vertebrae.

***Treatment of Pott's Disease.*** This consists mainly of complete immobilization of the spinal column by an orthopedic surgeon. In addition, dietetic and physical treatment for tuberculosis should be prescribed, with plenty of rest and sunshine.

## LATERAL CURVATURE OF THE SPINE

***Causes of Lateral Curvature.*** This disorder differs entirely from Pott's disease. Lateral curvature of the spine is a deformity of the body caused by a permanent bending of the spine to one side, so that instead of being straight it assumes somewhat the shape of the letter S. Not only is the spine bent to one side, but it is turned, to some extent, on its axis. In the beginning this distortion of the spinal column is not usually brought about by disease of the spine itself, although sometimes, in children with rickets, the softer bone makes the child liable to favor the deformity. It arises from causes which tend to pull the spine out of line more or less constantly. Since it occurs at an early age, when the spine structures are very pliable, permanent distortion results, with gradual changes in the structure of the bones of the spine (vertebrae).

It is very important, then, that this condition should be discovered before actual structural changes occur, because the disease may be overcome, and in this way incurable and lasting deformity can be prevented.

Among the predisposing causes are all sorts of circumstances leading to faulty positions of the body, such as improper arrangement of school desks; carrying of heavy weights constantly in one hand or one arm, as when children carry books; certain occupations; effects of clothing; difficulties, such as faulty sight, requiring bending of the head and body to see. Other causes are paralysis of muscles on one side of the body, loss of one arm, rapid growth, rickets, etc.

***Symptoms of Lateral Curvature.*** Lateral curvature is much more frequent in girls than boys; but it may be seen in robust boys who practice special exercises. While the deformity often begins in young children, it does not commonly become obvious until a later period (from eight to fifteen years of age), when growth is rapid. The bending in the upper part of the spine is usually to the right, while the left shoulder is lowered and the left hip is raised as compared with these areas on the right side of the body. The condition can best be observed by marking the line along the bony projections of the spine down the back.

There are frequently no unpleasant symptoms. Sometimes, however, there are fatigue from slight causes, general irritability, and pain on the left side, if the bending of the spine is toward the right. More often no pain is produced. Occasionally the disease may closely resemble angular curvature, already described, but the fever, pain on movements, and stiffness of the back are absent.

***Treatment of Lateral Curvature.*** In children, this deformity of the spine may sometimes be corrected by properly selected exercises or by orthopedic apparatus. Special knowledge and skill are required for this purpose, so that the physician should be informed as soon as any evidence is found of lateral deformity.

## HIP-JOINT DISEASE (HIP DISEASE)

***Causes of Hip Disease.*** The disease of children commonly called hip disease is usually an inflammation of the hip joint, caused by the germ of tuberculosis. It begins slowly, lasts from several months to many years, and sometimes may apparently be traced to an injury, such as a fall or blow.

***Symptoms of Hip Disease.*** The first symptom which attracts attention to the disease in the child is usually a slight limp and stiffness of the affected limb in the morning. This stiffness may pass off after a while when the child is playing. Sometimes there may be periods of weeks when this disappears, only to return in a worse form. More often, however, it is constantly present and grows worse.

Along with the lameness, or a little later, pain appears. But the pain at first is not as a rule in the diseased hip joint, but in the toe, calf of the leg, or knee. This is naturally apt to mislead parents into thinking the condition is due to the misnamed "growing pains," to rheumatism, or to weakness in the knee. This error must be avoided. At night the child often cries out in pain.

The position in which the child holds the affected leg is often typical. The lameness increases in severity, and the weight is chiefly borne on the sound limb, while the diseased limb is bent slightly at the thigh, and the toes and limb are turned outward. At the same time the crease, naturally present under the buttocks, is less noticeable on the leg of the affected side.

***Treatment of Hip Disease.*** The constitutional treatment is that of tuberculosis elsewhere in the body. The local treatment consists in the provision of complete rest for the joint by means of special orthopedic measures, such as traction, braces, plaster of Paris cast, and sometimes surgery.

If the physician's attention is drawn to it in the beginning, almost every case can be cured by rest in bed, splints, and apparatus of various kinds. If neglected till late, abscess about the joint, years of suffering, permanent crippling and lameness, loss of the limb, or even death may result.

## MALFORMATIONS IN CHILDREN

Any deformity that a child has should be corrected as soon as possible. A club-foot, for example, can be corrected if treated early enough, whereas if the condition is neglected, the child may be lame for life.

To neglect physical defects during the first year in the hope that the child will outgrow them is unwise. During this year of rapid growth, defects grow rapidly worse.

***Cleft Palate.*** In a newborn infant with a cleft-palate, for example, the objective of greatest importance is to maintain the child in a condition of good nutrition. The difficulty arises from the fact that the infant cannot grasp the nipple. This makes a cleft-palate a far more serious condition for the infant than for the child later on. The condition is remediable by plastic surgery.

***Bowlegs and Knock-Knees.*** These deformities are usually caused by rickets, but a hereditary factor must be assumed in some patients. Bowlegs are relatively rare, but knock-knees are seen daily in spite of the use of anti-rachitic (rickets) remedies. Overweight is a cause. To prevent knock-knees, the heavy child should lose weight and receive large doses of concentrated cod liver oil. It is important that he wear shoes that fit properly. Severe cases of the disease require orthopedic treatment, but if the deformity is recognized early, prescribing a proper diet or ordering the proper shoes may be curative.

## INVOLUNTARY PASSAGE OF URINE (BED-WETTING IN CHILDREN)

Inability to hold urine is normal in infants. Control of the bladder is acquired only after a certain development of the nervous system. In highstrung and nervous children, bed-wetting is a common occurrence at a later age than in others.

***How to Train the Infant.*** Most infants can be trained to control the bladder some time between the fifteenth and eighteenth month, if intensive training is carried out. Either in the morning or afternoon the infant is placed on the chamber for a minute or two every fifteen minutes for about an hour. He soon learns to urinate in the chamber and is accordingly praised, or rewarded, or both. If this training is persisted in for a week or two, with the usual praise, and there is no condemnation for failure to carry out instructions, he will in time realize what is expected of him. In this training, be certain that the child is fully awake when you place him on the chamber during the night.

***What Causes Failure in Training.*** In general it should be realized that if bed-wetting persists after three years of age, the condition may be abnormal. As a rule no physical cause can be found, and the disorder is attributed to bad habits. Certain factors, however, play a part, such as drinking too much water in the evening. Psychological factors may also be present. In a certain number of children, the condition is the result of local disturbances and malformations of the urinary tract and certain diseases of the nervous system.

***Treatment of the Condition.*** During the day the child should receive plenty of milk and water, but fluids should be restricted after 4 or 5 P.M. This holds true also for semi-solid foods, such as applesauce and stewed fruits. A thirsty child at night may receive small pieces of apple or orange. The infant should be awakened a few times at night to pass urine. Gradually the intervals at night are lengthened. The child should be kept well covered with blankets in the winter. (Bed-wetting frequently disappears during a hot summer when a child perspires freely.)

Punishments or scoldings are no curative measures—in fact, they sometimes work harmfully. Sometimes a child who has acquired control will wet the bed following an illness. This, however, is only a temporary condition.

## BOWEL DISTURBANCE (ACID DYSPEPSIA)

***Causes of Bowel Disturbance.*** This disorder often begins about two or three weeks after birth. The cause is unknown, but may be owing to milk too rich in fat or to infection of the intestinal tract.

***Symptoms of Bowel Disturbance.*** The baby cries—sometimes continuously—and does not sleep. Severe attacks of colic occur soon after nursing. The infant may stop nursing. His abdomen is distended. The stools are frequently thin, watery, containing much mucus and often full of bubbles.

***Treatment of Bowel Disturbance.*** The main objective is to try to maintain maternal nursing. When the infant is on artificial food, the disorder may be cured by withholding all food, except weak tea, for twenty-four hours. An ounce of barley water is given before feeding, and a mixture of paregoric and atropine, prescribed by the doctor.

## INTESTINAL COLIC

***Causes and Symptoms of Intestinal Colic.*** The swallowing of air with milk frequently causes a large air bubble to form in the infant's stomach. This distresses the infant after a full meal. He should be "burped," that is, given a chance to belch, by putting him on his stomach and gently patting his back.

***Treatment of Intestinal Colic.*** The treatment consists of giving an enema of warm water once or twice a day, giving peppermint or cinnamon water, and application of a warm water bottle to the abdomen.

## DIARRHEA

***Causes of Diarrhea.*** Diarrhea is only a symptom. The causes are many. They are usually classified as mechanical, toxic, chemical, nervous, metabolic, and infectious. There are various kinds of diarrhea. In fermentative diarrhea, there are frequent, offensive and sour-smelling stools. Specific diarrhea of infants may occur in newborn infants who often have a looseness of the bowels even when breast-fed. Giving too much sugar water during the first milk period may cause intestinal fermentation. Artificial feeding sometimes starts the episode, when the food is too concentrated or fed in large quantities. There is also summer diarrhea, a condition which may be caused by bacterial toxins in the milk—food poisoning. It arises principally from contaminated and decomposed cow's milk.

***Symptoms of Diarrhea.*** The symptoms sometimes begin with fever and vomiting. Convulsions may occur. Thirst is a prominent symptom. The stools are fecal (formed) at first, but soon become watery and have an offensive acid odor. There are small curds and mucus in them. Greenish or slightly yellowish stools are noted. The infant may have as many as fifteen to twenty bowel movements a day.

***Treatment of Diarrhea.*** For mild diarrheas (three or four movements daily) solid foods should be omitted and the quantity of milk reduced to half by the addition of water or barley water.

To prevent this disorder it is important to purchase the freshest and cleanest milk obtainable and to boil it during the summer *even if it has previously been pasteurized.* The bottles and nipples must also be kept scrupulously clean.

During an attack, the milk should be excluded from the feeding. Plenty of sweetened and salted barley water should be given—at least a quart daily. The infant is kept in the coolest part of the house and sponged a few times during the day with alcohol and water.

## DYSENTERY

***Causes of Dysentery.*** This disease usually appears in the summer months, mainly in infants and older children. It is caused by a group of bacilli.

***Symptoms of Dysentery.*** There are vomiting and high fever, abdominal pain, and diarrhea. There is quick loss of weight and even early prostration. Convulsions are common at the beginning. The stools are full of pus cells.

The mortality is high during hot weather.

***Treatment of Dysentery.*** The purity of the milk and water must be safeguarded.

The child or infant is kept in a cool room. No adult who is suffering from any kind of intestinal trouble should be permitted to come near the patient. In the summer, mosquito netting should be used over the child's crib, because the germ may be carried by flies.

The milk must be discontinued for a number of days. In infants, sweetened and salted cereals, boiled until they are soft, should be freely given. Plenty of water, sugar, and some salt will prevent a severe loss of fluids from the body. Every effort should be made to maintain a normal balance in the body fluid.

Vitamin C is added to the feeding in the form of orange or lemon juice as soon as possible. Vitamin B is included by giving some juice of vegetables. Milk is gradually added to the diet in the form of whole buttermilk or powdered protein milk. In some instances one to three pounds of ripe, peeled, and grated apples are given daily. Another form of treatment consists in giving fruit juices early, and banana pulp.

The following prescription is often beneficial:

Chalk mixture ............... 3 ounces

Give two teaspoonfuls every two hours. In older children the following prescription often gives relief:

Bismuth subnitrate ........... 2 drams
Phenyl salicylate .............15 grains
Cinnamon water ............. 2 ounces

Mix. Shake and give a teaspoonful every two hours.

Sulfathiazole or sulfaguanidine is used on the physician's prescription as an intestinal antiseptic in all examples of infectious inflammation of the intestine.

Sulfaguanidine is used especially for the treatment of dysentery caused by bacilli, for ulcerative colitis (in adults), and for stomach and intestinal disturbances in children.

To control the diarrhea, irrigation of the bowels with normal salt solution is sometimes necessary. Bismuth, kaolin, and charcoal powders diminish the intestinal fermentation, but should be given only on a doctor's prescription.

## CONSTIPATION

As a rule the infant is considered constipated if he does not have at least one bowel movement a day. The term is also used when the stools are firm and dry.

The disorder often occurs in breast-fed infants.

***Treatment of Constipation.*** The breast-fed infant should be taught early (at six months) to sit on a vessel supported by the mother, to strain, and to start his bowel movements.

A mild soap or glycerin suppository can be used at first. In bottle-fed infants the constipation can be overcome by adding a fermentable carbohydrate to the milk. The most effective are sorghum molasses and honey. Corn syrup also has a laxative effect.

In severe constipation, a teaspoonful of milk of magnesia may be added to a single bottle.

The pulpy fruits, stewed, such as prunes, pears, apples and peaches, may be prescribed even for young infants—one tablespoonful daily, an amount which can be increased. The addition of an ounce of prune juice to the diet may prove effective. Enemas—not too frequently—may sometimes be given.

In older children it is best to diminish the quantity of milk and increase the pulpy fruits and vegetables in the diet. Sorghum molasses should be substituted for the sugar. Malt extract in tablespoonful doses, two or three times a day, has a laxative effect. Whole-grain cereals (Wheatena, for example) are useful in the relief of constipation in infants over three months old.

## TEARS AT THE ANUS (FISSURES)

A single tear at the anus may be caused by the passage of a constipated stool or laceration by some foreign body. There is sharp, stabbing pain in the anal region during and after moving the bowels. It is often so acute that the act is deliberately postponed, with consequent constipation. The condition should be treated by a physician.

## INFANTILE SCURVY

In general, infants and older children who have been inadequately fed are likely to develop scurvy or rickets, or both. The child getting the disease is usually about eight months old, and is rarely a breast-fed infant. The cause of scurvy is an inadequate amount of citrus fruit juices—vitamin C—in the diet.

***Symptoms of Infantile Scurvy.*** There are collections of fluid in the body cavities and swellings in the tissues beneath the skin.

Restlessness at night and increasing pallor are the first general symptoms. The earliest symptom noted, as a rule, is that the infant cries when diapered. It becomes obvious that the pain is caused by certain movements, especially of the lower extremities. The gums show a characteristic change. A bluish spongy swelling appears around the upper central incisor teeth, if they are present. A swelling along the bones is found usually above the knee or the ankle, which are tender to pressure. Occasionally a bleeding tendency is noted in the urine and in the substance that has been vomited.

There is a "beading" of the ribs (appearance of nodules where the ribs join the cartilage).

It is often thought mistakenly that the infant suffers from "rheumatism."

***Treatment of Infantile Scurvy.*** The infant should be put on a diet of fresh milk and meat juice. Orange juice or grape juice should be given, at least one ounce daily. An older child should receive two or three ounces daily.

If tomato juice is substituted for orange juice, twice the quantity must be given, because tomato juice contains less vitamin C. Tomato juice or canned tomatoes are less expensive than orange juice. (The juice poured off from canned tomatoes should be used rather than canned tomato juice; the latter contains condiments and other substances that may sometimes upset an infant's digestion.)

Certain varieties of tomatoes contain double the quantity of vitamin C of others grown in the same soil under the same conditions. Tomatoes increase somewhat in vitamin C content as the fruit ripens.

Pure vitamin C tablets can be purchased at drug stores.

When an infant is on a mixed diet and receives other raw fruit (apples, peaches, cantaloupe) the amount of orange juice may be reduced. During the summer, the fruits which a child is fed should be varied to include: raspberries, strawberries, tomatoes, peaches and apples. (Raw cabbage is a good source of vitamin C, and can be given to older infants.) When tomato juice or orange juice is not tolerated on account of vomiting or diarrhea, banana pulp, scraped apple, or fresh peach juice may be given.

Dry cereals and legumes (peas, beans, etc.) of all varieties contain no vitamin C. Butter, eggs and cheese contain no vitamin C. Bread and most of the prepared infant foods do not contain vitamin C. The exclusive use of these foods for several months almost invariably results in latent or obvious scurvy, unless the necessary vitamin is supplied by an accessory diet of fruit juice.

Milk is the most nearly perfect food and the food one can least do without. Even so, the vitamin C content of commercial milk, raw or pasteurized, is not dependable and should never be relied upon to supply the requirements. Loss of vitamin C, owing to pasteurization, aging, reheating and diluting, such as usually occurs in preparing a formula for babies, results in a formula extremely low in scurvy-prevention value.

## MEASLES

***Causes of Measles.*** Measles is an acute, contagious disease marked, over a period of a few days, by a slowly rising fever, symptoms of a "cold," and a rash which appears about the fourth day. The disease is caused by a filterable virus. It is one of the most contagious diseases known.

***Symptoms of Measles.*** The child appears to have a "cold." His eyes are congested; he sneezes, and a cough develops. By the fourth day there is high fever–104° F. or more–and a dry "barking" cough. An eruption appears in the mouth. The rash develops first behind the ears, on the forehead and on the neck. It soon spreads all over the body and becomes profuse on the face and neck. The fever now declines unless there are complications.

Complications are frequent in infants and young children; of these the most serious are broncho-pneumonia and ear infections.

During an epidemic, practically all susceptible children who have been exposed get measles after an incubation period of ten or eleven days.

***Treatment of Measles.*** The child should be isolated, and kept in bed in a darkened room, since there is usually great sensitiveness to light. The bowels must be kept open, and there should be a bland diet till temperature goes down. Give copiously of fluids–water, fruit juices, and milk.

There is no specific drug for measles, but lung and other complications, owing to secondary bacterial invasion, must be dealt with by the appropriate antibiotics (antibacterial substance) and sulfonamides. Where the sulfonamides are used, some secondary infections may be held in check.

## SCARLET FEVER (SCARLATINA)

***Causes of Scarlet Fever.*** Scarlet fever is an acute, eruptive, contagious disease caused by the streptococcus scarlatinae. Formerly, the disease was usually a serious one, but of late years it seems to have lost much of its severity, and the grave form of the disease is now exceptional.

***Symptoms of Scarlet Fever.*** Scarlet fever begins suddenly with high fever, vomiting, and sore throat. The eruption usually appears within twenty-four to forty-eight hours as a red flush, first upon the neck and chest. It then spreads rapidly. The rash consists of minute red points closely packed together. Fine brown scales form after a time. The cheeks are flushed, and a pale circle of skin is noted around the mouth and nose. The eruption lasts for two or three days.

No disease of childhood produces so many and such serious after-effects as scarlet fever. Of these, involvement of the neck glands, ears, and kidneys are the most common.

***Immunity to Scarlet Fever.*** A physician can determine whether a child is susceptible to the disease by the use of what is known as the Dick test. If the child is found susceptible, he can be made immune to the disease.

Immunity (resistance to development of the disease) may be conferred by injecting increasing doses of the Dick toxin. However, the reaction is sometimes so severe that the method has not been widely adopted. The danger of a severe reaction may, however, be avoided by using a smaller dose, and increasing the number of injections from five to eight. Normal human or convalescent serum may also be used to increase the resistance of children who are susceptible. Sulfonamides may aid in preventing the disease when given for five to seven days after exposure.

***Treatment of Scarlet Fever.*** Prompt isolation is extremely important. The quarantine should be rigidly enforced for three weeks in mild conditions and for six to seven weeks in severe ones.

In the severe form of the disease, scarlet fever antitoxin should be promptly injected and the injection repeated in twenty-four hours.

In the treatment of the gravely ill infant, immune serum from an adult may be used.

In mild conditions, the serum may be omitted and the disease controlled by sulfadiazine.

Penicillin has been found effective in preventing complications. The drug should be given intramuscularly.

In scarlet fever the throat needs special attention. An ice-collar may be worn part of the day if the neck glands are enlarged and tender.

In some instances the patient continues, even after recovery, to harbor hemolytic (blood-destroying) streptococci in the nose and throat. Penicillin is then more efficient than antitoxin in reducing the number of disease carriers as well as in decreasing toxicity (poisonousness) and preventing complications. The urine should be carefully watched for several weeks after convalescence. There is danger of a chronic Bright's disease coming on later.

## GERMAN MEASLES (RUBELLA)

***Causes of German Measles.*** This disease is an acute, eruptive, contagious disorder which is marked chiefly by enlarged neck glands and a rash. (German measles have no relation whatsoever to measles.) The cause is unknown.

***Symptoms of German Measles.*** The rash appears first on the face and neck, and then spreads over the body in twenty-four hours. It consists of rose-red macules or discolored spots on the skin, which are not elevated above the surface.

There are mild catarrhal symptoms of the upper respiratory tract during the stage when the spots come out.

***Treatment of German Measles.*** The treatment is directed at the symptoms. The patient stays in bed, away from others who may contract the disease. The diet should be bland.

## CHICKENPOX (VARICELLA)

***Causes and Symptoms of Chickenpox.*** Chickenpox is an acute infectious disease in which an eruption appears, marked by successive crops of tiny blisters. These later dry, to form scabs that are brownish in color. General bodily symptoms may be entirely absent, but they are usually moderate. There is an irregular fever which persists for a few days. The disease is produced by a virus.

***Treatment of Chickenpox.*** Bed rest and isolation are important until all the minute crusts have fallen off. Bathing should be discontinued for a week or ten days. Carbolated ointment, or a 1 per cent ointment of thymol iodide, may be used effectively on the small open sores. Scratching should be avoided to prevent secondary infection and permanent scarring.

## WHOOPING COUGH

***Causes of Whooping Cough.*** This is an acute, infectious, and contagious disease of the respiratory tract, caused by the pertussis bacillus, which is found in the sputum. The disease is characterized by violent fits of coughing with apparent strangling, ending in a whoop. The infection is most rapidly spread in the first stage before severe coughing has begun. An attack confers lifelong immunity to the disease.

No age is exempt, but most cases occur in children under five.

Whooping cough used to spread epidemically in the spring and summer. Whooping cough causes more deaths in children under two years of age than any other acute infection, except pneumonia and the diarrheas.

***Symptoms of Whooping Cough.*** The time from exposure to the development of symptoms (incubation period) is estimated variably from three to fifteen days. The beginning stage (catarrhal stage) resembles an ordinary cold. Sneezing, redness of the eyes, and slight fever are present. A short, dry, irritating cough arises and persists. The first phase ordinarily lasts two weeks before the secondary symptoms of more severe coughing develop.

***The Cough in Whooping Cough.*** The occurrence of a characteristic cough reveals the transition to the second stage. The paroxysm of coughing is often brought on by some act, such as swallowing, crying, or gagging. The child gives a series of short, explosive coughs without stopping to take a breath. His color, first red, changes to blue; his eyes water and become congested. Saliva dribbles, his tongue protrudes, and the veins of his neck are distended. When at last the cough stops, the child takes a long breath, with the characteristic whoop, and temporarily holds his breath. The process is sometimes repeated a number of times, and when the paroxysms finally end, a small pellet of sticky mucus is expelled.

The spells occur at irregular intervals, sometimes in rapid succession, and sometimes at several-hour intervals. Vomiting usually follows immediately after the coughing spell, particularly if food has been recently taken. The disease may last from six to eight weeks. Ordinarily, after a few weeks, the intensity and frequency of the spells gradually subside, and only a slight cough of a non-paroxysmal character remains.

***Diagnosis of Whooping Cough.*** Whooping cough in the second stage can hardly be mistaken for any other illness. The diagnosis is made by hearing the characteristic cough. In the early stage the bacillus responsible for the infection may be grown from special culture plates exposed to the patient's cough.

***Treatment of Whooping Cough.*** In the early stage and until the more severe coughing spells have abated, rest is important. Later the child does better in the open air, but he should be kept from other children to prevent spread of the disease. Sedatives and codeine mixtures are useful in decreasing the number and severity of the coughing paroxysms. Steam inhalations may be prescribed. If secondary pneumonia develops, penicillin is frequently given with good results, but penicillin has no direct effect on the pertussis bacillus. Recently encouraging results have been published suggesting that aureomycin may shorten the course and severity of whooping cough.

***Prevention of Whooping Cough.*** Effective artificial immunity can now be produced by pertussis vaccine. It is usually given by the pediatrician sometime in the first year of life in a series of injections. Most often it is combined with diphtheria and tetanus toxoid. Booster doses are given yearly for the first few years by many physicians. Widespread immunization in the infant has greatly reduced the incidence of the disease and mortality from it.

## DIPHTHERIA

***Causes of Diphtheria.*** This throat infection is most prevalent from the second to the twelfth year of life. It is most dangerous in late infancy and early childhood. Predisposing causes are chronic tonsillitis and other inflammatory conditions of mouth and throat. Diphtheria occurs the year round; but is most frequent in autumn and winter, when nose and throat infections make persons more susceptible to the disease.

***Symptoms of Diphtheria.*** The incubation period is usually two to four days. The disease sets in, often quite suddenly, with a mild sense of illness, sore throat, and fever (100° to 102° F.), with a disproportionate degree of prostration and illness. The pulse is usually rapid. A membrane gradually forms on the tonsils, which are swollen and inflamed. By the third day the membrane may cover the tonsils and uvula, the fleshy lobe hanging down in the middle of the back of the soft palate. This membrane varies in extent and is greenish or grayish. The glands of the neck are swollen. The membrane may grow down the throat, cover the tonsils completely, enter the nose, larynx and trachea, and bring about death by suffocation.

***Complications.*** Bronchopneumonia is a common and dangerous complication of diphtheria, and a frequent cause of death. Heart failure and paralysis are apt to occur in the second or third week of convalescence.

***Immunization Against Diphtheria.*** The average child under eight is susceptible to diphtheria, and all children should be immunized. The Schick test is a specific skin reaction for the purpose of finding out whether and how much a person is susceptible to diphtheria. Another test, the Moloney, determines susceptibility to the toxoid (the injected substance capable of producing antibodies). If this test

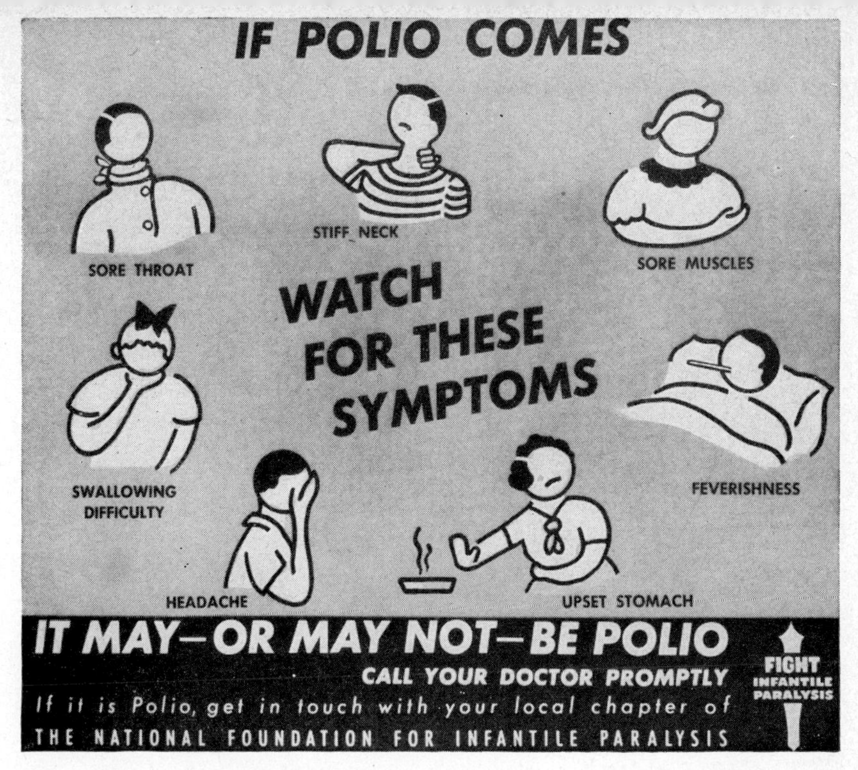


## WHAT CAUSES POLIO (INFANTILE PARALYSIS)

Polio is caused by a tiny organism known as a virus. The polio virus attacks the spinal cord and brain, injuring or destroying the nerve cells. Polio is transmitted by close personal contact. *(Below)* Little girl, Kathleen, runs high temperature, has sore muscles and other symptoms. Mother calls doctor at once.

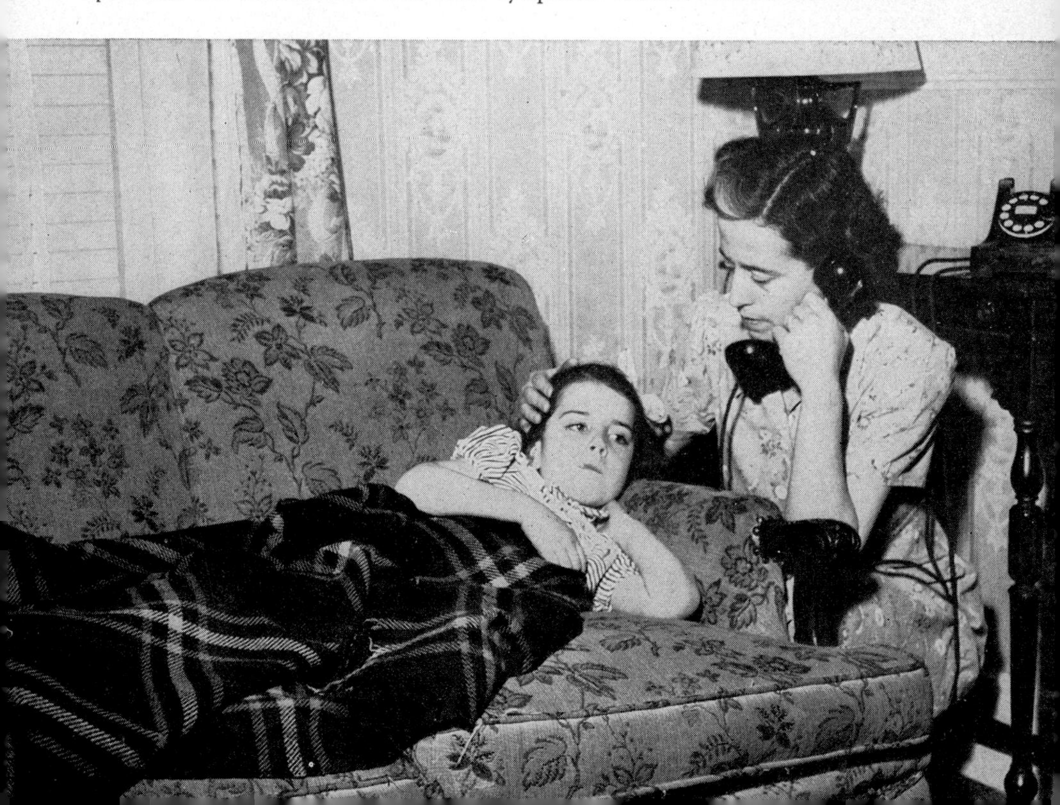

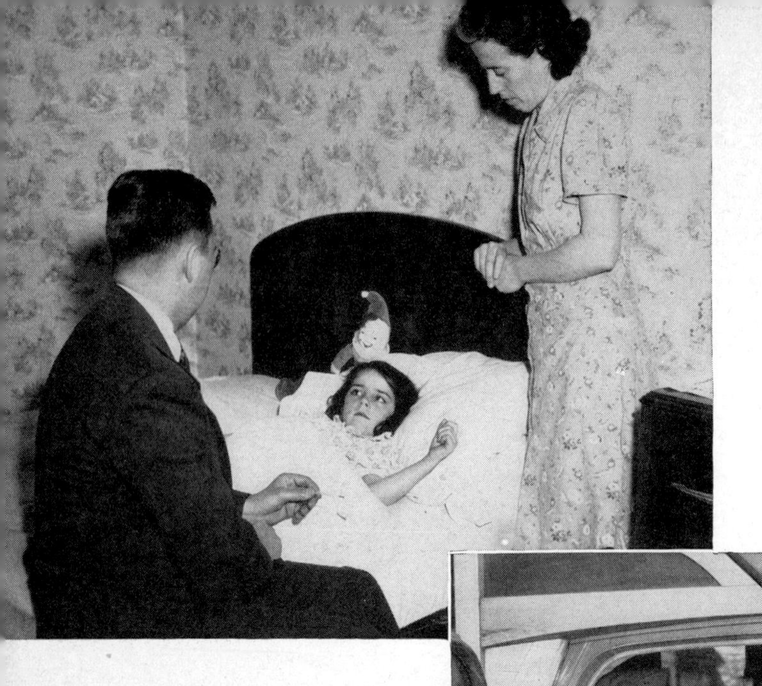

## AVOIDABLE

Kathleen's case has been definitely diagnosed as polio. Disease is often escaped by carefully observing these precautions: (1) avoid new groups; (2) don't get overtired; (3) don't get chilled; (4) keep clean.

## HELP FOR POLIO

Kathleen is rushed to hospital in Red Cross ambulance driven by local representative of National Foundation for Infantile Paralysis. This organization stands ready to aid all in fighting the disease.

## IN THE HOSPITAL

Kathleen is hot-packed by nurse in the hospital. This helps to relieve pain and muscle "spasm." Nurse checks Kathleen's temperature, pulse, and respiration often, notes changes.

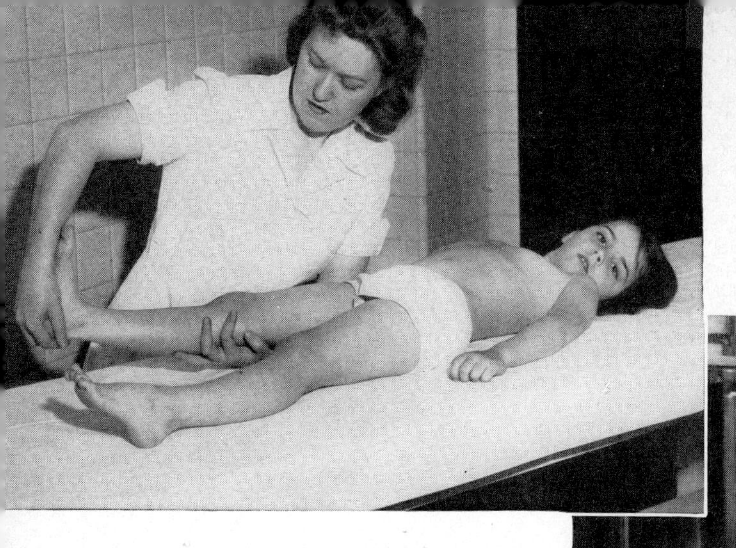

CARING FOR WEAK MUSCLES

Physical therapist exercises Kathleen's weakened muscles and stiffened joints to strengthen them and bring them back to normal again.

HOMEWARD BOUND

It is a happy day for Kathleen's mother when she takes daughter home. Thanks to prompt treatment, the recovery is complete.

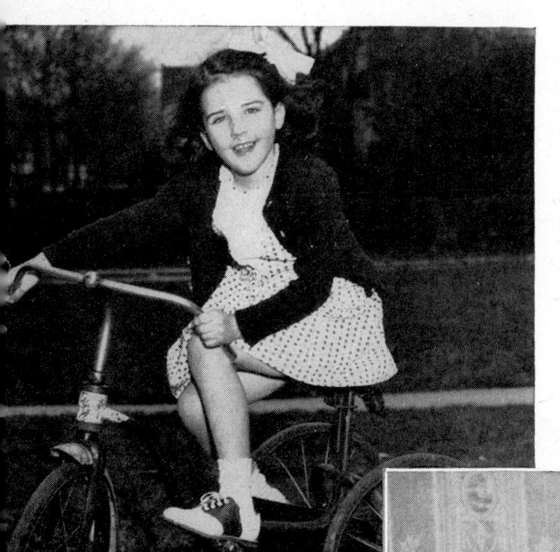

STRONG LEGS AGAIN

Kathleen, last traces of polio gone, rides her tricycle as she did before the disease struck.

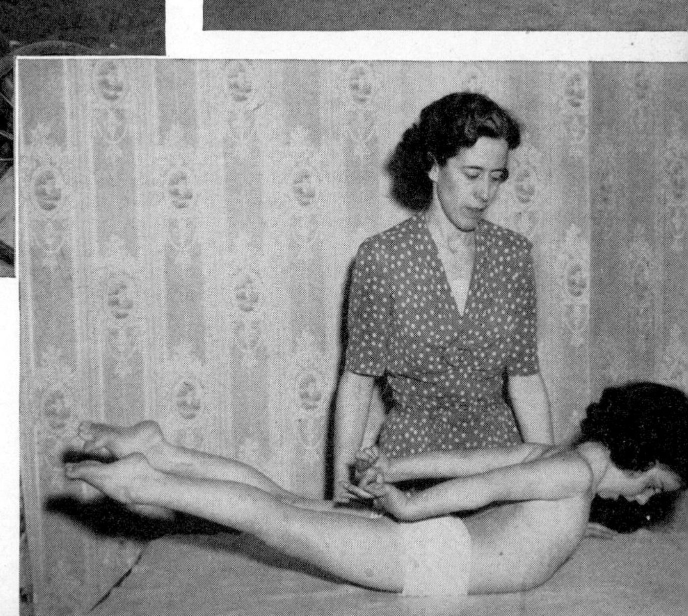

HOME TREATMENT

Mother must continue therapy during the convalescence.

## IRON LUNG

Sometimes breathing difficulties develop in cases of polio, and iron lung must be used. About 75 per cent of all polio patients make satisfactory recoveries.

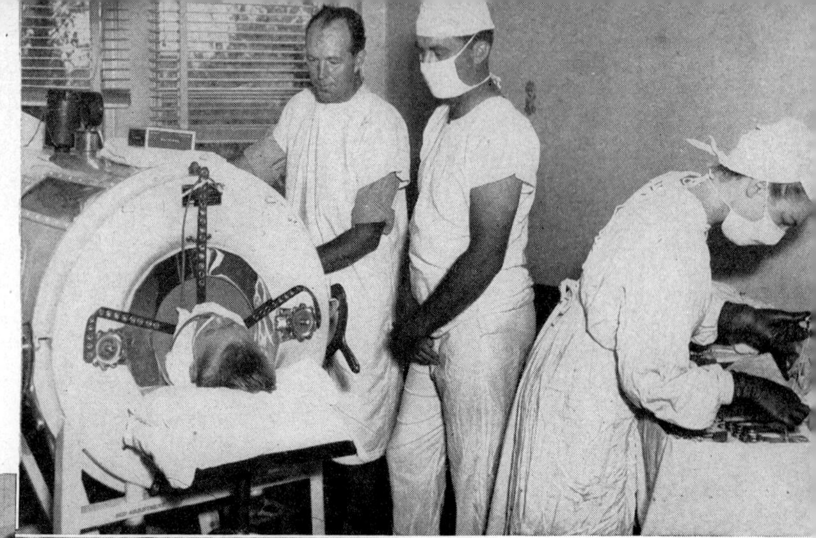

## WATER THERAPY

A skillful teacher encourages this young child to use his weakened muscles. Swimming pool therapy was a favorite of late President Franklin Delano Roosevelt, victim of polio.

## MAKING FINGERS AGILE

Polio - weakened hand muscles learn to work again by manipulating ordinary household items on gadget board. Cheerful frame of mind and parents' encouragement will help child to make recovery.

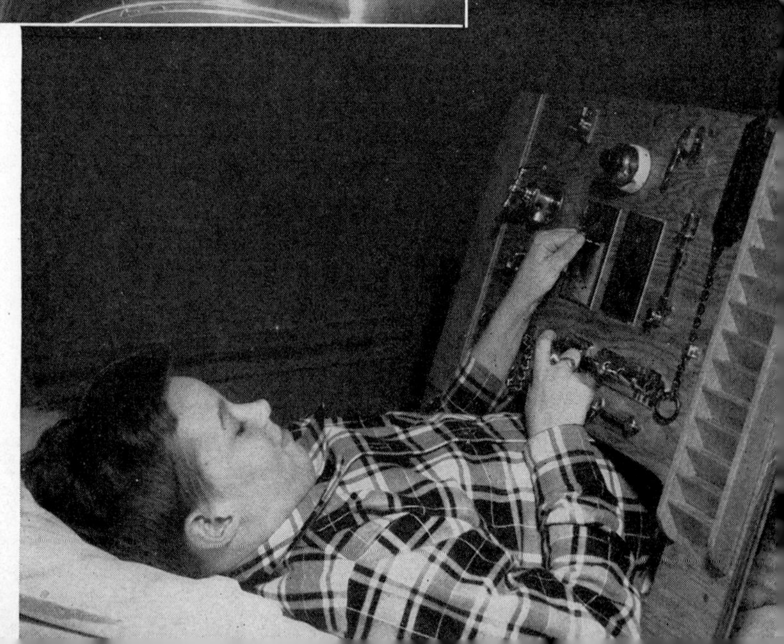

is positive, it is an indication that the injections of diphtheria toxoid, formed by treating the diphtheria poison with physical or chemical agents, should be given gradually.

In epidemics, Schick-positive or susceptible people, i.e., those who give a local skin reaction to injection of the diluted toxin directly *into* the skin, should be immunized by three weekly injections of a substance called diphtheria prophylactic toxoid antitoxin. In epidemics, and in persistent sore throats, cultures of the throat and nose should be taken, since it is the mild, unknown infections that spread the disease.

***Infant Vaccination.*** Vaccination of infants at six months generally makes the child immune during the months when he would be most susceptible and the disease most dangerous. There are a number of methods of immunization against diphtheria. The most satisfactory, apparently, is to immunize infants against diphtheria, tetanus, and whooping cough all at the same time.

***Treatment of Diphtheria.*** The patient suffering from diphtheria must remain in bed in a well-ventilated room. He must be isolated for four to six weeks, until he has had three successive negative throat swab reports on alternate days after the disease has "died out." He must be kept in bed for at least three weeks after the throat has cleared. Then gradually he may be permitted to sit up and finally to walk. The diet must be liquid.

Every doubtful condition must be treated as diphtheria, until it has been disproved. A culture of the nose and throat must be taken at the earliest possible opportunity.

***Giving Antitoxin.*** By far the most important factor in the success of antitoxin treatment is the time factor. The amount of antitoxin needed varies according to how severe the infection is and how long it is since it began.

Therefore, antitoxin must be given as early as possible. The earlier it is injected, the greater the prospect of a quick recovery. Usually the dose is given under the skin or in the muscles, and repeated in twenty-four hours, and again, if necessary. A rash frequently appears soon after the injection, but soon disappears. In severe forms of the disease, half of the dose is given in the muscles and the other half by way of a vein.

***Use of Drugs.*** The administration of vitamin C is valuable. The sulfa drugs have no curative effect on the disease, but penicillin seems to be of value in shortening its duration. For the average patient, antitoxin alone is adequate, but for the gravely ill the use of penicillin is vitally important. When antitoxin and penicillin are both given, the results are often miraculously effective.

## TRUE CROUP (LARYNGEAL DIPHTHERIA)

***Croup and Diphtheria.*** True croup is a different disease from what is ordinarily referred to as croup. The latter is a form of catarrhal laryngitis, whereas true croup is a form of diphtheria. Its cause is the diphtheria bacillus. It is most likely to occur in children under two years of age. Children at birth, and most adults, are immune. Formerly the disease had a high mortality, but nowadays it is readily controlled. It is most common in the autumn and winter.

***Symptoms of True Croup.*** The disease may affect the larynx primarily, or it may be secondary to a similar involvement of the nose or pharynx, or both. It begins treacherously with only a slight temperature, cough, and moderate hoarseness. The cough is croupy (hoarse and ringing). Loss of voice, as time goes on, is accompanied by shortness of breath and a bluish tinge to the skin. Later, breathing becomes harsher, with increasing evidence of obstruction in the larynx. This obstruction may be mechanical, caused by the presence of a membrane (see Diphtheria); or it may be reflex, the result of spasm of the larynx caused by inflammation of the muscles of the larynx.

***Treatment of True Croup.*** The treatment is, in general, the same as for diphtheria. The sooner the disease is treated the less danger. If diphtheria antitoxin is given promptly, the patient recovers. The membrane loosens, small pieces are coughed up, and respiration becomes easier and finally normal. The condition is sometimes so severe that a tube is inserted in the larynx to enable the child to breathe. If the proper instruments for this are not available, the trachea may have to be opened from the outside for the same purpose.

It is best to hospitalize a child suffering from true croup.

## NASAL DIPHTHERIA

***Symptoms of Nasal Diphtheria.*** This condition occurs mostly in children. Its beginning is similar to that of the common cold, with little or no fever, but a sense of illness. A more or less chronic nasal discharge, on one or both sides of the nose, soon becomes bloody and irritates the upper lip. Nasal bleeding may be severe and frequent.

***Treatment of Nasal Diphtheria.*** A culture of the nasal discharge should be taken. It will reveal the nature of the condition. The specific antitoxin must be administered.

## TETANUS

This is a disease caused by the tetanus bacillus, which occurs especially in the earth. Accordingly, tetanus is liable to follow wounds contaminated with ground dirt. Of these, punctured wounds are the most dangerous.

***Symptoms of Tetanus.*** The incubation period is about ten days, as a rule. The disease sets in with stiffness of the neck and jaws, which eventually enter into a state of lockjaw. Gradually the spasm invades the whole body.

***Prevention.*** Immunization should be carried out at about the sixth month of life. This should be repeated every two or three years, and additionally a booster dose of toxoid should be given if the child receives an injury which is contaminated with dust, soil, animal excretion, or other materials which are likely to contain the germ.

***Treatment of Tetanus.*** If the disease becomes evident, tetanus antitoxin is given. If there are convulsions, the physician also uses avertin.

## MUMPS

***Causes of Mumps.*** Mumps is an acute infectious disease, caused by a virus which occurs in the saliva during the first six days of illness. Severe swelling of one or more of the salivary glands occurs. There is a tendency for other glands to be involved, particularly the testes or ovaries in adults.

The condition is rare in children under four. It occurs chiefly between the ages of five and fifteen. Although not highly communicable, mumps may occur in epidemic form, when large groups of susceptible persons are living in close association, as in army barracks.

***Symptoms of Mumps.*** The average incubation period is eighteen days, with extreme limits of eight and thirty days. The disease sets in with headache, chilly sensations, loss of appetite, and tenderness of the affected glands. Several glands may be involved in succession, the first to enlarge usually being one or both parotids (glands in front and below the ears). The temperature ranges between 100° and 104°F., with a relatively slow pulse.

Mumps in itself, while painful, is not fatal, both fever and glandular swelling subsiding in a few days. However, complications, chiefly in the years after adolescence, may be serious. Atrophy of the testicles occurs in about 6 per cent of hospitalized boys and young men, though it is extremely rare in childhood.

***Treatment of Mumps.*** The treatment is directed toward the symptoms. Adults must have absolute rest in bed.

## SMALLPOX (VARIOLA)

***Causes of Smallpox.*** Smallpox is an acute infectious disease occurring in epidemics. It attacks people of all ages. Infection is carried by the excretions and exhalations, particularly the dried scales which occur on the skin of convalescent patients.

Three varieties of the disease are found: discrete smallpox, confluent smallpox and hemorrhagic smallpox.

***Symptoms of Smallpox.*** The discrete variety sets in acutely, with chills, severe headache, acute pain in the back, and vomiting. The pulse is rapid. The temperature rises quickly to 103° or 104°F. The rash appears on the third day as small, red shotlike papules (slight elevations) on the forehead at the hair margin, and on the wrists; later it spreads to the face and extremities. On the sixth day the papules become blisters. On the eighth day they contain pus.

The initial symptoms in the confluent variety are more severe. The rash appears earlier and is more thickly set. The pustules combine and form superficial abscesses. The temperature may rise to 105°.

In hemorrhagic smallpox the symptoms are extremely severe. As the term denotes, hemorrhages occur in the skin.

***Prevention.*** Smallpox vaccine virus should be administered at the sixth month of life or shortly thereafter. This should be repeated at six and twelve years. Re-vaccination is carried out when the child is likely to be, or to have been, exposed to the infection.

***Treatment of Smallpox.*** The patient must be isolated, and most careful disinfection of all things used or touched by the patient should be carried out. The nursing must be extremely careful. Complete bed rest is required.

The skin should be kept clean with mild antiseptics. Local itching should be controlled with soothing lotions. The light in the sickroom should be subdued. Boric acid solution should be used for the conjunctivitis (inflammation of the eyelids) that occurs. Medicine for relief of headache and backache should be given. The maintenance of fluid balance and general nutrition, plus a vitamin supplement, is recommended.

Vaccination of all persons in the immediate vicinity is essential.

Drug treatment is useless against the virus. However, penicillin for three or four days appears to be of great value in the pustular stage, resulting in profound improvement in the general condition, rapid drying of the pustules, and minimal pockmarking. Aureomycin may be substituted for penicillin.

## CEREBROSPINAL MENINGITIS

***Causes of Cerebrospinal Meningitis.*** This disease occurs in epidemics and also in isolated cases. It is commoner in the later winter months than in spring.

The disease is caused by a germ called the diplococcus intracellularis. The source of the infection is obscure, as a rule. It is known, however, that many persons may harbor the germ in the nose and throat. It is believed that these germ carriers are the principal source of the infection and that dissemination takes place by contact. Contrary to general belief, the disease is rarely spread in schools.

***Signs and Symptoms of Cerebrospinal Meningitis.*** The incubation period is one to five days. There is an abrupt beginning, with headache, vomiting, fever, and frequently convulsion. There is general irritability and stiffness of the neck; the head is bent backward and cannot be moved forward. There is also sensitiveness to light, noise, or passive motion. A general muscular rigidity is often detected.

In examining patients showing suggestive signs and symptoms (convulsions, stupor, retracted neck, general hypersensitiveness), the physician looks for two signs of cerebrospinal meningitis which are obtained by passive movement: the inability to extend the leg when the thigh is bent on the abdomen and involuntary bending of the thighs when the head is bent forward. These signs confirm other signs.

The diagnosis rests on the fever, headache, vomiting, stupor, rigidity of the extremities, and the position of the head. When the spinal fluid is examined, it is found to be turbid and to contain white blood cells, as well as the germs.

***Treatment of Cerebrospinal Meningitis.*** The treatment by administering sulfonilamides and antibiotics (penicillin) is regarded as the best. As soon as the diagnosis is complete, the physician makes injections into the spinal canal.

## INFANTILE PARALYSIS (POLIO)

***Prevention.*** In its brochure entitled "Doctor, What Can I Do About Infantile Paralysis?" The National Foundation for Infantile Paralysis states:

"Since there is no specific means of warding off the disease, such as medical science has provided for diphtheria, typhoid fever, smallpox, and many of the other communicable illnesses, prevention, for the present, depends on avoidance of exposure. This is exceedingly difficult, if not even impossible, in most cases. During an epidemic many carriers and persons with the mild undiagnosable forms of poliomyelitis infection unintentionally and unknowingly spread the virus.

"There is yet no practical way to detect these carriers. All that can be done is to prevent unnecessary contact with others. During epidemics, avoid having children come in contact with new groups of people. Since this disease comes from other infected persons, the less the number of contacts, the less the chance of being infected. Even rigid confinement of a child to his home, however, will not always prevent the disease from being carried to him.

"See that children—and all other members of the household—take nothing into their mouths that could have been soiled by the discharge from the bodies of others.

"Screening of the house against flies may be an important preventive measure as this insect may be capable of carrying the virus from known cases or undetected carriers. . . .

"Hard and fast rules cannot be formulated relative to attendance at schools. In most communities, this and similar problems will be carefully considered by the health officer. In cities, the child actually makes fewer new and intimate contacts in school than out of school. In cities, children are drawn from a relatively small area. In the country, the reverse may at times be true, for here the children may travel long distances, and to them the school may add new hazards and new exposures.

"Swimming may be an important factor during an epidemic. Swimming itself is not thought to be harmful, but if the water is contaminated by sewage and human pollution a definite danger is introduced. If the child meets new people and is exposed to new crowds, swimming may be a menace even though the water itself is safe. Chilling and fatigue are to be avoided.

"All children with fever should be isolated in bed pending diagnosis. Avoid undue fatigue and exertion during the polio season.

Avoid unnecessary travel and visiting in areas where polio is known to be prevalent. Nose, throat and dental operations, unless required as an emergency, should *not* be done in the presence of an increased incidence of the disease in the community."

All patients and those with symptoms suggestive of infantile paralysis should be promptly reported to the local health officer.

***Symptoms of Infantile Paralysis.*** These depend upon the severity of the infection, and vary in different patients. The mild variety may start with very slight symptoms such as irritability of the child, some redness of the throat, and maybe nausea or vomiting. The temperature may be only 100° to 101°F. These findings, at the bedtime hour, may be all that there are. By morning, the temperature instead of being lower, has risen to 103° to 104°F. Then there is definite soreness of the muscles of the back and legs, and, of special importance, "stiffness" of the neck. This symptom, together with the others mentioned, is almost a sure sign of the disease.

The other type, or malignant form, of the disease is violent in its beginning. There are nausea, vomiting, sudden rise in fever to 105° to 106°F., bending backward of the head, extreme tenderness of all the muscles, marked prostration. Within six or eight hours, paralysis has set in. This may be confined to the legs or also the breathing apparatus.

If during an epidemic any of these symptoms develop in a child, be prompt in calling your doctor. A few hours delay may mean the difference between life and death or crippling for life.

***Treatment of Infantile Paralysis.*** In the acute stage, there is little that can help. A serum is used, but it is not specific, since the exact cause of the disease is not known. Care is thus directed mainly toward the symptoms.

If there is paralysis, various orthopedic measures are carried out to prevent shrinking of the muscles, regardless of how mild the condition may be, because weakened backs and extremities, if not supervised, may result in permanent injury.

Moist heat, massage, and early gentle exercises are the only means of restoring potential polio cripples to normal life and of helping the stricken to adjust themselves to their handicaps.

***Use of Artificial Respiration.*** In severe attacks of polio it is sometimes urgent to give artificial respiration. This is done by what is termed an "iron-lung." Another machine about the size of a portable radio is used where the "iron-lung" proves ineffective and cumbersome. It is also cheaper than the iron-lung.

The respirator induces rhythmic controlled breathing by means of an electric current carried into the phrenic nerve at the base of the neck. This is the nerve that causes the diaphragm to contract and draw the air into the lungs. The electric charge is controlled by a timing device that decreases the current automatically from time to time, thus causing the diaphragm to relax and force out the air.

## INTESTINAL WORMS

Cleanliness of person is the first requisite in the avoidance of parasites. Children are more apt to be attacked by worms, as they are much less clean in their habits than adults.

***Causes and Prevention.*** Children suck their fingers, and handle dogs and cats from which they may acquire the eggs of the worms. They are also apt to scratch themselves about the exit of the bowel. In this way, if they are suffering from worms, the eggs may again be returned to the bowels, through the child's fingers and mouth. As many as three thousand worm eggs have been counted in a piece of excrement as large as a single grain of wheat. Worms are often conveyed, too, in the form of eggs, in drinking water contaminated with human excrement. Uncooked vegetables may also be infected, in backward and undeveloped areas, by human or other manure.

The common varieties of tapeworm are acquired by human beings through eating raw or imperfectly cooked beef, pork, or sausage. Dogs may contract tapeworm from eating the offal of slaughtered sheep and cattle.

The greatest care must be taken to destroy tapeworms and other parasites by fire, and to keep the rectum clean. In the case of pinworms, after their removal by treatment, the bedclothes should be boiled, children's toys burned, carpets cleaned, and floor and furniture washed, in order to avert a return of the disease through eggs which may be attached to these objects.

***Symptoms of Worms.*** To hear the opinions of many mothers, it might be supposed that worms are among the most common causes of disease in children, and that, together with teething, they account for the chief part of infantile illness. Both are enormously overrated as sources of trouble. The only proof of the presence of worms in the body is their appearance in the excrement, or in vomited matter, or in or about the patient.

All symptoms are very indefinite and uncertain, even to the physician, as, with the exception of pinworms, they often produce no trouble whatever. There are a great number of possible symptoms of worms in children. They include weakness, peevishness, nervousness as shown by fidgets, twitching, crying out or grinding the teeth when asleep. Also, picking the nose, fever, convulsions, uncertain—sometimes ravenous—appetite without gaining weight, pain and uneasiness about the navel, foul breath, vomiting, constipation, and diarrhea. These symptoms, however, are often merely the result of debility and have no connection with worms.

In the presence of pinworms, there is almost always great itching about the bowel, in the early night especially. The worms may indeed often be seen about these parts. In girls the worms may wander into the vagina, causing inflammation with swelling and discharge from the sexual organs. The local irritation of the pinworms in the lower bowel may also lead to bed-wetting, masturbation, fainting, and sleeplessness in children.

Tapeworms in adults also produce very indefinite symptoms, such as nausea, diarrhea, discomfort in the bowels, pallor or anemia, and, in nervous persons, sometimes melancholy.

***Treatment for Pinworms.*** In this condition tablets of methylrosaniline chloride, which can be procured on a physician's prescription, bring about a cure. Two tablets are to be taken immediately before meals three times a day for eight days. After an interval of a week, the medication is repeated. If a child suffers from pinworms, the entire family should be treated at the same time.

Another drug, which should be used with great caution and only under strict instructions of a physician, is remarkably and quickly effective in the cure, without the necessity of a few days' abstention from the drug. It is oil of chenopodium. For a child, as many drops of the oil are given on a piece of lump sugar as the child is years old. The dose is repeated in two hours, followed by the use of castor oil.

### Round Worms

These are from four to ten inches long, pointed at the ends like earthworms, but of a yellow-white color or tinged with red. They naturally inhabit the upper parts of the bowels, but wander about and often are vomited from the stomach. They may thus be found in the nose or throat. They are ordinarily seen in the excrement, and a white, mucous discharge from the bowels is occasionally mistaken for them.

***Treatment of Round Worms.*** Santonin is one of the most ancient drugs used for the cure of round worms. It is tasteless and non-irritant, and easily administered to children. It is the most effective remedy. It is also used for the removal of pinworms. It is prescribed by the physician with calomel. For children the small crystals can be used with sugar.

### Tapeworms

The common tapeworms are of two varieties: beef and pork tapeworms, caused by the eating of the raw or imperfectly cooked meats. If raw beef is very finely minced, or if the juice is squeezed out of raw beef and strained, the danger of tapeworm is averted. There is great danger of children with tapeworm conveying some of the eggs from the parts about the rectum to their mouths, through sucking their fingers. In this event the immature tapeworms enter the body and attack other organs, thus endangering the life of the patient. The ordinary tapeworm is from twenty to fifty feet long, made up of white, flattened joints or segments. The head is the size of a pinhead, and the neck is not much thicker than a thread, but the middle and lower part of the body is from a quarter to half an inch wide. The presence of the worm is recognized by the escape of pieces of it in the excrement every few days.

***Treatment of Tapeworms.*** The treatment should be given only by a physician. He administers a drug which has a specific action on the tapeworm.

## CHAPTER 16

# THE SKIN

Excessive Sweating ... Sunburn ... Run-Around, and Whitlow or Felon ... Erysipelas ... Itching ... Itching at the Anus ... Lice Infestations ... Chafing and Chapping ... Prickly Heat ... Hives ... Acne (Pimples and Blackheads) ... Freckles ... Cold Sores (Fever Blisters) ... Shingles ... Ringworm ... Athlete's Foot ... Psoriasis ... Impetigo Contagiosa ... Boils ... Carbuncle ... Ivy Poisoning ... Eczema ... Warts ... Corns ... Calluses and Cracks of the Skin ... Baldness and Dandruff ... Excessive Hair and the Epilating Needle ... Ingrowing Hairs ... Gray Hair, etc.

Most of us probably give some thought to our internal organs from time to time, possibly because they carry some mystery with them, being hidden from sight. But it is a safe venture to guess that rarely do we think about the important role of the skin with its estimated two and one-half million sweat glands!

The skin is the largest organ of the body and has the greatest contact with environmental irritants. It is a shock organ of the body, the only organ that is constantly and directly exposed to the elements.

Rich in blood and nerve supply, the skin contains these millions of sweat glands throughout its area, except at the margins of the lips. These tiny glands are more numerous in the armpits and on the palms and soles.

***Perspiration.*** Ordinarily, when we speak of perspiration we mean sweating, but, scientifically, perspiration indicates the elimination through the skin of all gaseous and fluid matter except that thrown out from the air passages. Water is also discharged in the form of vapor. This is insensible and invisible, and is fairly uniform over the whole body. Of the physiologic factors that influence the rate of perspiration, the blood circulation is especially of importance.

*Sweating.* The elimination of water from the skin by the activity of the sweat glands is what is meant by sweating. Its amount is influenced by mental and sensory nerve factors as well as by high temperatures. The amount also depends upon the severity and duration of muscular exertion. It differs with different individuals and depends greatly upon the individual's physical condition. The total quantity varies, the average in twenty-four hours being approximately one to one and one-half quarts. This roughly equals the urinary secretion and is of importance in the body's water balance. For perfect health, the amount of fluid taken in and the amount excreted should almost balance.

***What Sweat Consists Of.*** The chemical analysis of sweat shows 99 per cent water and 1 per cent salt and various acids to be found only in a trace. Seven-tenths of the 1 per cent is salt. Although the salt is found only in this small amount, salt balance in the body is of importance for perfect health. As much as forty-five grains of salt can be drawn from the system per quart of sweat. Such quantities, of course, are encountered only under stress of high tropical temperatures or intense muscular exertion. To counteract excessive sodium chloride (salt) loss, salt is taken by mouth. This will be a familiar statement to ex-service men who were stationed in the tropical areas.

***The Role of Sweating.*** The chief functions of the process of sweating are regulation of body temperature, elimination of poisonous substances during muscular exertion, and the protection of the skin against infection.

***Bacteria of the Skin.*** The normal skin is almost entirely covered by bacterial flora composed of potential pus-forming germs. These are what are called the staphylococci. They get their name from their microscopic grouping in "grapelike" bunches. It is generally believed that the surface acids of the skin derived from sweat have a bacteria-killing action. It has also been found that the various molds (fungi) which are often found in the skin pores are destroyed by the acid reaction of the sweat. In certain skin diseases due to fungi (ringworms), the sweat is found to be alkaline.

***Sweating Produced by Exercise.*** This is a common and purposeful manifestation of sweating. The temperature of the blood is not appreciably increased; indeed, the prevention of a rise in temperature is the very purpose of increased sweating.

***Nerve Factors Influencing Sweating.*** These originate in the brain and the sympathetic nervous system. Stimuli arising in the brain are usually associated with severe shock, when the individual is said to be in a "cold sweat," a common occurrence. The sympathetic stimuli are usually emotional. A common example is embarrassment, with "blushing," accompanied by or followed by profuse sweating of either the face or the entire body. The so-called "hot flushes" of both the male and female change of life (climacteric) are probably a body surface occurrence due to hormonal imbalance.

***Drugs That Influence Sweating.*** There are drugs that both increase and decrease sweating. The most important one that increases sweating is pilocarpine, and the one most often used to decrease sweating is atropine. The use of these is often of great value in certain diseases, especially when it is desirable to increase sweating in order to reduce the burden of overworked or diseased organs. Such is the case in certain heart and kidney diseases.

## EXCESSIVE SWEATING

***Causes and Symptoms of Excessive Sweating.*** This condition is called hyperidrosis. It can be a very annoying condition. It is either local or general and is independent of the usual physiologic causes. It is limited usually to the armpits, the palms and the soles. Persons so afflicted are very unhappy, and many are forced to change their clothing or shoes several times a day. The hands often drip the sweat when held up. The causes of most cases are not determinable. Sometimes the cause is found to be symptomatic of general malnutrition. The results are uncertain.

***Treatment of Excessive Sweating.*** The condition, whether local or general, may spontaneously disappear, may recur, may promptly respond to treatment, or may prove obstinate to all treatment. The X-ray has been found to give the best results, but it must be used by an expert or severe burns may result.

## SUNBURN

***Causes of Sunburn.*** There is a difference between "burning" and "tanning." In the process of burning, the cells of the outer layers of the skin are injured by the ultra-violet rays of the sun, according to the depth of the burn. The microscopic, tortuous ducts of the sweat glands swell, and sweating is diminished or even ceases in all areas exposed. The body may suffer shock, with very severe illness following in a few hours. This is readily understood when we consider what was said earlier about the importance of sweating.

Tanning is another process. It is achieved by exposure in broken doses. The sensitivity of the skin and its glands diminishes with each successive exposure and there is a deposit of pigment in the skin.

***Prevention of Sunburn.*** There are many preparations on the market that are said to be protective against the undesirable effects of sunburn. Most of these do not live up to their advertised value. Some are harmless and may offer a degree of protection, but not too much reliance can be put in any preparation.

Here is a simple formula for a suntan oil to be prepared by your druggist:

Menthyl salicylate........................10%
Sesame oil................................50%
Liquid vaseline...........................40%

***Treatment of Sunburn.*** For acute illness following a severe burn, apply a calamine lotion or zinc ointment, drink a great deal of water, and rest in a cool spot.

## RUN-AROUND, AND WHITLOW OR FELON

***Causes and Symptoms of Run-Around.*** "Run-around" consists of an inflammation of the soft parts about the fingernail. It is more common in the weak, but it may occur in anyone, owing to the entrance of pus germs through a slight prick or abrasion which may pass unnoticed. The condition begins with redness, heat, tenderness, swelling, and pain of the flesh at the root of the nail. The pain extends all about the nail and may be slight and soon subside. There may, however, be great pain and increased swelling, with the formation of "matter" (pus). It may result in the loss of the nail, particularly in the weak.

***Treatment of Run-Around.*** "Run-around" is treated by iodine, cold applications, and, if inflammation continues, by hot poulticing and incision with a knife; but poulticing is often sufficient. Attention to the general health by a physician will frequently be of service.

***Causes and Symptoms of Felon.*** Whitlow or felon is a much more serious trouble. It begins generally as a painful swelling of one of the last joints of the fingers on the palm side. Among the causes are a blow, scratch, or puncture. Often there is no obvious cause, but in some manner the germs of inflammation gain entrance. The end of the finger becomes hot and tense, and throbs with pain that may sometimes be almost unbearable. If the inflammation is chiefly of the surface there may be much redness. If mainly of the deeper parts, the skin may be but little reddened or the surface may be intensely pale. There is usually some fever, and the pain is made worse by permitting the hand to hang down. If the felon is on the little finger or thumb, the inflammation is likely to extend down into the palm of the hand, and from thence into the arm along the course of the tendons or sinews of the muscles. Death of the bone of the last finger joint, requiring removal of this part, stiffness, crippling, and distortion of the hand, or even death from blood poisoning may ensue if prompt surgical treatment is not obtained.

***Treatment of Felon.*** At the very beginning it may be possible to stop the progress of the felon by keeping the finger constantly wet by means of a bandage continually saturated with equal parts of alcohol and water. At night, keep it moist by covering with a piece of oil silk or rubber. If after twenty-four hours the pain increases, it is best to apply hot poultices to the finger, changing them as often as they cool. If the felon has not begun to subside by the end of forty-eight hours, immediate attention by a surgeon is required.

## ERYSIPELAS

***Causes of Erysipelas.*** A very acute and dangerous infection of the skin, erysipelas originates at the site of some kind of an infection or any crack of the skin—usually on the face. It is often first noted at the junction of the skin and mucous membrane of the nose. It is due to a very virulent germ called the streptococcus.

It is not as prevalent as it was many years ago before surgical antisepsis was developed as highly as it is today.

It can prove rapidly fatal in the aged. A prompt diagnosis is vital.

***Symptoms of Erysipelas.*** An area of redness appears on the skin, a sort of suffusion, so to speak. It grows in size. There is a sudden rise in temperature, perhaps preceded by a chill.

***Treatment of Erysipelas.*** Do not lose any time in calling a doctor. He will immediately give an intra-muscular injection of streptomycin. Local wet alcoholic applications are also used. Keep all children away from the case. Also any pregnant woman. The infection is highly contagious.

## ITCHING (PRURITUS)

Itching is not a distinct disease by itself, but a symptom or sign of other disorders. The disorder may involve one or several areas of the body or even the entire skin. In persons with temperature sensitiveness, exposure to heat or cold will excite an attack. In the variety known as "bath pruritus," for example, burning and itching come on immediately after the bath.

Occasionally itching must be treated as if it were a separate disease. This is when no cause can be discovered. Such itching may occur about the opening of the bowels (anus), the external female sexual parts (vulva), the scalp or when it attacks the skin generally, but is not accompanied by any skin eruption except that caused by scratching.

***Causes of Itching.*** Among the causes of the itching are changes which occur in the skin in old age, jaundice, overactivity of the thyroid gland, diabetes, pregnancy, intestinal parasites, and intolerance to certain drugs—opiates, for example. Some of the local causes include fungi, roundworms, constipation, piles, fissures (tears), and medication. Allergy in any form may provoke itching. Gases and dusts may act by absorption in breathing as well as by contact. Certain kinds of soap, clothing (wool, silk, fabric finishes), or cosmetics (including scented talcum and nail lacquer) are often the basic causes.

***Treatment of Itching.*** Every effort should be made to discover the cause, for which appropriate treatment can then be prescribed. In the main, the diet should be simple and nutritious, and it may be wise to avoid alcohol and coffee.

External treatment is of great importance in all varieties of itching. The underclothing must be soft and non-irritating. Cotton and linen are preferable. In laundering, all soap should be thoroughly rinsed out. Frequent bathing, particularly in hot soapy water, is to be avoided. A sulfonated oil should be substituted for soap. Bran, starch and alkaline baths are sometimes helpful in widespread pruritis. Carbolized calamine lotion is effective. Vaseline or mineral oil is preferable to cold cream or olive oil.

## ITCHING AT THE ANUS (PRURITIS ANI)

***Causes of Itching at the Anus.*** This condition may be caused by skin infections, rectal tumors, pinworms, piles, fungus, infection about the anus, or many other factors. Lack of cleanliness is an important cause. Many cases result from nervous exhaustion, falling in the large group of functional diseases for which no organic cause can be found.

***Symptoms of Itching at the Anus.*** The most prominent symptom is an intolerable itching of the anus and surrounding area. In severe conditions the itching is more or less continuous and is associated with smarting and burning sensations. In the chronic variety, itching is intermittent, and usually occurs after a bowel action, or soon after the patient has become warm in bed.

***Treatment of Itching at the Anus.*** The skin around the anus should be cleansed with absorbent cotton and mineral oil or wet toilet tissue. Calamine liniment is applied locally.

If these remedies fail and the condition becomes intolerable, resort must be had to a physician.

## SCABIES (THE ITCH)

The most frequent infectious and contagious skin disease is known as scabies, or "the itch," and causes intense itching and burning. The disease is spread by contact with an infected person, his bed, or his personal clothing or belongings.

***Causes and Symptoms of Scabies.*** There is a single cause—a parasite which burrows its way into and out of the skin. The itching is worse at night. The burrows made by the parasite are found between the fingers and along the wrists, along the front of the armpits, on the lower abdomen, buttocks and genitals. The face usually escapes attack. In infants the palms and soles are frequently infested.

***Treatment of Scabies.*** The most reliable treatment for scabies consists of the application from the neck down of 10 per cent precipitated sulphur and 10 per cent balsam of Peru in equal parts of petrolatum and lanolin. Four ounces of the ointment are used, one third of which is applied at night after a hot soap bath. On the next day, without bathing, one third is applied in the morning and the remainder at night. On the following morning, a hot soap bath is followed by spreading a generous amount of talcum powder over the entire body. Fresh underclothing and bedding must be used and all infested members of the family must be treated to prevent reinfestation.

For a child of five to twelve years, the strength of sulphur and balsam of Peru is reduced to 5 per cent. For younger children it is reduced to 2½ per cent and the amount of the ointment is cut in half.

## LICE INFESTATIONS (PEDICULOSIS)

When there are head lice, the hair should be soaked in a mixture of half-and-half kerosene and vinegar. This treatment should be given several times, and the hair combed with a fine comb frequently soon afterward. Tincture of larkspur is also used.

Pubic lice—lice in the pubic hair—are treated with ammoniated mercury, under the supervision of a doctor.

If there are body lice, all you need do is remove them and sterilize the clothing, in which they live.

## CHAFING AND CHAPPING

***Causes of Chafing.*** Chafing occurs when two opposing skin surfaces rub together and are irritated by sweat, as in the armpits, under the breasts, between the thighs and buttocks, and beneath overlapping parts of the abdomen of obese people. The same result follows irritation brought on by discharges touching the skin, as is seen in infants from the presence of urine and bowel discharges. The irritation caused by saliva when the lips are frequently licked is commonly called chapping, but it is proper to consider chafing and chapping together, since the treatment is the same for both.

Chafing occurs more often in hot weather and after violent exercise, such as rowing, riding, or running, and is aggravated by the friction of clothing or of tight shoes. It may, on the other hand, appear in persons who sit a great deal.

***Symptoms of Chafing.*** The parts affected are hot, red, and tender, and emit a disagreeable odor when secretions are retained. The skin becomes soaked with retained sweat, and may crack and bleed. The same kind of redness and tenderness is seen in the chapping of the face and lips, or other skin surfaces.

***Treatment of Chafing.*** In chafing, the first requisite is to avoid soap and water. Calamine liniment is helpful.

## PRICKLY HEAT (MILIARIA)

This is a common eruption which afflicts adults in hot weather. It frequently attacks children. It consists of a fine, pointed red rash or tiny blisters, and occurs on parts of the body covered by clothing, frequently on the chest.

***Causes and Symptoms of Prickly Heat.*** The eruption is caused by much sweating, which leads to congestion and swelling of the sweat glands. Burning, stinging, and itching accompany the disorder, which must be distinguished from contagious skin eruptions. The latter conditions are accompanied by fever, sore throat, backache, headache, and general sickness; in prickly heat there is no general disturbance. There is no fever, unless the eruption comes out in the course of a fever, and then it is of significance only as one of the indications of fever.

***Treatment of Prickly Heat.*** The treatment of this hot-weather complaint consists of avoiding heat as much as possible, and sponging the body with cold water, then dusting it with some simple powder—starch or flour, or better, borated talcum. An effective measure to relieve itching is sponging with limewater or a saturated solution of baking soda (as much as will dissolve) in water. Bran baths, made by tying one pound of bran in a towel, which is allowed to soak in the bath, are helpful, as is calamine liniment.

## HIVES OR NETTLERASH (URTICARIA)

***Causes of Hives.*** Hives is an allergy that may result from many different causes. Certain unusual foods may be a provocative factor; on the other hand, some simple article of diet, such as eggs or berries, may be the principal cause. Food hives or urticaria is usually discovered in childhood.

An attack may be brought on by physical agents, such as light, heat, and cold, or by scratching. Some injected foreign proteins, especially serums and bacterial products, produce hives in susceptible persons. Hives may also result from the inhalation of pollen, from insect bites, from the fur or saliva of domestic animals, or the taking of various drugs, including aspirin, morphine, codeine, barbiturates, iodides, bromides, quinine, atropine, belladonna, sulfa drugs, and phenolphthalein.

Chronic urticaria is sometimes caused by certain foods, by focal infection, or by animal parasites, but is usually caused by nervous exhaustion.

The allergy may be of obscure origin, and in some cases many factors may be involved.

***Symptoms of Hives.*** Hives is characterized by the sudden appearance of hard round or oval lumps in the skin, varying in size from a pea to a silver dollar. They are pinkish-white, or white in the center, and often surrounded by a red blush. The rash is accompanied by itching, burning or tingling, especially at night when the clothing is removed.

The eruption may affect any part of the body, but the lumps do not run together. Scratching the skin often brings out lumps in a few minutes. The swellings may last a few minutes or hours; they may suddenly disappear, to reappear in some other place. The whole trouble usually continues only a few days, although at times it becomes a chronic disorder.

***Treatment of Hives.*** The treatment of hives requires the services of a physician. Chronic recurrent urticaria is not easily treated, and search should be made for the cause. Relief is sometimes sudden, following extraction of a decayed tooth. Histamine desensitization is sometimes of benefit. Histaminase may be taken by mouth in coated capsules, if the physician prescribes it. The condition is also frequently alleviated by the use of benadryl or pyribenzamine in tablet form.

Most chronic urticarias are caused by nervous exhaustion. The exhaustion is treated by a daily nap, daily exposure to natural sunshine or a home model (R-S or Sperti) sunshine lamp, mild sedation, a vacation of four weeks, and correction where possible of irritating social factors.

For itching, the following substances are used with varying degrees of relief: sodium bicarbonate baths; starch baths; calamine and zinc lotion containing 1 per cent carbolic acid; cold applications; applications of heat; anti-itching ointments; adrenalin, injected under the skin by a physician; or ephedrine by mouth. In severe cases of the disease, calcium lactate, calcium gluconate, or calcium chloride may be given in the veins.

Usually in urticaria attacks a saline cathartic is necessary.

## ACNE (PIMPLES AND BLACKHEADS)

***Causes of Acne.*** Pimples and blackheads are both caused by inflammation around the glands of the skin which secrete oily material. The mouths of the glands become plugged, thus retaining the oily secretion and causing the blackheads. If these glands are then invaded by germs producing pus, a pimple results. Constipation and indigestion favor the occurrence of pimples and blackheads; also a poor state of the blood, or anemia.

***Symptoms of Acne.*** Acne appears chiefly on the face, but often also on the ear, the back, shoulders, and chest. It is a disorder which is seen mostly in young people of both sexes at about the age of puberty. "Blackheads" appear as slightly elevated black points, sometimes having a yellowish tint, from which a little, thin, wormlike mass can be pressed. Conical elevations of the skin, from a pin head to a pea in size, form an eruption which is often reddened and tender on pressure, and with a tendency to form matter or pus, as shown by a yellow spot in the center of the pimple. After three to ten days this matter is discharged, but red elevations remain, which later become brown and disappear without scarring, except in rare cases.

***Treatment of Acne.*** The bowels must be moved daily. The blackheads should be squeezed out with an instrument made for the purpose, not with fingernails. Pimples containing matter should receive an application of iodine or rubbing alcohol, then emptied after being pricked with a sterilized needle.

Do not use complexion brushes and creams. If there is redness of the skin and irritation associated with pimples, bathe the skin with very hot water and green soap three times daily, and apply calamine lotion or lotio alba at night. When the skin is not sensitive, and zinc or mercury has not been used, a treatment with sulphur soap and hot water at bedtime (allowing the suds to dry and remain on the face during the night) is recommended. An ointment consisting of one-half teaspoonful of precipitated sulphur with one-half ounce each of powdered starch and vaseline applied each night, and hot water used on the face three times daily, are also effective.

A highly successful technique in the treatment of acne consists of the use of what is known as a polysulphide. Vaccine therapy and injections of vitamin B are occasionally beneficial.

The various sulphur products have been combined with neutracolor (a mixture of betonite and oxide of iron powder) to produce a lotion closely resembling the color of the skin. It can be filled at the drug store.

Shake and apply to the face after treatment with sulfated oil.

***Diet for Acne.*** The diet should consist principally of vegetables, fruit, milk, eggs in moderation, and meats (only once a day, unless engaged in active physical exercise). Drink at least six to eight large glasses of water daily.

*Omit*—pastries, pies, cakes, ice cream, soda fountain drinks, jam, jellies, fried foods, gravies, alcoholic drinks, iodized salt, peanut butter, nuts, chocolate, cocoa, sugar, potatoes, rice, macaroni, noodles, spaghetti.

*Limit*—fats, meats, bread, cheese.

*Cereals*—cereals, hot or cold, may be eaten with milk (or cream) and a *limited* amount of sugar, two or three times a week.

*Eggs*—poached, soft boiled, scrambled, or in omelet. Not more than once a day.

*Soups*—all soups or broths. Avoid overseasoning.

*Meats*—all meats except pork and veal. Meats may be boiled, broiled, or stewed, but not fried.

*Vegetables*—all vegetables, fresh or canned, cooked or raw, except potatoes.

*Bread*—whole-wheat and graham bread, preferably toasted; hard rolls, corn and bran muffins.

*Desserts*—fruits only, preferably stewed.
*Beverages*—tea, coffee, milk, buttermilk.

## FRECKLES

Freckles appear as small, yellowish-brown spots on the face, arms, and hands, following exposure to the sun in the summer. They generally fade away almost completely in winter. However, they do not always disappear in winter, and they do occur on parts of the body covered by clothing. Freckles are generally seen on red-haired persons, rarely on brunettes, and never on the newborn.

Prevention of freckles is secured by not exposing the unprotected skin to the sun—though it is doubtful whether the end gained is worth the sacrifice, if carried so far as to avoid the open air and sunlight whenever possible.

***Treatment of Freckles.*** Their removal is accomplished by the use of agents which cause a flaking off of the superficial layer of discolored skin, but after a few weeks the discolorations are apt to return.

Boric acid, sixteen drops to one ounce of water, is absolutely harmless and useful for removing skin discolorations. The skin may be freely bathed with it night and morning. The following lotion (prescription to be filled by the druggist) is also effective:

| | |
|---|---|
| Zinc oxide | 30 grains |
| Powdered starch | 30 grains |
| Kaolin | 60 grains |
| Glycerin | 2 drachms |
| Rose water | 2 ounces |

Shake, paint over spots, and allow the preparation to dry; wash it off before each fresh application.

A saturated solution of sodium hyposulphite, if dabbed on the skin and repeated nightly, often removes freckles.

## COLD SORES (FEVER BLISTERS)

***Causes of Cold Sores.*** Fever blisters are caused by a certain virus infection. They often occur in the course of fever, including the common cold, influenza, pneumonia, malaria, and meningitis. Windburn or sunburn are often responsible for them, and indigestion is a common cause.

***Symptoms of Cold Sores.*** The sores, usually a few in one place, form on the face, generally around the mouth. The inner surfaces of the lips are sometimes affected. The sores contain a watery fluid.

*Treatment of Cold Sores.* Picking and scratching are very harmful, and cigar or pipe smoking must be stopped. Painting the sore with collodion, by means of a camel's hair brush, as is often done, is poor treatment in the early stages. In the earlier stages it is better to use spirits of camphor, and afterwards, if there is much itching or burning, to dab the eruption with calamine liniment to relieve the discomfort. A 5 per cent solution of silver nitrate, applied lightly once a day, will help in the healing process.

In a patient with fever the mouth must be kept as clean as possible. Clean it before and after eating. Lubricate the tongue and lips with equal parts of lemon juice and glycerin, using cotton-tipped swabs.

## SHINGLES (HERPES ZOSTER)

*Causes of Shingles.* This is an acute inflammatory skin disease. Its typical sign is the appearance of small blisters along the course of some superficial sensory nerve. Evidence seems to show that it is essentially an acute inflammation of the posterior spinal ganglia, and is caused by a virus, at times that of chickenpox.

*Symptoms of Shingles.* The disease attacks all ages, and is common in those who are overworked or ill. It appears, as a rule, only on one side of the body, with a discharge of serum and formation of blisters. There is intense pain. This may persist in old persons and be very troublesome. An attack usually confers immunity.

*Treatment of Shingles.* It is important to keep the blisters dry in order to prevent reinfection, because the virus of zoster is present in the blister-fluid. Locally, calamine liniment is a useful dressing.

Among the remedies the physician uses which often work miraculously are injections of pituitrin (surgical), cobra venom, ethyl chloride spray, dry heat, and thiamin chloride. Injection of sodium iodide into a vein on the first, third, fifth and seventh day diminishes the pain and hastens healing. Other pain-killers are also used.

## RINGWORM

*Causes and Symptoms of Ringworm.* Ringworm is an infection of the skin, hair, or nails, caused by various fungi. On the body it attacks the neck, face and hands. It appears first as small, red, scaly spots which may spread into a circular patch as large as a dollar, with a red ring of small, scaly pimples on the outside. The center may exhibit healthy skin, or may be red and thickened. There may be several patches of ringworm near each other, and they may run together, or there may be only one patch.

***Treatment of Ringworm.*** Any one of the following ingredients, when applied in a base, is usually curative: thymol (0.5 per cent); sulphur (2 to 15 per cent); sodium thiosulphate and salicylic acid (of each, 2 to 10 per cent); resorcinol (1 per cent); ammoniated mercury (5 to 10 per cent). If the condition is persistent, it requires a physician's attention.

***Ringworm of the Scalp.*** This is a disease usually confined to children and is difficult to cure. It is contagious and may be acquired from children with the disease, or from fondling and handling cats and dogs who have ringworm. Preventive care is necessary when there is an epidemic. The hair should be closely clipped, and the scalp should be washed with non-medicated soap and water once a day, or once in two days. A child suffering from ringworm of the scalp should wear a skull cap, and have brush, comb, towels and wash cloths carefully reserved for his personal use.

The following solution may be used for washing the scalp in ringworm of the scalp, or for ringworm of the body proper. It is dispensed by the druggist.

| | |
|---|---|
| Precipitated sulphur .......... | 1 drachm |
| Betanaphthol .................. | 20 grains |
| Medicinal soft soap ........... | 1 ounce |

Use like soap in cleansing the scalp.

The condition is sometimes helped by applying compresses of hot boric acid solution to the affected areas for fifteen to twenty minutes several times a day. Following each application, a 5 per cent salicylanilid ointment should be thoroughly rubbed into the affected areas. In ringworm of the scalp caused by a human type of fungus, temporary removal of the hair by X-rays is sometimes necessary.

### Athlete's Foot (Ringworm of the Feet)

This is the most common variety of ringworm. The feet should be washed with soap and water each night, rinsed well, and scaly accumulations wiped away. The toes should be dried carefully after bathing. A preparation of boric acid, tannic acid and zinc oxide in equal parts is then used.

Blisters should be opened with a sterilized needle, and the area painted with a 10 per cent watery solution of silver nitrate.

The feet should be soaked in some antiseptic foot bath, such as 1:8000 potassium permanganate or 1:10,000 bichloride of mercury, either of which can be had at a drug store. The soaking should last at least ten minutes, from two to eight times a day, using lukewarm water. Sulphur-salicylic acid ointment is helpful.

## PSORIASIS

***Causes and Symptoms of Psoriasis.*** Psoriasis is a chronic infection of the skin, of unknown origin. Reddish, rounded patches appear. They are usually dry and covered with silvery, overlapping scales. The disease affects persons of either sex and any age. It is commonly first found in early adult life as an eruption which involves the outer surfaces of the joints in the limbs, particularly the elbows and knees, the scalp and sacral region. When a scale is scraped or torn off, minute droplets of blood ooze out.

***Psoriasis of the Scalp.*** The scalp is often the first site of the disease. There are no bodily symptoms, but itching is exceptional and the affected areas are usually dry. Once established, the disorder persists, on and off, for many years. The eruptions may disappear during the summer, to reappear in the winter or spring. Hair loss does not result when the scalp is affected. The disease is only slightly infectious, if at all.

***Treatment of Psoriasis.*** In mild cases, ammoniated mercury with or without 2 per cent salicylic acid, applied night and morning, is frequently effective. Chrysarobin is also used. One teaspoonful may be mixed with two tablespoonfuls of vaseline—this constitutes a 12 per cent chrysarobin ointment, to be used twice a day. Take care to avoid the eyes, and keep the ointment away from clothing to prevent staining.

If the irritation is severe, it can be counteracted with 1:3000 water solution of potassium permanganate, procurable in any drug store.

Sun bathing is recommended, either natural or with a home model bulb. Ultra-violet light in daily increasing doses is best for those who tan easily—but never for the acute disease. X-ray treatment is beneficial for a short time, especially if used on localized patches.

Rest (mental and physical) is essential in the treatment of psoriasis.

## IMPETIGO CONTAGIOSA

***Causes of Impetigo.*** Impetigo is one of the most common skin diseases of children and is caused by germs, the streptococci or staphylococci. It is spread by direct contact or through the use of infected towels, and is often acquired in barber shops.

***Symptoms of Impetigo.*** Impetigo usually occurs on the face and scalp and rarely on the limbs or body proper. Blisters form. When they break, they produce yellow "stuck-on" crusts. The fresh crusts are yellow but later turn brown; when mixed with blood they may turn black. Itching is severe.

***Treatment of Impetigo.*** Treatment by a physician soon clears up this condition. The crusts are removed with forceps by the physician and the residual base is touched with an appropriate antiseptic. Bacitracin or aureomycin is applied in ointment form. In mild varieties of the disease ammoniated mercury ointment is prescribed.

## BOILS

***Causes of Boils.*** Boils are the result of an inflammation which has its beginning in an infection of a hair-sac. A pustule surrounds the shaft of the hair, and the pus-infected boil develops. Boils are usually found on the neck, armpits, face, buttocks, and legs, although no area of the body is exempt. The basic infection is caused by staphylococci, which are germs.

***Treatment of Boils.*** Formation of a boil can sometimes be prevented by the early application of tincture of iodine or mercurial plaster. If this fails, you can bring the boil "to a head" with the aid of dry heat.

Mild antiseptics may be applied. A good plan is to paint the boil once daily with diluted tincture of iodine or 1 per cent gentian violet in alcohol; then apply a large gauze pack (hot) moistened with half-and-half glycerol and alcohol. Physicians often prescribe bacitracin or aureomycin ointment.

It is unwise for anyone but a physician to cut into a boil, and it is seldom necessary. Infected hairs should never be pulled out. Also, the boil should never be squeezed out.

## CARBUNCLE

***Causes of Carbuncle.*** A carbuncle is similar to a boil in cause and structure. It is, however, usually a much more serious matter, since it has a tendency to spread at the sides and involve the deeper layers of the skin. It occurs most frequently on the neck, back, or buttocks. It is particularly dangerous when attacking the back of the neck, upper lip, or abdomen. It is commonly a disease of old persons, or those prematurely old or worn out.

***Symptoms of Carbuncle.*** Carbuncle often begins as a pimple, with a chill and fever, but increases rapidly in size to form a hot, dusky red, rounded lump which may grow until it is from three to six inches in diameter. Occasionally it runs a mild course, remains small, begins to discharge pus and dead tissue at the end of a week, and heals rapidly. More commonly, there is pain of a burning, throbbing character, which soon becomes intense, and the carbuncle continues to enlarge for a week or ten days; then it softens and breaks open at various points, discharging shreds of dead tissue and pus.

The skin over the whole top of the carbuncle dies and separates from the underlying matter, leaving an angry-looking excavation or crater-like ulcer. This slowly heals from the edges and bottom, so that the whole period of healing takes from a week to two months or even six months. The danger depends largely upon the exhaustion which follows the pain and continuous fever—also upon the possibility of blood poisoning. The more prominent signs of blood poisoning are sweating, chills, and fever which gets higher at night.

***Carbuncles Compared with Boils.*** Carbuncles differ from boils in their much larger size, in having rounded or flat tops instead of the conical shape of boils, in having numerous, sievelike openings, in the occurrence of death of the skin over the top of the carbuncle, and in the intense pain and high fever which accompany them.

***Treatment of Carbuncle.*** Carbuncle should be treated by a physician. The urine and blood should be examined to ascertain the presence or absence of sugar, since diabetes is often associated with carbuncle. Carbuncle demands incision by a surgeon as early as possible, since it is only by cutting it freely open, or even removing the whole carbuncle as if it were a tumor, that the best results are obtained. However, when no surgeon is available, the patient's strength should be sustained by feeding every two hours with beef tea, milk, and raw eggs, and with wine and alcoholic liquors.

Physicians often find penicillin and/or aureomycin of great value in controlling the infection.

## IVY POISONING

***Causes of Ivy Poisoning.*** Poison ivy, like poison sumach and poison oak, causes inflammation of the skin in certain persons who touch it. In some cases, even approaching within a short distance of the plants sets up the inflammation. The plants contain a poisonous oil, and the pollen blown from them by the wind may convey enough of this oil to poison susceptible persons. Signs and symptoms may appear within four to five hours, or in as many days after exposure to the plant.

There is a common belief that ivy poisoning recurs at about the same time each year. This belief has no foundation in fact.

***Symptoms of Ivy Poisoning.*** The skin of the hands or other affected parts becomes red, swollen, painful, and itchy. Soon little blisters form, and scratching breaks them open so that the parts are moist and then become covered with crusts. The poison is conveyed by the hands to the face and other parts of the body and, in men, to the sexual organs, so that these areas soon partake of the same trouble. The face and head may become so swollen that the patient is almost unrecognizable.

***Treatment of Ivy or Oak Poisoning.*** Ten per cent sodium perborate in a protective ointment base protects successfully if applied to exposed parts of the body before contact with poison ivy. Clothes and equipment must be decontaminated after exposure.

If you touch poison ivy, take a hot bath and rub the body thoroughly with soap. In mild ivy poisoning, some relief is obtained from swabbing the parts with 2 per cent potassium permanganate solution and carbolized calamine lotion. Burow's solution (aluminum acetate) may be tried as a healing, wetting agent. This may be made up with prepared tablets. Keep the solution in a bottle labeled "For Poison Ivy." Use it as a wet dressing for not more than ten minutes; after that, daub on a little if the itching returns, and let it dry.

The affected parts may also be bathed for a few minutes at a time in water just hot enough to be uncomfortable—paradoxically giving comfort. Dry heat is just as good.

An effective formula for poison ivy treatment consists of the following medical ingredients in the proportions given. It can be made up by the druggist, and is applied locally, as a lotion.

|  |  |
|---|---|
| Castor oil | 21.5 |
| Olive oil | 21.5 |
| Lanolin (without water) | 21.5 |
| Diglycol stearate | 12.9 |
| Paraffin, refined | 8.6 |
| Boric acid | 2.0 |
| Sodium perborate | 10.0 |
| Duponol W. A. Pure | 2.0 |

## ECZEMA

Eczema is an inflammation of the skin, of uncertain cause, marked by blisters, watery discharge, and the formation of scales and crusts. Fluid is concealed beneath the surface or appears on the surface after the skin has been irritated. There are many varieties, and they are classified according to whether they are of internal origin or of external origin, caused by occupation, climate, or by certain glands of the skin.

***Eczema of Internal Origin.*** This form of the disease almost invariably appears on both sides of the body at once, as for example, on both cheeks, or both arms, or both thighs. Its border shades into the surrounding skin; it is dotted with papules (or heads) filled with fluid, and its surface is clean and not greasy. Exhaustion plays a prominent role. Among the drugs producing it is cod-liver oil.

***Eczema of External Origin.*** Occupational eczema occurs first on exposed parts—the hands, arms, face and neck—of those who handle irritant dyes, sugar, formalin, etc.

Climatic eczema includes the "winter itch" common in the north temporate zone, appearing on wrists and ankles in the form of clean, scaly patches, often ringed.

The seborrheic variety caused by the oil glands of the skin spreads from the scalp to the folds of the skin. Its borders are sharply defined, its crusts and scales yellowish and greasy. It spreads from a center in all directions at once.

***How to Treat Eczema.*** The treatment of eczema is puzzling to the physician. As a rule, only specialists in skin diseases are able to diagnose easily the subacute or chronic forms. It may appear different, and require different treatment, almost from day to day; consequently only general suggestions can be made for home management of the disease. However, the outlook is always good; and even in the case of weak patients, there is excellent chance of cure. Soap must be religiously avoided. Where there are pustules, a 2 per cent watery solution of gentian violet is of value. The germ-killer, bacitracin solution or ointment, is often effective in the treatment of pustular eczema. Eczema with secondary infection is improved by local treatment with this drug.

If itching is pronounced, remove crusts and scabs after soaking with olive oil, and dust borax, finely powdered, on the surface. If the itching is not controlled in twenty minutes, wipe off the borax with a cloth moistened with olive oil.

The following three eczema prescriptions are often helpful:

*Powder for Eczema*

| | |
|---|---|
| Boric acid | 2 drachms |
| Zinc oxide | 1 ounce |
| Purified talc | 4 ounces |

*For Pustular Eczema*

| | |
|---|---|
| Boric acid | 10 grains |
| Bismuth subnitrate | 1 drachm |
| Pine tar | 20 grains |
| Rose water ointment | add to 1 ounce |

Apply to the pustules.

*Ointment for Chronic Eczema*

| | |
|---|---|
| Salicylic acid | 1 drachm |
| Pine tar | 1 ounce |
| Vaseline | 4 ounces |

After removing all crusts in the affected areas, apply this ointment freely once a day.

## WARTS

Warts are flattened or rounded outgrowths from the outer and middle layers of the skin, varying in size from a pinhead to one-half inch in diameter. Warts most commonly appear on the hands of children, but they may be present on any part of the body and at all ages. They may disappear quickly or remain indefinitely and are not communicable from one person to another. There are several varieties, among which the following are common:

***Seed Warts.*** These have numerous, little fleshy projections over their surface, which are enlarged normal structures (papillae) of the middle layer of the skin, together with the thickened, outer, horny layer.

***Threadlike Warts.*** These are found along the edge of the nails, on the face, neck, eyelids, and ears. They are formed by the great prolongation and growth of the projections, or papillae, of the middle layer of the skin.

***Flat Warts.*** These warts are raised but slightly above the surface. They are more common in young people.

***Moist Warts.*** These are present when softened by secretions of the body, as in the region of the external sexual organs (in connection with their diseases), and about the anus, or natural opening of the bowel. They are white, pink, or red, and consist of numerous, little fleshy projections, usually covered with an ill-smelling secretion.

***Treatment of Warts.*** Many warts disappear by themselves in time. Warts can sometimes be removed by painting them frequently with acetic acid, or with tincture of iodine. These remedies are harmless, but somewhat slow and not always effective. Application, morning and evening, of a saturated solution of "washing soda" (impure bicarbonate of potash) will often remove a wart.

Warts are readily removed by physicians, who may use caustics, surgery, or other methods. The administration by mouth of 100,000 units of vitamin A daily for from two to three months will cure many warts.

## CORNS

***Causes and Kinds of Corns.*** Corns are slightly elevated thickenings of the horny layer of the skin, varying in size, shape and consistency. They occur on the toes, or other places exposed to friction and pressure, usually from ill-fitting shoes. A corn is distinguished by the presence of a horny core, the deep end of which presses on the tender cutis (dermis, or "true" skin). Hard corns occur on exposed surfaces; soft corns develop between the toes.

***How to Treat Corns.*** Comfortable shoes are the first requisite; they should be well-fitting, neither tight nor loose. Pressure may be taken off the corns by surrounding them with felt rings or corn plasters. To remove the corn, the foot should be soaked for a long time in warm water, in which washing soda has been dissolved. Then the surface of the corn is gently scraped off with a clean, sharp, sterilized knife, and an antiseptic applied. Another useful method is to paint the corn with a preparation which can be made up by the druggist from the following formula:

| | |
|---|---|
| Salicylic acid ................ | 30 grains |
| Tincture of iodine ............ | 10 drops |
| Collodion ..................... | 4 drachms |

Shake the preparation before using it. The corn should be painted night and morning, for five days, and the preparation left on. After the final application, soak the corn for some time in warm water. The corn will come off in the coating that has been formed.

## CALLUSES AND CRACKS OF THE SKIN

***Causes and Symptoms of Calluses.*** A callus consists of round or irregular, flattened, yellowish thickenings of the upper or horny layer of the skin. The skin becomes thick as the result of intermittent pressure from tools, shoes, etc. The whole palm or sole may be the seat of a widespread callus. It is not harmful, except in leading to cracks of the skin near the bend of joints; also, rarely, in causing irritation, heat, pain, and even the formation of pus in the skin beneath, from secondary infection. Callus usually disappears when the exciting cause or pressure is removed.

***Treatment of Calluses.*** Calluses can be temporarily removed by applications of 20 per cent salicylic acid in an ointment, or by careful shaving with a sterilized blade, after applying an antiseptic. Cracks in the skin can be made to heal by the application of tincture of benzoin, followed by a protective layer of collodion, held on by a few strands of cotton.

## BALDNESS AND DANDRUFF

In most cases of baldness the condition is inevitable, and follows a pattern set by heredity. However, baldness may be the result of other causes—burns, for example, erysipelas, emotional shock, glandular disturbances, sterility, etc. It may be patchy or widespread. The condition is sometimes due to seborrhea of the scalp (overly active oil glands), which is probably caused by microbes, and consists of an inflammation of the skin, with great increase of dandruff of a thick, greasy variety. Excess of oily food, particularly milk, cream, butter, chocolate, is a predisposing factor. The patient should be put on a low fat diet.

For mild dandruff, a good preparation to be dispensed by the druggist is the following:

Phenol (carbolic acid) .............10 drops
Mercuric chloride ................ 1 grain
Euresol (resorcinol monoacetate).... 2 drachms
70 per cent alcohol ................add to make 8 ounces

Rub into the scalp several nights a week, especially after each shampooing, and shampoo every two weeks. Use no brush, unless it can be sterilized satisfactorily. Use a cheap new comb after each shampoo, to avoid infection, and then discard it. Shampoo at home after each haircut.

In severe dandruff, a salve is more effective than the above. For this have the druggist make up 4 per cent salicylic acid and 6 per cent precipitated sulphur in a greaseless ointment base that washes out easily.

## EXCESSIVE HAIR (HYPERTRICHOSIS)

Abnormal hairiness from any cause may be hereditary or acquired. The areas commonly affected are the cheeks, chin and upper lip, and occasionally the forearms and legs. Various glandular (endocrine) disturbances greatly influence the growth and distribution of hair. Use of the epilating needle is the safest and best means of destroying the follicles.

## INGROWING HAIRS

It is common for one or several hairs of the beard to be set obliquely and to pierce the epidermis. These hairs are usually surrounded by pustules. Close shaving may predispose to the condition. Papules (small solid elevations of the skin) containing ingrowing hairs should be pricked with a sterilized needle and the hair pulled out, using clean hands and sterilized instruments, and touching the wound afterward with a suitable antiseptic.

## GRAY HAIR

While usually hereditary, sometimes this is a symptom of a special condition. It occurs in disturbances of the endocrine glands, thyroid diseases, or Addison's disease. The use of hair dyes, which may contain silver nitrate, pyrogallic acid, or paraphenylen diamine, is sometimes injurious.

## CHAPTER 17

# CARE OF THE COMPLEXION AND HAIR

**Use of Cold Water and Soap . . . Do Mud Baths and Other Special Baths Help? . . . Creams for the Skin . . . How to Make Your Own Cold Cream . . . Lanolin Massage Cream . . . Cleansing the Face . . . When to Use Sulfonated Soap . . . Disease and the Hair . . . Treatment of the Scalp . . . How to Shampoo the Hair . . . Treatment for Dry Hair . . . Dyeing Gray Hair . . . Use of Hair Tonics . . . How to Brush and Comb the Hair, etc.**

THE COMPLEXION is an index of general health. A good complexion is the reward of hygienic living. Any internal derangement may affect the hue and texture of the complexion.

The skin is intimately related by way of the nervous system with the emotions. Slight skin conditions frequently clear up when the patient is relieved of anxiety or worry.

One of the most common causes of all skin disorders is the suppression of the secretions of the sebaceous glands and of the perspiratory fluids. If these secretions and fluids are not removed, they may cause inflammation of the skin.

***Use of Cold Water and Soap.*** Cold water is better than warm for the complexion and for the skin in other parts of the body. It improves the tone of the skin of the face and gives it color.

The habitual use of soap on the face is not absolutely necessary except in the case of oily skins or a soiled face. There is a vast deal of nonsense in the popular idea that great care must be exercised in the selection of a toilet soap. One toilet soap is about as good as another in regard to special beneficial or injurious action on the skin. The countless toilet preparations made for application to the face may afford some pleasure to the users, but, actually, a few simple medicaments will suffice.

Medicated baths, mud baths, vapor contraptions, and Turkish baths have no special value, contrary to popular belief.

***Cold Cream for the Skin.*** Cold cream protects the skin from dirt, softens it, and prevents it from becoming dry. Many women believe that certain advertised varieties of cold cream "nourish the skin." They do not. The skin is nourished through the digestive tract, the sun, and the sebaceous glands. And, despite the many claims, there is no cream which "reduces large pores."

So-called "theatrical" cream is a good variety. Irradiated or hormone creams are best avoided because they may contain certain drugs that should not be used except under medical supervision.

A good cold cream is composed of the following ingredients, all of which may be obtained at a drugstore:

| | |
|---|---|
| White wax | 1 part |
| Spermaceti | 10 parts |
| Oil of sweet almonds | 10 parts |
| Rose water | 6 parts |

Melt the first three ingredients together over a low flame; remove from the heat. Then stir in rose water and beat the resultant mixture with an egg beater until it "jells." A little oil of rose may be added to scent the product.

A camphorated cold cream is made as follows from ingredients to be had at any drugstore:

| | |
|---|---|
| Oil of sweet almonds | 4 ounces |
| Spermaceti | ½ ounce |
| White wax | ½ ounce |
| Camphor | ½ ounce |
| Powdered borax | 2 teaspoonfuls |
| Rose water | 2½ ounces |

The spermaceti and white wax are melted together over a low flame. Dissolve the camphor with the oil of sweet almonds by gentle heating. Add this to the melted spermaceti and wax. Then dissolve the borax in the rose water and slowly pour this solution into the prepared hot mixture. Stir or beat thoroughly until the cream is cool.

A good lanolin massage cream consists of the following ingredients, to be procured at any drugstore.

| | |
|---|---|
| Anhydrous lanolin | 2 ounces |
| Coconut oil | 2 ounces |
| White wax | 1 ounce |
| Spermaceti | 1 ounce |
| Oil of sweet almonds | 4 ounces |
| Orange-flower water | 2 ounces |
| Tincture of benzoin | 6 drops |

Melt the lanolin with the coconut oil, white wax, spermaceti and oil of sweet almonds in a porcelain container over a low flame. After removing this mixture from the heat, stir in the last two ingredients. Beat rapidly until the cream thickens.

## CLEANSING THE FACE

Care of the complexion is a varied process. Take the matter of cleansing, for example. The chin and nose, with their great number of oil glands, should be washed often with soap and water and cleansed with an alcohol lotion. The cheeks, which are not so oily, require less washing but are likely to require extra care with cold cream. At times, as in adolescence, the face in its entirety may become too oily. The excess of oil induces the formation of blackheads, which may become infected and result in pimples. This, as is common knowledge, is a source of great anxiety and of a sense of inferiority to most girls and many boys. The treatment is given later in this chapter.

The proper steps in cleansing the face may be outlined for women as follows:

***Before Bedtime.*** Tie a band around the hair face-line; wash the face with warm water and a bland pure soap. Then, rinse the face with warm water; follow with splashes of cold water. Dry with a soft bath towel.

***In the Morning.*** Tie a band around the hair. Next, apply a cleansing cream with a light upward stroke (from chin to forehead), using the fingers and palms of both hands. Next, apply cream to the neck with an upward stroke. Wipe off all the cream.

It has been estimated that the public outlay for cosmetics and skin preparations is well over a billion dollars a year. Accordingly, face creams, toilet soaps, skin lotions and powders offer a tempting field for adulteration as well as for the compounding of injurious imitations. Above all, beware of the many quacks who practice "face-peeling"—a so-called rejuvenating treatment.

## USE OF SOAP ON THE SKIN

Soap is a combination of an alkali with a fat. Potash soaps are soft soaps. They contain a large amount of water and are made more or less in the form of a jelly. Ordinary soaps are made with soda. They contain a small amount of water and are known as hard soaps. The better class of toilet soaps contains vegetable oils or lard.

Sulfonated soap is valuable for those persons whose dry skin is sensitive to ordinary soap. For persons with oily skin, the use of hot water and soap is best followed by a cold shower.

Price is no indication of the value of a soap. So-called medicated soap, transparent soap, and castile soap possess no unusual antiseptic features. Persons who are sensitive to coconut oil should not use hard-water soap because it often contains a large amount of oil.

## CARE OF HAIR AND SCALP

***The Hair.*** Hair, like other living things, is formed of cells. It breathes, in a sense. It receives blood, and therefore nourishment, through the skin. Like the rest of the body, hair grows to maturity, then to old age, and dies.

When any single hair has attained its natural limit of growth, and fallen out, it is replaced by a young, new hair. On the scalp the natural life-expenctancy of a hair has been variously estimated at eighteen months, two, four or six years. (The life of an eyelash, incidentally, is about 150 days.) Various diseases bring about profuse hair fall. When a hair has fallen out, the new one that replaces it normally is observable on the scalp in about six to ten weeks.

Hair is a modification of the growth of the upper skin. Hair owes its color to the different proportions of the chemicals which form its pigment. This accounts for the different shades of color which the use of some hair dyes often causes.

Living tissue, whether it is that of the skin, eye, nose or throat, is easily injured. Hair is no exception, and the effects are evident in various diseases. The greatest injury is suffered by the hair of the scalp. It is a vast storage space for bacteria of all degrees of virulence that have been deposited on it by the dust and soot.

***Effect of Food on Hair.*** Certain foods appear to influence the health of the hair. Experiments with animals prove that a loss of fur occurs when they are given a diet poor in protein, quantitatively and qualitatively. To a certain extent, vitamin A determines the quality of hair texture and its degree of oiliness or fragility.

Poor blood makes poor-quality hair just as improper food, inadequate food, or both, make unhealthy bodies. Many examples of dry, lustreless hair, for example, are caused by anemia. The condition of the hair is therefore largely a matter of physical and mental health. However, certain characteristics are the result of fastidious care and cultivation. Neglected hair can absolutely not be beautiful; in nothing is personal neglect more obvious.

### Treatment of the Scalp

The scalp should be treated gently. It should, as a general rule, be washed twice a week. This does not injure the hair. With the right variety of soap, thorough rinsing and drying, and the application of a little oil to hair that tends to dryness, shampooing will not dry the scalp secretions, destroy hair growth, or increase dandruff. Instead, the dirt, dust, scales, grease, and infectious agents that are present are displaced and removed, and the blood circulation of the scalp is improved.

In the main, hair is composed of a nitrogenous substance—keratin. Keratin is soluble in alkalis. It is this property which exposes it to destruction from the chemical action of any minerals that there may be in soaps, dyes and bleaches. It is therefore advisable to use a superfatted soap on the hair because such soap has no free alkali.

## HOW TO SHAMPOO THE HAIR

When the hair and scalp are thoroughly wet, soap is rubbed in until a thick lather forms. This is kneaded into the scalp with the fingertips.

Rinsing carries the detached matter from the hair; it should therefore be thorough, with alternate applications of hot and lukewarm water until every particle of soap is removed.

After the final rinsing with hot water, cold water is applied for its stimulating effect on the blood circulation of the scalp, and to close the opened pores.

The hair is then dried immediately with towels or warm towels if desired. It is good practice to shake the hair while drying. The use of the super-heated electric drier following shampoo or for permanent waves is most harmful. It reduces the life of the hair and causes splitting and breaking off of many of the hair filaments.

## TREATMENT FOR DRY HAIR

The white of an egg rubbed into the hair (or added to the shampoo water) increases its gloss and helps to prevent dryness. Extremely dry hair may be rubbed with olive, almond or coconut oil, or odorless castor oil and perfume. A cream of lanolin, glycerin and rose water in equal parts is also good for this purpose. Hair that is exceptionally greasy may be rubbed with cologne water, and quickly dried.

Where the only water obtainable for the shampooing is hard water and there is no hard-water soap, silicate of soda should be added to the shampoo water.

When hair is thin and oily, it is necessary to cleanse it more often than when the scalp is dry and the hair is coarse.

It is often difficult to dress the hair after washing with soap and hard water. This explains the often-heard plaint: "I can't do a thing with my hair after washing." Washing with soft water gives a different effect, because it leaves no deposit to be rinsed away. The removal of a deposit is aided by adding a little diluted acetic acid or lemon juice to the rinsing water.

***Preparations for the Hair.*** Hair tonics are usually valueless. Hair removers should be used only on the advice of a physician. Soapless shampoos are likely to have a drying effect on the scalp because, as a rule, they dissolve the natural oil. Avoid preparations for dry cleaning the hair. Many of them contain inflammable isopropyl alcohol. This is just as toxic as wood alcohol. It dissolves the oils of the hair and scalp. Some dry cleaners for the hair contain carbon tetrachloride, which has a poisonous effect.

The treatment of dandruff is discussed in the preceding chapter.

It is best to do nothing about gray hair. Moreover, the use of metallic hair dyes is risky. Aniline hair dyes are best avoided because they contain irritating coal-tar products. Vegetable dyes, such as henna, may be used safely. (White henna is a bleach which contains hydrogen peroxide.)

## BRUSHING AND COMBING THE HAIR

The purpose of combing and brushing the hair is to remove the scales and to stimulate the blood circulation in the scalp. Brushes and combs should be selected with care. Stiffer brushes are required for one head of hair than for another. Don't use wire or metal brushes.

Individual combs and brushes are as essential as separate toothbrushes. A good rule is: neither a borrower nor a lender be, in the matter of combs, brushes or hairpins.

A brush should have firm and well-spaced bristles. The bristles should be variable in length and graded so that the longest are in the center of every group. This permits more even and deeper penetration through the hair to the scalp. It is advisable to use two brushes—

a stiff one for removing scales and stimulating the scalp, and a softer one for smoothing and glossing the hair.

Too-pointed teeth in a comb, or those of uneven length, may injure the scalp.

There is an art in using the comb. Do not use the comb in the petulant way some harried mothers have of yanking it through the tangled locks of their offspring. The brush should not be used until all snarls have been carefully disentangled with the comb, aided at times by the fingers. Begin carefully combing below the snarl.

Force should never be used when brushing or combing. When the hair is extremely long or thick and when it is tangled, when it becomes too dry (as with certain kinds of "permanent waving") and when it is falling profusely, the brush should not be drawn rapidly and forcibly down in one long stroke. Rather, you should bend over and brush the hair gently from the scalp to the hair ends.

The hair should be brushed at such an angle that the stroke draws the hair from the scalp. This forces the separate hairs to be "individualized." The ordinary method of brushing the hair from the top of the head toward the shoulder is poor.

CHAPTER 18

# CANCER AND OTHER TUMORS

**Difference Between Benign and Malignant Tumors... What Causes Cancer... Cancer in Children... Heredity and Cancer... Is Cancer Contagious?... Warning Signs of Cancer... How Cancer Is Treated... Hormones and Radioactivity... Cancer of the Lung... Cancer of the Breast... Cancer of the Stomach... Cancer of the Lower Bowel and Rectum... Benign Tumors of Rectum and Anus... Cancer of the Womb ... Cancer of the Bladder and Kidneys... Cancer of the Prostate Gland... Cancer of the Lip... Cancer of the Tongue... Malignant Moles... What to Do About Small Growths... Wen or Ganglion, etc.**

FOR MANY YEARS a great number of agencies have been investigating cancer from every angle. Much has been accomplished by way of treatment, particularly where the disease has been diagnosed early. The present intensified interest will undoubtedly yield even greater results.

We can further decrease the amount of cancer to a considerable degree by educating people about the value of early diagnosis. In this connection, the periodic physical examination is of outstanding importance. Every man and woman over forty should have a complete physical examination every six months. A competent physician will detect early signs of cancer or any other disease, and either further advance will be prevented or the disease will be eradicated.

## BENIGN AND MALIGNANT TUMORS

The word "tumor" originally meant a swelling. As commonly used, it means a new growth or enlargement of a part, which is not directly caused by injury or inflammation. In other words, tumors are new formations in tissues. They tend to grow and extend locally and reproduce their own likeness in different parts of the body. They often appear without apparent cause; they persist; and fulfill no function. Chronic and long-continued irritation, with or without infection, may be a common forerunner of a tumor.

There are two kinds of tumors—benign and malignant. In general, benign tumors grow only slowly, or remain stationary. They are not necessarily harmful, and seldom become malignant. Warts and polyps are examples of benign tumors. These we shall discuss later in this chapter.

The malignant tumors progress slowly and without pain. It is in their later stages that they become painful. They do not move about freely but become fixed to the neighboring or underlying parts. Their growth is more rapid than that of benign growths; they often have no well-defined borders; they frequently return after removal.

Malignant tumors are divided into cancers (carcinomas) and sarcomas. Cancer is much more common than sarcoma, and occurs more often in persons over thirty years of age.

***What Sarcoma Is.*** Sarcoma is a malignant growth which has its origin in the connective tissue. It is often seen in the young and well-nourished; it is rarely found in adults. Heredity has no relation to its development.

Sarcoma grows very rapidly. The skin usually does not adhere to the tumor. There is generally no pain. The victim, in many cases, does not appear pale and with the peculiar complexion which physicians describe as "cachexia" (ill-looking, or morbid). It appears most often in the muscles, bones, glands of the neck, and brain, but is found also in many other tissues.

If diagnosed early, most cases of sarcoma can be cured by the combined use of radium and X-ray.

## THE NATURE OF CANCER

Cancerous tumors vary greatly in their appearance and rate of growth. Cancer of the skin may exist for many years without causing death; yet there are some skin varieties that are much more rapid in their growth. Cancer never disappears by itself. It may for a time seem to have grown somewhat smaller, but it will go on relentlessly if not interfered with. Death from cancer is not caused by a poison from the tumor. It is due to some interference with the normal functioning of the body. If a cancer decays, as it not infrequently does, it may ulcerate; then germs get into it and set up a general infection. Death follows as a result of the infection.

## CAUSES OF CANCER

There are many factors that can cause cancer—X-rays and ultraviolet rays of the sun, for example, and such substances as hormones, arsenic, chromium, cobalt, and asbestos. Cancer can be traced to such varied causes as smoking, some viruses, tar, and creosote. It has been shown that certain chemicals, as, for example, hydrocarbons, can produce a certain variety of cancer.

Some investigations have indicated that apparently cancer is a virus disease, but there is no general or final agreement on this subject. "Excessive stimulation" by sex hormones may induce prostate gland cancer in men and breast cancer in women. On the other hand, some chemicals temporarily arrest cancers.

## CANCER IN CHILDREN

Unfortunately cancer is not so rare in children as most people believe. Mortality figures have shown that from the third to the tenth year, cancer and related diseases are second as a cause of death in children. The two most common forms of cancer in children are those of the eyes and of the kidneys. Both may be congenital, that is, dating from birth, or they may be constitutional.

## HEREDITY AND CANCER

Today no scientist believes in the hereditary influence of cancer. There is no proof of any direct inheritance of this dreaded disease, except in certain rare types which may develop in the early years of life, but in such cases it is never found in the mother; therefore it really cannot be considered as having been acquired from the mother.

It is often said that cancer runs in such and such a family. A daughter, a mother, a grandmother even, all have had cancer—let us say, cancer of the breast. We will analyze this.

There are many types of breast cancer. Some are no larger than a hazelnut, some grow rapidly and grow much larger. Some increase in size very slowly, even taking years. Some types remain localized, others drop off small particles which get into the circulation of the blood and lymph stream; these particles may start to grow in some remote part of the body.

Some malignant tumors (cancer) are quickly destroyed by exposure to X-ray or radium; others are cured by surgical removal, and then there are still others which are highly resistant, especially if neglected.

Now we will go back to the three generations who had cancer of the breast. In the average case, it will be found that the grandmother's, for example, was of slow growth and developed in old age. The mother's cancer was noted at the time of menopause and was completely dissolved by either X-ray alone or in combination with radium, or it may have been noted early enough to be removed by a simple local anesthetic procedure, or maybe even a more formidable operation. In any event, there was a complete cure, one which remained permanent. But the daughter, at sixteen, had a more malignant variety and because of her youth it was not noted early enough, so that she succumbed in a short time.

Now what does all this add up to? The breast tumors in the three generations are quite evidently no more related than three cases of some disease of the kidneys, one a late complication of scarlet fever, one associated with high blood pressure, and the third an infection.

## IS CANCER CONTAGIOUS?

It was formerly thought that any malignant tumor was contagious. It is definitely proved that this is untrue. There is no record of a surgeon having gotten cancer from operating on a patient. Nor has a nurse ever gotten cancer from a patient. Cancer is not a germ disease. It is a cell disease. Therefore, there can be nothing to the stories concerning cancer houses or districts. These myths arise from the fact that in certain areas all the young people have gone away, leaving the old folks behind, and, since the frequency of cancer increases with age, naturally such areas have a higher cancer death rate.

## SIGNS OF CANCER

The parts of the body where cancer most commonly develops are the breast and womb in women, and the lip and stomach in men. In cancer of the lip, the neighboring glands become enlarged, as shown by the lumps which form under the jaw. In cancer of the breast, they may be felt sometimes in the armpit or breast. In cancer of the womb, there is unexplained vaginal bleeding. However, these are late signs, and the growth should never be permitted to remain long enough for them to develop. Paleness, weakness, and loss of strength and weight often accompany the development of cancer, but many persons in the early stage of the disease do not show these symptoms.

***Warning Signals.*** Everybody should beware, and seek medical advice when: (1) a sore does not heal, particularly about the nose, tongue, mouth or lips; (2) a painless lump or thickening is observed, especially on the breast, lip, tongue or nose; (3) irregular bleeding or discharge from the nose or any body opening occurs; (4) progressive change appears in the color or size of a wart, mole or birthmark;

(5) persistent indigestion is noted; (6) unexplained cough hangs on, or hoarseness, or difficulty in swallowing; (7) any prolonged change takes place in the normal bowel habits.

## HOW CANCER IS TREATED

In most cases, early surgery is the only treatment to be considered for cancer. Delay and neglect are suicidal in malignant disease. Cure is successful just in so far as the operating is done early enough. If fear of operations were not so common, the results of cancer removal would be immeasurably better. The common bad results of operation—that is, return of the growth, and the consequences—are chiefly owing to the late stage at which surgeons are compelled to operate because of the reluctance of the patient and, strangely enough, sometimes of his family physician. Cancer should be removed in such an early stage that its true nature can often not be recognized until the tissue is examined under the microscope after its removal.

X-ray is useful in the case of superficial growths which are limited to the skin, or when directed against the scar left by removal of a cancer. Although the growth may disappear during the treatment, it recurs in many patients. When tumors are so far advanced that surgery is impossible, other means often give great relief from suffering. In many cases they may prolong life for a very considerable period. Demerol and methadon have been found useful in allaying the intense pain of the later stages of the disease.

## HORMONES AND CANCER

It has been thought that absence of ovarian hormones has some relation to breast cancer. Indeed, the improvement shown by women of sixty years of age or a little older when they are treated with female sex hormones (estrogens) appears to confirm this view. The treatment must be confined to women sixty years and over. It may be dangerous for others.

Male hormone (testosterone) may be given to women with primary cancers which have gone too far for operation, or with recurrent breast cancers, at any age. The dose is given in the muscles three times a week for eight to ten weeks. Women with breast cancer which has spread to the bone are relieved of pain after receiving the male sex hormone, so that they are able to sleep without the aid of sedatives and narcotics. For such patients, the hormone appears to be more beneficial than X-ray treatment.

To a certain degree, what is true of breast cancer holds true of cancer of the prostate gland.

It has been shown repeatedly that if the normal proportions of androgens and estrogens in adult men and woman are upset, notable changes occur in the secondary sexual glands, including the breasts. Thus, if the estrogenic substance known as stilboestrol is given to a man in sufficient amount and over an adequate period of time, there is a tendency to reduce the size of the major part of the prostate, and a few associated parts, and the cancer as well.

## RADIOACTIVITY AND CANCER

Radioactive isotopes are being used in the treatment of certain varieties of cancer. Radioactive iodine, for example, is used in cancer of the thyroid gland. About 15-20 per cent of all thyroid cancer absorbs radioactive iodine, and by the use of so-called tracer doses it is often possible to detect and localize the disease. If the tumor picks up iodine, therapeutic doses of the radioactive element can be given by mouth.

## PRIMARY CANCER OF THE LUNG

Primary cancer of the lung is a fairly frequent condition, apparently on the increase, which accounts for 10 per cent of cancer deaths. It is seen more often in males and usually does not arise before the age of forty. It arises from an abnormal site of growth somewhere in the membrane lining the bronchial tree.

***Symptoms of Lung Cancer.*** Cough is the most common initial symptom. At first it is dry, but later mucoid sputum is produced. Bloody sputum as a rule follows. If secondary infection occurs, fever may be present and the sputum grows purulent. Breathlessness may be striking and sometimes wheezing is present. At times swelling of the face, neck, and arms may be seen, due to interference with the circulation by pressure of the growth and its extensions. Chest discomfort, not severe, but a tight feeling, is experienced fairly often. Sharp pleural pain may be felt if the disease extends to the lung cover. Involvement of the laryngeal nerves may give rise to hoarseness.

***Diagnosis of Lung Cancer.*** In any person over forty if there is a change in the cough habit, unexplained chest discomfort or wheezing, or bloody sputum, the possibility of cancer of the lung should be investigated. The diagnosis is made by physical examination, X-ray and bronchoscopy (direct investigation of the larger bronchial tubes by a lighted cylindrical instrument).

***Treatment of Lung Cancer.*** As with cancer elsewhere, the most important phase of treatment is early diagnosis. Cancer of the lung can be cured if the trouble is recognized before great extension or spread of the disease has taken place. Cure is by surgical removal only. This has become less difficult with improvement in surgical technique, advances in anesthesia, and the modern drug treatments for infections.

## SECONDARY (METASTATIC) CANCER OF THE LUNG

Spread to the lungs from cancer elsewhere in the body is unfortunately frequent if the primary growth is not removed. The cancer may spread by invasion of the lymph and blood vessels or by direct extension. Secondary cancer commonly arises from cancer of the breast, stomach, kidneys, uterus, prostate, thyroid, and pancreas. X-ray is the principal diagnostic aid. The condition may be widespread before becoming symptomatic. Cough, breathlessness, and chest pain eventually develop. No curative treatment is possible.

## CANCER OF THE BREAST

***Symptoms of Cancer of the Breast.*** This begins as a lump, which is usually found to the outside of the nipple. It may, however, develop in any part of the breast. It may or may not be painful at first, but the skin becomes attached to it, and sooner or later the nipple is drawn in. It occurs in women over forty, as a rule.

Lumps in the breast which date from the nursing period are often caused by inflammation alone, and usually have no relation to cancer, unless they persist for a long time. Any lump which appears in the breast without apparent cause, or which remains for a considerable period after an inflammation ceases, should be promptly removed by a surgeon, since without microscopic examination the most skilled examiner is unable to distinguish absolutely between a harmless and a malignant tumor. Since even so-called benign tumors (for example, inflammatory lumps in the breast, warts, moles, etc.) may become cancerous, all tumors, wherever situated, and no matter what their apparent nature, should be removed at once.

The tumor may be noticeable as a swelling over one part of the breast. Commonly it is in the upper, outer quarter-section; the next most frequent location is just below the nipple. Later the nipple is drawn back or lifted, and the skin becomes puckered. In an examination of the breast, it is important to observe: whether the two nipples are on the same level and are facing in a normal direction; whether there is any deformity in the natural shape of the breast; and whether there are enlarged veins on the chest, or a pink shade to the skin.

The following points suggest a breast cancer: the tumor is hard and knobby; its limits are not well defined; and it cannot be moved independently of the rest of the breast. Also, the skin over the tumor may be dimpled, or the nipple drawn in; and there may be blood-stained discharge from the nipple.

***Treatment of Cancer of the Breast.*** The treatment is surgical, and should be undertaken as early as possible, except in cases where only X-rays or radium can be used in an attempt to stop the progress of the disease.

## CANCER OF THE STOMACH

***Symptoms of Cancer of the Stomach.*** Cancer of the stomach is observed most often in men over forty. It usually begins gradually, showing as its symptoms loss of appetite, nausea, or vomiting. There may be vomiting of blood, pain in the stomach, and loss of weight and color. Where sudden obstruction to the outlet of the stomach takes place, pain and vomiting may be the first obvious symptoms.

***Treatment of Cancer of the Stomach.*** Improved methods of surgery have made early operation for cancer of the stomach a hopeful measure. Even when cure does not result, life is prolonged and much suffering is saved.

## CANCER OF THE LOWER BOWEL AND RECTUM

The rectum is one of the commonest sites of cancer, the greatest number of cases occurring in men, between the ages of fifty and sixty years. The cause, as of cancer in other organs, is still unknown.

***Symptoms of Cancer of the Lower Bowel and Rectum.*** Fairly persistent constipation is usually a characteristic feature. In the later stages of the disease, symptoms vary with the position of the tumor. The stools may be tinged with blood, and there is sometimes considerable mucus. Pain is not an early symptom. As in all other kinds of cancer, it is most important to recognize the disease promptly.

In all adults with prolonged constipation, or other rectal symptoms, the patient must be thoroughly examined for cancer before being treated for any other rectal condition. The disease is treacherous in its beginning and early progress. A person may have cancer of the rectum for six months or more before the symptoms are serious enough to make him go to the doctor. The period of constipation is often followed by diarrhea, which in its early stages occurs only after meals. Sooner or later certain other signs appear.

Even when they are very small, cancers in the anal canal cause great discomfort during the early stage of the disease. After the bowels move, there is a sensation of incomplete relief. Pain is experienced while the action of the bowels goes on, and it persists for some time afterward.

***Treatment of Cancer of the Lower Bowel and Rectum.*** The method used in treatment is surgery. X-ray and radium treatment also prove valuable.

### Benign Tumors of Rectum and Anus

Benign tumors of the rectum and anus occasionally form, showing the same characteristics as similar growths elsewhere in the body. They develop slowly; they do not spread to other parts of the body; and usually they do not come back after removal. Benign tumors of the rectum itself grow slowly. They may be present for many months or years before they cause symptoms indicating their presence. The common variety are known as polyps. When small, they may be present for some time without giving pain. As the growths increase in size they become more and more irritated during the passage of bowel contents, especially in cases of constipation, when scratches of the rectal lining often occur and cause bleeding. The passage of blood from the rectum in children always suggests tumors. A careful examination of the rectum must be made by a physician or proctologist (a specialist in disorders of the rectum or anus), who will remove any new growth.

## CANCER OF THE WOMB

Sixty of every one hundred women with cancer go to doctors when it is too late for adequate treatment. In order to effect a cure, the condition must be discovered when only extremely early symptoms are present, and before bloody vaginal discharge, or contact bleeding, appears. On theoretic grounds, it may be said that all cancers can be cured if the diagnosis is made early enough and treatment is started immediately. Early detection is the key to the control and possible cure of cancer.

***Signs of Cancer of the Womb.*** An irregular or persistent bleeding from the vagina should at once be studied by the family physician, or by a specialist in women's diseases (gynecologist). Women, particularly those who are elderly, who suffer from unexplained irregular vaginal bleeding must undergo an early and thorough examination of the genital tract; also X-ray examination of the bones.

***Prevention of Cancer of the Womb.*** The only possible preventive measure of cancer of the womb is to treat any chronic irritation of the genital tract. Above all it should be kept in mind that pain is a late symptom, occurring as a rule only in the advanced stage of cancer.

***Biopsy Technique.*** An important early means of detecting cancer is through what is known as "biopsy," that is, removal and microscopic examination of a piece of tissue from a living person. This technique is advisable whenever there is a growth which suggests a tumor, in a location where it can be reached.

***Cell-Smear Examination.*** This technique has been shown to be a valuable way of detecting cancer cells. It involves microscopic examination of various secretions obtained from the genital tract.

The smear method has a wide range of usefulness. It may be used to show how the ovaries are functioning. It is also a good indicator of the presence of some dangerous development in the genital tract—for example, by showing an increased number of separated cells from a tumor. Because it may show the presence of cancer cells in secretions from the vagina and from the mouth of the womb (cervix), it is of use in the diagnosis of early womb and cervical cancer. In the same manner, it is of aid in determining the effectiveness of treatment by X-rays, radium, and surgery.

The examination of cell-smears was first done in the study of uterine cancer. It gives promise of being a most valuable aid in the early diagnosis of cancer in other parts of the body. For example, in cancer of the male and female urinary tract, smears from the tube which leads from the urinary bladder and sediment from treated urine have been found to contain loose cancer cells. The same holds true in cancer of the bladder, prostate, and kidney. The smear tests do not replace the long and well-established methods for the diagnosis of womb cancer, among which biopsy is the final test. The smear tests are used mostly for screening all women coming for a check-up or a routine physical examination.

***Scheller Test.*** This is another important means of early diagnosis of cancer of the mouth of the womb. Dr. Scheller discovered that the glycogen (a carbohydrate) in the normal superficial cells of the cervix (mouth of the womb) stains brown with iodine, but that the areas of early cancer are without glycogen and therefore do not stain brown. This procedure enables the examiner to find the area which should be cut into for a sample for microscopic examination.

***Treatment of Cancer of the Womb.*** Cautery, X-ray, and radium are of value only in advanced cases. Even then, they serve merely to relieve the symptoms, although they may also retard the advance of the disease. Surgery is the only genuinely effective method generally used. This fact emphasizes again the need for early diagnosis.

## CANCER OF THE BLADDER AND KIDNEYS

***Signs of Cancer of the Bladder and Kidneys.*** A blood-stained urine is the most important sign. If the kidney is involved, there may be some pain extending from the kidney region in the back toward the front and down toward the bladder. If the bloody urine (hematuria), when voided, is intimately mixed, has no clots and has no pain associated with it when voided, then the preponderance of evidence is that the bleeding is from the bladder. This diagnostic point holds for both sexes.

There are other causes of blood appearing in the urine, but attacks of marked hematuria, occurring closely together, mean a tumor of either the bladder or one of the kidneys.

***How the Diagnosis Is Made.*** In no other branch of medicine or surgery can so rapid a diagnosis be made as in the urinary tract. However, this demands about two days in the hospital. What is called a cystoscopic examination is made. This is accomplished by passing into the bladder an electrically lighted metal tube equipped with visual lenses. The bladder is dilated by filling it with water when the inside can be clearly seen by the examining physician. The openings of the tubes (ureters) which carry the urine from the kidneys to the bladder can be seen. X-ray examination is done at the same time and the diagnosis is made as soon as the bladder findings are compared with the X-rays. This kind of an examination is performed painlessly under local anesthetic, but it must be done by a urologist, that is, one who specializes in diseases of the urinary tract.

***Treatment of Cancer of the Kidney.*** As soon as the diagnosis is made, no time should be lost in removing the kidney. This is the only means of saving a life with this disease. The results after early operation are excellent. If the tumor has not broken through the capsule of the kidney—and this should not be if it is diagnosed early—the life span will not be shortened.

Some people think that the loss of one kidney shortens life. That is not true. Many who have lost one kidney have lived into old age.

The convalescence is only about five days, when the patient can leave the hospital. Of course one must be guarded in some ways after losing a kidney. Care must be taken not to catch cold in the wintertime. It is better not to drink too much hard liquor, but an occasional drink will do no harm. Otherwise one can lead a perfectly normal life.

***Treatment of Cancer of the Bladder.*** This is also surgical. If the tumor is small, then it is removed by means of the cystoscope. This is accomplished by means of an electric wire being attached to the instrument, and the small growth is cauterized. However, if the cancer is large, say the size of a pigeon's egg, then it is better to open the bladder and use a very powerful cautery.

The stay in the hospital is longer than after the kidney removal. It averages two to three weeks. In early cases the outlook is excellent.

## CANCER OF THE PROSTATE GLAND

***How Cancer of the Prostate Gland Develops.*** The prostate gland, present only in the male, lies at the neck of the bladder completely surrounding the urinary canal (the urethra). It is a sex organ. Its secretion gives activity to the sperm of the semen. Sixty-five per cent of men past fifty years of age have enlargement of this gland. Twenty per cent of these enlargements become malignant. At first glance this looks like a dismal picture, but it is not so black as it appears.

As a rule, cancer of the prostate is the least progressive in growth of cancers of any part of the body. Let us examine the development of a typical case, in a man of fifty with a prostate enlargement. He has some minor urinary difficulty for which he consults a specialist. Examination gives no evidence of a malignant tumor. He is told that he should have a checkup every three months. If, during the course of the next two years, a little suspicious nodule is felt by the examining finger in the rectum, he is watched very carefully. Conservative urologists with many years of experience defer operation until they are definitely certain that there is some progression. It must be remembered that this is a very serious operation, the mortality is high, and the possibility of stirring up trouble and sending some of the cancer cells from the prostate into a remote organ is not small. Death then occurs in a few months.

Since cancer of the prostate is slow growing, the patient has a better chance to advance into old age with very little prostatic difficulty.

***Symptoms of Cancer of the Prostate Gland.*** The first sign of a man having anything wrong with his prostate may be blood coming from the urethra. The blood may appear in only a few drops at the end of urination or there may be a considerable amount of blood mixed with the urine. It is more likely than not that there will be no pain. That is the time to hurry to the doctor. His examination will at once show whether there is an advanced stage of a growth of the gland or he may find nothing except an enlarged gland that is perfectly smooth. If there is a tumor present the surface will be nodular.

***Treatment of Cancer of the Prostate Gland.*** The decision may be very difficult to make as to the procedure that will be to the greatest benefit to the patient. Radical surgery has done little in these cases for prolonged good results. If there is an early diagnosis, then deep X-ray is better than any other procedure. Remember that at least half of these cases grow slowly, and there are many men who have had cancer of the prostate for many years and have died of some other cause.

If the case is far advanced and there is discomfort or much pain, then the administration of female hormones either by mouth or injection will give great relief from pain; it often reduces the size of the growth so that urination becomes easier. Up to the last several years it was thought that the removal of the testicles would greatly prolong the life of these patients by removing the excess of male hormones as a possible cause of cancer in the gland. This procedure has now been cast aside. As a last resort for palliative treatment, an opening is made in the urethra from either above or below. This is done to give relief from pain on urination.

Before consenting to any radical treatment it is better to get a second opinion. Two heads are always better than one.

## CANCER OF THE LIP

This arises as a small lump—like a wart, as a rule—on the lower lip, in men from forty to seventy. Sometimes it appears at first simply as a slight sore or crack which scabs over repeatedly but does not heal. Its growth is very slow, and it may seem like a trivial matter. However, any persistent sore on the lower lip of a man over forty demands the immediate attention of a surgeon. Early removal of cancer of the lip is highly successful.

## CANCER OF THE TONGUE

***Causes of Cancer of the Tongue.*** This is a common condition, mainly affecting men between the ages of forty and sixty. Conditions which may lead to cancer are: chronic superficial inflammation of the tongue; excessive pipe smoking, especially clay pipes; irritation from a decayed or sharp tooth, or sharp dental plate edges.

***Symptoms of Cancer of the Tongue.*** An early sign is the hardening of any part of the tongue; if ulceration is present, the edges are hard and raised and the base is hard and ill-smelling, bleeding readily. Painful swallowing may be an early symptom. Later the breath is offensive, saliva dribbles constantly, and movement of the tongue is limited and painful. There is often considerable pain, at first in the tongue, and later spreading out to the ear and side of the head.

***Treatment of Cancer of the Tongue.*** Like all malignant tumors that are on the surface of the body, cancer in this location is readily reached and cured by the application of radium. One point must be emphasized—the condition must be diagnosed early or before it has spread to the glands of the tongue and neck. Otherwise a cure is doubtful. But if treatment is given early, all cases are cured.

## MALIGNANT MOLES

Cancer sometimes forms in a mole. A colored mole should be removed if it is in a place where it may often be irritated, as in the shaving area of a man's face. This is also true of a colored mole which is obviously increasing in size. In general, darkly colored moles (particularly those covered by hair) may be left undisturbed. A bluish or slate-colored smooth mole which is only slightly raised must be removed without fail.

## WHAT TO DO ABOUT SMALL GROWTHS

There are, of course, many comparatively harmless or benign forms of tumors which do not return if removed, and which do not endanger life unless they grow to a large size. Among these are the soft, flattened, fatty tumors of the shoulders, back, buttocks, and other parts.

## WEN OR GANGLION

***Causes and Symptoms of Wen.*** This is a cystic tumor resulting from fluid retention following injury and inflammation of either the tendons of the hands or wrist, and the scalp. These cysts may vary in size from that of a bean to a hen's egg. They are painless and movable and never do any harm except to offend the eye.

***Treatment of Wen.*** The only rational and permanent cure is to dissect out the sac under local anesthesia. The old-fashioned and brutal method of "dropping a window" on the cyst or giving it a terrific blow with a book is reprehensible. This barbaric procedure may rupture the cyst but may also fracture one or more bones of the hand or wrist.

CHAPTER 19

# RHEUMATISM AND ALLIED DISEASES

**Rheumatic Fever (Inflammatory or Acute Rheumatism) . . . Heart Disease as a Complication . . . How the Disease Affects Children and Adults . . . Cortisone and Other Treatment . . . Muscular Rheumatism (Myalgia) . . . Lumbago . . . Stiff Neck . . . Chronic Rheumatism and Arthritis . . . Rheumatoid Arthritis . . . Atrophic Arthritis . . . Hypertrophic Arthritis . . . Gout . . . Acute and Chronic Gout . . . Synovitis and Bursitis . . . Water on the Knee . . . Bursitis of the Shoulder . . . Chronic Shoulder Bursitis, etc.**

## RHEUMATIC FEVER (INFLAMMATORY OR ACUTE RHEUMATISM)

RHEUMATIC fever is also known as inflammatory or acute rheumatism. Its exact cause has not been established. In general, it attacks young adults and children. However, extremely young children are usually exempt.

Rheumatic fever is a disease of late winter and early spring; it is also a disease of the slums. It is more prevalent in cities than in rural areas, and the greatest number of cases appear where persons are subjected to the most crowding. Conditions favorable to its development are dampness, cold, and tonsillitis. Poor diet also favors it, as well as lack of warm clothes, and poor heating in homes.

The greatest damage in rheumatic fever occurs in the heart and arteries. The fever for which the disease is named may play only a minor part in its course.

The disease involves every part of the heart, as a rule—cover (pericardium), muscle, and lining of the heart and valves. The more severe the rheumatic infection in early youth, the more extensive, as a rule, is the damage to the heart. When, as frequently happens, all parts of the heart are involved, the term "pancarditis" is used by physicians to describe the condition.

***Rheumatic Heart Disease.*** Rheumatic heart disease is the most serious aspect of rheumatic fever. It may include acute, subacute, or chronic involvement of the heart. There are several varieties of rheumatic heart disease: mild, where the heart symptoms are the least severe; ordinary grade, where the child is ill, pale and thin, the pulse rate is raised, the respiratory rate is somewhat raised, and fever up to 102°F. is present; and severe inflammation of the heart, where the child is extremely ill, the heart functions badly, and the child is pale. In this variety, the lips tend to be bluish, there is shortness of breath, especially at night; the pulse is rapid and feeble, the temperature is between 102° and 104°F.; there is also pain over the heart; and vomiting may be troublesome.

Rheumatic heart lesions are described as active or inactive, depending on whether inflammation is present, or there is merely scar tissue resulting from previous inflammations. An extremely serious variety noted in childhood results in death from cardiac (heart) failure.

***Signs and Symptoms of Rheumatic Fever.*** The attacks may vary greatly, depending on how severe the general symptoms are, and the extent of involvement of the joints. The disease usually follows acute tonsillitis or an acute upper respiratory infection, and there is ordinarily a quiescent period of from ten to twenty-one days. The beginning is sudden, with moderate fever and sometimes with a chill. The patient complains of severe pains in one or more joints.

An important indication of the disease is the increased heart rate, but it may not rise in proportion to the rise in fever. There may be pain and palpitation in the heart area. When the infection is severe there may be shortness of breath, and a heart murmur, which is discovered by the physician. Rheumatic nodules (lumps under the skin) indicate a severe infection. The electrocardiogram (graphic record of heart action) shows various indications that suggest the disease.

In childhood, acquired heart disease virtually means rheumatic inflammation of the heart. The rheumatic state in childhood, as previously mentioned, is almost unknown under two years of age, and rarely under three, but becomes more common from then on up to fifteen years. The pulse rate is very important. Records are kept of the pulse in the waking and sleeping state. In the early acute conditions the pulse rate is usually rapid.

***Immunity.*** An attack of rheumatic fever gives no immunity. Indeed the opposite is actually true: each recurrence tends to inflict further damage on various structures of the heart.

### How the Disease Affects Children

In children, infection of the joints is usually slight and may be absent, but the heart is frequently attacked. The only obvious evidence of an active rheumatic infection may be so-called "growing pains," tonsillitis, or St. Vitus's dance. The doctor, stethoscope, and electrocardiogram are necessary to detect the heart disease.

In dealing with the symptoms of rheumatic inflammation of the heart in children, two points are of fundamental importance. First, with the exception of pain caused by friction of the heart-cover, all the heart symptoms are the result of involvement of the heart muscle. As the heart muscles becomes more and more diseased it fails to maintain the blood circulation sufficiently, at first during exertion, but later even when the child is at rest. Second, the beginning of heart symptoms in a rheumatic child always denotes fresh, active inflammation of the heart.

It must be borne in mind that irregular beating of the heart is definite evidence of disease of the muscle part of the heart.

As a rule, the symptoms are only moderately severe. Pain over the heart, palpitation, rapid heart action, and shortness of breath are present. Among the signs of active change in rheumatic fever, showing that the disease is still smouldering, are the following: fever, aches and pains in the joints and limbs, weakness, rheumatic nodules, and frequent, spontaneous nose bleeds. There are also vanishing skin eruptions, failure to gain weight. There is persistent increase in the white blood cells. Changes in the heart action are shown by the electrocardiogram tracings.

### Difference Between Rheumatic Fever in Children and in Adults

Rheumatic fever is liable to be overlooked in childhood. It may, as Dr. Osler once said, "lick the joints, but bite the heart." It is important to bear the following distinctions in mind: in adult life, arthritis is the chief way in which rheumatic infection appears. It is considered to be the characteristic attack, and the heart involvement is regarded as a complication. In children, on the other hand, arthritis is often only slightly in evidence. It may even be entirely absent. Infection of other parts is more frequent and overshadows the remaining features of the disease. For example, the disease is sometimes limited to the tendons or the fascia (sheets of tissue which surround and connect the muscles) or to the joints (synovial membranes).

Another point is that while inflammation of the heart may occur in an acute form in children, it more often appears in a subacute form. Often there is a complete absence of symptoms felt by the person involved, or if they are present, they are masked by other signs and symptoms of rheumatic fever. Weakness, pallor, fatigue, loss of appetite and irritability are the usual symptoms.

It therefore becomes obvious that when there is even the supicion of rheumatic infection in a child, *that child should be put to bed at once* and the most thorough examination of the heart made daily, including electrocardiograms.

In the absence of complications, the fever and acute symptoms subside in about ten days. In the subacute form the duration may be long. Relapses are frequent. In children, rheumatism tends to attack all the parts that make up the heart; in adults, the heart cover often escapes damage. For this reason rheumatic heart involvement in children has a much more serious outlook than in adults.

### Complications of Rheumatic Heart Disease

The three most important complications of rheumatic heart disease are: congestive heart failure (overfulness of blood vessels); inflammation of the inner lining of the heart; and changes in the upper chambers of the heart (auricles). Inflammation of the heart muscle is present to a greater or lesser extent in the majority of children who are affected. Inflammation of the cover of the heart (pericardium) occurs in 10 per cent of afflicted persons. It may affect the lungs, their blood vessels and covering (pleura).

### Treatment

Medical management has a number of aims: First, to arrest the progression of the active rheumatic process, and to prevent recurrent attacks and heart damage, as far as possible; second, to prevent psychic disturbances resulting from chronic, prolonged illness. The treatment varies with the stage of the disease. The care of the acutely ill child can usually be given best in a hospital, though in special circumstances the child may be adequately treated at home.

There are a number of suggestions that may prevent serious impairment of the heart during an attack of rheumatic fever. These should be followed under a competent physician's direction. The child should be confined to bed until the heart rate is normal and all signs of fatigue are gone. Later all foci (centers) of infection should be removed; and adequate doses of salicylates should be administered. The affected joints, if any, should be wrapped in absorbent cotton soaked in oil of wintergreen. The limbs should be "cradled" under a frame made to support the weight of bedclothes and keep them from pressing on the joints.

***Drugs.*** There is no known successful specific remedy in the treatment of rheumatic fever. Drugs are of value only in certain phases.

During the active stage of the disease, salicylates are the most important drugs. They help to reduce fever, swellings of the joints, muscle pains, and other symptoms. For example, sodium salicylate or aspirin is given. In correct doses these give much relief from the pain.

***Cortisone Treatment for Rheumatic Heart Disease.*** Cortisone is a hormone (internal secretion) from the adrenal gland near the kidney. It holds considerable promise of effectiveness in rheumatic fever, as in rheumatism in general. On account of the scarcity of the drug, its use has been limited to institutions with adequate facilities for investigation and clinical control.

The giving of cortisone has certain disadvantages. Whenever a new drug with astonishing effects is discovered and tried out by the medical profession, conservative physicians give considerable thought to the question of whether the benefits that follow its use may not be associated with harmful effects that are worse than the original affliction itself. After cortisone administration, symptoms appear that suggest overdosage or intolerance.

The major importance of cortisone treatment in acute rheumatic fever is the fact that it throws a blanket, as it were, around the patient, between him and the disease, and thus protects him from some of its ravages. This pertains especially to the changes in the heart muscles and heart valves. The cortisone helps to defend the heart while the infectious process is running its course. The evidence so far is that the largest share of patients have their hearts spared when the attacks have passed over.

***Diet for Rheumatic Fever.*** The diet should be based on the following principles: The food should be simple, well-cooked and easily digested. Moreover, the total quantity should be small and served three times a day, with the largest meal at noon. A light evening meal should be served early enough to insure complete digestion before retiring. If food is insufficient, light "snacks" in mid-morning or mid-afternoon should be given; fluids should be restricted to a quart or 1 1/5 quarts in twenty-four hours.

To be avoided in the diet are: foods that are bulky, or fried, those causing fermentation, highly seasoned foods, pastries, elaborate desserts, condiments and relishes.

Above all, the sick person should avoid overeating, especially at night.

### Convalescence

When a physician decides that it is safe for the patient to get up, it must be done gradually, starting with a short period each day out of bed in a chair, and later, more and more frequently, walking about and taking mild exercises. There is a strong indication that removal of a patient to a tropical or subtropical climate affects the condition favorably.

### Prevention of Rheumatic Fever

There is general agreement that preventive measures must continue as long as relapses are likely—that is, until adolescence. Preventive treatment is not begun until the acute attack of rheumatic fever has subsided; it is, however, necessary to wait until certain tests are made. In the hope of preventing throat infections, particularly those caused by streptococci, tonsillectomy has been carried out extensively, after attacks in rheumatic patients. Reports as to results have been conflicting. There should be avoidance of damp or chill and avoidance of dietary deficiency, notably in protein, iron, calcium and vitamin A. Progress has been made in prevention of rheumatic fever. There has been administration, every winter for a period of several years, of hemolytic streptococcal filtrates to patients known to have had rheumatic fever. This has reduced the number of attacks of the disease.

Living conditions should be the best that circumstances permit. When feasible, change of residence to a warm, equable climate is desirable, either permanently or at least during winter and spring.

## MUSCULAR RHEUMATISM (MYALGIA)

In this disease there is pain in the muscles, which may be constant, but is more pronounced on movement. Exposure to cold and wet, combined with muscular strain, frequently brings on an attack. On the other hand, attacks do occur during hot, dry, fine weather. Attacks usually last only a few days, but they may be prolonged for weeks. The pain may be dull, as if the muscle had been bruised, but it is also often very sharp and cramp-like. Commonly, there is no fever and no general disturbance of health. The following are the most common varieties of muscular rheumatism:

### Lumbago

This attacks the muscles in the small part of the back. It comes on often with great suddenness, as on stooping or lifting. It may be so severe that the body cannot be moved, and the patient may fall down and be unable to rise, or even to turn in bed. In less severe conditions the pain "catches" the patient when attempting to straighten up after stooping. Pain in the back is often attributed by non-medical persons to Bright's disease, but it is rarely felt in that disorder. It is much more often caused by rheumatism.

The patient should rest in bed and avoid muscular efforts. Heat and massage should follow the acute stage. For pain, aspirin or other salicylates can be given.

### Stiff Neck

This is a very common variety of muscular rheumatism, and is seen more especially in young persons. It may appear very suddenly, as on awakening. It attacks the muscles of one side and back of the neck. The head is held stiffly to one side, and to turn the head the body must be turned also, because moving the neck causes severe pain. Sometimes the pain is agonizing when the neck is moved suddenly, or placed in certain positions; yet when it is held in other positions a fair amount of comfort can be secured.

Application of dry heat and occasional doses of aspirin usually relieve the condition within a few days.

## CHRONIC RHEUMATISM AND ARTHRITIS

Arthritis, commonly called rheumatism, ranks first among the disabling diseases. It includes a large group of diseases, with a great variety of signs and symptoms, the cause of which is often unknown. They are, however, grouped together because of their tendency to involve the bony structures of joints. The term "chronic arthritis" refers primarily to involvement of joints. It is somewhat incorrect since the view is widely accepted that this is a systemic (general bodily) disease, not a local manifestation which involves only the joints. There are many large groups of arthritis, and physicians differentiate between them.

Many muscle and tendon diseases are mistaken for chronic arthritis. If there is disturbance in one or more joints it must be determined by a physician whether the involvement is part of a general systemic disease or is a complication of some injury, disturbed surface blood circulation, tumors, cysts, loose bodies (fragments of cartilage) in the joints, bone disease next to the joints, or of any other condition.

### Types of Arthritis—According to Cause

All arthritic joint conditions may, for convenience, be divided into two classes: those whose causes are known, and those whose causes are not known. In the known-cause group, there is the infective arthritis in which the bacteria have been identified; the infective invasion of the joint may occur from within or from outside the body. The germs which cause arthritis in this category are those of gonorrhea, tuberculosis, scarlet fever, influenza, diphtheria, measles, streptococci, staphylococci, viruses, etc.

Arthritis may also be caused by injury and disturbances of the physiologic function. In the latter group the cause is to be found in scurvy (adult and infantile), rickets, loss of bone substance, sprue, beriberi, diabetes (mellitus). Other forms of arthritis result from various diseases of the spinal cord, and leprosy. Serum sickness sometimes causes arthritis. Then, again, tumors within or outside of joints may bring on arthritis, as well as loose bodies (cartilage fragments) within the joints. Strange forms of arthritis sometimes follow emotional strain, especially hysteria.

A large number of arthritis cases are secondary to diseases of the bone—infection, injury, Paget's disease (joints deformed), and tumors. Endocrine disturbances cause arthritic manifestation.

A great number of arthritic manifestations, as previously noted, are of unknown cause. In this large group of chronic sufferers the signs in the joints are of primary importance, and the existing general diseases are of interest only secondarily. Examples are: rheumatoid arthritis, degenerative joint disease, gout, arthritis of rheumatic fever, non-specific infective arthritis, and non-articular rheumatism.

## RHEUMATOID ARTHRITIS

Rheumatoid arthritis is usually chronic but commonly starts as an acute attack, generally in persons of middle age or after. It is seen more commonly in poor, hard-working persons who have been exposed to cold and damp, as, for example, laborers and washerwomen. Deficiencies in diet are common. There are two forms of chronic arthritis of this type, rheumatoid and hypertrophic arthritis.

## Atrophic Arthritis

This term does not describe the beginning of the disease, which is commonly an acute attack in one or more joints. It may follow an injury, especially if the patient has been in poor health or is suffering from a throat or upper respiratory infection. It may resemble an acute rheumatic fever but tends to linger in one joint longer before a second joint becomes involved, and the first joint does not tend to clear rapidly at this time as it does in rheumatic fever. This joint condition usually flares up and down for a time and then gradually improves. The improvement may be over weeks or recur and flare up over a period of months or years.

There may be very acute swelling with severe pain, and often there is an accumulation of fluid in the joint which can be determined by tapping the joint or noticing its increased size. It is usually not as red as the acute disease and, as a rule, does not respond to salicylates or aspirin. It may involve any joint in the body—knees, elbows, ankles, wrists, fingers, spine, jaw, and hips are the commoner ones. Under the influence of stress and strain or any acute infection, it may commonly flare up, with symptoms more or less like the original attack, but it clears up less and less with subsequent attacks.

A great progressive change usually develops in the tissues about and in the joint and finally involves the cartilage and sometimes the bone. These changes result in some deformity of the joint and limitation of motion. There are great variations in the amount and time of improvement or extent of damage. In some individuals, after a stormy attack and with careful living, the changes clear up, leaving little trace behind. The common course is that they progress, leaving a good deal of deformity. This is one of the greatest sources of disability known to medicine.

After a joint has been involved for some time, there is limitation of movement, and this results in poor nutrition, not only of the individual as a whole, but of the muscles that move the joint. Lime salts are absorbed from the bone. There is one form called Still's disease, which affects children. This is very progressive and leads to great disability, with swollen joints with fluid in them, especially in the wrists, fingers and knees. There is usually an associated anemia, with bouts of fever, and commonly an enlarged spleen. It is very resistive to treatment. Since the tissues about the joints, and often between them, undergo wasting or atrophy, it is given the name atrophic arthritis, although in many instances, especially in the minor cases, there is little atrophy but usually some weakness or lack of certainty in the movements at the joint.

### Hypertrophic Arthritis

This is an extremely common condition which results in a bony thickening along the margins of joints, especially in the last joint of the fingers and in the spine. In many instances, the individual is entirely unconscious of it. About 75% of men and women who reach the age of fifty experience some change in the last joint of the fingers which may result in periods of tenderness or a mild degree of stiffening and commonly a slight thickening of bone in the margins of the joints. Since it is a great source of worry, it should be remarked that it rarely develops very far. It may, however, progress to produce a great deal of thickening and deformity, with twisting and bending of the finger joints.

The other susceptible area is the joints of the spine, in which little spicules are found in both men and women past the age of fifty or sixty. These are usually discovered only on X-ray, and frequently when a person is being X-rayed for another purpose. They, too, are usually with few symptoms but may progress and produce marked deformity.

Both the fingers and the spine are susceptible to having imposed upon them the changes associated with pain and tenderness that we find in the atrophic form. It seems that women use their last finger joints more than men and it is the stress associated with sewing, scrubbing, dishwashing, piano playing and typing that is responsible. In men, the spine seems to carry the load. Another form of hypertrophic arthritis occurs in the spine, chiefly the lower spine in young people, and commonly follows some strain associated with infection. It tends to become progressive and, without proper treatment, leads to progressive stiffening of the spine, which may extend up to the neck. Any disorder of the spine that in any way resembles this description should be treated quickly and adequately and, therefore, hopefully.

### Treatment of Rheumatoid Arthritis

There are several methods of treatment: induction of fever, either with or without the use of sulfonamides, or penicillin for those resistant to the sulfa drugs. The patient is put to bed and the joints placed in splints. Fever is lessened by the salicylate drugs. Sulfathiazole is given by the physician in full doses every three or four hours day and night. At least ten glasses of water should be drunk daily. Treatment may be continued for from two to three weeks after the symptoms have subsided, but the dose of the drug is diminished.

The medical profession is hopeful that cortisone will bring relief.

***Treatment with Gold.*** Gold has been used in the treatment of arthritis—gold sodium thiosulfate or gold sodium thiomalate. The treatments are not without danger and should be carried out by a physician. In the relief of arthritic pain, amidone is superior to morphine, which was formerly used.

## GOUT

***Causes of Gout.*** Although gout is one of the oldest known diseases, having been described by ancient Greek medical writers two thousand years ago, its exact cause is still unknown. It is fairly common in the United States, but it frequently remains unrecognized.

Although the cause of the gouty state is not known, certain factors may start an attack where there is a predisposition—emotional upsets, blood diseases, and various medicinal and chemical agents.

***Symptoms of Gout.*** Gout occurs almost entirely in middle-aged males. It is rare in women. There is a difference between what is termed gout and gouty arthritis. It is possible to suffer from gout due to metabolic (bodily) changes and all its complications, without having arthritis. Gout appears to be caused by defective kidney excretion of uric acid. At recurring intervals uric acid is retained in the blood, partly free and partly as a sodium salt. When this concentration reaches a certain level, an unknown factor starts the depositing of sodium monourate crystals into and around the joints and tendons, which constitutes an acute attack of gout. In the blood of gouty persons the uric acid content is usually above the normal.

### Acute Gout

Acute attacks of gout frequently occur at night. The first attack of gouty arthritis appears suddenly, lasts a few days or perhaps a week or two, and then disappears completely. In the majority of patients the main joint of the big toe is the first to be affected, and in 90 per cent of patients either the big toe, heel, ankle or instep is involved in the first attack. Later attacks may include the joints first affected, or may involve the knees, hands or elbows. The pain becomes excruciating. Patients describe it in different ways. Some speak of it as intense and burning, others as grinding and crushing, and still others as toothache-like in nature.

The early attacks, though very severe, are of relatively short duration. In those which occur at night, the pain usually disappears by morning. At this stage the joint is usually red and swollen. The engorged (congested) veins often give a purplish tinge to the overlying skin. There may be severe recurring attacks each night for several nights before the symptoms disappear. Following the acute attack there is usually a complete absence of symptoms for a period of months, or even years, after which other attacks may begin.

### Chronic Gout

After many repeated episodes with acute gout, chronic gout develops. It may occur from three to even forty years after the first attack. Unlike acute gout, the remissions or periods of relief are incomplete or absent. The pain is less severe than in acute gout, but the joint may be swollen and tender. At this late stage there may be notable deformity of the affected joints. In about 50 per cent of patients, small hard deposits (tophi) appear as yellowish areas in the deep red inflamed joint.

### How to Prevent and Treat Gout

Proper diet is extremely important in the prevention as well as in the treatment of gout. The diet should be regulated in two particulars. First, the total caloric intake should be such as to achieve and maintain normal weight. Second, the intake of nucleoprotein (a combination of nucleic acid with simple proteins) must be controlled. Nucleoprotein yields the substances that are converted into uric acid. Foods to be avoided include meat, fish, chicken, and all internal organs. Fruits, vegetables, milk, eggs, cheese, nuts, butter and bread are recommended. Fats tend to raise the blood uric acid and should be avoided as much as possible; also condiments and spices. Alcoholic beverages, especially fermented liquors, such as wines, beer and ale, should be strictly forbidden. No value has been proved for mineral water in the treatment of gout, and the use of plain drinking water should be encouraged. In many patients who are overweight, a diet suitable to proper weight reduction is often sufficient.

## SYNOVITIS AND BURSITIS

This condition may affect any joint membrane. If the joint is involved, it is called a synovitis; if the tendon sheath is involved, it is called teno-synovitis. A bursa is a small sac that secretes a fluid which acts as a lubricant to the joint. Some bursae are nearer the surface than others; these are the ones usually involved. The two bursae most commonly affected are those of the knee and the shoulder, and when a bursa is inflamed the condition is known as bursitis.

### Water on the Knee

***Causes and Symptoms of Water on the Knee.*** Inflammation of the knee bursa may come on without any apparent cause, in which case there is swelling but slight pain. Water on the knee has another name—"housemaid's knee." This term has its origin in the presumed injury during scrubbing of floors when the maid is on her knees. The swelling is especially below the kneecap, on each side in front of the joint, and also may be above the kneecap. Pain is present as a rule only on movement of the joint.

***Treatment of Water on the Knee.*** This varies according to the severity of the symptoms. If the pain is marked, the leg should be completely rested and heat applied. The use of a cane will often greatly relieve the pain when walking. Most orthopedists advise against immobilization—that is, the use of bandage, adhesive tape or splint. If the joint is made immobile, there is danger of adhesions forming and permanent stiffness resulting.

### Bursitis of the Shoulder

***Symptoms of Shoulder Bursitis.*** Involvement of this bursa is always a terrifically painful condition, especially in the acute stage. The patient cannot get any relief in any position. There is seldom any swelling or redness present, but the tenderness on touch just over the shoulder joint in front is very great.

***Treatment of Shoulder Bursitis.*** The patient may require codeine or morphine on account of the severe pain. This, of course, will have to be prescribed by a physician. No layman can obtain any opium in any form without a doctor's prescription. Rest in bed and the application of either heat or cold is used. Some prefer an ice bag; others will not tolerate the application of cold. It is the counter-irritation that is effective, so it makes no difference whether heat or cold is used. Avoid massage or the application of salves. Massage is harmful and ointments are useless.

### Chronic Shoulder Bursitis

Bursitis of the shoulder usually runs a chronic course. After the acute stage subsides, which may take three or four weeks, great care should be taken not to break up the adhesions which usually form. These are part of the healing process. Tennis, swimming, handball and golf are strictly forbidden. The shoulder should be protected from cold. A shoulder cap made of wool material or felt should be worn. Sleeping with the arm raised over the head is often of value for comfort in this chronic stage.

Very often, after some months of discomfort, an X-ray will show a deposit of calcium in the sac. Some orthopedic surgeons advise the removal of this calcium by surgery. The conservative surgeon says, "No, leave it alone," and he is probably more often correct.

Intermittent pain, according to the use of the shoulder and inclement cold weather, may persist for years. Exposure to the rays of the hot sun is of value at this stage.

CHAPTER 20

# THE URINARY SYSTEM

**Parts of the Urinary System . . . What the Kidneys Do . . . How Urine Is Formed . . . What Normal Urine Is Like . . . Signs and Symptoms of Urinary Disease . . . When Urine Increases or Diminishes . . . Examination of the Urine . . . Casts, Blood Corpuscles, Albumin, Blood, Fat, and Pus—Why They May Be Found in the Urine . . . Uremia . . . Inflammation of the Bladder (Cystitis) . . . Frequent Urination . . . When Urine Cannot Be Passed . . . Acute and Chronic Forms of Bright's Disease (Nephritis or Inflammation of the Kidneys) . . . Stones in the Kidney, Ureter, and Bladder.**

***How We Get Rid of Body Waste.*** The excretory system is a mechanism by which our bodies get rid of waste material. Some of this waste matter consists of water and salts eliminated through the skin in the form of sweat secreted by the sweat glands. Another kind of waste matter consists of the feces, products of the digestive system, eliminated after the food has passed through the entire digestive tract. Still another waste product is the urine. It contains various waste substances derived partly from food and partly from the processes of building up and breaking down tissue, which go on constantly in the body.

***Our Urinary System.*** The urinary system consists of two kidneys, each of which secretes urine into a closed space, the pelvis of the kidney; two tubes, the ureters, which conduct the urine from the kidneys to the bladder; the bladder itself; and a canal, the urethra, which carries the urine from the bladder to the outside. The kidneys, which are bean-shaped, about the size of the palm, are situated in the upper back part of the abdomen. They are made up of a mass of glomeruli (the filtering mechanism) and tiny tubes held together by connective tissue.

***What the Kidneys Do.*** The kidneys are essentially filters. Their basic job is the excretion of certain substances present in the blood. In the main, the kidneys keep the composition of the blood constant by excreting into the urine any excess of substances normally present in the blood, such as salt or sugar; also other substances which are not normal parts of the blood, and waste matter, such as urea and uric acid. As regards water, the kidneys eliminate all that is not absorbed through the stomach and intestines, or lost through the lungs and skin. They thus help keep a normal water balance in the body.

A certain excess of water is necessary for our kidneys to work properly, since dissolved in the urine are substances which are poisonous if they are not eliminated. Therefore we take more water in daily than we lose by the above channels, so that there will be an adequate amount to permit excretion of urine.

## THE URINE

***How Urine Is Formed.*** Urine is derived from blood. It enters the kidney under high pressure and leaves under low pressure. Almost everything which is present in the urine has first been present in the blood.

***How Much Urine Is Secreted.*** The kidney secretes between one and two quarts of urine daily. Diet, the fluid intake, environmental temperature and humidity, posture, exercise, mental excitement, disease or drugs, weight, age and sex—all are factors which affect the volume of urine passed. The amount may be limited by loss of fluids through hemorrhage, vomiting, diarrhea, and excess perspiration. Illness involving high temperature, or disease of the kidney, decreases the amount of urine.

### What Normal Urine Is Like

Normal urine varies in color, specific gravity, odor and reaction from a clear, transparent, pale straw liquid to a cloudy, opaque, deep yellow one. It has a very characteristic odor. The precise color, odor, and reaction depend upon diet, fluid intake, weather conditions, etc.

The average composition of the urine is 96 per cent water and 4 per cent solids, half of which is urea. In addition to solid substances in solution, the urine also contains gases—carbon dioxide, nitrogen, and oxygen in solution.

The color of the urine is almost entirely due to a pigment called urochrome, though it also contains other pigments. Blue urine is caused by taking methylene blue into the stomach; greenish-yellow urine is noted in jaundice. Certain dyes color urine—for example, eosin (used in sweets) produces pink urine; pyramidon causes the urine to appear reddish-orange, if acid; santonin makes it look yellow (pink, if alkaline); senna and rhubarb, reddish brown (pink, if alkaline).

## SIGNS AND SYMPTOMS OF KIDNEY DISEASE

The chief signs and symptoms of kidney disease are: frequent urination, burning and/or pain on urination, decreased output of urine, and discomfort in the flanks. There may also be swelling of the feet and eyelids, high blood pressure, blood in the urine (hematuria), pus in the urine (pyuria), and finally coma in the later stages of the disease.

### When Urine Increases

This may come from any of several causes, including the taking in of large quantities of fluids, certain drugs (diuretics), diabetes, certain kidney diseases, or hysteria.

### When Urine Diminishes (Oliguria)

Causes of this condition are acute inflammation of the kidneys, stone in the kidneys or ureters, acute fevers, or hysteria. It may also exist as a result of rectal operations, profuse sweating, severe shock, tumors, or poisoning with lead, phosphorus, or turpentine.

### Examination of the Urine

The examination of urine is one of the physician's most important methods of ascertaining not merely the condition of the kidneys, but also of the body as a whole. When an organ does not work properly, this fact is frequently shown by the urine.

### Casts in the Urine

Casts represent destroyed kidney tissue, and can be seen in the urine only by means of a microscope. Their significance depends chiefly on their number, variety, and associated conditions. The hyaline (glassy) variety may appear in normal urine and in nephritis (inflammation of the kidneys). Epithelial casts (from the delicate cuticle of internal cavities) may mean acute inflammation of the tubule cells, and they occur most commonly in acute toxic nephritis. Granular casts occur in acute and chronic nephritis.

### Red and White Blood Corpuscles in the Urine

These corpuscles often are found microscopically. The presence of one or both is an indication that some disease is present.

### Albumin in the Urine

The meaning of this abnormality in the urine varies with the condition of the patient and with other signs. Albumin is sometimes discovered in the urine during adolescence, and in what is known to physicians as cyclic albuminuria. Under these circumstances it has no great significance. Albumin may appear for a time after violent exertion or a heavy meal. In some persons it appears at certain hours of the day or only when they lie down. Albumin in the urine is regarded as important from the viewpoint of life insurance, but if there are no signs of arterial or heart disease the outlook is most favorable.

Albumin is sometimes discovered in the urine of patients with fever and in certain diseases of the nervous system, such as apoplexy and epilepsy. The most common appearance of albumin in the urine is in organic disease of the kidney—namely, in all varieties of Bright's disease. Many other abnormalities, such as acute infections, tuberculosis, tumors, etc., may cause albuminuria if there is destruction of kidney tissue or blood in the urine. In many cases the change is reversible if the disease is treated in time.

### Blood in the Urine

Blood may be present in the urine due to injury of any part of the urinary or genital tract or nearby organs. It may also occur in blood disorders and in some general diseases. Blood is also found in the urine in the following conditions: kidney conditions of all varieties, especially acute inflammation; when there are tumors, stone or stones; blocking of the arteries by a clot; early kidney tuberculosis; poisoning by mercurials, turpentine, carbolic acid, cantharides ("Spanish fly"); or when certain medications have been taken. There may also be blood in the kidneys in disease of the urinary passages when a specific fever, scurvy, high blood pressure, or leukemia is present.

If the first urine voided (passed) is blood-stained, and the remainder clear, it is probable that the blood is coming from the tube which leads from the bladder to the outside. On the other hand, if the last urine voided is blood-stained and the rest is clear, it is strong evidence that the blood is coming from the bladder. If the urine is evenly stained throughout, it is probable that the blood is coming from the kidneys. When bleeding in the bladder is profuse, the urine is stained throughout.

### Fat in the Urine

Urine sometimes contains drops of fat (lipuria). This condition is extremely rare; however, it may be noted in fracture of the long bones, diabetes and tumors of the kidney.

### Pus in the Urine

Pus is found in the urine in acute infections or inflammations of any part of the urinary tract. The common cause for infection in the lower canal (urethra) is gonorrhea. Cystitis (inflammation of the bladder) is very common in women, less so in men. It is frequently caused by transmission of infections from the vagina to the bladder directly or through the lymph passages. Often the bladder infection is associated with infections elsewhere in the body, as in the throat or ear. Sometimes it occurs by extension of infection from the kidney, and transmission from the colon (large intestine). The bacteria are often those found normally in the colon or those found in the adjacent genitals. The usual symptoms of these inflammations of the lower part of the urinary tract (bladder and urethra) are frequent voiding, both day and night, burning on voiding, frequent desire to void, and often blood in the urine, especially at the beginning of the disorder. There is often tenderness to pressure over the pelvic bone and slight elevation of temperature.

Pus in the urine arising from infection in the kidney usually causes the above symptoms plus chills and fever and pain in the back. This infection may be due to causes similar to those in bladder infections, or to stones or tumors in the kidney or kidney tube. This condition of pus in the kidney is called pyelitis.

## UREMIA

Uremia is a toxic state which results when the kidneys do not perform. Often it arises as a result of inflammation of the kidney. The beginning may be abrupt (acute) or insidious (chronic). The symptoms vary greatly in different persons. Thus there may be a sudden appearance of twitchings, convulsions, headache, foul breath, contraction of the pupils, blindness, and coma, or a slow beginning with anemia, drowsiness and shortness of breath—what is termed kidney asthma. Again, mental symptoms may be the most striking feature, such as dullness, delusions and hallucinations, or actual mania. Immediate treatment by a physician is called for.

## INFLAMMATION OF THE BLADDER (CYSTITIS)

***Causes of Inflammation of the Bladder.*** Inflammation of the bladder is common in women, but not infrequent in men. It is the result of infection by virulent germs. Before the germs can produce inflammation in men, one of the following conditions must be present: obstruction to the proper emptying of the bladder; the presence of stones (calculi) or foreign bodies; the presence of malignant growths, or absence of proper nervous control of the organ. In women, acute bladder infections often arise from infections in the vagina and neighboring organs. The disease appears in acute and chronic forms as well as various intermediate stages.

***Symptoms of Inflammation of the Bladder.*** Pain and frequency in passing of urine are constant features. Urine is passed at frequent intervals through the night. In severe conditions, there is loss of bladder control. Pain may be not only local but in the thighs and abdomen as well. Low-grade fever, with or without bloody urine, is the rule; it is, however, often absent unless the infection has spread to the kidneys.

***Treatment of Inflammation of the Bladder.*** In the acute stage there should be rest in bed. Fluid intake is increased to help "wash out" the germs. Hot sitz baths, fifteen minutes each, should be taken every four to five hours. If the pain is severe it will be necessary to call a physician to prescribe an analgesic. The physician will usually also prescribe a medicine, often a sulfa drug, to cure the infection. The diet should be bland, and alcohol should be excluded. If an acute attack does not subside within a week or ten days, it is possible that the infection is coming from the kidney.

***Treatment of Chronic Conditions.*** If, after the usual time for the cure of an acute attack, the symptoms persist, the condition is called chronic. This is often treated by bladder irrigations, and X-ray examination of the kidneys is made to determine whether or not one or both kidneys are involved. Do not delay seeking professional advice if the symptoms last longer than a few days.

## FREQUENT URINATION

***"Irritable Bladder."*** In only prolonged mental strain is there likely to be a diminution in the production of urine. The emotions, on the other hand, usually cause a marked increase in the amount of the urine. Prolonged nervous strain, fright, anger, or great joy will have telling effect upon the kidneys. This increased need for emptying the bladder is not a disease but merely an annoying symptom. It is often called "Irritable Bladder."

### Urine Production in Health

The normal amount of urine passed in twenty-four hours averages, for the healthy individual, from one to two quarts. As stated earlier, the amount varies according to fluid intake, temperature, climate and numerous other local conditions. The rate of secretion also varies in different persons.

The average bladder capacity is about one pint, a trifle more in females than in males. There may be wide variations in this capacity, reaching as high as one or two quarts, yet these may be normal for a given person. Increased bladder capacity is seen often in chronic beer drinkers. One should not consider it a sign of prowess to be able to hold the urine for a long period of time; although the bladder is a very elastic organ it can be overstretched by resisting the urge to empty it. This may cause a temporary paralysis or sudden loss of control.

The frequency of urination may be considered normal when it occurs every two hours by day and not more than once at night. Sometimes a large amount of water or alcoholic drinks is taken around the bedtime hour. This will naturally disturb the bladder rest because the amount of urine entering the bladder is increased.

Coffee and alcoholic drinks are common offenders. Many persons cannot tolerate even small amounts of alcohol or coffee without having to empty their bladders at an increased rate. These individuals will notice that within a few minutes after the taking of one or more cocktails or highballs, they will have to answer the call of the bladder. This may be likewise true after one or more cups of strong coffee.

***Causes of Frequent Urination.*** The kidneys, like many of our other vital organs, are involuntary, and all nerve control of the involuntary organs is from the highly sensitive sympathetic nervous system. Therefore, emotional upsets and instability produce an irregularity of kidney activity. On the other hand, under normal conditions the bladder is a voluntary organ, and even though the kidneys may secrete at an increased rate without any voluntary control, the bladder usually receives this increase under complete control. What, then, is the irritable bladder that annoys so many men and women? That which is considered under this caption is not the case of true bladder disease, such as infection, or stone; here we have to deal with cases that may be divided, as to cause, into three headings—nervous irritability, changes in the chemical reaction of the urine and mechanical pressure on the bladder wall. The first we have already discussed.

***Changes in Urine Reaction.*** The normal urine is either neutral in reaction or slightly acid. The change to a highly acid reaction or, as is less frequent, an increase in the alkalinity, will produce an irritation of the mucous membrane of the bladder neck and urethra. This in turn will be responsible for the frequent desire to urinate every few minutes and often lack of control. What causes this chemical change? It is due either to the intake of irritating fluids, or to errors in diet.

The use of certain mineral waters that contain a high percentage of calcium salts may be very harmful and is quite unnecessary at all times. The foods that may cause this same condition are concentrated proteins in excess—meats and eggs; certain vegetables—tomatoes and asparagus; and, among the fruits, berries with seeds. The reaction to these articles of diet may be allergic, or possibly due to changes in acidity.

***Mechanical Disturbance.*** We now come to a consideration of the third of our classifications—mechanical influences that cause frequency of bladder activity. In women this condition is often due to pressure on the bladder resulting from relaxed abdominal muscles, as seen in obesity, or to relaxed support of the roof of the vagina, which is usually caused by improper repair of tears resulting from childbirth. The presence of such mechanical defects causes one of the most pronounced forms of bladder irritability and occasionally completely incapacitates the individual.

In the male, mechanical disturbance is usually due to enlargement of the prostate gland. It should be emphasized that this enlargement more often than not is inflammatory or congestive and not the true enlargement found in men of advanced age. Young men therefore may have bladder disturbance due to pressure by the prostate, but not as commonly as the older ones.

***Treatment of Frequent Urination.*** The first need is: Do not ignore the symptom. Consult a physician, who will examine the urine. If the urine reaction is markedly changed from what it normally should be, this increased acidity or alkalinity is brought back to normal by the elimination of the foods and drinks which are found to be the offending articles of the diet. If the bladder disturbance is found to be purely nervous in origin, then a capable psychiatrist must be consulted. He will determine what the troublesome factors are—the condition is usually minor—and institute corrective measures.

In women who have the mechanical type of bladder distress, nothing but a plastic operation by a capable gynecologist will relieve the patient. This operation is without any danger, and requires usually about ten days' hospitalization.

In men in whom the prostate is enlarged, a competent urologist will determine the type of enlargement and will outline necessary treatment whereby the size of the gland will be restored to normal. The bladder will consequently resume its normal action.

One final caution—do not ignore the symptom of bladder distress; it may be a warning of a serious bladder or kidney disease which can be stopped if diagnosis is made early enough.

## WHEN URINE CANNOT BE PASSED (RETENTION OR STOPPAGE OF URINE)

When the urine has been accumulating in the bladder for a considerable time—over twelve hours—and cannot be passed, the condition is described as retention or stoppage of urine.

***Causes and Symptoms of Retention of Urine.*** Retention may follow an obstruction from disease, to which is added temporary swelling and nervous contraction of some part of the urinary passage; or it may be caused by spasms and closure of the outlet, as in injuries and surgical operations in the vicinity of the sexual organs, the rectum, or other parts of the body. Tumors of the urinary tract or adjacent organs, as of the prostate in men and the womb in women, may block the passage and lead to retention. Occasionally, stones or strictures, either in upper or lower portions of the canal, will produce obstruction. Various general diseases, such as severe fevers, unconsciousness, and other disorders of the nervous system, are frequently accompanied by retention of urine. Finally, it may also be due to hysteria.

In retention of urine there is often an escape of a little urine from time to time, and not necessarily entire absence of outflow. This is serious, since infection is almost always the result of stagnation of the residual urine. Over-distention of the bladder from failure to pass water for a long time may lead to a condition where urination becomes an impossibility for some time.

***Treatment of Retention of Urine.*** Treatment naturally varies with the age and condition of the patient, and the cause of urinary retention. It is usually necessary for the doctor or nurse to pass a narrow rubber tube (catheter) into the bladder to remove the urine, which flows out from the rubber tube by itself. This must be done with sterile technique in order to prevent infection. The cause of the difficulty must then be determined by studies and X-rays of the urinary apparatus. Treatment may be surgical in case of tumors, etc., or medical if due to infection or disease of the nervous system.

## ACUTE BRIGHT'S DISEASE (ACUTE INFLAMMATION OF THE KIDNEYS)

Bright's disease may be acute or chronic. Its presence can be definitely determined only by chemical and microscopic examination of the urine. However, acute Bright's disease, coming on in persons previously well, may present certain symptoms by which its presence may be suspected even by the layman.

***Causes of Acute Bright's Disease.*** Acute Bright's disease is often due to exposure to cold and wet with resulting infection of the nose and throat. Damage to the kidneys may be produced by swallowing bichloride of mercury, turpentine, large amounts of the cheap flavoring extracts, carbolic acid and "Spanish fly."

Certain drugs, taken without careful instruction, may also damage the kidney. This may result in a condition similar to acute Bright's disease.

The contagious germ diseases are frequently the cause of acute Bright's disease, either as a complication or a sequel. Thus, scarlet fever is the most frequent cause; but measles, smallpox, chicken-pox, yellow fever, typhoid fever, erysipelas, diphtheria, cholera, and malaria may also be causes.

***Symptoms of Acute Bright's Disease.*** Acute nephritis, as acute inflammation of the kidneys is also known, may occur in one of two forms: insidious or sudden. In the first variety, symptoms may be slight or absent at the beginning. Following the subsiding of a respiratory infection, for example, the urine may reveal albumin, red blood cells, and casts. The second variety may manifest itself at a later date as a sequel of infection.

Acute Bright's disease may develop suddenly, with pallor and puffiness of the face, due to dropsy (swelling caused by accumulation of fluid). The eyelids, ankles, legs and lower part of the abdomen are apt to show dropsy most. There may be nausea, vomiting, pain and lameness in the small part of the back, chills and fever, loss of appetite, and often constipation. In children convulsions sometimes appear.

The urine is small in amount, perhaps not more than a cupful in twenty-four hours. Occasionally complete suppression of urine takes place. It is high-colored, either smoky or of a porter color, or sometimes a dark or even bright red, from the presence of blood.

Stupor and unconsciousness may occur in severe conditions.

Recovery usually occurs, in favorable cases, within a few weeks, with gradually diminishing dropsy and increasing secretion of urine; or the disease may end in a chronic disorder of the kidneys. If acute Bright's disease is caused by, or complicated with, other diseases, the probable result becomes much more difficult to predict.

***Treatment of Acute Bright's Disease.*** Obviously only a physician is competent to treat this condition. The patient must be confined to bed, and his diet for the first few days must consist of nothing but glucose water or orangeade—two cups of glucose in one pint of water, or the juice of one orange. Total fluids must not be more than one and one-half pints in twenty-four hours. After a few days, when the urinary output has increased, one-half pint of milk, with thin bread and butter, and coffee may be taken. Salt must be avoided, and fluid intake restricted if the swelling still persists. The protein intake should be reduced to about three to four tablespoonfuls a day. The patient should be kept in bed until the daily output of albumin in the urine remains at a stationary level. Maintenance of body temperature by the use of warm bedding is of great importance.

The patient must be followed closely by his physician for months to come in order to determine the extent of the damage.

## CHRONIC BRIGHT'S DISEASE

This includes several forms of kidney disease. The usual types are due to chronic infection, acute nephritis (acute Bright's disease) which has not cleared up, or changes in the vessels of the kidney. The symptoms are often very obscure, and the condition may not be discovered or suspected by the physician until an examination of the urine is made. Accidental discovery of Bright's disease during examination for life insurance is common. The disease may be present for years without serious impairment of health.

***Symptoms of Chronic Bright's Disease.*** Often the disease develops very slowly. Thus it may be unnoticed for a long time. The first symptoms are mental and physical fatigue, severe headache, loss of weight, anemia, and loss of appetite. There may be giddiness, passage of large quantities of water, and failure of sight. Swelling of the face and extremities is found in only one form of chronic nephritis, and is not a common symptom until marked damage has occurred. Noises in the ear are frequent and troublesome symptoms in later stages. Vomiting occurs in later stages. When the disease is well developed, the urine is pale and increased in amount; when the urine is examined, it usually contains albumin and granular casts. Uremia develops toward the end, and is often noted by a "frost" on the face.

***Prevention and Treatment of Chronic Bright's Disease.*** Preventive measures must, of necessity, be of a general nature. These include avoidance of exposure to the elements and to infection, and the proper care of infection once it has begun. The diet should be light, and only a little meat should be eaten. The bowels and the skin must be kept active. In general, the tendency in the past has been to cut the protein intake too drastically; it should be varied to suit the patient. Cheese, as a high protein food, can be used as a substitute for eggs or meat. In the main it is best to consult a physician regarding the diet. The patient must live a quiet, regular life and abstain from excesses of any kind.

Where symptoms are marked, treatment resembles that used for the acute form.

Medicines will no more cure Bright's disease than they will cure old age. Out-of-door life in a dry, warm, and equable climate has the most favorable influence upon chronic Bright's disease. If the patient shows uremic symptoms he must be under the immediate care of a physician.

## STONES IN THE URINARY TRACT

***Diet As a Cause.*** There are many indications that diets too rich in calcium and uric acid may produce stones. This is, however, probably very rare and needs merely to be mentioned. Diets which are deficient in certain vitamins, particularly vitamin A, have also been suggested as causes of stones. In general, however, if an individual eats the usual three meals a day with plenty of green vegetables, milk and average amounts of protein and carbohydrates (such as meat and potatoes), there is little chance of diet being a factor in the formation of stones.

***Infections, the Commonest Cause.*** Infections in the kidney are probably the greatest cause of stones. To form a stone it is necessary to have a nucleus or "beginning." Accumulations of pus and bits of infected tissue commonly form this nucleus. Therefore, it is important that infections be treated early.

***Fluid Intake.*** This factor is also extremely important, especially in hot weather, when much fluid is lost by perspiration. This gives the kidney little to work on and, consequently, the urine becomes concentrated and there is little flow. As a result of this condition, particles accumulate, forming a nucleus for a stone.

***Other Conditions Causing Stones.*** Other conditions in the urinary tract may act as contributing factors in the cause of stone formation. These include any mechanical interference with the free flow of urine from the kidney and extrusion from the bladder, such as strictures or narrowing of the ureter or urethra in either sex. These conditions are mainly surgical. Any mechanical interference usually causes the infectious type of stones.

### Prevention of Stones

***Role of Drugs.*** Before the recent advent of sulfonamides and streptomycin, infections of the kidney and bladder easily gained headway in their destructive processes and stone formation was a common result. Today, if early diagnosis is made, these drugs will promptly destroy the bacteria and stop the infection, and thus no stones will be formed.

***Recommended Diet.*** Follow two simple dietary rules: Do not overeat at any time, and eat a well-balanced meal at least once daily, well-stocked with vegetables, which should overbalance the amount of meat and other protein intake.

***Weakening the Urine Concentration.*** Water dilutes the urine and eliminates the tendency to the formation of the uric acid variety of kidney stones. When the average person is asked how much water he drinks in a day, he will say either that he does not know or that he drinks very little. It is true that fluid intake is often in the form of other liquids, such as coffee and tea, and, of course, all foods contain varying amounts of water. However, only pure water, unadulterated by other substances, is essential for proper kidney balance and dilution of the solid content of the urine. The amount of water should average eight to ten full glasses in twenty-four hours. Great emphasis must be placed upon this.

The best time to drink water is the first thing in the morning and between meals. Less favorable is during meals, as this may retard digestion, and in the evening, as one may have to get up at night to empty the bladder.

***Taking Mineral Water.*** Some mineral waters are reputed to dissolve kidney stones and stones in the gall bladder. This is absolutely not true. The only constituent of a mineral water that is of value is the water itself. If it contains properties that act upon the bowels and is taken copiously, it is likely to set up an irritation of the lining of the intestines and cause colitis. If its constituents act upon the kidneys, it may cause irritation of these organs and the urinary bladder. Continued use of large quantities of water rich in calcium may produce kidney and bladder stones if there is abnormal calcium metabolism. Such cases have been observed rarely.

### Locations of Stones

Stone formation in the urinary tract may take place in one of three places: the kidney, the ureter (tube that carries the urine from the kidney to the bladder), and the bladder. The symptoms and treatment vary according to the location of the stone. There are two different kinds of stones. Both have chemical formation. One may be due to abnormal metabolism of calcium due to tumor of parathyroid gland, and the other to pus, around which calcium deposits.

### Kidney Stone

***Symptoms of Kidney Stone.*** Kidney stones are divided into the so-called "silent" and the actively moving stones. The "silent" type may have been present for many months without the patient's having any knowledge of its presence. The stone may have been discovered when the patient had an examination for some other condition.

If the stone is of any considerable size, there is usually a dull, aching pain in the back on the affected side; this pain is more pronounced when the patient is up and about, but it does not entirely disappear when he is lying down. Tenderness can be caused when making pressure over the kidney. Blood and pus are found upon urinalysis. This varies in quantity according to the size of the stone and whether its origin is due to infection or to chemical changes in the urine. The taking of an X-ray film usually completes the diagnosis. About 5 per cent of the stones are radio-lucent (do not show on X-ray).

***Treatment of Kidney Stone.*** Never let anyone tell you that there are any drugs or medicines of any kind that dissolve urinary stones. There are no such things, unfortunately. In an occasional case, a solution can be injected into the kidney which will dissolve a "soft stone." If a large stone is diagnosed, one that is too large to pass down the ureter, which would mean not any larger than a small pea, an operation for removal of the stone is indicated, and the longer the delay the more danger of further destruction of the kidney and recurrence of other stones.

### Ureteral Stone

***Symptoms of Ureteral Stone.*** Stones do not form primarily in the ureter. They are said to be ureteral when they are small enough to pass from the kidney into the ureter. If a stone passes into the ureter it produces colic, which is one of the most painful happenings in the human body. The pain doubles up the patient and may last for many hours, or after medication there is some relief; then the colic will again start. The colic is due to the movement of the stone down the ureter. When you consider that the ureter is about twelve inches in length and that the progress of the stone may be delayed for even days or months by catching in a fold of mucous membrane, then you realize what an ordeal this is to go through.

There is always blood present in the urine, especially during the most active movement of the stone. There is marked tenderness along the course of the ureter down the groin and into the scrotum and testicles in the male and into the vagina in the female.

***Treatment of Ureteral Stones.*** There are two ways to handle these cases. It all depends upon whether there is infection present. If there is infection with chills and fever, this infection must be treated first. Surgical removal of the stone may be necessary if the infection cannot be controlled and the stone does not move into the bladder. This is a very delicate operation and should be attempted only by an experienced urological surgeon.

Whether there is infection or not, the use of opiates to relieve the pain is indicated. A very hot bath may help by relaxing the muscles. When no infection is present, the progress of the stone is watched by repeated X-rays. If after a period to be determined by the doctor there is no progress of the stone, then there is a procedure that can be performed, but again only by an experienced doctor. This procedure is called a cystoscopic examination. An instrument is passed through the urinary canal (urethra) into the bladder, and through this instrument the doctor can see the openings of the urinary tubes. A catheter is passed into the ureter and some oil is injected beyond the stone. The stone will often pass into the bladder, from which it is usually voided in the urine.

### Bladder Stone

***Symptoms of Bladder Stone.*** There are two types of bladder stones, primary and secondary. If the formation of the stone takes place in the bladder, it is primary; but if a ureteral stone passes into the bladder, it is then a secondary bladder stone. Either stone can grow to the size of an orange. Of course there are very unpleasant symptoms associated with large bladder stones. There are always blood and pus in the urine, and the desire to empty the bladder is so frequent that the patient is completely incapacitated; with each urination there is much pain. X-ray will show the stone.

***Treatment of Bladder Stone.*** There is only one thing to do—that is surgical removal. This can be done in one of two ways, either by crushing with a special instrument which is introduced into the bladder, or by opening the bladder and taking out the stone. If there is considerable infection, then the latter procedure is better. It takes an expert to crush a stone without doing injury to the bladder wall. Of course all these procedures can be performed only in a hospital.

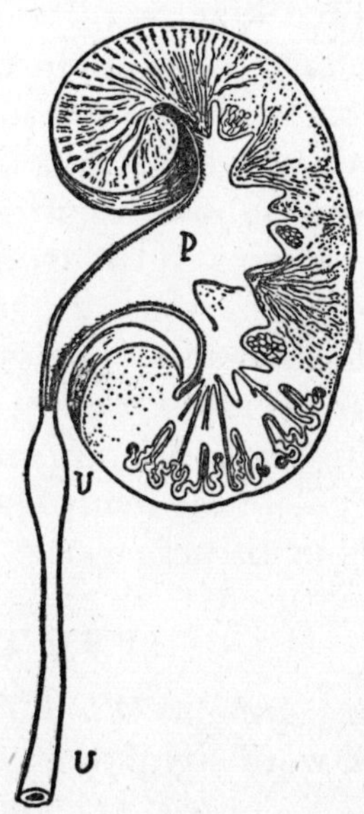


THE KIDNEY
The human body has two kidneys. In the inner part of each is a pelvis (P), from which the urine passes into the ureter (U).

CHAPTER 21

# NUTRITION AND GOOD HEALTH

**Things We Need for Nourishment . . . Proteins and What They Do . . . The Role of Fats . . . Carbohydrates . . . Minerals . . . Water . . . The Indispensable Vitamins—Why We Need Them and Where to Find Them . . . Vitamin Deficiency Diseases . . . Beriberi . . . Pellagra . . . Sprue . . . Rules for Selecting and Cooking Foods . . . Meaning of a Balanced Diet . . . Calories and Energy . . . Your Daily Calorie Needs . . . Normal Daily Diet . . . Caloric Values of Food . . . Your Normal Weight . . . Importance of Weight Control after Thirty . . . Height and Weight Charts.**

NUTRITION means nothing more nor less than the nourishment of our bodies. Through good nutrition we provide for the proper growth, maintenance, and repair of our body tissues. Nutrition, in this sense, makes us what we are. It is our "internal environment."

Health does not have to be graded as just normal or average, but may also be above average, or buoyant and vigorous. It is now definitely known that merely adequate dietary amounts will afford protection against any important deficiency disease and will give average grades of nutritional well-being, growth, body structure, and functioning. But it is also clear that more than the minimum amounts give substantial benefits in improved well-being and superior general health. An abundance of the right food will also give something of equal importance—a reserve to draw upon. If you eat wisely and keep to a balanced diet, as recommended in the pages that follow, you will find it easy to maintain this reserve and to enjoy vigorous good health, from a nutritional standpoint.

The things we need for nourishment include water and a vast variety of chemical substances, which are grouped into classes. These classes are the proteins, carbohydrates, fats, minerals, and vitamins. We need the proteins, minerals, and water for the construction and maintenance of our tissues. The carbohydrates and fats are the chief providers of our energy. Protein provides energy also, although this is not its essential task. Water, minerals, and the vitamins serve to promote and regulate the many chemical reactions of the nutritional processes of all our tissues.

## PROTEINS

***What Proteins Are and What They Do.*** The name protein comes from the Greek word signifying "that which is of first or prime importance." Proteins occur in all living material, and are the most abundant solids present. They are found in plant and animal matter. Proteins differ from carbohydrates and fats in that they contain nitrogen in addition to carbon, hydrogen and oxygen.

The main value of proteins is that they provide the nitrogen, in the form of amino acids, which is essential to the upkeep of every part of our body structures. They are of primary importance as the material of which protoplasm (living substance) is made.

The child needs relatively more protein than the adult. There is no storehouse for protein in the body, so protein must be given daily. The proteins in milk contain all the essential amino acids.

Proteins in foods vary as to quality and value to the body. The differences in value among proteins depend upon the amino acids of which they are composed. Although there are only about twenty or so amino acids, a great number of proteins are formed from them.

All amino acids essential for bodily use are believed to be supplied in one or other of the following forms: milk albumin, beef protein, egg albumin and glutenin of wheat. Good basic sources of protein are fish, beef, veal, lamb, poultry, mutton, pork, milk, eggs, butter, cheese, nuts, corn, beans, peas, and grain. All meats should be lean.

In general, the amount of protein desirable should measure 10 to 15 per cent of the total number of calories consumed daily.

## FATS

***The Role of Fats.*** Fats are chemical substances found in plant and animal matter; like carbohydrates, they contain carbon, hydrogen, and oxygen. They are the most concentrated forms of energy, providing more than twice as many calories as carbohydrates.

Meals containing insufficient fat lack so-called staying power, with the result that hunger is experienced sooner than with meals containing considerable fat. Also, fat is important in the diet for the palatability it imparts to other foods. Fats reduce the rate of discharge of the stomach contents and are absorbed from the intestine at a slower rate than the carbohydrates, which is desirable in the process of digestion.

Fat is needed in the structure and functioning of all tissues, in particular of the nerves and brain. That may be one reason why overweight persons are more evenly tempered and less nervous as a group. As a padding, fat holds body organs, blood vessels, and nerves in place and rounds out the contour of the body structure. Under the skin, fat serves as an insulator for retarding loss of body heat. Body fat deposits constitute the most important source of energy for use in periods of food privation.

Dairy products (milk, butter, etc.) are rich in fats. Fat can be obtained also from nuts, vegetables and animal foods (meat, poultry, fish, lard, etc.).

FAT CONTENT OF SOME COMMON FOODS

| *Low in Fat (Less than 2%)* | *Medium Fat Content (2 to 10%)* | *Rich in Fat (Above 10%)* |
|---|---|---|
| Vegetables | Cream soups | Salmon |
| Most fruits | Milk | Tuna |
| Cereals | Veal | Lamb |
| Bread | Chicken | Pork |
| Egg white | Turkey | Duck |
| Buttermilk | Lean beef | Goose |
| | Crab meat | Egg yolks |
| | | Cheese from whole milk |
| | | Bacon |
| | | Nuts |
| | | Chocolate |

## CARBOHYDRATES

These are, in general, the various types of sugar—fruit, cane, or beet; milk and malt—and the starches. They contain carbon, hydrogen, and oxygen, but usually no nitrogen.

VEGETABLES ARRANGED ACCORDING TO CONTENT OF CARBOHYDRATE
*(Fresh or Canned, without Added Sugar)*

| *1-3%* | *3-5%* | *10%* | *15%* | *20%* |
|---|---|---|---|---|
| Lettuce | Tomatoes | String beans | Green peas | Potatoes |
| Cucumbers | Watercress | Brussels sprouts | Artichokes | Shell beans |
| Spinach | Cauliflower | Pumpkin | Parsnips | Baked beans |
| Asparagus | Eggplant | Turnip | | Green corn |
| Rhubarb | Cabbage | Squash | | Boiled rice |
| Endive | Radishes | Okra | | |
| Marrow squash | Leeks | Beets | | |
| Sorrel | String beans (young) | Carrots | | |
| Sauerkraut | Broccoli | Onions | | |
| Beet greens | French artichokes | Green beans | | |
| Celery | Summer squash | | | |
| Mushrooms | Kohlrabi | | | |

Essential vitamins and minerals found in foods containing carbohydrates are to a great extent removed when the foods are refined. The most striking examples are refined flour, polished rice, and pure sugar, as these are commonly used in bakery products, confectionery, soft drinks and dessert type foods. Using brown rice, bread made with enriched flour, and brown sugar makes up for this shortcoming, at least on three items in the list.

Potatoes are rich in carbohydrates, as are cake, candy, macaroni, spaghetti, and similar foods. Carbohydrates should be taken only sparingly in weight reduction.

## MINERALS

Many mineral elements are required in the diet. About nineteen of these mineral elements have been found in the human body and all of them are present in food materials.

***Calcium and Phosphorus.*** Calcium, the building material of the skeleton, is perhaps the most important. Approximately 98 per cent of the calcium in the body is contained in the bones, where, combined chiefly with phosphate, it gives strength and rigidity.

Bone is a living tissue which is most susceptible to nutritional disturbances during the early periods of growth. Even in adult life, however, inadequate nutrition over a long period may lead to the bones' being porous.

Smaller amounts of calcium are essential for such work as building strong teeth, maintaining the sensitivity of nervous tissue and muscle, and making blood clot when there is a wound. From the viewpoint of nutrition, the problem is to insure an adequate intake of calcium and phosphorus, together with the necessary vitamin D to promote their assimilation in the tissues. Milk is an excellent source of calcium; it is also found in fruits, meats, green vegetables, whole grains and meats. These will also provide phosphorus, for which other good sources are fish, dried beans, nuts, and cheese.

***Iron and the Blood.*** Iron is another important mineral. It is vital to the health of the red corpuscles in our blood, and is needed to prevent anemia. Good sources are green vegetables, fruits, dried beans, egg yolk, lean red meat, and whole-grained cereal.

***Iodine and Where We Get It.*** Iodine, for which the body has only a small need, is essential for the health of the thyroid gland and for the prevention of goitre. Iodized salt is a good source. Too much, however, should not be used. Seafood and vegetables grown in soil rich in iodine, if eaten regularly, will provide an adequate supply of iodine for the body's needs.

***Other Necessary Minerals.*** Other minerals required by the body are sodium, potassium, sulphur, lithium, chlorine, copper, silicon, barium, and manganese. These are generally provided in a good balanced diet.

## WATER

Water is an essential constituent of all living matter. It is important for many reasons. It is an excellent solvent for food. It is the most important chemical constituent of the body, not only in amount—it makes up two-thirds of the body's weight—but also because of the activities it takes part in. It helps regulate body temperature, it bathes all our cells and tissues, and is the basis of all our vital fluids and secretions. The fluid intake must be maintained in the body, even if the intake of other dietary constituents is not maintained, for the body can withstand lack of food better than lack of water.

## VITAMINS

Few fields in medicine have developed more rapidly or given rise to a greater volume of literature than that of the vitamins. The first vitamin was discovered in 1912 by Doctor Casimir Funk. A vitamin may be described as an organic substance that is present in most foods in small amounts. Vitamins are necessary for the normal functioning of the body—for its normal growth and health.

With the discovery, isolation, and manufacture of the several vitamins, there has evolved the concept of vitamin deficiency diseases. We are here concerned with the *prevention* of these diseases by emphasizing the need of body protection against a reduced amount of these vitamins.

Vitamins are nutritionally essential. Small amounts of them exert powerful physiologic effects. The individual vitamins are fairly widely distributed in various natural foods. Their toxic potentialities are very limited even in extremely large dosage. The normal requirements for the individual vitamins are from small to very minute amounts.

Our estimated total lifetime intake of all vitamins is but twenty to thirty teaspoonfuls in an estimated total of seventy tons of food that we take into our bodies.* Yet, without this amount, small as it is, we would die of insufficiency starvation.

If one is constantly reminded that "perfect health" can be maintained by uninterrupted well-balanced diet, there will be no cause for worry which of the various vitamins should be considered as essential. In fact, all are essential, and all are supplied in adequate amounts in the emphasized balanced diet.

***Vitamin Preparations.*** The indiscriminate wholesale distribution for sale of the various commercial vitamin combinations is unnecessary and is to be decried as an economic extravagance.

When vitamins as such are to be prescribed, let your physician decide what you need, and be guided solely by his recommendations.

## VITAMIN A

***Why We Need Vitamin A.*** Vitamin A is valuable to us because it promotes normal growth, especially in children, and is helpful in preventing infections, particularly of the respiratory tract. It aids keenness of vision, prevents night blindness, and is necessary to maintain normal skin condition. This vitamin is frequently given in pregnancy, prematurity, tuberculosis, ulcerative colitis, infantile eczema and other conditions.

Vitamin A is rapidly destroyed if exposed to air and high temperatures. It is not destroyed by heating in a tightly closed container. Its absence leads to lowered resistance to infection, especially of the mucous membranes.

***Good Animal Sources.*** Liver oils, kidneys, liver, roe, salmon, whole milk, cream, butter, cheese, eggs, fish liver oils.

***Good Fruit Sources.*** Apricots, cantaloupes, mangoes, peaches (yellow), prunes.

***Good Vegetable Sources.*** Asparagus, beans (green), beet tops, broccoli, Brussels sprouts, carrots, celery (green), chard, Chinese cabbage, collards, corn (yellow), dandelion greens, endive, kale, leeks, lettuce, mustard greens, okra, onions (green), parsley, peas, peppers, potatoes (sweet), pumpkin, spinach, squash (Hubbard or summer), tomatoes, turnip greens, watercress.

***Vitamin A and Vegetable Colors.*** Color may be used as a guide to how much vitamin A is contained in vegetables. Green vegetables are richer than yellow; and yellow vegetables are richer than red. Vege-

* *Living Should Be Fun,* by Carlton Fredericks, head of the National Research Institute.

tables of deep colors are usually better sources than those of pale colors.

## VITAMIN $B_1$ (THIAMINE)

***Why We Need Vitamin $B_1$.*** This vitamin is not only essential, but it also helps maintain appetite and is necessary for carbohydrate utilization. It is essential for both proper nerve function and one's best muscular work. It prevents the disease beriberi, a form of neuritis. It is also used medically during fever conditions and in cases of overactivity of the thyroid gland.

Vitamin $B_1$ is injured by cooking in neutral or alkali solutions. Heating in acid such as tomato or citrus juice contains will cause it little damage.

***Good Animal Sources.*** Beef, chicken, eggs, fish (fresh), ham, lamb, liver, lobster, oysters, pork, roe, sweetbreads, veal, whole milk.

***Good Fruit Sources.*** Avocados, bananas, cantaloupes, figs (fresh), gooseberries, oranges.

***Good Grain Sources.*** Breads (enriched or whole grain), enriched five-minute Cream of Wheat, rolled oats, barley (whole), rice (brown).

***Good Vegetable Sources.*** (Thiamine dissolves in water. Therefore save and serve the cooking water in soup or gravy, at the same meal if possible.) Artichokes, asparagus, beans (kidney, lima, Navy, string), beet greens, broccoli, Brussels sprouts, cabbage (fresh), carrots, cauliflower, collard, corn, dandelion greens, kale, leeks, lentils, mushrooms, mustard greens, parsnips, peanuts, peas, potatoes (sweet and white), spinach, tomatoes, turnip greens.

## VITAMIN $B_2$ (RIBOFLAVIN)

***What Vitamin $B_2$ Does for Us.*** This vitamin promotes growth and increases adult vitality. Vitamin $B_2$ is one of the antipellagra vitamins. It is necessary for the well-being of the eyes. It is also used medically for sore tongue and lips and in cases of retardation of growth.

***Good Animal Sources.*** Liver, milk, beef (lean), brains, cheese (Cheddar and cottage), eggs, finnan haddie, haddock, ham, hearts, kidneys, red salmon.

***Good Grain Sources.*** Stabilized wheat germ.

***Good Vegetable Sources.*** Beans (kidney, lima, Navy, and soy), beet greens, broccoli, collards, escarole, kale, lettuce, mustard greens, peanuts, peas, spinach, turnip greens, yeast.

Vitamin $B_2$ is not affected by heat, but is destroyed by light. The vitamin $B_2$ content of milk is affected by sunlight, for example. Pasteurization and drying do not injure $B_2$.

## VITAMIN C (ASCORBIC ACID)

***Why We Need Vitamin C.*** This vitamin prevents scurvy. It is necessary for good teeth and gums, speeds healing of wounds, and helps formation of normal bones, cartilage, and muscles. It also aids the blood in forming cells in bone marrow.

***Good Fruit Sources.*** Apples (fresh), avocados, bananas, blueberries, cantaloupes, cherries, cranberries, currants, gooseberries, grapefruit, lemons, limes, oranges, peaches (fresh), pineapple, red raspberries, rhubarb, strawberries, watermelon. The citrus fruits are the best sources.

***Good Vegetable Sources.*** Artichokes, asparagus, beans (lima, soy, string), beets, beet greens, broccoli, Brussels sprouts, cabbage, carrots, celery, chard, corn (yellow), eggplant, kale, kohlrabi, leeks, lettuce, mustard greens, okra, onions, parsnips, peas, peppers (green), potatoes (sweet and white), radishes, rutabagas, spinach, tomatoes, turnips, turnip greens.

## VITAMIN D

***What Vitamin D Does.*** Vitamin D prevents rickets and is especially important for tooth formation in young children. The body needs it to make proper use of calcium and phosphorus.

***Good Animal Sources.*** Cod-liver oil, halibut-liver oil, other fish oils, irradiated milk and evaporated milk, salmon, sardines, clams, cream, liver, oysters.

Vitamin D is given as viosterol for children, and is important in the prevention of infantile rickets (page 268).

## VITAMIN E

The requirements have not been definitely established. It is known to be of great value in reproductive disorders in the male and female.

***Uses of Vitamin E.*** Vitamin E active substances have their use in the treatment of habitual abortion.

***Sources of Vitamin E.*** The best source is wheat germ oil. Other sources are butter, green leafy vegetables, milk, most meats, peanuts, whole grain cereal, wheat germ.

## VITAMIN K

The normal amount of vitamin K is usually found in a good diet. However, a mother who has an inadequate supply of vitamin K in late pregnancy may produce a baby with hemorrhage disease or jaundice. The mother should take extra liver in her diet, and spinach, cabbage and soy beans, which contain small quantities. Although vitamin K does not stop hemorrhage, it may help to prevent it. In emergencies, intramuscular injections may be given either to the mother or child.

There is no evidence that vitamin K has any significant effect in the prevention of bleeding caused by an injury, wound or shock. It may, however, reduce the extent of bleeding from such a cause during the first few days of life. It might be advisable to give vitamin K to all premature infants, to all full-term infants with bleeding from whatever cause, and to those who for any reason require surgery during the first six days of life. Vitamin K is also of use for infants and children with certain gall bladder tract or liver disturbances.

## VITAMIN DEFICIENCY DISEASES (AVITAMINOSIS)

We have seen that if our systems do not get the proper amounts of each kind of vitamin we need, deficiency diseases may occur. Some of these are highly important and so we shall sum them up here. Fortunately these diseases can be promptly cured by the increase of the particular missing vitamin.

Probably the most widely known of the deficiency diseases is rickets. This is found only in young children, and is due to absence of sufficient vitamin D (page 268). Scurvy, which was formerly so prevalent among sailors, is caused by reduction of vitamin C (page 280). Beriberi is found among the Asiatics, rarely in this country, and occurs because of the absence of vitamin $B_1$ in the diet. Pellagra, a subtropical disease, is at times prevalent in the Southern states of this country. It is due to deficiency in vitamin B-complex (thiamine, riboflavin, and niacin).

Two conditions of the eyes are sometimes found when there is a deficiency of vitamin A in the diet. One is called "night blindness," and the other is an inflammation of the eyelids called "xerophthalmia."

### Beriberi

***Causes of Beriberi.*** This disease occurs where the staple diet is polished rice and wheat, from which thiamine or vitamin $B_1$ has been removed by machine milling.

***Symptoms of Beriberi.*** The beginning of the disease is characterized by nerve pain of the extremities, with muscular wasting, weakness, constipation, nausea, disordered sensory impressions, heart weakness and shortness of breath.

***Treatment of Beriberi.*** The disease has largely been eliminated by substituting unpolished rice or enriched flour in the diet. Treatment requires a well-balanced diet with added quantities of vitamin $B_1$.

### Pellagra

***Causes of Pellagra.*** This is a nutritional disorder of subtropical areas. It is widespread in the southern United States. Pellagra mainly affects persons living chiefly on maize. It is caused by absence of niacin, and may be accompanied by lesions due to lack of vitamins $B_1$ and $B_2$. The disorder is rare in infants but it often affects young children. It has a tendency to recur in the spring.

***Symptoms of Pellagra.*** The disease begins gradually, without striking symptoms. In a poorly nourished child, or an adult, repeated attacks of redness of the skin suggest the presence of pellagra, especially if associated with a tendency to diarrhea or constipation. The redness which encircles the neck is often more intense.

The skin becomes thickened, rough, scaly and dry. A sign of importance for diagnosis, after the redness has subsided, is the brownish pigmentation of the skin. There is nausea and anemia, and sometimes mental symptoms—dementia in the severe forms.

***Treatment of Pellagra.*** The principal treatment is dietetic. Fresh meat, milk and eggs are given. Extract from the germ of wheat or yeast should be given daily to supply the deficiency in vitamin B. Niacin (nicotinic acid) tablets given two or three times a day seem to have a definite effect in improving the condition.

### Sprue

This is another of the deficiency diseases. It is rarely found in other than tropical regions. Some of our soldiers were affected with it during World War II.

***Symptoms of Sprue.*** This is primarily a disease affecting the mucous membrane of the mouth and tongue. These become red and swollen. There are also intestinal symptoms such as diarrhea and gas formation.

***Treatment of Sprue.*** A well-balanced diet containing full measure of vitamins will promptly correct this condition and restore the patient to normal.

## HOW TO SELECT AND COOK FOODS

The following rules * should be of particular interest and value to the housewife as a guide to the selection and cooking of food:

***Give Naturally Colored Foods Your Preference.*** The outer green leaves of vegetables, such as cabbage, broccoli, and lettuce, should not be discarded. These are filled with vitamins and minerals from the direct rays of the sun. Avoid bleached celery and endive. Use brown sugar instead of white; polished rice is without vitamins, so use only the brown unpolished variety. Use whole wheat or rye flour. White flour, unless enriched, has all the vitamins removed in the process of refining. Prefer yellow turnips to white, buy sweet potatoes more often than you usually do. Color in food, that is, natural color, is often the sign of its vitamin value.

***Eat Raw Food.*** Twice daily, one should consume raw vegetables and uncooked fruit.

***Choose Cooking Methods Wisely.*** For the preservation of vitamins and minerals in food, by far the best utensil is the pressure cooker. Avoid frying, use broiling or *slow* boiling, always keep the cooking utensil covered.

***Undercook Rather Than Overcook.*** With the exception of pork, dried beans, and peas, it is advisable to sacrifice some tenderness to save vitamin content.

***Eat Your Cooked Food Promptly.*** Leftovers are usually greatly reduced in vitamins.

***Do Not Use Soda in Cooking Vegetables.*** It is a common custom to add soda to make vegetables greener. This will completely *destroy* the vitamins. Rapid cooking, especially in a pressure cooker, will keep the green color.

***Do Not Discard Cooking Water.*** Sometimes the juices left after cooking vegetables contain more vitamins than the cooked vegetables themselves.

* From *Living Should Be Fun,* Carlton Fredericks' book.

## A BALANCED DIET

The energy requirement of the body is influenced, as we have observed, by the person's activities. The more active a person is physically, the more carbohydrates, fats and proteins he must have to supply the energy for his work. The diet must also be varied, because the different foods serve us in different ways.

All the essential foods in the required amounts can be provided in each day's diet by using the following as a guide:

Milk—one quart; vegetables—a potato and two portions of leafy green or colored vegetables; fruits—orange, grapefruit or tomato juice and two servings of raw fruit or vegetables; eggs—one a day or at least four a week; meat, fish, poultry—one portion; cereals—two servings of whole wheat bread or cereals; butter (or enriched margarine)—three times; dessert, if needed, to complete the energy requirements; cod-liver oil, if ordered by a physician. Vitamin D milk can be used and cod-liver oil will be unnecessary.

## CALORIES AND ENERGY

Just as the amount of fuel needed to run an engine can be calculated, so can the amount of energy-providing food necessary for the

YOUR DAILY CALORIE NEEDS

| | | *If engaged in:* | | |
|---|---|---|---|---|
| *Weight in Pounds* | *Sedentary Occupation* | *Light Exercise* | *Moderate Exercise* | *Hard Work* |
| 104 | 1,560 | 1,768 | 1,976 | 2,288 |
| 108 | 1,620 | 1,836 | 2,052 | 2,376 |
| 112 | 1,680 | 1,904 | 2,128 | 2,464 |
| 116 | 1,740 | 1,972 | 2,204 | 2,552 |
| 120 | 1,800 | 2,040 | 2,280 | 2,640 |
| 124 | 1,860 | 2,108 | 2,356 | 2,728 |
| 128 | 1,920 | 2,176 | 2,432 | 2,816 |
| 132 | 1,980 | 2,244 | 2,508 | 2,904 |
| 136 | 2,040 | 2,312 | 2,584 | 2,992 |
| 140 | 2,100 | 2,380 | 2,660 | 3,080 |
| 144 | 2,160 | 2,448 | 2,736 | 3,168 |
| 148 | 2,220 | 2,516 | 2,812 | 3,256 |
| 152 | 2,280 | 2,584 | 2,888 | 3,344 |
| 156 | 2,340 | 2,652 | 2,964 | 3,432 |
| 160 | 2,400 | 2,720 | 3,040 | 3,520 |
| 164 | 2,460 | 2,788 | 3,116 | 3,608 |
| 168 | 2,520 | 2,856 | 3,192 | 3,696 |
| 172 | 2,580 | 2,924 | 3,268 | 3,784 |
| 176 | 2,640 | 2,992 | 3,344 | 3,872 |

body's vital processes. The energy value of foods is measured in the unit of heat energy, or calorie. A calorie is the amount of heat energy required to raise the temperature of one gram of water one degree Centigrade. In terms of actual food, a calorie is equal, for example, to four grains of sugar.

The amount of energy-providing food necessary to a resting man depends, of course, on his size; for instance, a man of five feet ten inches needs about 1790 calories a day. Theoretically, he could obtain the energy he needs by consuming a pound of sugar a day, or its equivalent in other forms of food. Actually, of course, he needs a varied diet, with all the different food elements we have been discussing.

If, for example, a person needs about 2400 to 2500 calories a day, they can be provided (among many other ways) as follows:

## NORMAL DAILY DIET

*(Approximately 2400 Calories)*

| | *Calories* |
|---|---|
| *Breakfast* | |
| Full-sized glass of orange juice | 100 |
| Cereal | 50 |
| For cereal | |
| Thin cream, ¼ cup | 120 |
| Milk, ¼ cup | 40 |
| Toast | 150 |
| Butter | 100 |
| Cream for coffee | 50 |
| *Lunch* | |
| Pint of milk | 320 |
| Crackers (2 ounces) | 200 |
| Baked apple with cream | |
| Apple | 90 |
| Sugar | 75 |
| Cream | 65 |
| *Dinner* | |
| Tomato juice | 25 |
| Toast or bread | 150 |
| Butter | 100 |
| Steak, ham or chops | 200 |
| Potato | 100 |
| String beans | 50 |
| Butter for potato and string beans | 50 |

## CALORIC VALUES OF FOOD

*(In Portions of 100 Calories Each)*

| *Foods* | *Portions* |
|---|---|
| Apple | 1 large |
| Apricots (canned) | 3 large halves (2 tablespoonfuls juice) |
| Asparagus (canned) | 15 large stalks |
| Asparagus (fresh) | 20 large stalks |
| Bacon | 4-5 small slices |
| Bananas | 1 large |
| Beans, Kidney (canned) | ½ cup |
| Beans, Lime (dried) | 3 tablespoonfuls |
| Beans, Navy (canned) | ½ cup |
| Beans, String | 2⅓ cups |
| Beef, Corned, Lean | 4 x 1½ x ⅚″ |
| Beef Kidney | ⅞ to 1 cup |
| Beef, Lean | slice 2¾″ x 1½″ x ¾″ |
| Beets, Sliced | 1-1⅓ cups |
| Bluefish | piece 3″ x 2½″ x 1″ |
| Bread, Rye | 1⅓ slices |
| Bread, Wheat | 2 slices |
| Butter | 1 tablespoonful |
| Buttermilk | 1½ cups |
| Cabbage | 2½ cups, cooked; 4-5 cups, shredded |
| Carrots | 4 or 5 young |
| Cauliflower | 1 head (4½″ diameter) |
| Cheese, American | 1⅛th cube |
| Cheese, Cottage, Skim | 5 tablespoonfuls |
| Cheese, Cream, Full | 2″ x 1″ x ⅛″ |
| Cheese, Whole Milk | ¾″ cube |
| Chicken | ½ small |
| Codfish | piece 3¾″ x 2½″ x ¾″ |
| Corn (canned) | ⅓ cup |
| Corn on Cob | 2 ears |
| Cornflakes | ¾ cup |
| Cream | 1¼ cup, scant |
| Eggs | 1½ |
| Farina | ¾ cup |
| Graham Crackers | 2½ |
| Grapefruit | ½ medium |
| Grapes | 1 large bunch |
| Griddle Cakes | 1 cake |
| Ham (boiled) | 1 slice |
| Herring | piece 2½″ x 1″ x 1″ |
| Ice Cream | ¼ cup |
| Lamb Chops (broiled) | one |
| Lamb, Leg Roast | slice 3½″ x 4½″ x ⅛″ |
| Lard | 1 tablespoonful, scant |
| Lentils, dried | 2½ tablespoonfuls |
| Lettuce | 2 large heads |
| Macaroni | ¾ cup |

| *Foods* | *Portions* |
|---|---|
| Malted Milk | 5/6th ounce |
| Milk, Condensed | 1½ tablespoonfuls |
| Milk, Cow's, Whole | 5/8 cup |
| Milk, Evaporated, Unsweetened | 4½ tablespoonfuls |
| Milk, Human | ¾ cup |
| Onions | 3-4 medium |
| Orange | 1 large |
| Orange Juice | ¾ cup |
| Peaches (canned) | 1 whole (3 tablespoonfuls juice) |
| Pineapple (canned) | ⅓ cup, shredded; 1 slice (3 tablespoonfuls juice) |
| Pork Chops | 1 small, medium fat |
| Potatoes | 1 medium |
| Prunes, stewed | 2 or 3 tablespoonfuls juice |
| Rice, steamed | ¾ cup |
| Rolled Oats | ½ to ¾ cup |
| Salmon (canned) | ½ cup, scant |
| Shredded Wheat | 1 biscuit |
| Spinach | 2½ cups |
| Squash (mashed) | 1 cup |
| Steak, Sirloin | slices 2" x 1½" x ¾" |
| Strawberries | 1⅓ cups |
| Tomatoes (canned or fresh) | 2 cups or 2-3 medium |
| Tuna (canned, oil) | ¼ cup |
| Turkey | slice 4" x 2½" x ¼" |
| Turnips | 2 cups or ½" cube |
| Veal, Breast | slice |
| Veal Chop | 1 small |
| Veal, Leg Roast | slice, medium |

## YOUR NORMAL WEIGHT

Your normal or standard weight is given in the accompanying tables. If you have a very light body frame, you may deduct seven pounds from the figure shown for your height and age in the tables. If you have a very heavy body frame, then add seven pounds. The result can be considered your "ideal" weight.

In general, you are all right as long as you are not more than 15 per cent above or 10 per cent below standard weight. Around the age of twenty, you can afford to be heavier if you wish—at that age you are likely to be more active. After thirty, and particularly during the change of life, it is safer to stay below your standard weight. Anyone over thirty should stay as close as he can to the normal weight given in the tables for thirty. If your weight is too high or too low, a later chapter presents advice on losing or gaining weight.

## Height and Weight Tables *

### for Women

| Height | Age 19 | 20 | 21-22 | 23-24 | 25-29 | 30-34 | 35-39 | 40-44 | 45-49 | 50-54 |
|---|---|---|---|---|---|---|---|---|---|---|
| 4 ft. 10 in. | 104 | 106 | 108 | 110 | 113 | **116** | 119 | 123 | 126 | 129 |
| 4 ft. 11 in. | 106 | 107 | 109 | 112 | 115 | **118** | 121 | 125 | 128 | 131 |
| 5 ft. | 112 | 112 | 113 | 115 | 117 | **120** | 123 | 127 | 130 | 133 |
| 5 ft. 1 in. | 116 | 116 | 116 | 118 | 119 | **122** | 125 | 129 | 132 | 135 |
| 5 ft. 2 in. | 118 | 118 | 119 | 120 | 121 | **124** | 127 | 132 | 135 | 138 |
| 5 ft. 3 in. | 120 | 121 | 122 | 123 | 124 | **127** | 130 | 135 | 138 | 141 |
| 5 ft. 4 in. | 123 | 124 | 125 | 126 | 128 | **131** | 134 | 138 | 141 | 144 |
| 5 ft. 5 in. | 126 | 127 | 128 | 129 | 131 | **134** | 138 | 142 | 145 | 148 |
| 5 ft. 6 in. | 130 | 131 | 132 | 133 | 135 | **138** | 142 | 146 | 149 | 152 |
| 5 ft. 7 in. | 135 | 135 | 135 | 137 | 139 | **142** | 146 | 150 | 153 | 156 |
| 5 ft. 8 in. | 138 | 138 | 139 | 141 | 143 | **146** | 150 | 154 | 157 | 161 |
| 5 ft. 9 in. | 142 | 142 | 142 | 145 | 147 | **150** | 154 | 158 | 161 | 165 |
| 5 ft. 10 in. | 144 | 144 | 145 | 148 | 151 | **154** | 157 | 161 | 164 | 169 |
| 5 ft. 11 in. | 146 | 147 | 149 | 151 | 154 | **157** | 160 | 164 | 168 | 173 |
| 6 ft. | 150 | 152 | 154 | 156 | 158 | **161** | 163 | 167 | 171 | 176 |

### for Men

| Height | Age 19 | 20 | 21-22 | 23-24 | 25-29 | 30-34 | 35-39 | 40-44 | 45-49 | 50-54 | 55-59 |
|---|---|---|---|---|---|---|---|---|---|---|---|
| 5 ft. | 111 | 112 | 114 | 118 | 122 | **126** | 128 | 131 | 133 | 134 | 135 |
| 5 ft. 1 in. | 116 | 117 | 118 | 121 | 124 | **128** | 130 | 133 | 135 | 136 | 137 |
| 5 ft. 2 in. | 122 | 123 | 124 | 125 | 126 | **130** | 132 | 135 | 137 | 138 | 139 |
| 5 ft. 3 in. | 127 | 128 | 128 | 129 | 131 | **133** | 135 | 138 | 140 | 141 | 142 |
| 5 ft. 4 in. | 130 | 131 | 132 | 134 | 135 | **136** | 138 | 141 | 143 | 144 | 145 |
| 5 ft. 5 in. | 134 | 135 | 136 | 137 | 138 | **140** | 142 | 145 | 147 | 148 | 149 |
| 5 ft. 6 in. | 139 | 140 | 141 | 142 | 143 | **144** | 146 | 149 | 151 | 152 | 153 |
| 5 ft. 7 in. | 142 | 143 | 144 | 145 | 146 | **148** | 150 | 153 | 155 | 156 | 158 |
| 5 ft. 8 in. | 147 | 148 | 149 | 150 | 151 | **152** | 155 | 158 | 160 | 161 | 163 |
| 5 ft. 9 in. | 152 | 153 | 154 | 155 | 156 | **158** | 160 | 163 | 165 | 166 | 168 |
| 5 ft. 10 in. | 155 | 156 | 157 | 158 | 159 | **162** | 165 | 168 | 170 | 171 | 173 |
| 5 ft. 11 in. | 159 | 160 | 161 | 162 | 164 | **166** | 170 | 174 | 176 | 177 | 178 |
| 6 ft. | 163 | 164 | 165 | 166 | 168 | **172** | 176 | 180 | 182 | 183 | 184 |
| 6 ft. 1 in. | 167 | 168 | 169 | 171 | 173 | **178** | 182 | 186 | 188 | 190 | 191 |
| 6 ft. 2 in. | 171 | 172 | 174 | 176 | 179 | **184** | 189 | 193 | 195 | 197 | 198 |
| 6 ft. 3 in. | 175 | 175 | 178 | 181 | 184 | **190** | 195 | 200 | 202 | 204 | 205 |
| 6 ft. 4 in. | 178 | 180 | 183 | 186 | 189 | **196** | 201 | 206 | 209 | 211 | 212 |
| 6 ft. 5 in. | 183 | 185 | 188 | 191 | 194 | **201** | 207 | 212 | 215 | 217 | 219 |

Your weight is found where height and age meet. Weights given in *pounds*.

* The above tables are based upon Weight Tables prepared by Baldwin & Wood, and upon Life Insurance Tables, published by Bureau of Publications, Teachers College, Columbia Univ., N. Y. C., 1925.

In ascertaining height—measure yourself in shoes; stand erect, and press measuring rod down against scalp. Weigh yourself in indoor clothing and shoes. If shoes have sensible heels, subtract one inch for height; if heels are "high," subtract two inches.

CHAPTER 22

# HOW TO LOSE OR GAIN WEIGHT

**What Causes Overweight . . . Dangers of Overweight . . . Overworking the Vital Organs . . . High Blood Pressure and Excessive Weight . . . How the Physician Can Help . . . Proper and Improper Dieting . . . Why Psychiatric Aid May Be Advisable . . . Disadvantages of Exercise in Weight Reduction . . . What to Eat in Dieting . . . Facts about Proteins, Carbohydrates, and Fats . . . Planning Your Diet . . . How to Accomplish Moderate Reduction . . . 1200-Calorie Diet . . . How to Overcome Underweight . . . Foods You Should Eat in Order to Gain Weight . . . 3000-Calorie Diet, etc.**

OVERWEIGHT is commonly caused by too much food and too little exercise, not by a glandular disorder. When food is consumed and not used immediately by the body, it is stored as fat in amounts which can easily become excessive. Normally, about 10 per cent of the body weight consists of fatty substances. Fat is present in the cells of every organ and tissue. In addition there are fat deposits inside the body. Most fat, however, is deposited under the skin. It is the average thickness of the fatty layer which determines whether a person is obese, thin or normal.

Fat distribution differs in the bodies of men and women. In women it is deposited mostly around the hips, lower abdomen, breasts, buttocks, and upper parts of the arms and legs. Fat in men is deposited mostly around the abdomen, shoulders and limbs.

***Dangers of Overweight.*** Overweight is a serious liability to health. The danger of excessive weight increases with age and with the degree of overweight. A simple but impressive way of expressing this is the old adage: "For every inch by which a man's waist measure exceeds his chest measure, subtract two years from his life expectancy."

Everyone has noticed the puffing and blowing of an obese person on physical exertion. There are several causes for this. First, the fat person must exert more effort in moving his excess, useless weight. Then, there is less freedom of movement of the diaphragm, which is held up by the abdominal-wall fat and abdominal organs. This restriction of the movement of the diaphragm is even more increased in women by the compression of the abdomen and its contents by tight, so-called "foundation garments." Fat cannot be compressed out of existence. Something has to give way, usually the diaphragm, causing cramping of the respiratory movements, and shortness of breath. Bronchial troubles, too, are more common in overweight persons.

In the obese person, the vital organs must work harder. This is especially true of the heart, which must overexert itself in order for the body, carrying extra "dead" weight, to perform the same work as it does for the normal-weight person. In addition there is an extra load on the heart in supplying blood for maintenance of the life processes of the excess tissue, the fat deposits.

In the long-time obese person, the heart may become dilated, flabby and weak. Frequently fatty deposits penetrate into the heart tissues, thus further reducing the efficiency of the heart. Sometimes there occurs enlargement of the heart, with thickening of the muscular wall as an effect, to compensate for the excess blood that must be carried.

It is commonly observed that the pulse is faster in obese persons. This, too, is owing to the heart's effort to compensate for the strain of a continuously present excess load.

High blood pressure tends to develop more often in the obese. However, the blood pressure often drops towards normal on reduction of excess weight.

## HOW THE PHYSICIAN CAN HELP

Reducing by means of an erratic diet or drugs taken at one's own responsibility is definitely a dangerous practice. Excess weight can be lost by a safe and simple reducing diet, as described later, or, where overweight is serious, under a physician's controlling care. The physician first carries out a complete physical examination to determine the cause of the overweight and how it should be treated. His examination includes blood count, analysis of the urine, and measurement of basal metabolism rate. Since the substance thyroxin produced by the thyroid gland regulates this rate, the physician is able to determine whether the body needs more of it. In such a case the physician prescribes certain forms of iodine.

The physician will also take into consideration the psychologic viewpoint of the patient, in order to aid him to overcome the desire for excessive food. Sometimes the appetite for food is a substitute outlet for physical and emotional satisfactions which are suppressed or unfulfilled. For example, a girl at the age of adolescence may suddenly realize that she is homely, and her personality development may subconsciously suffer as a consequence. She may tend to withdraw into herself, substituting appetite and excessive eating for normal social pleasures. In such cases the physician can give appropriate guidance or can help the patient obtain psychiatric help if it is needed.

## EXERCISE AND WEIGHT REDUCTION

In attempting to lose weight, discretion is necessary in carrying out physical exercises. Excessive fat, we have seen, throws a heavy load upon the heart and circulatory system, and it may be dangerous to increase this still more by strenuous exercise. Another disadvantage of exercise is that it increases appetite and so makes food restriction more difficult. Moderate general exercise such as walking and calisthenics, which make use of the muscles of the abdomen and back, are useful to give a sense of well-being and to increase the tone of the tissues.

## WHAT TO EAT IN DIETING

What you should or should not eat in dieting is a very simple matter if you will always remember that there are three classes of food, proteins, carbohydrates and fats—and that fats and carbohydrates are the two classes that add to your weight and that protein foods are the least fattening. But you must also remember that it is not so much *what* you eat that is fattening as *how much* of fattening foods you do eat. It is further essential to remember that the amount of physical exercise you do also determines the quantity and quality of your diet. For example, the laborer must eat fattening food and more of it than the man who spends his day behind a desk. The same is true of the female. Those who lead a sedentary life require less food and less fattening food. Then, one more thing to remember is that you must not give in to the habit of indulging yourself in certain foods because you just prefer them—you should always eat what is called a "balanced diet." That means that you should have some of each of the three classes of food with every meal.

***Protein Foods.*** These are milk, eggs, all the meats, fish, fowl, cheese of all kinds, and nuts (especially peanuts). Under this class there is flour—consequently bread is also highly protein. Then there are certain vegetables, the legumes, that are high in protein—these are lentils, soy beans, and dried beans.

*Comparative Table of Protein Equivalents*

One ounce of meat is equal to:

- 2 tablespoonfuls of cottage cheese
- 1 ounce of fish
- 1 ounce of fowl
- 1 cup of milk
- 1 egg (raw)

***Carbohydrates.*** These are all the starches and sugars. Unless you can burn these up by muscular activity, be careful not to include too many if you want to reduce your weight. It is estimated that the average American consumes 116 pounds of sugar per year. The starches are breads, all kinds of pastries, and other forms of desserts. Corn, barley, wheat, and rye are the cereals that contain a high percentage of carbohydrate. The sugar products that are very fattening include syrups, candy, and soft drinks.

***Fats.*** These are concentrated in calories. There are animal fats and vegetable fats. The principal animal fats are butter and that of all the meats. The vegetable fats are olive oil, cottonseed and corn oils, and peanut oil. Fats provide more than twice the fuel value of starches and sugars. But a reducing diet must not be devoid of fats. A fat-free diet would cause a very irritable disposition since on such a diet the nerve sheaths lose their protection.

## PLANNING YOUR DIET

Your dieting must have a plan. Even if you are going to eat less, what you do eat must still provide you with enough proteins, carbohydrates, vitamins, and minerals to provide energy for your daily activity and to keep you healthy. Skipping meals or omitting essential health-protecting foods will lower your resistance to many illnesses.

First of all, you must determine the normal weight for your height, age, and frame. This you can do by consulting the tables on page 387. If you are not overweight by these tables, you do not need to go on a diet. If you are overweight, then find out how many calories you need for the kind of work you do, by looking at the table on page 383. If you eat food containing fewer calories than this number every day, you will lose weight.

Moderate reduction of weight usually can be accomplished merely by reducing to a minimum foods of high caloric value. The quantity of food necessary to satisfy the appetite can be made up by fruits, vegetables and lean meats. A reduction of 500 calories in the daily diet should result in the loss of about a pound a week. Cut out 1,000 calories, and you will lose twice as much. Under no circumstances go below an 1100-calorie daily diet.

To count your calories, consult the list starting on page 385.

If you want to lose weight very gradually, you might follow a moderate diet like the one that follows. Notice the presence of the skim milk, the emphasis on fruits and vegetables. And do not add a cocktail to the dinner—alcoholic drinks are very rich in calories.

## REDUCING DIET

*(1200 Calories)*

*Breakfast*
Fruit, medium serving
1 egg
2 thin strips crisp bacon
1 glass milk, partly skimmed
1 thin slice toast
Coffee
2 tablespoonfuls cream
or ½ square butter
½ grain tablet of saccharine

*Lunch*
1 cup clear broth
1 tablespoonful cottage cheese
Vegetable, generous serving
1 square butter
½ thin slice bread
1 glass milk, partly skimmed or buttermilk
Fruit, medium serving
Coffee or tea without cream or sugar

*Dinner*
Lean meat or fish, 2½ ounces
Vegetable, generous serving
1 square butter
1 thin slice bread
1 glass milk, partly skimmed
Fruit, medium serving
Coffee or tea, clear

## HOW TO OVERCOME UNDERWEIGHT

Underweight may result from improper eating habits, inadequate food, functional disturbances of the body, or actual disease. If the basic cause is disease, the underweight may be a valuable first symptom. Hence the only intelligent way to start on a program for gaining weight is to have a thorough physical examination. If the underweight is found to be only a dietary problem there are two general principles to be followed to gain weight: one is to eat more food, particularly of high caloric value; the other is to use up less energy.

A moderately active woman of average size uses up about 2500 calories a day. For such a person to gain weight, a diet of 3000 to 4000 calories should be provided. However, before starting your gaining diet, you should determine the actual number you need for the kind of work you do (see page 383).

In order to gain a pound a week a diet must be increased by approximately 500 calories a day. The support of greater weight, however, requires greater energy expenditure, so for continued gain the diet must be increased still more.

Fat and carbohydrates yield more energy, weight for weight, than any of the other foods. See the table starting on page 385 for the actual calorie value of different foods.

In this, as in other food problems, a balanced diet should be maintained. This calls for plenty of leafy green and yellow vegetables, meat, eggs, milk, butter, cheese, and fresh fruit.

### HIGH CALORIE DIET

*(3000 Calories)*

*Breakfast*

1 serving fruit
Cereal, cooked, 2/3 cup
2 slices bacon
1 egg
1 slice bread
2 squares butter
1 tablespoonful sugar
Jam or jelly
½ glass cream (for coffee and cereal)
½ glass milk
Coffee or tea
10 A.M.—1 glass fruit juice or 1 glass milk

*Lunch*
1 serving egg or substitute
1 small serving potato or substitute
2 vegetables
1 tablespoonful salad dressing (oil)
1 slice bread
2 squares butter
¼ glass cream
¾ glass milk
3 P.M.—1 glass fruit juice or milkshake of ice cream

*Dinner*
1 serving meat
1 small potato
1 serving vegetable
1 serving salad, fruit
1 slice bread
2 squares butter
1 serving dessert

CHAPTER 23

# SPECIAL DIETS

**Diets for the Sick . . . Liquid Diet . . . Bland Diet . . . Soft Diet . . . Light Diet . . . High Vitamin Diet . . . Diets for Child and Adult with Fever . . . Low Caloric Diet . . . High and Low Protein Diets . . . High Carbohydrate and Fat Diets . . . Fat-free Diet . . . Low-fat Diet . . . Salt-restricted Diet . . . Diet for Patients with Heart Disease . . . Anemia . . . Constipation . . . Acne or Pimples . . . Diarrhea . . . Acute Indigestion . . . Chronic Stomach Ulcer . . . Flatulency . . . "Acid Stomach" . . . Arthritis . . . Diabetes . . . Gallbladder Disease . . . Allergy Diet . . . Diets for Elderly and Aged Persons . . . Diet in Convalescence . . . How to Prepare Special Foods for the Sick and Convalescent—How to Make Beef Juice, Barley Water, Porridge, etc.**

## DIETS FOR THE SICK

THERE are a number of routine diets for the sick. These diets include the liquid, soft, solid, bland, convalescent, and others that we shall explain in this chapter. Your physician will tell you which one is most suitable for a particular condition. Whatever diet is recommended, in selecting the specific foods you must keep certain considerations in mind. The food should in general be varied, so that the patient will find it tasty. It should provide him with the energy and strength he needs. This means, where there are no special restrictions, that he should receive a good balance of proteins, carbohydrates, and fats, as well as ample vitamins, calcium, iron, phosphorus, and other essential ingredients of the diet.

The patient's food should be neatly and attractively served on his tray. Do not set the foods on it in unplanned order, but arrange them for the convenience of the patient in eating. A pleasing tray does much for the patient's appetite and morale.

Foods with a strong flavor, such as onions, cabbage, cauliflower and turnips, should seldom be used. Excessively sweet foods, such as jams, jellies, preserves, candies and very sweet desserts should be given sparingly. Condiments and spices should be used as little as possible. Obviously, irritating foods should never be served.

Foods may be more quickly and easily digested if they are given in liquid form, such as milk, broths, raw eggs, fruit juices, and cereal gruels. Solids should be finely divided—by scraping or chopping meat and by chopping or mashing vegetables. Foods should be given in bland form—by straining out cellulose and large particles from such foods as cereals and vegetables; also by using finely milled, rather than coarse, cereals. All foods should be properly cooked, with proteins and cellulose softened and fats not decomposed by excessively high temperature.

Diet in convalescence, and how to make a variety of recipes for sick and convalescent persons, will be explained at the end of this chapter.

## LIQUID DIET

The diet consists of liquid foods only and is, as we have said, the most easily digested of all the diets. Liquid foods are usually served often and in small amounts. Feedings may be given every two or three or four hours, with two night feedings if the patient is awake.

Foods allowed include:

Beverages—tea, coffee or coffee substitutes.

Cereals—thin gruels and cereal waters.

Dessert—plain ice cream and sherbets made from strained fruit juices; custards, junkets and plain gelatin desserts; concentrated sweets—small amount of sugar; concentrated fats and cream.

Eggs—well-beaten eggs in beverages.

Soups—all clear soups; strained, vegetable soup, or milk soups made with sieved vegetables.

Vegetables—strained vegetable juices and small amounts served in cream soup.

## BLAND DIET

This diet consists of non-stimulating and low-residue foods. No irritating fruits, vegetables, or unnecessary condiments are allowed.

***Breakfast.*** Fruits—stewed or canned prunes, peaches, pears, apricots; no pineapple or fruit salad; baked apples wtihout skin; applesauce (without cinnamon); orange juice, one-half strength. Cereals—cooked, such as farina, Cream of Wheat, Wheatena, oatmeal; dry cereals—cornflakes and puffed wheat. One egg, soft boiled, or poached. Bread—one slice of toasted white bread with butter; marmalade or seedless jelly, if desired. Beverages—milk, weak Postum, Kaffee-Hag, very weak tea, or Sanka coffee.

***Lunch and Dinner.*** Soups—cream soups and plain vegetable soups cooked without meat stock; chicken soup occasionally, if skimmed; noodles or rice. Main dishes—chicken, steak, lamb chops (broiled), chopped meat balls, broiled calves liver; haddock, pike, flounder, cod, halibut, striped-bass, whitefish, trout, baked or broiled—never fried or boiled; baked macaroni and cheese; soft-boiled or poached eggs; spaghetti without sauce; potatoes, boiled or mashed; mashed or strained asparagus tips, carrots, squash, beets, spinach. Salads—tender lettuce, chopped fine with a dab of mayonnaise. Bread—one slice white bread, preferably toasted; no rye. Beverages—milk, malted milk or weak tea, Sanka coffee once daily. Desserts—simple puddings, custard, plain jello, stewed fruits, canned fruits, ice cream, baked apple, applesauce, sponge cake, and ripe banana; no pineapple.

At 10 A.M. or 3 P.M., eat any of the following: two crackers and a glass of milk; custard; cooked cereal with cream; jello with cream; tea, with buttered toast or zwieback; vanilla ice cream.

### Sample Bland Diet

***Breakfast.*** Fruit or fruit juice; cereal with milk or cream and sugar; egg, if desired; toast or white rolls; butter; jelly; beverage.

***Lunch or Supper.*** Soup, fruit juice, etc., if desired; main dish; vegetable; white bread or rolls; butter or other spread; dessert; milk.

***Dinner.*** Meat or fish; potato; vegetable; white bread or rolls; butter or other spread; dessert; beverages.

## SOFT DIET

This soft diet consists of feedings every three hours of any of the following: any liquid food; cream soups; buttermilk; cereals (oatmeal strained); cottage cheese; stewed fruits without skin and strained if seedy or coarse; boiled rice; baked potato; custards; milk toast with butter; ice cream or ices; milk; soft cooked eggs; junkets; gelatin.

In addition, the following may be given:

Breadstuffs—enriched white, zwieback, plain crackers.

Cereals—enriched white, macaroni products, rice.

Cheese—pot cheese, cream cheese.

Desserts—cornstarch, custards, tapioca, sponge or angel cake.

Eggs—coddled, scrambled, poached.

Fruits—juices, cooked purées, ripe banana.

Vegetables—juice and purées, baked or boiled mashed potato.

Butter and sugar may be added to make foods palatable.

## LIGHT DIET

Feedings are arranged with intermediate light nourishment. The following may be added to the foods in the soft diet (just given):

puréed vegetables; broiled lamb chop; tender, broiled, scraped beefsteak; bread and crackers; roast lean leg of lamb; baked whole chicken meat; jellies or preserves.

## HIGH VITAMIN DIET

Here are a number of suggestions for diets high in specific vitamins:

Vitamin A—fish-liver oils, deep-green leafy vegetables, carrots, sweet potatoes, apricots, butter, cheese, egg, milk, tomatoes, cantaloupe.

Vitamin $B_1$ (thiamin hydrochloride)—whole-grain or enriched bread; whole-grain, restored or vitamin-fortified cereals, such as whole wheat flakes; beans, egg yolk, fish, liver, milk, peanuts, peas, lean pork, potatoes, tomatoes, yeast.

Vitamin $B_2$ (G) (riboflavin)—beans, cauliflower, cheese, yellow corn, eggs, fish, beet greens, liver, lean meat, milk, peas, peppers, wheat, whole grains, yeast.

Vitamin C (ascorbic acid)—broccoli, cabbage, cauliflower, cantaloupe, grapefruit, green peas, oranges, strawberries, tomatoes, turnip greens.

Vitamin D (anti-rachitic factor)—fish-liver oils, egg yolk, cream, whole-wheat flakes and other D-vitamin-fortified foods.

Vitamin D may be produced in the body by exposure of the skin to direct sunshine.

## DIET FOR CHILD WITH FEVER

At first, no solid foods should be given. Fruit juices, preferably orange juice, pineapple juice in water, prune juice, grape juice; weak tea with sugar; milk; semi-solids as fever declines.

## DIET FOR ADULTS WITH FEVER

Formerly, patients with fever were almost starved to death. However, since all body processes are accelerated during fever, more food than normal is required. A diet with a high food value is needed. Food should be given in small quantities at frequent intervals.

## LOW CALORIC DIET

Beverages—one pint skim milk or buttermilk daily, coffee or tea without cream or sugar, unsweetened fruit juices.

Bread—one-half slice dark bread or one small bran muffin per meal.

Cereals—small servings whole-grain or bran cereals with skim milk.

Cheese—cottage cheese as substitute for milk or meat.

Desserts—fruit, fresh or water packed.

Eggs—one daily, prepared without fat.

Fats—about one level teaspoonful butter or margarine per meal.

Fruits—see Desserts.

Meat—two portions daily of any lean meat, fish, turkey or chicken prepared without fat or gravy.

Soups—clear soups and broths, if desired.

Vegetables—two servings of cooked vegetables and one raw vegetable prepared without fat or sauce daily. Vegetables allowed: asparagus, broccoli, Brussels sprouts, cabbage, carrots, celery, chard, kale, mushrooms, onions, beans, spinach, tomatoes, turnips.

Salad Dressing—lemon juice or vinegar.

### Sample Low Caloric Diet

Here is a sample of a low caloric diet:

***Breakfast.*** Fruit or fruit juice: small serving whole-grain or bran cereal with skim milk; one-half slice toasted dark bread or small bran muffin; butter or margarine; beverage.

***Lunch or Supper.*** Soup or fruit juice, if desired; small serving lean meat, fish, turkey, chicken or egg; cooked vegetable; raw vegetable; one-half slice dark bread or small bran muffin; butter or margarine; fresh fruit; beverage.

***Dinner.*** Meat or fish or egg; small potato, baked or boiled, if desired; cooked vegetable; vegetable or fruit salad; one-half slice dark bread or small bran muffin; butter or margarine; fresh fruit; beverage.

Vitamin supplements only as prescribed.

## VARIOUS SPECIAL DIETS

***High Protein Diet.*** Regular diet plus extra meat, eggs, cheese, custards.

***Low Protein Diet.*** Regular diet, omitting meat and all but one egg daily, plus portions of vegetables and fruit.

***High Carbohydrate Diet.*** Regular diet, omitting meat and eggs; extra portions of vegetables and fruit, rice, macaroni, puddings.

***High Fat Diet.*** This is used in epilepsy and urinary infections, and should be supplied by the physician to suit individual needs.

***Fat-free Diet.*** This includes only foods with no fat content, such as fruits, vegetables, and cereal products, 1200 to 1600 calories a day.

## LOW-FAT DIET

This is for use in liver and gallbladder diseases.

Beverages—tea, coffee, skim milk, fruit juices.

Bread—no restriction, except for high-fat hot breads.

Cereal—ready-to-eat whole-grain or restored.

Dessert—plain desserts made without fat and egg; jams, jellies, hard candies, fruit ices.

Eggs—restricted to one daily, prepared without fat.

Fats—*none.*

Fruits—all fruits except melons.

Meat—lean beef, liver, veal, lamb, chicken, turkey, fish.

Soup—skimmed meat, chicken or vegetable broths.

Vegetables—all bland vegetables, fresh or cooked. (Avoid broccoli, Brussels sprouts, cabbage, cauliflower, corn, onions, parsnips, turnips.)

Vitamin A supplement, if needed.

### Sample Low-Fat Diet

Here is a sample of a low-fat diet:

***Breakfast.*** Fruit or fruit juice; ready-to-eat cereal, whole-grain or restored; skim milk; sugar; egg, prepared without fat; toast; jelly; coffee or tea with skim milk and sugar, if desired.

***Lunch or Supper.*** Soup, fruit juice, etc., if desired; meat, fish or other main dish; vegetables, cooked and raw; bread and jam; dessert; tea or coffee, if desired.

***Dinner.*** Soup, fruit juice, etc., if desired; meat, fish or other main dish; potatoes, prepared without fat or sauce; vegetables, cooked and raw; roll or bread and jam; dessert; beverages.

***In-between-Meal Nourishment If Desired.*** Fruit juices, fresh fruit, bread and jelly sandwich, ready-to-eat cereal with skim milk, hard candy.

## SALT-RESTRICTED DIET

This is used in acute kidney trouble and high blood pressure.

*Use no salt in food preparation—no table salt.*

Beverage—milk, milk drinks, fruit juices.

Bread—salt-free bread or rolls.

Cereals—ready-to-eat or home-cooked without salt. (Shredded wheat is processed without salt.)

Cheese—unsalted cottage cheese.

Dessert—puddings, gelatin desserts, fruits.

Eggs—one daily.

Fat—unsalted butter, other salt-free fats.

Fruits—fresh or canned.

Meat—lean fresh meat, fresh-water fish, chicken and turkey. (Exclude salted and smoked meats, salt-water fish.) For high blood pressure, it is often preferable to obtain protein from milk and eggs.

Soups—cream soups.

Vegetables—all kinds, raw and home-cooked. (Avoid all commercially canned vegetables and relishes, unless prepared without salt.)

Salad Dressings—home prepared (no salt).

### Sample Salt-Restricted Diet

Here is a sample salt-restricted diet:

***Breakfast.*** Fruit or fruit juice; salt-free cereal with milk or cream and sugar; egg, if desired; toast, muffins or rolls; unsalted butter or other spreads; jam or marmalade; beverages.

***Lunch or Supper.*** Meat, fish or other main dish; vegetable; salad; rolls or bread; unsalted butter or other spread; dessert; milk.

***Dinner.*** Fruit juice or soup, if desired; meat, fish or other main dish; potato, vegetable; rolls or bread; unsalted butter or other spread; dessert; beverages.

## DIET FOR PATIENTS WITH HEART DISEASE

This diet is based on the following principles: The food should be simple, well-cooked, and easily digested. The total quantity should be small and served in four daily meals. The heavy meal should be served at noon. The evening meal, a relatively light one, should be served sufficiently early to insure completion of stomach digestion before retiring. If the caloric content should be insufficient when meals are taken as indicated, mid-morning and mid-afternoon nourishment may be allowed. Restrict fluids to four to five tumblerfuls in twenty-four hours.

Foods allowed are:

Beverages—milk, buttermilk, milk shakes, malted milk, eggnog, tea or coffee allowed once daily.

Bread—day-old, well-baked white or brown bread, toasted rolls, toasted zwieback.

Cereals—cooked or prepared.

Meats—tender rare beef, lamb (roast or chops), poultry, fish (baked), oysters.

Eggs—any except hard boiled or fried.

Vegetables—asparagus, string beans, beets, beet greens, carrots, celery, eggplant, lettuce, mushrooms, okra, potatoes, spinach, squash, tomatoes.

Fruits—apples, apricots, blackberries, cherries, figs, grapes, huckleberries, oranges, peaches, pears, pineapple, plums, prunes, raisins, raspberries, strawberries.

Salads—simple fruit or vegetable, with plain mayonnaise, French dressing, or boiled dressing.

Desserts—cereal puddings, custards, fruit desserts, jello, plain ices, ice cream, sponge cake.

Miscellaneous—cream and cottage cheese.

The patient must avoid the following foods: bulky foods, fried foods, foods causing fermentation (such as starches), highly seasoned foods, pastries, elaborate desserts, condiments and relishes. *Above all, the patient must avoid overeating and eating at night.*

## DIET FOR ANEMIA

The diet must contain a variety of foods which aid the body to store hemoglobin and red blood corpuscles. For this purpose, iron is absolutely necessary. Therefore, the diet should contain a liberal amount of foods having a high iron content, such as liver, kidneys and other organ meats. Other foods valuable for the anemic person are: meat, eggs, green leafy vegetables, cabbage, potatoes, prunes, raisins, and whole-grain cereals.

## DIET FOR CONSTIPATION

The diet for the relief of constipation must supply material which will be absorbed in the small intestine to only a limited extent, which will largely pass on into the colon, and which will add bulk. Thus, it should include adequate amounts of fruits and vegetables. In addition, the intake of adequate amounts of fluids, at least 2½ to 3½ quarts daily, is of great importance. Because it is difficult for many persons to include adequate amounts of fruits and vegetables to provide bulk, it may be necessary to add a variety of auxiliary foods to the diet. Such bulk substances include agar-agar, kelp, acacia, tragacanth, psyllium seeds, methyl cellulose, and many others.

Foods particularly good for supplying bulk include all vegetables, especially green vegetables, such as cabbage, spinach, celery, lettuce and tomatoes. Fruits of all kinds are valuable not only for the cellulose they contain but for the fruit acids, which are laxative. Dried fruits are good for the purpose. The skins of all fruits should be eaten.

Bread and cereals made of whole grain and containing bran are good aids to overcome constipation. Other valuable foods are honey and molasses, because they tend to ferment, thus causing gas formation, which acts as a slight stimulant to the bowels. Their use must be restricted, however, for too much of either honey or molasses causes digestive disturbances.

The constipation of some adults has a long history, extending back to childhood. It may not respond to proper diet and hygiene. Even in these cases continued proper diet and hygiene, adequate fluid intake, physical and mental relaxation and continued encouragement will result in conquering the difficulty in almost every instance.

Water is valuable because it keeps the food masses in semi-solid condition.

## DIET FOR CONSTIPATION IN HEALTHY ADULTS

Here is a sample of a helpful diet for constipation.

*Breakfast.* One orange, cut oats, cream, wheat germ muffins and honey, cup of milk or buttermilk, cup of bouillon.

*Lunch.* Scalloped corn, biscuit, baked apple.

*Dinner.* Vegetable soup, roast beef, spinach (large serving), baked potato (including skin), cabbage salad (large serving), whole-wheat bread, stewed figs.

Another sample diet for constipation consists of:

*Breakfast.* Stewed prunes; shredded wheat and wheat germ, cream; tomato omelet; whole-wheat toast; cup of milk.

*Lunch.* Pork and baked beans, Boston brown bread, sliced pineapple, oatmeal macaroons.

*Dinner.* Boiled mutton with sauce, stewed onions (large serving); lettuce salad, French dressing (large serving); bran wafers, lemon jelly, whipped cream.

## DIET FOR ACNE OR PIMPLES

The diet should be simple and should include plenty of fruit and vegetables. Pastry, fried food, nuts, gravy, cream, chocolate, cocoa and other oily foods should be avoided. It is important to prevent constipation by regulating the diet.

## DIET FOR DIARRHEA

The most important rule in diarrhea is that all foods of high residue must be stopped as soon as symptoms occur. Limit the amount of water and nutritive beverages, such as clear broth, as well as tea and coffee. The diet is gradually increased. Soft-cooked eggs, toast, chicken or beef jellies, well-cooked cereals (Cream of Wheat or Cream of Rice), milk, junkets and soft custards, later followed by tender meat, make a good diet.

The diet, in the main, depends on the cause of the disorder.

## DIET FOR ACUTE INDIGESTION

In this condition, it is best to go without food for at least twenty-four hours. During this time much water must be taken. The next day, some beef or lamb with boiled rice, butter and sugar, or a little cream, may be served.

## DIET FOR CHRONIC STOMACH ULCER

The rule is that feedings should be small in quantity and intermeal feedings given. A standard diet is the following:

***Breakfast.*** Cooked cereals—only those of the oatmeal, farina type; two eggs, poached or soft boiled; milk, postum or decaffeinated coffee; white bread or lightly buttered toast; strained orange juice well diluted with water, at the end of breakfast.

***Lunch.*** Vegetable or milk soups—avoid all thick or creamed soups;

carrots, squash, peas, spinach, boiled or mashed potatoes, string beans must all be puréed or strained; white bread or buttered toast; shredded lettuce with cottage cheese, pot cheese or farmer cheese; such desserts as cooked pears, baked apples, applesauce, rice pudding, tapioca pudding, junket or gelatin desserts; milk, postum, decaffeinated coffee or buttermilk.

***Dinner.*** Vegetable or milk soups—avoid all thick or creamed soups; broiled, baked or roasted beef, lamb, liver, chicken, turkey; baked or cooked fish, such as flounder, pike, perch, cod, halibut; vegetables may be served with this (from the above Lunch list); white bread or toast (lightly buttered); shredded lettuce, with cottage or pot cheese; cooked fruits, cooked pears, baked apple, rice pudding, chocolate pudding, tapioca pudding, blanc mange; milk, postum or decaffeinated coffee.

One glass of sweet milk between meals.

***Foods to Avoid in Chronic Stomach Ulcer.*** Canned, salted, spiced meats and fish; oysters, clams or lobsters; raw fruits and vegetables; cabbage, cauliflower, cucumbers, onions, peppers; whole wheat and whole wheat cereals; all gravies; spices; sauces; alcoholic and carbonated drinks; pastries; cakes; jams; thickened or creamed soups.

## DIET FOR FLATULENCY (GAS IN THE STOMACH AND INTESTINES)

All the following foods are to be avoided:

Beverages—carbonated water, highly sweetened drinks, malt beverages, soft drinks, sparkling wines.

Soups—meat broths, especially stock soups containing any of the following gas-forming vegetables: beans, dry; broccoli, Brussels sprouts, cabbage, cauliflower, cucumbers, garlic, lentils, lettuce, onions, peas (dried), peppers, radishes, turnips.

Desserts—all sweet foods, candy, clear sugar, honey, jam, maple sugar.

Also avoid cold fried foods, condiments, excessively salted foods, extremely hot and cold foods, nuts, spices; apples, fresh; cantaloupe, raisins, watermelons; all highly fermented cheeses.

## DIET FOR "ACID STOMACH"

The diet list for persons with hyperacidity may be selected from the following articles:

Meats—in hyperacidity, meats are used sparingly, and are best given boiled or roasted, and without fat or gravy. Beef, minced lamb, chicken, or turkey are suitable. Broiled or boiled fish, such as bass, cod, halibut, white fish or other lean variety served with a simple cream or egg sauce may be eaten. Also oysters, which may be taken with a little lemon or very little salt.

Soups—may be either creamed or puréed from vegetable stock. Tomato soup is best avoided. Meat stock should not be used.

Vegetables—should be chosen from the soft green varieties, such as beans, beet tops, celery, peas, spinach. Rice may be used. Potatoes may be cooked in any way without the use of fat.

Cheese—any mild variety, such as cottage, cream or Swiss.

Desserts—cream and egg desserts of all sorts; custards, blanc mange, Bavarian cream, junkets, soft rice or bread puddings, without rice sauces; gelatin desserts, not highly flavored, and with very little sugar.

Breads—toast, stale bread, hard rolls. It is best to use sweet butter.

Cereals—all varieties, if well cooked, with cream and very little sugar; spaghetti and macaroni.

Eggs—in any simple form, except fried or hard boiled.

Fruits—usually forbidden in severe examples of the condition, but in milder varieties where there is obstinate constipation, soft stewed fruits may be used in moderation. The fruits should be stewed with very little sugar. No fruits with seeds or tough skin, such as figs, blackberries or prunes, should be eaten.

Foods to Be Avoided—sour spiced foods or those with condiments, salt foods, pickles, jellies, raw vegetables, very hot or cold food or drinks, sweets of all kinds, fried foods, all alcoholic drinks, coarse, hard foods, seeds, skin of fruits or vegetables, corn, pies, pancakes, or hot breads, syrups, marmalades, honey.

### Sample Menu for "Acid Stomach"

***Breakfast.*** Cream of Wheat with cream; boiled or poached egg; toast and butter; weak coffee or coffee substitute, with hot milk or cream.

***Mid-Morning Lunch.*** Milk with crackers.

***Luncheon.*** Cream of asparagus soup; small portion of broiled lean beef or lamb, or fish, or chicken; mashed or boiled potato with butter; baked squash; toast and butter; small portion of fresh or stewed fruit.

***Mid-Afternoon Lunch.*** Milk with crackers.

***Supper.*** Soft-boiled or poached egg on toast; puréed vegetable, spinach or peas; toast and butter; fruit or custard dessert with whipped cream.

***Bedtime.*** Milk with crackers.

### Another Menu for "Acid Stomach"

***Breakfast.*** Cream of Wheat (or any simple cooked cereal without much cellulose residue); cream, but no sugar; melba toast with butter; soft-boiled or poached egg, or omelet; applesauce; coffee or coffee substitute with milk, but no sugar.

***Lunch.*** Baked or broiled or mashed potato; butter; chicken or fish; puréed vegetable; toast with butter; custard with whipped cream; milk and cream, one glass.

***Supper.*** Cream vegetable soup; cottage cheese; toast with butter; baked egg; tender lettuce with mayonnaise or oil dressing (no pepper or spices in preparation).

## DIET FOR ARTHRITIS

Fruits, vegetables, a moderate amount of meat and only a moderate amount of carbohydrates should form the basis for a diet in arthritis.

## DIET FOR DIABETICS

The treatment of what is commonly known as diabetes (mellitus) is based upon the adjustment of diet, insulin and exercise to the requirements of the specific patient. Diet is the basis of treatment. Insulin (from a source outside the body) is used when necessary.

The average diet calls for approximately two-thirds of the carbohydrate commonly used in a normal diet. This was not the case in the past. In special instances, as, for example, when heavy physical labor is required, this proportion may be increased. More protein is given, too, than formerly. Fat is used to complete the desired total caloric value.

### Calorie Requirement in Diabetes Diet

The total caloric value for the diet is determined in the following manner. First we figure how many calories are required when the patient is at rest. This figure is based on the height and age of the patient, and the average normal weight for that specific height and age, or for what is considered the best weight for the patient. Then, from one-quarter to one-half, depending upon the patient's activity, is added to this figure. We now have the approximate number of calories needed to keep the patient comfortable. Special allowance is made for growth in children, varying with their age.

The diabetes is controlled by having the patient consume the necessary diet. What diet is necessary is shown by periodic examinations of urine and blood sugar-level. The closer these are to normal, the better the assurance we have of maintaining the patient's current health and protecting his future welfare.

The basic necessary foods must be included in the diet—fruits, vegetables, cereals and milk, and different sources of protein, such as meat, fish, fowl, cheese and eggs. The value of food ordered by the physician (minus the value of whatever interval or bedtime feedings are prescribed) is divided equally among three meals.

If satisfactory control of the diabetes and balance between diet and insulin are to be maintained, the total caloric value and sugar value of the diet must not vary 10 per cent above or below what has been determined as the best from day to day.

A bedtime feeding of milk is included for the patient who is taking protamine zinc insulin. The carbohydrate of this feeding is subtracted from the total amount of carbohydrate allowed for the three meals. It is difficult to figure the carbohydrate for each meal exactly, so a variation of two grams in either direction is permitted. It is also impossible to figure the total diet exactly as prescribed; therefore a variation of five grams above or below the prescribed amount of carbohydrate, protein and fat, is also permitted.

In using the fixed weight diet plan, which is carefully explained to the patient by the physician, the patient decides what foods he wants to eat. These he selects from tables, which also show the percentage of carbohydrate in various fruits and vegetables. He is given special diabetic recipes for other foods. He then weighs on a scale the amount indicated in the grams column. Though he is taught the food value of ordinary foods he need not, as a daily routine, figure the carbohydrate, protein and fat.

## DIET FOR GALLBLADDER DISEASE

In diseases of the gallbladder, the patient should remain on a low-fat and low-residue diet and one which is free from highly seasoned foods and pastries. If the patient is obese, the caloric content should be reduced.

Eggs as well as all egg preparations should be omitted from the diet; also cream, cream sauces, and ice cream. Fatty fish must not be in the diet. Salmon, shad, tuna, herring, sardines, mackerel and pompano should not be eaten. Fish must be baked or broiled, not sautéed.

***Breakfast.*** Ripe fruits, skim milk or plain milk; cooked cereals are preferable; milk.

***Lunch.*** Consomme and purée soups (without cream); vegetables prepared by rapid boiling and not in deep fat. Brussels sprouts, cabbage, and cauliflower may be given in small amounts and without cream sauces, but no parsnips, radishes or turnips. No French dressing or mayonnaise. When lemon juice alone is not satisfactory, a good French dressing can be made with lemon juice and mineral oil flavored with salt and pepper and a dash of mustard. Desserts—ices, junkets, gelatin preparations, stewed or ripe fruits.

***Dinner.*** No fatty meats are allowed. Lamb, lean beef, hamburg steak, roast beef and all poultry can be taken; also sea bass or filet of sole, baked or broiled.

## ALLERGY DIET (EGG-, WHEAT-, MILK-FREE)

For those with allergies, the following diet should prove helpful:

Beverages—coffee, tea (without cream or milk), cocoa made with water, fruit juice. Avoid cereal beverages and malted milk.

Breads—rice biscuit, Ry-Krisp, whole rye bread, all made without wheat, eggs, or milk; no white bread, graham bread, crackers, cakes, cookies, macaroni, spaghetti, noodles.

Cereals—corn flakes, Rice Krispies (with fruit juice), hominy, rice, tapioca, oatmeal, cornmeal, rye flour, barley, barley flour, potato flour, rice flour.

Desserts—fruit ices, fruit tapioca without milk or eggs, gelatin desserts, cookies or pastries made with special flour (listed under cereals) and without milk, butter or eggs.

Fats—olive oil, Mazola, Wesson oil, bacon fat, lard, meat drippings; no mayonnaise or cooked salad dressing; no butter or margarine.

Fruits—all kinds—canned, stewed, raw; serve without milk or cream.

Meats—all meats, fish or fowl, prepared without milk, wheat or eggs. Avoid prepared sausage or any type which may contain wheat cereal filler.

Soups—homemade broths, clear or with vegetables. Avoid canned soups.

Vegetables—all kinds—canned, cooked or raw, prepared without butter or cream sauce.

## DIETS FOR ELDERLY AND AGED PERSONS

Older persons often have poor appetites, and it is therefore desirable to arrange surprise dishes for them. This may make a great difference in their appetites. They should be allowed to eat foods which they like and are accustomed to, unless the family physician specifically advises against it. Provide food that does not require prolonged chewing, because the teeth of many elderly persons are few or defective. Meat can be cut up in small pieces, vegetables can be put through a coarse strainer or food grinder, or the canned strained or chopped vegetables prepared as baby foods may be used.

## FOODS FOR THE AGED

Here are some recommended foods:

Milk—served hot or cold, in weak cocoa or ice cream, custards, cereal puddings, or cream soups.

Lean Meats and Fish—these should be eaten at least once a day. Bacon is also allowed, as are clear soups and broths. If there is a tendency to intestinal putrefaction, it is best to exclude meat of all kinds.

Eggs—prepared in all ways, except fried.

Cereals—thoroughly cooked.

Bread—preferably toasted; freshly baked bread and hot breads of all kinds should be excluded.

Vegetables—almost any kind unless they are found to upset the person. Beans, cooked cabbage, onions, and turnips are likely to cause gas in the stomach or intestines, and are therefore best excluded. An excellent way to serve vegetables is as purées.

Fruits—mild ripe, fresh or thoroughly cooked.

### Sample Diet for Patient with Deficient Chewing

A typical diet may consist of:

***Breakfast.*** Orange juice, one tumblerful; soft-boiled or poached egg, or plain or jelly omelet; tea or coffee with cream and sugar; two slices of soft white bread with square of butter; serving of well-cooked, diluted, warm breakfast food—farina, oatmeal or Wheatena, with cream and sugar.

***Lunch.*** Soup, well-seasoned, made either of vegetable or meat stock; two soft meat croquettes; mashed potatoes; puréed peas or beans; tender asparagus; chopped fruit salad in gelatin with dressing; ice cream, or other frozen dessert, or junket or custard.

***Supper.*** Macaroni and cheese; or cottage cheese with syrup; puréed vegetable or vegetable cooked very tender, dry or with butter sauce; custard with cream and sugar; soft white bread, with butter if desired; tea or coffee with cream and sugar, or glass of milk and cream.

## DIET IN CONVALESCENCE

A simple mixed diet is suitable for convalescence. Foods recognized as difficult of digestion should be excluded from the diet. Emphasis should be placed on milk, eggs, toast and well-cooked cereals. Foods allowed for convalescents include:

Soups—any kind, except those made with dried beans, dried peas and onions.

Meat, Fish and Poultry—broiled or baked lamb chops, chicken, turkey, fish, rabbit, liver, sweetbreads, and scraped or ground beef.

Eggs—in any form except fried.

Milk and Milk Products—milk in all forms, cream, butter and mild cheese.

Vegetables—any cooked vegetable, except strongly flavored and gas-forming vegetables, such as dried beans. Raw tomatoes and tender hearts of lettuce may be included.

Fruits—any cooked fruits; raw citrus fruits (one or more servings), ripe banana, pears, peaches and strawberries.

Salads—any salad made from fruits and vegetables allowed; avocado, gelatin and cheese may be served with salad dressings.

Cereals—any kind except bran products; preferably cooked, whole-grain or enriched; also plainly cooked macaroni, spaghetti or noodles.

Breads—any kind except bran products; preferably whole grain or enriched.

Desserts—any kind except rich pastries and steamed puddings.

Concentrated Sweets—a small amount of sugar, fruit jams and jellies, honey and syrup.

Concentrated Fats—butter and cream and other vegetable or animal fats, including bacon.

Beverages—tea, coffee, or coffee substitutes.

### Sample Menu for Convalescent Person

Here is a sample day's menu for a convalescent:

8 A.M. Orange, cereal with milk, toast, coffee.

10.30 A.M. Milk or eggnog or fruit beverage.

12.30 P.M. Soup, crackers or toast; broiled halibut or chicken; baked potato; stewed tomatoes; bread, butter; tapioca pudding.

3.30 P.M. Milk or eggnog or fruit juice.

6.30 P.M. Cream potato soup, crackers; peas; lettuce salad; bread, butter; applesauce.

10 P.M. Milk with crackers or toast.

## HOW TO PREPARE SOME FOODS FOR THE SICK AND CONVALESCENT PERSON

***How to Make Beef Juice.*** There are two ways to prepare beef juice:

*Hot Process.* Take one pound of ground, lean round steak. Sear it in a hot pan long enough to start the juices. Press out the juice in a special press. Season with salt. Serve either cold or hot.

*Cold Process.* Place one pound of ground, lean round steak in a jar. Add 1½ cups of cold water and a pinch of salt. Cover the jar and chill for five or six hours, or overnight, shaking occasionally. Strain the juice through coarse muslin. Season and serve either hot or cold.

In heating beef juice, use a double boiler.

One-half cup, scant, contains thirty calories; protein five grams; fat one gram.

***How to Make Barley Water.*** Mix one tablespoonful of barley flour with one pint of water. Cook for twenty minutes. Strain

***How to Prepare Barley Milk.*** Ingredients—one pint of milk, a quarter pound of pearl barley, half a pint of water, one dessertspoonful of sugar.

Boil the barley in one pint of milk and half a pint of water for two hours. Sweeten with one dessertspoonful of sugar. Serve it while it is just warm.

***How to Prepare Barley Porridge.*** Ingredients—two ounces of pearl barley; rind of one lemon, sugar, one quart of water.

Wash the barley thoroughly. Boil it for a quarter of an hour in half a pint of water. Strain off the water and add a quart of fresh boiling water. Let it boil until only half the quantity of liquid remains.

Strain off, add the rind of one whole lemon, and a little sugar. Let the gruel simmer for five minutes, then pour it into a jug or basin to cool. When cold, take out the lemon rind. Serve.

***How to Prepare Rice Water.*** Use one tablespoonful of rice (washed) to one pint of water. Cook for two hours in a saucepan or double boiler. Strain.

***How to Prepare Albumin Water.*** Cut the white of an egg with sterile scissors into a number of small parts. Add cold boiled water (five ounces for an adult and eight to ten ounces for a child), but do not strain. Albumin water may be flavored with a little lemon juice.

***How to Prepare a Milk Shake.*** Ingredients—one cup of milk, one tablespoonful of sugar, one-quarter teaspoonful of vanilla.

Put in shaker or glass fruit jar with chipped ice and shake vigorously until it is frothy. Serve immediately.

***How to Prepare a Malted Milk.*** Ingredients—three-quarters of a cupful of hot water or milk, one heaping tablespoonful of malted milk in powder or tablet form. The proportions may be varied in accordance with the patient's taste.

Mix a little of the water or milk with the dry powder to make a smooth paste. Add the remaining hot water or milk and a dash of salt and serve.

***How to Prepare an Eggnog.*** Ingredients—one egg, three-quarters of a cup of milk, one teaspoonful of sugar, one-quarter teaspoonful of vanilla or three-quarter tablespoonful of brandy, whisky or sherry; nutmeg, if desired.

Beat the white of egg until it is stiff; add the yolk and beat together well. Add sugar, milk and flavoring, beat well and put in glass. If nutmeg is used, sprinkle it lightly over the top.

***How to Make Chicken Broth.*** Ingredients—one chicken, two quarts of cold water, one teaspoonful of salt.

Cut chicken in small pieces; put cold water in kettle; add chicken and salt. Cover and bring to boil slowly. Lower flame and simmer for three hours. Skim off fat and strain.

***How to Prepare Porridge.*** Thin porridges can be made from flour or other finely ground grain products, with either water or milk. They are cooked for a long time to insure that the starch is changed to soluble starch or even partly dextrinized. Time for cooking should therefore be carefully watched.

By passing the material after it is cooked through a cheesecloth or sieve, the coarser, undissolved parts are removed and the smooth product does not irritate weakened digestive organs. This method of preparation is therefore desirable for invalids and young children.

In cooking all cereal products, observe the following points: Use a double boiler; be sure to use the correct proportions of cereal, water and salt. Cook at boiling temperature (212° F.). Additional food value may be added by using sugar or lactose and butter. The cereal itself may be cooked in milk.

***How to Make Scraped Beef.*** Wipe a small piece of beefsteak, cut from the round. Lay it on a meat board and with a tablespoon or back of a knife scrape off the soft part until there is nothing left but the tough stringy fibers. Make into "pats" and cook in a pan over the direct flame, or in a broiler, for about two minutes. Use only enough fat to keep the scraped beef from sticking to the pan. Season with salt and pepper.

***How to Make Junket.*** Ingredients—one pint of milk, pinch of salt, one-half tablespoonful of granulated sugar, two teaspoonfuls of Fairchild's essence of pepsin, or liquid rennet, or one-half of a junket tablet dissolved in water.

Warm the milk. Add salt, sugar, and the pepsin or other ingredient. Stir for a moment. Then allow it to stand at the temperature of the room for twenty minutes or until firmly coagulated; place in refrigerator until thoroughly cold. This can be seasoned with grated nutmeg.

CHAPTER 24

# EXERCISES FOR GOOD HEALTH

**Amount of Exercise You Require . . . Dangers of Excessive Exercise . . . Exercise for Infants and Children . . . Proper and Improper Exercise for Adults . . . Recommended Sports . . . Exercise for Persons with Tuberculosis, Heart Impairment, and High Blood Pressure . . . Why Good Posture Is Important and How to Achieve It . . . Healthful Exercises . . . Developing and Reducing the Waistline . . . Correcting Pendulous Abdomen . . . Reducing the Buttocks . . . Developing the Muscles of the Back, Chest, Thighs, and Legs . . . How to Develop the Muscles of the Neck, etc.**

OUR RESPONSIBILITIES to ourselves and to those around us demand that we keep physically fit. We can achieve this by physical culture. But if we become too carried away and indulge in exercise to excess, the routine may become monotonous or harmful. The underlying principle is simply the proper use of every part of the body—regular, sensible exercise. Elasticity and movement are the keynotes in maintaining every part of the body.

***Amount of Exercise Required.*** To get the full benefit of exercise you should perform it with regularity. *Form the habit of exercise.* The amount of exercise needed in a day varies with different persons because they react differently to similar amounts of exercise. Some require more than others. An adequate amount produces the sensation of having been physically active without causing undue fatigue. Other factors are the speed of performance and the amount of strength required. Exercises that require much speed or those that require powerful muscular exertion should be relatively short in duration.

***Excessive Exercise.*** In excessive exercise the heart is apt to suffer. If the strain is sudden, the heart becomes dilated and weakened. If excessive exercise is engaged in continuously, the heart is apt to become an enlarged and overgrown muscle, so that it is too strong and powerful for existence in ordinary life. Not having enough resistance to overcome in sedentary occupations, the heart may cause great distress by beating tumultuously and irregularly. The enlarged heart and thickened heart may weaken in time if the condition does not disappear. The valves of the heart are also sometimes so strained that they give way or are otherwise damaged.

Eating immediately after severe exertion, and severe exertion immediately after eating, are both inadvisable, since the necessary supply of blood for digestion is apt to be diverted to the muscular system.

## EXERCISE FOR INFANTS AND CHILDREN

Exercise should be started in infancy. A baby begins to exercise even before birth. From birth on, a baby exercises by kicking, by waving his arms, by attempting to lift his head and by crying. For at least twenty minutes daily, but not directly following the bath, he should be placed on a big bed, in a comfortably warm room. He should not be played with at this time. He should be left to exercise as he wills. The only garment necessary is a diaper. His movements should not be restrained by clothing. His position should be changed occasionally so that he may use different groups of muscles as he lies on his back, on his abodmen, and on each side.

At about the ninth month the child usually begins to crawl. He seems to like to lie on a rug on the nursery floor and to drag himself along. This is good exercise. The child should not be encouraged to try to walk until he is over a year old. No violent exercise is good for infants. They should never be rocked vigorously in their carriages or jolted up and down, or tossed up and down.

In older children, all varieties of outdoor exercise should be encouraged. However, excessive exercise or the overuse of particular muscles must be avoided.

## EXERCISE FOR ADULTS

If there is any doubt about it, fitness for a particular exercise should be determined by a physician.

Competitive sports should not be indulged in by persons over 35 years of age unless they were regularly active in such sports in their younger years. At about this age an adult may engage in exercises requiring moderate endurance only.

Accordingly, if a person must exercise, he should at least be reasonably certain that he is healthy enough to undergo the strain. He should keep in mind—above all—that the fact that he feels well is no proof that he is well. A thorough annual physical check-up is the only way of knowing for certain.

The ability to recover quickly from the effects of exercise is a good index of whether it is suitable or not.

Besides the outdoor exercises which favor general development, such as rowing, swimming, tennis, golf, and riding, it is well to promote special development of any parts which are naturally deficient,

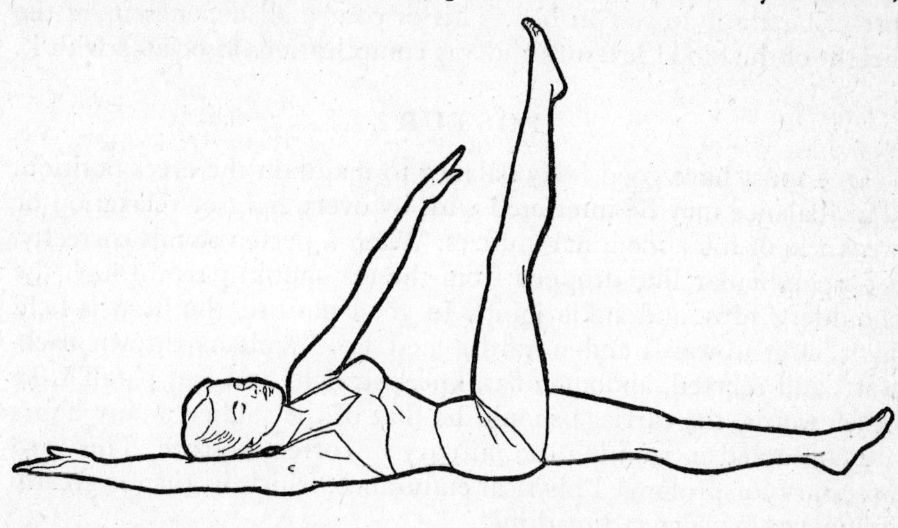

EXERCISE FOR THIGH MUSCLES

Lie on your back with arms outstretched above your head, both feet touching the floor. Now raise your right leg, without bending at the knee, and try to touch the toes with the fingers of your left hand. Do this a number of times, alternating right and left.

by means of so-called setting-up exercises (calisthenics) which can be adapted to special requirements.

Exercise should be adapted to age, sex, occupation, climate and the individual person.

## EXERCISE AND DISEASE

***Tuberculosis.*** In order to properly help the healing of a tuberculous area, especially in the lungs, it is most imperative that the entire body be at rest until the process is healed. For that reason exercise is absolutely forbidden in any form. The tuberculous patient is kept in bed for an indefinite period.

***Heart Impairment.*** Particularly in any disease of the heart muscle or advanced valvular disease the patient must be kept at rest. This is also true for a long period following a blood clot formation (coronary thrombosis) in the blood vessel to the heart. After marked improvement and prolonged rest in bed, the patient will be allowed some mild form of exercise such as a short walk.

***High Blood Pressure.*** There is a difference of opinion on the question of exercise for high blood pressure patients. Some medical authorities advise mild exercise in the form of a short slow walk; others prescribe absolute rest in bed. This of course all depends upon the height of the blood pressure and any complications associated with it.

## POSTURE

One must have good body balance to maintain the erect position. This balance may be interfered with by overweight or relaxation or weakness of the abdominal muscles. When a person stands correctly, a perpendicular line dropped from the ear should pass through the shoulders, hips, and ankle joints. In good posture, the head is held high, chin upwards and inwards, chest up, shoulders thrown backward and relaxed, abdomen flat, knees straight and feet parallel. In other words, the carriage should be that of the soldier. Many hours are consumed in training the military in correct posture. This is so necessary for prolonged physical endurance, which in turn is greatly influenced by correct breathing.

## HEALTHFUL EXERCISES

***To Develop the Waistline.*** In a sitting position, extend both arms and legs as far apart as possible, twist your body from the waistline, touch your right toe with your left hand, then twist your body in the opposite direction and touch your left toe with your right hand.

Start in a standing position. Your weight should be evenly distributed upon both feet. Raise your arms over your head and lower them. Now reach up with the right arm as if to pick up a small object from a place higher than your head. At the same time, keep your left side completely relaxed. Now, use your left arm and relax your right side, but really reach, so that you can feel the stretch deep down in your abdomen. Repeat this several times. Then reach up with your chin. Next, stand on tiptoe, so that you feel every muscle in your legs stretching.

Now quit and relax. Make your arms limp and shake them vigorously, but without tension. Next, relax your right leg and shake it vigorously, avoiding tension. Repeat with your left leg. By now your entire body will be glowing and yet you will feel completely relaxed.

***Exercise for Pendulous Abdomen.*** The best correction for the pendulous abdomen is to reach toward the skies. Bend forward until you feel a slight pull. As a starter, repeat this ten times.

***Reducing the Waistline.*** Stand with your weight evenly distributed on both feet. Bend to the right, running your right arm down alongside your right leg; your left arm should be crooked over your head,

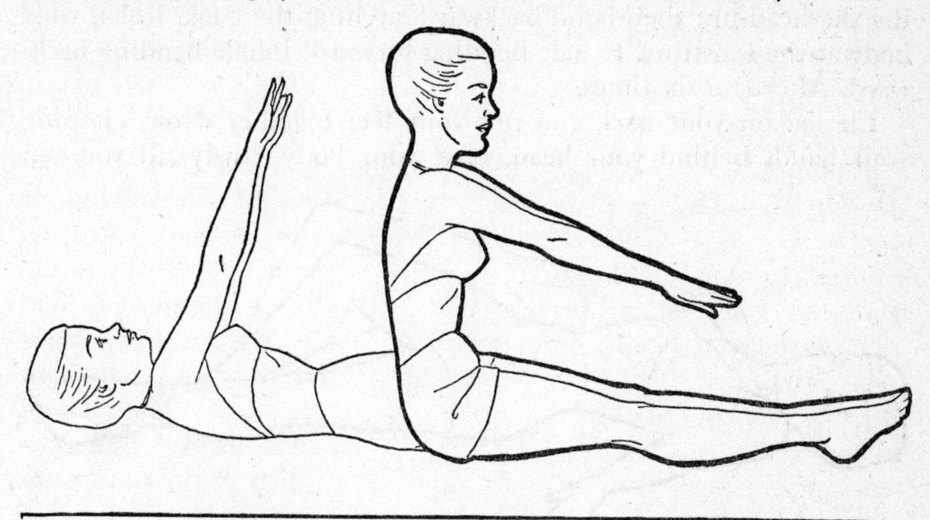

EXERCISE TO REDUCE WAISTLINE

Lying flat on the floor, raise both arms and then your trunk. Now reach forward and touch your toes with your fingertips without bending the knees. With practice this will become an easy exercise to do.

with your left hand touching your right ear. Bend until you feel a good pull. Then reverse this procedure. Again relax and take a few good breaths.

Lie down on the floor and relax. After a few minutes' rest, raise your legs and support your buttocks with your hands, elbows resting on the floor, then ride "the bicycle" for a few laps. After you have accomplished this, straighten out your knees and try to touch your toes to the floor over your head; then lower your legs slowly back to the floor and at the same time sit up slowly. This will tighten the muscles of your abdomen and give you a flat belly.

***Reducing the Buttocks.*** Sit tailor fashion on the floor. Rock from right to left, shifting your weight from side to side. Do this regularly to reduce and harden the buttocks.

The basic rule of this system is stretch and reach, reach and stretch, then completely relax.

***To Develop the Muscles of the Back and Abdomen.*** Spread your legs and arms outward at right angles to the body. Twist your body from the waistline to the right; bend forward, touching the floor with your left hand, your right arm extending upward. Repeat with your right arm touching floor. Exhale bending forward; inhale coming up.

With hands on hips, legs together, bend your body forward, keeping the head up; then bend backward, arching the back. Relax your body at the waistline. Exhale bending forward; inhale bending backward. Alternate six times.

Lie flat on your back and put your feet together. Now, clasping your hands behind your head, raise your body slowly till you can

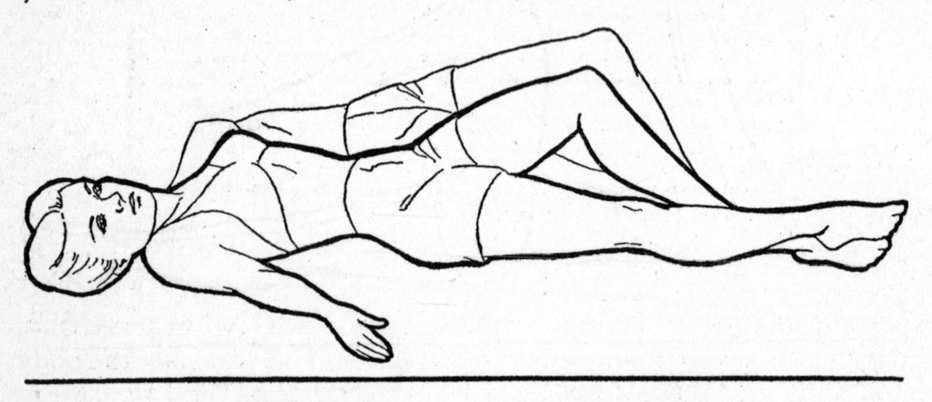

EXERCISE TO DEVELOP BACK

To start, assume a position like the one shown in darker outline—one foot crossed over the other and one leg raised. Now, relying solely on your back and arms, raise your body to the position shown in light outline, with feet still crossed. Alternate the leg raised and do the exercise a number of times.

rest your elbows on your knees. Now return to your original position slowly. Bend forward and exhale; inhale going backwards.

***To Develop the Muscles of the Back, Chest, Thighs, and Legs.*** Stand with your legs wide apart, your hands clasped over the head. Keeping your knees rigid, twist your body to the right, bend over and touch your right foot; then rise to your original position. Alternate to the left. Exhale bending over; inhale coming up.

Stand with your hands on hips, legs together. Now stoop to a squatting position and sit on your heels with your body weight evenly balanced on the balls of both feet. Keep your knees together and your back arched. Exhale stooping, inhale coming up.

***To Develop the Muscles of the Neck and Spine.*** Lie flat on your back with your legs together, your hands placed at your sides, palms down. Raise your legs upward and over your head till your toes touch the floor, keeping legs straight, then back to your original position. Exhale going over; inhale coming back.

CHAPTER 25

# COMMON SIGNS AND SYMPTOMS OF ILLNESS

**Your Periodic Health Examination and Why It Is Important . . . Common Symptoms of Illness . . . Mechanical Headaches . . . Functional Headaches . . . Toxic Headaches . . . Reflex Headaches . . . Headache Remedies . . . Anatomical Backache . . . Low Backache . . . Backaches Caused by Posture Defects and Flat Feet . . . Low Backache in Women . . . Mechanical Backache from Enlarged Prostate Gland . . . Reflex Backache . . . Bleeding . . . Kinds of Hemorrhages and Their Care . . . Localized Pain . . . Reflex or Referred Pain . . . Vomiting . . . Coughing . . . Fear and Depression . . . Sleeplessness (Insomnia) . . . Coma . . . Fever and What Causes It, etc.**

## YOUR PERIODIC MEDICAL EXAMINATION

GOOD HEALTH is the greatest of all blessings. Good health makes possible the greatest enjoyment of life. It consists in keeping the body and mind at the best level. It provides each person with the ability to study his powers, learn his needs, exercise his abilities, improve his resources, develop his mind and body and thus be prepared for the daily needs of life and be ready to meet emergencies as they arise. A healthy man finds joy in play, satisfaction in work, and inspiration in service.

To this end it is necessary for every man, woman and child to have health examinations at least twice yearly. Such examinations should begin in infancy and continue through childhood, puberty, and adult life. Each period has its special problems.

When a man dies at seventy of apoplexy, the changes in his arteries which brought about the condition began twenty to thirty years before. If he had had periodic examinations, his stroke might have been prevented.

The examinations are best carried out by the family physician, who is qualified to make use of the conditions he has found in the patient in health, comparing them with those that develop in disease.

The work must be well done in order for it to be successful. The idea of health examination is not new, but today, with the dawn of Preventive Medicine, the profession is equipped to recognize danger signals to prevent the development of many diseases.

The procedure must be twofold. It must be thoroughly carried out and each person considered on an individual basis; and the patient in turn must cooperate conscientiously with the doctor.

As part of the complete physical examination, the doctor looks into the patient's family history, the conditions of his environment, his occupation, and his habits as to food, sleep, and exercise. The condition of the respiratory, heart and circulatory systems comes in for first consideration. The eyes, nose, throat, teeth and glandular system must be thoroughly investigated.

We have learned that we should not wait for a toothache to drive us to a dentist; the same idea must obtain with all the other organs and structures of the body.

Those who are endowed with a robust frame, sturdy body, sound functions, and a strong constitution must also recognize that there is a limit to which the human machine may be driven without permanent harm.

One of the important lessons of life is to develop good inhibitions. This is fundamental for a temperate, normal life, which leads to longevity. To follow our instincts blindly would be to live on the plane of the lower animals. Persons who do this fall into grave error. Our sensations are not always to be trusted. We may feel tired, yet need exercise; we may be bursting with energy, yet need rest; we may not be thirsty, yet need water.

Man is too often ignorant of the fundamental factors which underlie the art of hygienic living. Although there are still many unsolved problems concerning diet, nutrition, work, play, exercise and rest, medical science has made great strides in the past decade in applying the principles of health as a foundation to battle disease.

The prevention of disease is a definite phase in personal hygiene which means correct living, whereby the individual protects himself against disease. Living to an advanced age is not enough in itself. Longevity without health and combined usefulness is a misfortune.

We must, then, have a constant inventory of our physical and physiological stocks. Your physician is the only one competent to make this inventory. He is your expert accountant. He will not only discover signs of conditions that may become serious in time; he will also give you fundamental instruction on how to live a long and healthy life.

## COMMON SYMPTOMS OF SICKNESS

By common symptoms of sickness we mean the variety of symptoms and signs one observes when a disease already exists, a disease is in the formative or incubation stage, or a disease has already reached its height and is on the decline. Such common symptoms include headache, backache, hemorrhage, pain, fever, vomiting, fear, depression, and sleeplessness. All of these symptoms have definite causes. They may occur singly, in pairs, or several at once.

Taken by itself, almost any one of the symptoms described in the following pages may not mean that anything is seriously wrong. However, each one contributes to a composite picture, which, when put together, makes a definite diagnosis. So always be accurate in telling your doctor exactly all the symptoms you have.

In this chapter, we shall examine these symptoms and what they may mean. A proper diagnosis, except in the most elementary cases, can and should be made only by a physician. The various diseases or disorders responsible for the symptoms are in general discussed in detail elsewhere in this book, and the index should be consulted.

## HEADACHES

More than half the patients that a doctor sees complain of headache. Headache is the reason given for a large percentage of absenteeism in industry. It has been estimated that there are over two hundred different causes of pain in the head. Headaches may be dull, severe, throbbing, intermittent, or constant. They may be classified as mechanical, functional, toxic and reflex.

### Mechanical Headaches

***Causes of Mechanical Headaches.*** This type of headache is associated with conditions within the head, that is, a pressure in the head, in most instances due to sinus infections in which the nose is blocked by swelling and the infected sinus discharges cannot escape. This condition can produce very severe aching or a constant dull ache. If the frontal sinus is involved, then the ache is in the forehead region; if the cheek sinuses (antrums) are the offenders, then the ache is over the cheekbones. As a rule, sinus aches are more severe in the mornings when there is more severe obstruction to the outflow of the pus which has accumulated during the night.

Changes in the pressure within the skull due to increase of the brain fluid between the brain coverings (meninges) may be the first sign of an inflammation of these coverings. This is known as meningitis.

***Treatment of Mechanical Headaches.*** There is little that one can do at home. Heat over the sinuses, rest in bed, in the sitting posture, and an aspirin or empirin tablet every three to four hours is about all the self-help possible. A good nose specialist can give great relief even if he cannot cure the condition. Living in a dry, uniform climate is about the only lasting cure.

If there is no sinus trouble and the ache grows worse rapidly, and especially if there is some stiffness of the neck, get a doctor quickly. This is particularly true in young children. This may be an early warning of impending meningitis. This is a fatal disease unless promptly diagnosed and treated.

A tumor of the brain is always associated with headache, even in its earliest stage.

Following an injury there will probably be considerable aching of the head. This is called concussion and may last many days. If the aching persists, an X-ray should be taken to make sure there is no slight fracture of the skull.

### Functional Headaches

The disease of some organs remote from the head often causes headache. Chief among the causes are diseases of the heart and blood vessels. High blood pressure usually is a cause of headache. Certain heart ailments, particularly those connected with the heart muscle, are frequent offenders. Rest in bed will give relief. If there is known to be some heart disorder, do not take any medicines without your doctor's prescription.

Instability of the nervous system is frequently associated with headache. Emotional upsets, hysteria, and nerve fatigue are all functional conditions in which ache in the head is more often than not a symptom.

Other neurologic functional causes of headache are chorea (St. Vitus's dance) and different types of neuralgia, especially involvement of the facial nerve. The application of heat to the face will give relief.

Chorea must be treated by a nerve specialist. This is a disease found only in children before puberty. In good medical hands, it is curable.

## Toxic Headaches

***Migraine Headaches.*** Chief under this caption is the so-called migraine or "sick-headache." Many causes have been said to be responsible for this common form of headache. Most physicians now agree that it is an allergic reaction to some form of food. There is a nervous element, undoubtedly, also present. There are many sufferers with this exasperating malady. Besides the ache in the head they experience nausea, vomiting, and, in severe cases, collapse. Every effort should be made to determine the cause. During the attack the patient should be in bed in a darkened and quiet room. Few drugs are of any value; the attack just has to wear off, which it usually does in a few hours.

***Other Causes of Toxic Headaches.*** Acute alcoholism, "the morning after the night before," too much coffee, smoking too much, certain drugs such as nitroglycerin, fumes of poisonous gases such as carbon-monoxide, sulfuric acid in industry—all these produce headache.

In children, as a preliminary symptom to most of the acute contagious diseases, there is a toxic headache. This is particularly true in measles, scarlet fever, and polio.

Influenza is usually ushered in by a headache. It may be the most prominent symptom in this common infection. In all these infections the headache is due to toxic absorption from the disease, which shows itself more markedly later.

The stomach and bowel may send forth poisonous substances which cause headache. This is true in indigestion and chronic constipation.

The most important danger sign during the latter months of pregnancy is headache. This may mean that the kidneys are not functioning properly, and the headache may be a first symptom of uremia (kidney poisoning). A specimen of urine should be sent to your doctor without delay. The urinalysis will promptly tell whether or not the headaches are from the kidneys.

Chronic and acute Bright's disease often have as a prominent symptom headaches. Again the urine must be watched very carefully.

Toxic headaches are of frequent occurrence with painful menstruation and as an accompaniment to the change of life in women (climacteric or menopause). Just why this occurs is not known, but it evidently has as its cause some disturbance in the hormone balance. Certain drugs are of value for painful menstruation (dysmenorrhea) and the hormones are given for severe headaches associated with the change of life.

### Reflex Headaches

In these, certain organs and disturbances not part of the head transfer, along the nerve paths, a symptom which takes the form of headache.

The most important of these conditions is eye-strain. This is usually due to defects of vision and can easily be corrected by properly fitting eye-glasses. Abuse of the precious eyes is very common; reading in a poor light or incorrectly adjusted light and overuse of the eyes will cause headache.

Arthritis involving the neck bones, cavities in the teeth, or a tooth abscess may cause headaches, as a reflex of these two conditions.

Overweight, often, is the source of headaches. The abdominal muscles cannot support the excess of fat, so the internal organs drop down; in so doing they pull upon the sympathetic nerves, resulting in headache, among other distressing symptoms.

Likewise, any abnormal conditions of the female genital organs, by reflex along the nerve tracks, will produce headaches, and severe ones too. The principal condition is "falling of the womb" due to tears during childbirth inadequately repaired or not repaired at all. A minor surgical operation will correct this, provided it is not allowed to persist over years. Then the operation becomes more difficult.

A common and little recognized cause of headache is hunger. The empty stomach sends direct nerve waves to the brain announcing its lack and need of food. The treatment? Eat.

### Headache Remedies

The number of headache powders and pills offered to the gullible public is almost as numerous as the different kinds of headache. Most of them contain dangerous ingredients and should never be used. Your doctor is again your adviser. If you do not consult a physician, or feel that it is not necessary, the simplest remedy is either aspirin or empirin. Such remedies as the barbiturates and the coal tar products, which are present in most "headache-cures," often cause drowsiness, toxic conditions, skin rashes, certain blood diseases, and heart disturbances. Do not use them.

## BACKACHE

At one time or another in nearly every one's life, backache is felt. It may be caused by postural defects, fatigue, overstraining, or definite abnormalities of the bony structure. Severity, duration, and treatment vary.

Backache is classified according to causes, as anatomical, mechanical, inflammatory, and reflex.

### Anatomical Backache

As the name implies, this condition is due to defects in the spinal column—the vertebrae (the spinal bones of the back) and the lower spine, which is the sacrum. Defect of these bones may have existed from birth and cause the deformity known as curvature of the spine. Curvature can also be acquired by infection with tuberculosis. This is called Pott's disease. Deformities can also result from injury producing fractures. When anatomical irregularities are noted, early correction by plaster casts will cure the condition. If Pott's disease is the cause, the treatment corresponds to that of tuberculosis elsewhere in the body, together with some form of mechanical support.

### Low Backache

Low backache is one of the most common varieties of pain in the back. The causes are numerous and are of a mechanical nature.

The main mechanical deviation is faulty posture, the next cause, in the order of frequency, is flat feet or fallen arches. Then follow obesity, relaxed abdominal muscles, misplaced female genital organs and, in the male, acute and chronic inflammations of the prostate gland.

Now, remember that we are talking about the nagging, low back pain and not the severe pain caused by the other diseases just mentioned. This nagging pain is usually present when one is on his feet; it is rarely experienced when lying down or during the sleeping hours. This is typical, and the pain rarely reaches the severe stages of the arthritic type. The mechanical variety is never relieved by drugs.

***Faulty Posture as a Cause.*** One must have good body balance to maintain the erect position. This balance may be interfered with by overweight or relaxation or weakness of the abdominal muscles.

When a person stands correctly, a perpendicular line dropped from the ear should pass through the shoulders, hips, and ankle joints. For good posture, the head is held high, the chin upwards and inwards, the chest is up, the shoulders thrown backward and relaxed, the abdomen flat, the knees straight, and the feet parallel. In other words, the carriage should be that of the soldier. Many hours are consumed in training the military in correct posture and it was rare during the training period in World War II that one heard any complaint of low back pain which could be traced to faulty posture.

With poor posture, unnatural stress and strain are thrown upon the chest and diaphragm muscles and ligaments which aid in support of the spinal column. These strains are most pronounced at the level of the lower column where it joins the sacrum.

***Diagnosis of Postural Backache.*** The diagnosis of mechanical backache of postural origin should be made only after careful evaluation of the patient's history and X-ray examination of the entire spinal column. The usual history is one of a gradual beginning of low back pain which commonly is localized to the sacral region; but not infrequently the patient complains of diffuse discomfort cross the entire lower back extending into the buttocks. The story is one of many years' duration, and although the patient may be incapacitated and unable to carry on, the pain is seldom severe. The history brings out definitely that the pain is rarely present in the recumbent position, but is aggravated by activity. Changes in the weather have no effect as they do in the various forms of arthritis and rheumatism.

***Treatment of Postural Backache.*** The condition can be relieved by certain simple procedures. The patient should sleep on a firm mattress, which prevents further strain on the muscles of the back. The application of heat is of great benefit, and the hot tub nightly for ten minutes brings relief. This is to be followed by a hot water bag or preferably the electric pad, but only used at medium and applied through the night. Gentle massage is very helpful but not necessary. Next in importance is a systematic and regular form of exercises in which the patient is carefully instructed. These exercises should be in writing and given to the patient for reference in carrying them out. The patient should be made to understand that evident improvement will not show for a couple of months since it will require that long before the back muscles gain strength. These exercises in detail are given in Chapter 24.

### Low Backache from Flat Feet

It is amazing how often the physician is consulted for low backache due to fallen arches of the feet. The patient approaches the doctor with fear in most instances, fear that his pain is due to some disease of the kidneys or a tumor, but having no idea as to the real source of his trouble.

***Causes of Flat Feet.*** It is manifestly impossible in a chapter of this type to go into the various kinds of flat feet. Suffice it to say: There are many varieties of flat feet and sufferers from the lack of support in the structures of the arches are many. Sufferers they really are. One who is never afflicted with fallen arches can never realize how fortunate he is. Many so afflicted are more or less incapacitated for their work. They more often than not give a long history, dating back years; in fact many feet have defective arch support from birth. Body weight is a big factor in producing relaxed arch support, but it is by no means unusual to find underweight or normal-weight persons suffering with pain due to relaxed arches.

***Back Symptoms of Flat Feet.*** The pain often is limited to the back, with little or no discomfort in the feet. It is naturally present only when one is on his feet. Relief always comes when sitting or lying down. On pressure over the calves of the legs, soreness is usually encountered and the ham-string muscles of the thigh are often tender.

***Who Makes the Diagnosis.*** The correct diagnosis should be made by an experienced orthopedic specialist, who will make a plaster cast of the feet, thus and only thus determining the degree of the flat feet; from this cast the physician will prescribe the correct type of arch support and shoes.

There are on the market many varieties of arch supports of different materials and many advertised arch-support shoes. Many are priced at out-of-proportion rates and are of no value to the individual in need of such correction. Only correctly adjusted appliances can bring the necessary relief to feet with fallen arches, and these appliances must follow the plaster cast from which the physician writes his prescription. After scientific correction is made, complete relief is immediate.

### Low Backache in Women

***Kinds and Causes.*** In those females who suffer from low backache, the condition is due to relaxed abdominal muscles. These are found usually in the overweight and in women who have had several children in rapid succession. There are three factors at work in such instances. One is dropping of the abdominal organs (ptosis), particularly the stomach and intestines, due to the pendulous nonsupporting abdominal wall. Then, there is the type in which the weight is normal, who also have insufficient abdominal support. In the third type, abdominal support is adequate but there is some malposition of the womb. It may not be possible to determine the cause of this type, but examination reveals the womb either tilted too far forward or backward.

***Treatment of Low Backache in Women.*** To relieve the backache of those women who have relaxed abdominal musculature, properly fitting supports are applied and certain exercises are advised. For the obese, reduction in the body weight is prescribed, and for the underweight, a high caloric diet is given. Above all, our young women must learn to space their pregnancies sufficiently far apart.

### Mechanical Backache from Enlarged Prostate Gland

The prostate, present in the male only, lies at the neck of the urinary bladder, where it completely surrounds the urethra. Normally the gland is about the size of a horse chestnut, but it may attain the size of an orange under certain pathologic conditions. When it is greatly enlarged, it makes pressure on the plexus of nerves that emerge from the lower end of the spinal column, and thus produces mechanical backache. It should be understood that prostatic enlargement may be inflammatory and may occur in young men, producing the same kind of pain that is experienced by any of the mechanical causative factors mentioned. The true prostatic enlargement of advanced age rarely causes backache; this is because the process of growth is upward and away from the nerve plexuses mentioned.

### Inflammatory Backache

Inflammation of the lower vertebrae (spondylitis) or of the sacrum (sacroiliac disease) will have pain more or less severe, somewhere in the region of the back. It may be confined to one side of the back or to both sides.

Different kinds of rheumatism localize in the back. This is usually accompanied by fever which in the acute stage may go as high as 103° F. or even higher.

***Lumbago.*** Severe body chilling may result in an inflammation of the back muscles. This is called "lumbago." In the acute stage this is usually more severe pain than an ache. The patient may recover from the acute attack in a few days or the attack may go into prolonged siege and become chronic. In the acute beginning, the pain may be so severe as to completely incapacitate the patient. Opiates may be necessary, which only the physician can give. Rest in bed and application of dry heat should be the rule. After the acute stage wears off, light massage may help to a more rapid recovery.

### REFLEX BACKACHE

This means pain or ache in the back, usually involving only the kidney area. It is due in most instances to some kidney disorder. Kidney stone is the most frequent cause, but any kidney disease, either medical or surgical, usually has backache as a symptom. The medical diseases are acute or chronic nephritis (Bright's disease). These diseases are discussed at greater length elsewhere in this book. See the index.

Remember that all back pains do *not* mean kidney disease as so many people think. If a backache persists after reasonable rest of a day or two, consult a physician. In such cases it may or may not mean anything serious, but don't take any chances by delaying.

## HEMORRHAGE (BLEEDING)

The presence of blood outside of the circulatory system, in any of the excretions or secretions, from any of the hollow organs, whether in small amounts or in profuse amounts, is to be considered as a hemorrhage.

One inviolable rule should ever be remembered: Any time blood appears from any source of the body, immediate professional consultation is indicated. It may save a life.

Until the doctor arrives, place the patient in a relaxed position. Avoid excitement. The application of heat or ice to external bleeding is the principle underlying first aid in minor cases. (See chapter on first aid.)

***Causes of Bleeding.*** The following sources and causes of bleeding are set down to acquaint the reader with them. Details of each are to be found in the chapters dealing with the special diseases of the organs involved.

***Nose Bleeding.*** Bleeding from the nose may be due to accidents, polyps, or associated with severe colds and forceful blowing of the nose. Picking at the mucous membrane, so often done by young children, may produce considerable bleeding. Profuse nasal hemorrhage often occurs with high blood pressure and is a blessing in disguise; otherwise the bleeding might occur in the brain.

***Throat Bleeding.*** This can occur as an accompaniment of severe fits of coughing. The bleeding is mechanical, due to injury of the mucous membrane of the throat.

***Mouth Bleeding.*** This may occur as part of infections of the mouth (stomatitis) or a condition of the gums (gingivitis) often found with scurvy, which is a vitamin deficiency disease. Following tooth extraction there may be considerable bleeding. Call the dentist.

***Lung Hemorrhage.*** This is associated with advanced tuberculosis or early tumor. In either case, get prompt medical aid. Pulmonary bleeding often is rapidly fatal.

***Stomach Hemorrhage.*** The cause of bleeding from this organ are ulcer and cancer. Bleeding may appear in vomit only, and usually comes on suddenly. Commonly, there have been stomach symptoms for a long time.

***Bowel Hemorrhage.*** Here again the causes are ulcer of the small bowel (duodenum) or malignant tumor of the large bowel. Early symptoms are always present. The bleeding may be slight and discovered mixed with the feces.

***Rectal Bleeding.*** The cause here is "bleeding piles" (hemorrhoids). It may become profuse following bowel movement, especially if constipation is present. This can usually be controlled by a very hot sitz bath for fifteen minutes. A sitz bath means sitting in the tub which contains just enough water to cover the buttocks. The legs should be drawn up; thereby the water-heat is concentrated on the rectal opening (anus), where the piles are protruding. A medicated suppository, well lubricated, if inserted into the rectum twice daily before the hot bath, will often relieve the condition and may cure it, provided the constipation is controlled. Cleanse with soft tissues after bowel movements.

***Suppositories for Piles.*** The following rectal suppositories have been found very helpful. Any druggist can make them. They do not need a doctor's prescription, as they contain no opium. Use one, twice daily before the bath.

Ichthyol ....................4.000 grams
Extract Belladonna ...........0.195 grams
Cocoa butter to make 12 suppositories

If there is no relief, surgery will have to be performed.

***Kidney Hemorrhage.*** Severe bleeding from the kidney occurs with malignant tumors and the passage of a stone from the kidney to the bladder. In the latter condition there is associated severe pain (kidney colic). There is also blood in the urine when there is an acute toxic nephritis (Bright's disease).

***Bladder Hemorrhage.*** Profuse bleeding from the bladder means there is a tumor. It is not necessarily a malignant tumor. Benign bladder tumors are common. They may cause considerable bleeding. Diagnosis is made by a specialist who will perform a cystoscopic examination. Occasionally a very severe infection of the bladder may cause blood to appear in the urine.

***Vaginal Hemorrhage.*** It is very important to have a definite diagnosis as to the exact source of blood coming from the vagina. Only a capable physician can determine this. Bleeding from the vaginal lining is secondary to infections, usually gonorrhea.

***Uterine Hemorrhage.*** If the blood is seen coming from the mouth of the womb, it is due to either tumor, benign or malignant; inflammation (endometritis); excessive menstruation (menorrhagia), threatened miscarriage, or abortion; or, if late in pregnancy, to a premature separation of the afterbirth (placenta).

It takes an experienced physician to make the diagnosis and it is vital that medical help be sought immediately.

***Hemorrhage from Diseases of the Blood and the Blood Vessels.*** Hemophilia is a congenital disease that is inherited by the son from the mother. Its cause is not exactly known. Its characteristic is bleeding from simple causes, a bruise or a slight cut.

Lowered clotting time may be the cause of hemophilia; there are other chemical causes of hemorrhage. Much help can be gotten by accurate laboratory tests done by an expert.

Another obscure blood disease which causes hemorrhages under the skin with painful nodule formation is erythema nodosum. This has some connection with rheumatic conditions.

***Hardening of the Arteries.*** This is called arteriosclerosis. Hemorrhage associated with this condition occurs by rupture of a small blood vessel, usually in the brain ("stroke" or apoplexy).

***Accident Hemorrhages.*** Following an accident, if there are no external signs and suddenly the person grows faint and pale, you must think of internal hemorrhages. Call the doctor, then place the patient in bed, keep him quiet, and put an ice bag on his abdomen.

Cuts involving the blood vessels are dealt with in our chapter on first aid.

## PAIN

The various kinds of pain are slight, severe, lancinating, dull, throbbing, colicky, intermittent, constant, local, and reflex. Pain may be either localized or referred.

### Localized Pain

If soreness or tenderness exists over some particular part of the body, such as a muscle, a bone, or in the region of a particular organ, the evidence thus obtained suggests an involvement of that structure or organ. For example, if a person complains of pain over the kidney region and, on examination, the muscle of that region is not painful, but deep pressure elicits pain, there is then enough evidence to suspect involvement of the kidney. Further examination then is carried on with the kidney in mind.

If tenderness is found and soreness is determined over the appendix region, which is on the right side at a point halfway between the navel and the prominence of the hip bone, then inflammation of the appendix is suspected. Of course all other symptoms connected with appendicitis must be taken into account.

Pain that is localized over the tip of the breast bone is suggestive of a stomach ulcer. But, again, all the other signs and symptoms must be added.

### Reflex or Referred Pain

This means that the pain travels along a nerve away from the source of the trouble. There are three particular organs in which this occurs—the heart, the gall bladder, and the kidney. Angina pectoris, or spasm of the artery that nourishes the heart muscle, sends the pain down the left arm to the finger tips. Inflammation of the gall bladder, which collects the bile from the liver, manifests iself by pain which travels toward the right shoulder blade. A kidney colic due to a stone passing downward will refer the pain to the bladder, testicles, or the ovaries. A curious manifestation in such cases is that the pain on one side may be due to the trouble of the opposite kidney. This has never been explained, but it occurs so often that it is given a name, renorenal reflex.

Again it must be pointed out that no single sign or symptom is ever conclusive in itself for the purpose of making an accurate diagnosis.

## VOMITING

The significance of this symptom is highly variable. What it means depends first upon the time of day the vomiting occurs, its relation to the intake of food, or whether it follows a spell of coughing. This last is of particular importance in children. They often vomit following a fit of coughing, which may be brought on by an outburst of temper. Then, again, vomiting may occur at the end of an attack of whooping cough.

If an adult woman says that she vomits after her breakfast, the first thing to suspect is that she is pregnant.

Vomiting in association with various diseases of the stomach, such as ulcer or chronic indigestion, is of common occurrence.

Vomiting with blood is a grave sign. It may mean cancer or a bleeding ulcer. On the other hand, blood in the vomit can be due to mere strain from the effort of the vomiting.

## COUGHING

This can have as its cause any abnormal condition that is present anywhere from the back of the nose to the base of the lungs. Acute colds that end up in the posterior nose or sinuses are probably the chief causes of coughing. Other simple causes of coughing are too many cigarettes, infected tonsils, and food going down the wrong way—that is, into the glottis instead of the gullet.

If the cough brings up blood, immediate complete examination is indicated to rule out tuberculosis.

## FEAR AND DEPRESSION

There can be no doubt that these two emotional disturbances are more often than not without any foundation. It is usually the things that we fear that never happen. We now know that fear may be the cause of ulcer of the stomach or intestine. If fear is persistent and without any cause in the outside world, it is known as anxiety, and may be a symptom of neurosis.

Depression may closely follow upon the presence of fear. The two are intimately related. Depression is sometimes felt because of weakness as a part of, or following, illness.

Encouragement and commonsense is the remedy for these mental states in their milder forms. If they are overwhelming, consultation with a psychiatrist is desirable.

## SLEEPLESSNESS (INSOMNIA)

If one cannot sleep at the correct time, then you can put it down as a fact that there is something wrong. The cause may be physical, but more often it is mental. Worry is a common offender. Of the simple causes, mention should be made of overeating before the bedtime hour, too much alcohol, too much excitement. Sleeplessness in children is definitely one of two things: either not having the correct diet or too much excitement.

## COMA

The state of coma is unconsciousness. It may be partial or complete. If it is partial the patient is said to be semicomatose; if completely unconscious then it is a state of complete coma.

***The Causes of Coma.*** Mechanical causes may be a blow upon the head (concussions), fracture of the skull, a fall from a great height, and apoplexy (rupture of an artery in the brain).

Comas also arise from toxic causes. These include acute alcoholism, and swallowing various chemicals. An overdose of medicines, usually sleeping pills, may be responsible, or taking opium in various forms, such as paregoric or cough mixtures that contain codeine. Sunstroke is often a cause.

Coma may also be secondary to some disease, like diabetes, kidney disease (Bright's disease), or an acute condition of the kidneys associated with pregnancy and called eclampsia. It may also follow a seizure of epilepsy.

***Diagnosis of Coma.*** This may be very difficult if the cause is not known. If there is a history of injury, then the diagnosis is clear that it is either a concussion or a fracture. If there is evidence of poisoning through finding a labeled bottle nearby, the diagnosis here too is clear. If the breath smells sweetish, then the cause probably is diabetes. If the coma is associated with convulsions, it is probably due to kidney disease.

***Treatment of Coma.*** The first thing to do is to call a doctor. If there is evidence of poisoning, get the patient up on his feet and try to get him to walk. If he can swallow, give an emetic. If there is evidence of a skull fracture, keep him quiet until the doctor comes. There is little else to do. If you are not able to get a doctor, then take the patient to the nearest hospital. Every minute is precious and no time should be lost obtaining expert medical attention.

## FEVER

The temperature of the human body is regulated centrally by specific areas in the base of the brain and also by the skin, which accomplishes temperature changes by the moisture given off through the process of perspiration.

The average normal temperature of the body is about 98.8 F. This is the mouth temperature, the rectal being about one degree higher. In very young infants the rectal temperature may average one-half to one degree higher.

***Causes of Fever.*** Increase in body temperature is always due to one of two factors: a disturbance of the central brain control or the presence of some infection in the blood. The infectious process is by far the more common. It is usually accompanied by some other symptom, even though the increase in the temperature may overshadow the other symptoms. The best example of this is to be seen in the beginning of the contagious and infectious diseases of childhood. When the temperature goes above normal the patient is said to have a "fever." A doctor should always be called as soon as the child develops fever.

***Signs of Fever.*** If no one knows how to take a temperature (page 451) and the face of the child feels hot, especially the forehead, and there is listlessness (that is, the child does not want to play but lies down and will not eat), you will know that something is wrong. The doctor may be able to give you enough information over the telephone so that you can watch for further developments. If there has been any injury of recent date, such as a cut of the hand, foot, or finger, look for an evidence of infection locally and note if there are any red streaks running up the arm or leg of the cut or bruised part. This is a danger sign of possible septicemia. Hurry and get the doctor then!

Frequently a fever is preceded by a sensation of chilliness or there may be a severe chill. Shortly afterward, there will be a rise in the temperature; in children this may go as high as 104° to 105° F.

Fever, as a beginning of one of the children's diseases, may keep up until a rash appears; then it will go down slowly.

***How Fever Disappears.*** There is one disease that is associated with a sudden drop in the fever (crisis). This drop is an accompaniment of the end of pneumonia and is often most dramatic in its suddenness. It can often be seen now, since we use the antibiotics for the treatment of all types of general and local infections. The other manner in which fever disappears is slowly (lysis). This is classical with typhoid fever, the different types of influenza, and malaria.

CHAPTER 26

# PROBLEMS OF OLD AGE



## MEANING OF AGING

What does "aging" mean? One school of thought considers aging to be an orderly, natural physical process which is revealed by inevitable changes of the cells, tissues, and fluids of the body. In that case, resistance to aging would mean the body's ability to put off or delay the changes which take place with the passage of time. The other school holds that the degenerative changes and impairments found in aged organs are due to unfavorable conditions proceeding from the environment. Such conditions include infections, injuries, and nutritional disturbances. In that case, resistance to aging would mean the ability of the body to withstand the microbic invasions and injuries to which it is subjected.

With our present methods of tissue inspection it is practically impossible to isolate the phenomena of pure physiological aging and those of pathological origin which are due to unfavorable environmental influences. As matters stand at present, all we can say is that the tissue changes commonly found in old people are doubtless brought about by combinations of constitutional and environmental factors. In some individuals the tissues are able to react more favorably, and in others less favorably, to environmental forces and injuries.

*Aging as a Normal Process.* In thinking of aging as a normal process we depend, as in many situations, upon what is conspicuously familiar. Throughout man's history the physical facts of birth, growth, maturity, old age, and death have been recognized and accepted. We may visualize this cycle as a curve with an initial upward slant representing the period of growth and a later downward slant representing the period of decline, with the period of maturity at the rounded peak of the curve. When we look at the whole of life in this way, aging becomes as much a part of existence as growth.

## TWO MAIN PROBLEMS OF AGING

There is a point beyond which human life does not extend even under the most favorable circumstances. At present this limit has tentatively been set at the century mark. It is a conspicuously familiar fact that very few individuals have lived or claim to have lived for more than one hundred years. It is common knowledge also that the human life span is very rarely completed and that the thousands of individuals who now come within one, two, or three decades of the century mark are not necessarily healthy, happy, and useful. So, for all practical purposes, the problems of aging resolve themselves into finding answers to these questions: What changeable influences operate to cut short the journey of life before its biologic age limit is reached? And what can be done to maintain physical, mental, and emotional competence for life as the years pass and to create along the upward path the interests and the capacities which will make life fruitful and happy going down?

## AGE, HEREDITY, AND ENVIRONMENT

Although man, by virtue of his physical organization, is capable of living to be one hundred years old, individual human beings vary greatly in their potentialities for long life. Upon the original quality of the fertilized egg from which each human being develops, depends in large part the ability to resist the hazards and the usual wear and tear of life.

However, heredity operates only within the framework of environment. Individual differences in the ability to resist infection, for example, may be attributed to variations in the hereditary pattern. But the infection itself proceeds from the environment. With a perfect environment, heredity might have a free hand to lead us to a full span of life, the latter part of which would be a gradual intensification of the process of aging. Yet heredity has never been given that free hand, and perhaps never will. No one in the course of a lifetime escapes unfavorable environmental influences, which result in injuries to various tissues and produce effects that complicate normal physiological aging.

## AGING VARIES WITH THE INDIVIDUAL

Time seems to have no constant impact on the tissues and their ability to resist age changes. For different individuals, and at different periods in the life of the same individual, the passage of time may flow at a different biological rate. Hence chronological age has varying significance for different individuals. Aging, or senescence, may occur in the relatively young, while youthfulness, or delayed aging may be found in the relatively old. Moreover, just as during the first part of life our growth and development take place in the different tissues and organs at different times and at different rates, so during the latter part the effects of age do not begin to make themselves felt on all organs and tissues at the same time. It is not possible in the natural course of events for the whole body to go to pieces all at once. We grow and develop, we mature and age, we even die piecemeal. When the body finally comes to a standstill many of its parts are still intact.

## LOSS OF RESISTANCE TO DISEASE

The progressive loss of resistance to disease often associated with advancing age may in part be accounted for by the waning of the body's natural defense mechanisms. The analogy of the ship and the storm has often been used: "The 'ship' in age is not as seaworthy as she once was and, too often, falls an easy victim to a 'storm' which, in her youth, she would have weathered with ease."

## CAN SERUMS LENGTHEN LIFE?

The most recent attempt to reactivate resistance to disease in the aging organism and so prolong life was the development of ACS (Antireticulo-Cytotoxic Serum) by the Russian scientist Dr. Alexander A. Bogomolets. He claimed that this serum, when injected under the skin, acts as an over-all stimulant on connective tissues, the health of which vitally affects the disease-fighting ability and efficient functioning of the whole body. A great deal of clinical and laboratory experimentation with ACS is now going on in this country, but reports on the serum's value in increasing resistance to disease and in retarding the aging process are not yet generally available.

## OUR INCREASED LIFE SPAN

Claims that the human life span can be extended beyond the century mark by ACS or by any other biologic stimulant have yet to be proved. On the other hand, there is dramatic proof that we have it in our power to extend considerably the mean length of life—that is, the average number of years lived by all persons born at a given period (expectation of life at birth). In 1945, life expectancy at birth for the whole American people reached a new height of nearly sixty-six years. This is sixteen and two-thirds years above the level prevailing at the beginning of the century. This spectacular progress has been made largely by following the path which leads to the conquest of types of illness, especially the infections, which are common in infancy, childhood, youth, and early maturity.

## CONQUERING THE DISEASES OF LATER LIFE

Only a bare start has been made on the other path, which leads in the direction of the chronic diseases and conditions of late maturity and old age. The big gains of the future will probably be made in the study of the aging process itself and its pathological complications. And it is not only in the lengthening of life expectancy at ages beyond the peak of maturity that progress in the control of the so-called degenerative diseases will prove of value. An infirm or embittered old age, stretched out through what Osler called "the cold gradations of decay" to the limit of its "stretchability," is not pleasant to contemplate. If medical research is to do mankind a service in permitting a closer approach to the limit of the human life span, it must include reasonable fitness for life in the older ages among its objectives.

## SOCIETY'S DUTY TOWARD THE OLD

Besides the special technical problems of aging which are definitely within the fields of biological research and curative and preventive medicine, there are the sociological and public health aspects, about which only a few persons have even begun to think seriously. Neither medicine nor public health nor industry nor the state has any carefully thought-out program of what to do about the vast population of older persons who are rising in our midst. This is not to be wondered at, because the scope of this problem has no precedent in human history, and the problem itself has come upon us within an incredibly short period of time.

Man individually does not have this excuse. In every generation he has known that in the long life he hopes for he cannot escape growing old. It is a curious fact, however, that the human mind is averse to accepting aging as a natural physiological process. In youth and in the period of maturity which lies on the upward slope of the curve of life we live as if there were nothing more than that side of the mountain. It is only when we get over the peak that we discover that growing old is, after all, only the other side of the mountain. Going up, we have what we need to make the grade—physical strength, agility, swiftness, exactness of motion, large reserves of energy, a wide margin of safety in body structure and function, dreams of what we are going to do and be when we reach the top. Going down, the essential characteristics of youth—strength, speed, and precision—decline, but in the climb up to and across the plateau of maturity, we have gathered information, learned to think and organize our emotional attitudes. From these mental activities wisdom is developed, or should be—enough to guide us to a sound outlook on old age. Of course, this is not always achieved.

Happiness and comfort in old age depend largely upon the recognition by society of the potential contribution to the advancement of humanity which is inherent in living long enough to acquire wisdom. This contribution, up to now, has been a mere dribble. One of the tasks laid on geriatric medicine—that branch of medicine concerned with the problems of old age—is to discover how to enable a progressively increasing number of older people to put their wisdom to work by helping them to maintain their physical and emotional competence for life. It is not too much to hope that the physicians and the aging patients of the future will work together on a design for living which takes into account both the assets and the liabilities which appear as the years pass.

## MAKING AN ADJUSTMENT TO OLD AGE

As individuals, our task is *to get over our emotional resistance to aging*. Adaptability to the passing years is essential to health and longevity. We cannot make too early a start during maturity at deliberately and consistently cultivating healthful habits of living and thinking and interests outside our work. By doing so we may hope to escape the preventable pathological conditions, the feeling of uselessness, the antagonisms, and the bitterness which so frequently complicate the aging process. In the world of tomorrow the cooperation of the public in efforts to get mental, emotional, and physical disorders of later life discovered in time to do something constructive about them, will probably be sought as eagerly through education as public support of efforts to control the acute infections is sought today. At present, the help of psychologists and psychiatrists should be used more fully than it is.

As for society, its biggest task is to institute the changes which will provide socially useful outlets for the wisdom which comes only on the downward slope of a life well spent.

## HABITS THAT RAISE RESISTANCE TO DISEASE

As we go through life we are often unaware of the perils we escape—sometimes, perhaps, through a fortunate combination of circumstances, often because of powers of resistance that we do not know we possess.

The idea that the human body has the ability to resist unfavorable influences is a very ancient one. In spite of all the wonder-working drugs, serums, organic extracts, and surgical techniques now available, physicians today, as in the days of Hippocrates, recognize the healing power of Nature as their ally-in-chief. This power we partly may compute because many of the methods by which the body heals itself or protects itself from specific dangers are known and measurable.

On the other hand, the mechanism of general resistance is vague. We really know nothing yet about the biochemical changes which are involved when general resistance is lowered. All we can say is that the soil is ready for the seed—that the person as a whole is ready to be ill. Yet the modern concept of the causation of disease as a combination of many different influences, classified by Stieglitz as "predisposing, provoking, and perpetuating," makes it necessary for us to take cognizance of many factors which, in ways not clearly understood, raise or lower resistance.

In advocating habits of living and thinking which seem to raise resistance we are going on everyday experience. We have no exact proof of their value as we have of sanitary measures directed against the spread of pathogenic agents, or of immunization against specific diseases. The respective roles of hereditary characteristics, accumulated fatigue, mild malnutrition, climatic changes, aging of the tissues, and distress of mind, for example, in predisposing a person to a disease or in perpetuating it are not nearly so well known as are the respective roles of microorganisms, toxins and allergens, psychic shock and physical traumas, and acute nutritional deficiencies in initiating or precipitating it.

## NEW MEDICAL OUTLOOK ON OLD AGE

The outlook of those who feel that a way of life based on a knowledge of physiology and other basic medical sciences will help to raise resistance against disease may seem visionary to others who would like to have mathematical confirmation of the value of their efforts. But gradually we are reaching the limit of the great gains which can be made in extending life expectancy by wholeheartedly doing the things which bring mathematically measurable results.

Now many physicians feel that much can be learned by going back over the lives of those who, in increasing numbers, are surviving to the older ages—seeking in the records of the earlier years clues to the infirmities of the later years—looking for leads to follow in efforts to make possible a closer, happier, and more comfortable approach to the biologic life span.

It may be by such methods of research or by some other method yet undeveloped that we shall find it possible to compute more exactly the relationship between habits of life and what is and what is not resisted. At present we are largely in the dark about what really happens inside to lower resistance when emotional maladjustments, for example, or mild nutritional deficiencies or accumulated fatigue seem to operate as predisposing factors in causing disease. But we do know that the body has certain definite needs, and we can rely on the trusty principle that resistance is highest when such requirements are met.

## ENJOYING THE LATER YEARS

All we have been saying is highly pertinent to the welfare of the older person, although it is rather generalized. Concrete advice can indeed be given to the man or woman who is eager for guidance about how to live healthily and happily in the later years. Much useful information is available on specific subjects in the various chapters of this book. The older person should, for example, read carefully the chapters on nutrition and losing weight. In middle age and beyond, a moderate, well-balanced diet, with avoidance of overweight, gains in importance. The older person, too, requires proper exercise. Walking and plenty of fresh air are recommended. He should develop a wide variety of hobbies, like painting, stamp collecting, carpentry, or even politics. These give pleasure and enrich leisure hours. Meeting with groups of persons in the same age range and sharing experiences with them provides a valuable and enjoyable stimulus. Taking an interest in other people—helping other people—is outranked by few pursuits as a means of making life worthwhile. The opposite is also true, for no one can be quite so unhappy as the person who concentrates on his own woes and problems. A cardinal rule of mental hygiene is to look outward.

Above all, the older person should visit his doctor regularly. From the doctor he will receive simple and sound guidance in health and hygiene, and careful examinations will reveal any conditions that are likely to result in trouble later on.

CHAPTER 27

# PRACTICAL NURSING AT HOME

**Management of the Sickroom . . . How to Equip a Sickbed . . . Other Sickroom Essentials . . . How to Make a Bed with a Patient in It . . . Moving the Patient . . . Preparing the Patient for Sleep . . . How to Take Temperature . . . Respiration and Health . . . How to Take the Pulse . . . How to Give Baths . . . How to Prevent Bedsores . . . How to Give an Enema . . . Use of Hot Water Bottle and Heating Pad . . . How to Apply Dressings . . . Compresses . . . How to Use an Ice Bag . . . Abdominal Binders . . . Vaginal Douches . . . Croup Steamer and Tent . . . How to Sterilize . . . Family Medicine Chest . . . Popular Measures . . . How to Give Medicine . . . Rules Everyone Should Follow . . . How to Make Various Solutions.**

## THE SICKROOM

THE IDEAL SICKROOM should have an adjoining bathroom, cross-ventilation, a sunny exposure, and a radiator or open fireplace. It should be as far as possible from noises and odors.

Since sunlight is essential to perfect ventilation, the room should be as sunny as possible, except in hot weather or in cases where the eyes are affected. If the sun is too bright, protect the patient's eyes with a shade, or use a screen around the bed—but let the sunlight pour into the room.

The sick person should be kept in the sunlight for brief periods each day. Direct sunshine is not only a germ killer, but it also contains ultra-violet rays, which form the highly important vitamin D in the skin—essential for growth and health.

Indirect sunshine is valuable, too, in warming and drying the air in the sickroom, especially if it contains overmuch moisture.

Excessive exposure, of course, is harmful, whether in the room or elsewhere. This is especially true if the patient is suffering from measles, because of the effect on the eyes.

***Ventilating the Sickroom.*** Artificial heat may cause dryness of the air in the room, but this condition can easily be relieved by keeping an uncovered basin of water on the radiator. The room should be aired regularly.

Open-window ventilation—natural ventilation—is the best means of providing motion and moisture in the air. Fresh air, being heavier than used air, should be introduced from below, while an escape for the impure air should be made above. This arrangement causes circulation of air.

When there are two or more windows, the one nearest the patient should be opened at the top to permit the escape of old air, while the one farthest from the patient should be opened at the bottom for the incoming fresh air. Windows on opposite sides of the room provide almost perfect ventilation without draught. If there is only one window, raise the bottom sash and lower the upper one. Regulate the spaces opened, above and below, according to the climate, the weather, or the condition of the patient.

The windows should of course be screened against flies and other insects.

***Room Temperature.*** The correct temperature for the sickroom must be judged according to the specific illness, the stage of recovery, and the patient's preference (within certain limits) concerning heat and cold. A room comfortably cool should have a temperature of 68° to 70°F.; a comfortably warm room, 75° to 80°F. For most sick persons a room temperature of 65° to 70°F. during the day, and 55° to 60°F. at night, is desirable.

## HOW TO EQUIP A SICKBED

The bed should be in such a position that the opening of a door does not cause a draught. A folding screen placed before the open window, or by the bed, may be used to keep such a current of air from the patient.

The bed should be large enough to permit the patient to rest in easy, relaxing positions. It should be fitted with a firm spring and a good mattress. If the bed is too low, it can be raised on wooden blocks about six inches high and four inches square—large enough so that there is no danger of their shifting position if the bed is moved slightly.

***Cotton Sheets.*** These should be sufficiently long and wide to tuck in well at bottom and sides.

***Blankets.*** These should be light, but sufficiently warm, and large enough to hang well over the sides of the bed, thus keeping air from getting in beneath the bedcovers. Woolen blankets, incidentally, are lighter than a mixture of cotton and wool.

***Pillows.*** The physician suggests the number of pillows which may be used. This depends mainly on the specific disease from which the patient is suffering, and his general physical condition. A patient with a heart or lung condition frequently requires a back-rest to make breathing easier. If necessary, this can be improvised with pillows supported by a small chair placed upside down in the bed.

Two or more pillows are usually needed. They should be light and soft, yet not too thin. Frequent shaking and occasional airing *in the shade* will keep them in good condition. Sunlight brings out the oil in the feathers and makes them heavy. Down pillows which are small and soft go far toward making the patient comfortable. The pillowcases should not be too large.

***Spreads.*** A cotton spread that needs no ironing makes the best cover for a sickbed.

## OTHER SICKROOM ESSENTIALS

***Smaller Equipment.*** In almost any sickroom, equipment should include: two basins, one for bathing and a smaller one for vomiting, etc.; a light-weight washable blanket; hand towels, bath towels and wash cloths; alcohol; powder; brush and comb; toothbrush and dentifrice; mouth wash; nail file and nail brush; orangewood sticks; soap; bed pan; toilet and face tissues; container of water and glasses; mouth and rectal thermometers; and drinking tubes; a call bell, if necessary.

***Light.*** There should be a good reading lamp at the bedside, above and behind the head for proper illumination, and placed where the patient can turn it on and off at will.

## HOW TO MAKE A BED FOR A PATIENT

1. Take all bed coverings off. Place the pillows and coverings on a chair.

2. Brush the uncovered mattress completely; then turn it either from top to bottom, or from side to side.

3. Place the mattress protector, if you have one, on the bed.

4. Place the bottom sheet on the mattress evenly and straight.

5. Starting at the foot, tuck the bottom sheet under the front of the mattress. Make a square corner at the head of the bed, at the side of the mattress, tucking the sheet in from head to foot.

6. Now start at the opposite side of the bed. Tighten the sheet so that it slightly bends the mattress. Now make a second square corner at the top of the mattress and tuck the sheet well under the mattress from head to foot.

7. Stand at the side of the bed and place the top sheet, wrong side up, with the large hem even with the top of the mattress. Tuck the sheet as far as it will go under the foot of the mattress. Draw the hem of the bottom sheet outward to tighten the sheet at the foot of the bed. Make square corners at the sides and tuck the sheet in.

8. Place blankets together, eight inches below the head of the mattress, fold their sides under at the foot and make square corners at the foot of the mattress. The spread covers the blankets from the top edge of the mattress, and spread and blankets are tucked under the mattress at the foot. Make square corners with the spread, on both sides at the foot of the mattress.

9. Turn the spread down over the top of the blankets and fold top sheet over the spread.

10. Put the pillows in place.

## HOW TO MAKE A BED WITH THE PATIENT IN IT

The easiest way to remake a bed is to lift the patient into another one alongside. If there is no other bed in the room, proceed as follows:

1. Take the blankets off the bed and put the top sheet over the foot of the bed. Cover the patient with a blanket, and turn him on his side facing you.

2. Loosen the bottom sheet. Push this next to the patient's back. Brush the top of the mattress, away from the patient.

3. Spread the top sheet (now to be used as the bottom sheet) right side up over the mattress, and beginning at the foot of the bed, tuck the sheet under the side of the mattress, making a square corner at the head and foot of the bed.

4. Roll the patient onto the clean sheet, on his back, and over onto his side, facing you.

5. Go to the opposite side of the bed again. Remove the old bottom sheet. Tighten the new bottom sheet and tuck it under the mattress, making square corners at the top and bottom of the bed.

Turn patient on his back. Continue as for an empty bed.

## MOVING THE PATIENT

***How to Help a Patient Into Bed.*** Assist the patient onto a footstool; he next sits on the side of the bed. Support the patient's shoulders with one arm, placing the other arm under his knees, and lift him into the bed.

***How to Turn a Patient.*** Ask the patient to bend his knees and press his heels against the mattress. Place one arm under his shoulders to the opposite armpit, the other hand under his knees. Request patient to lift his hips and help move himself at the same time that you lift him.

***Lifting a Heavy or Helpless Patient in Bed.*** In cases of injury, when the patient cannot move by himself, the help of two persons is required to move him. The two helpers stand on the same side of the bed, one placing an arm under the patient's shoulders, and the other arm under his hips. The assistant places one arm under the paitent's back, the other under his knees. The lifting is done by both at the same time.

***Moving a Patient to the Side of a Bed.*** Stand next to the bed, with one foot in front of the other; then bend your knees, keeping approximately at the level of the bed. Place your arms under the patient, and with his help, move him and yourself at the same time by the use of your arm and leg muscles. Always remember when lifting a patient to lift with your arms and not your back. This will protect you from back-strain.

***How to Prevent a Patient from Sliding Down in Bed.*** Place a pillow or folded blanket at the feet of the patient so that he can use it to brace himself when necessary. A padded box may be used for the same purpose. Also a roll-pillow (bolster) placed under the knees will prevent downward sliding.

## CARE OF THE PATIENT FOR NIGHT AND SLEEP

Wash the patient's face and hands, and brush his hair. Change his pajamas or nightgown. See that the sheets are not rumpled. Give an alcohol back-rub and dust with talcum powder. Air the pillows for a moment or two. Give mouth treatment, also bed-pan or urinal. Place an additional blanket at the foot of the bed for use in case of a change of temperature.

Place fresh water in the decanter. Dim the light in the room, and place a bell within the patient's reach.

***Mouth Care.*** Mouth hygiene plays an important part in protecting the general health of the patient. A toothpaste or powder need not be used more than once a day. It is the thorough brushing of the teeth and the rinsing of the mouth with plenty of water after every meal that does the work rather than pastes or powders.

Mouth washes are no more effective than water for cleansing purposes. The chief value lies in the pleasant taste they leave in the mouth. One-half teaspoonful of salt or one-half teaspoonful of baking soda in a glass of water makes a good, inexpensive mouth wash.

## HOW TO PLACE A PATIENT IN A WHEELCHAIR

Dress the patient in underwear, stockings, slippers, and bathrobe. Place the wheelchair at the foot of the bed. Raise the patient to a sitting positon, support his back with one arm, place the other arm under his knees, and draw his legs over the edge of the bed. Stand in front of him, place your hands under each of his armpits, and assist him onto the chair.

## HOW TO TAKE A PATIENT'S TEMPERATURE

The nurse should always wash her hands before giving any kind of nursing care. This is for the protection of both nurse and patient.

There are three ways to take a patient's temperature: (1) by mouth, with thermometer placed under the tongue, lips closed; (2) in the armpit; (3) in the rectum, inserted about one inch. Temperature taken by mouth is about a degree lower than when taken by rectum, and nearly a degree higher than when taken in the armpit.

***Normal Temperature.*** Mouth, 98.6°—two or three minutes; rectal, 99.6°—five minutes; armpit, 97.6°—ten minutes.

### How to Take Temperature by Mouth

Look at the thermometer to see just where the mercury is, hold it firmly with thumb and first two fingers (the hand slightly bent inward) and with a quick movement of the wrist downward and outward, shake it until it registers 96°F. or below. Place the thermometer under the tongue at the center, the end coming out at the corners of the lips in a slanting direction. Request the patient to close his lips and not to try to talk. Leave the thermometer in at least two minutes, even if it is marked "one minute." It will take a minute for the mouth to become even in temperature, and the other minute for the thermometer to register. Hold the thermometer horizontally between the thumb and first finger and rotate it slowly until you can see the line of mercury.

When taking temperature by mouth, be certain that the patient has had nothing hot or cold in the mouth for at least 15 minutes before the thermometer is put under the tongue; otherwise you cannot get an accurate reading. See that the lips are closed all the time the thermometer is in the patient's mouth.

Do not take temperature by mouth if the patient cannot keep the lips closed because of coughing, weakness, or difficulty in breathing; if the mouth is very dry; if he is mentally unbalanced, delirious, or unconscious; if he has had a mouth or nasal injury; if he is an infant, or a child not old enough to know how to hold the thermometer properly in the mouth. In all these circumstances, temperature should be taken in the rectum or armpit.

### How to Take Temperature in the Armpit

This is done when for any reason the mouth or rectum cannot be used. Wipe the armpit with a soft, dry wash cloth. Do not rub. Place the bulb in the center, with the end slanting toward the body, and request the patient to grasp the opposite shoulder with his hand. Prevent contact of the thermometer with clothing. Leave in place for ten minutes; then take out and read.

### How to Take Rectal Temperature

Taking the rectal temperature is the most accurate of all methods. The rectal thermometer differs from the mouth thermometer in that the bulb is usually slightly larger and is often colored. Oil the bulb of the thermometer, but never dip it directly into a jar of vaseline or oil. Let the patient turn on his side. Lift the upper fold of the buttocks with one hand while you gently insert the thermometer into the rectum about one inch. Leave the thermometer in for five minutes.

When taking the temperature of an infant or young child, hold the child on your lap face downward, lubricate the thermometer and insert it gently, slanting it toward the navel. Hold the thermometer in place for five minutes.

Do not take temperature by rectum if the patient has painful piles, or after a rectal operation.

### Care of Thermometer

Thermometers must be kept clean in some disinfectant solution such as 70 per cent alcohol. For this purpose a small glass is convenient, with a piece of soft cotton at the bottom on which to place the bulb.

After use, the mercury in the thermometer should always be shaken down, the thermometer washed with soap and *cold* water and replaced in the container.

## RESPIRATION AND HEALTH

Shallow respirations, in which little air is breathed in, are usually rapid, as in pneumonia and other diseases of the lung. Deep breaths are usually slow and are found in conditions affecting brain pressure, and in some forms of coma.

Sighing respiration may be a symptom of hemorrhage or faintness, when accompanied by other serious symptoms.

Crowing inspiration (breathing in) occurs in croup, bronchitis, and asthma and is often accompanied by wheezing.

***Rate of Normal Respirations.*** The rate of respiration is often a clue to a patient's condition. The patient's respirations should be counted when he is quiet and comfortable. Normally, his breathing should be full, easy, and without pain. Count the number of times the chest rises in one minute. Note the depth and rate of the breathing. The normal rate is: for men, 14-18 respirations in one minute; for women, 18-20 respirations in one minute; for children, 20-26 respirations in one minute; for infants, 30-38 respirations in one minute. If the respirations are markedly above or below the number normal for his condition, and there is no obvious innocent reason, notify your doctor.

## HOW TO TAKE THE PULSE

Before taking the patient's pulse, make sure his forearm and hand are in a relaxed position. Put the cushion ends of your forefinger and middle finger on the thumb side of the patient's wrist, making only as much pressure as is necessary to feel the rhythmic beat. Be sure to keep the pressure even while counting. Use a watch having a second hand; count the beat. Never use the thumb in counting the pulse beats.

In the adult the normal rate of the pulse beat will average seventy-two to seventy-five times a minute. However, many ordinary circumstances may cause increase of the rate. Thus, after eating or any excitement, the pulse beats will rise in number.

The child's pulse rate up to six months of age is normal up to 120. During the second year it averages 100; in the sixth year it averages 90. At puberty, the normal rate is about 80. A range of twenty above or below the average would not be considered abnormal unless there are other symptoms associated.

## HOW TO GIVE BATHS

Baths are given at varying temperatures from 45° to 110°F. In all instances the temperature should be taken by a thermometer and never gauged by the hand alone.

Recommended temperatures for the different kinds of baths are: hot–100° to 110°F.; warm–90° to 100°F.; tepid–80° to 90°F.; cool –65° to 80°F.; cold–45° to 65°F.

The full bath should not be given until *at least two hours* after a meal. The room temperature should be 75° to 80°, and free of drafts. In general, a face towel should be used for the face, ears and neck; a bath towel for the rest of the body.

In removing the patient's gown, take out an injured arm last. When putting on the gown after the bath, insert the injured part first.

### Bathing the Patient in Bed

Room temperature, as we have said, should be 75° to 80°F. The windows near the bed must be closed and screens placed around the bed. On a table near the bed, put a basin, soap, wash cloths, towel, alcohol and dusting powder, and a clean shirt or nightdress. Jugs of hot water and a pail should be at hand. Use two wash cloths–one for the face and arms, the other for the trunk and legs. Remove the bedclothes, leaving one blanket covering the patient. Put one bath blanket and rubber sheet (a shower curtain can be used) under the patient, and a second bath blanket over him. Remove his shirt or nightdress and the covering blanket.

Wash the face and neck, then arms and chest, following with the abdomen and legs, first one and then the other. Now turn the patient on his side and wash the back. Dry each part carefully and cover it before proceeding with the next, so that only the one part being washed is exposed.

Give special attention to cleansing the ears, nostrils, armpits, between the legs, and the navel. After the bath, powder all folds of skin. Keep the patient warm. Use an electric pad or hot water bottle during or immediately after the bath.

### How to Give a Tepid Sponge Bath

Tepid sponging is useful in relieving the restlessness resulting from fever. It also reduces the temperature, makes the patient feel fresh and more comfortable, and helps to induce sleep.

Required equipment: long rubber sheeting or shower curtain, two blankets, six to eight sponges, bath thermometer, electric pad or hot water bottles, bowls of tepid (lukewarm) water and ice. The water is gradually reduced from 90° to 70°F. by the addition of ice. First, take the patient's temperature. Then place him between blankets, with rubber sheeting or a shower curtain under the bottom blanket, and the hot water bottle or electric pad at his feet. Apply cold to his head. Wring out a large flat sponge and put it on his head, or wrap his head in a cold wet cloth. Place another cold wet cloth on the nape of the neck, and one in each arm-pit.

Sponge and dry the face; have the patient lightly clasp another sponge to cool the hand. Sponge the arm in long rhythmic strokes from the shoulder. As the sponge gets warm, cool it by putting it in iced water. Sponge the other arm in the same way; then sponge the hands in the basin. Leave the body somewhat exposed to dry by evaporation. Next, sponge the chest and abdomen with long strokes. Remove the sponges from the arm-pits, cool them in the iced water and place them in the groins. Put other sponges in the spaces behind the knee-joint.

Expose each limb in turn, and sponge first the thigh and then the leg. To sponge beneath the limb, bend the knee and support it. Lift the feet into the basin one at a time and sponge them. Do not let the patient exert himself, even to assist when you turn him over. Sponge the back with long rhythmic strokes on both sides of the spine. Sponge the shoulders and hips with semicircular strokes. Sponge the back with alcohol, and dust it with powder.

During the sponging, take the patient's temperature. The treatment should not last longer than twenty minutes and is adequate if the temperature is found to have dropped 2°F. Keep a careful watch on the pulse and on the color of the patient's face. Stop the treatment if he shivers or turns blue, or if the pulse weakens. Have brandy ready in case it is needed.

When the treatment is finished, turn the pillow and cover the patient with a cool sheet and one blanket.

### The Tepid or Lukewarm Bath (80° to 90° F.)

This has no special effect apart from cleansing. It is suitable for invalids, the elderly, convalescents, and those who do not react well to cold baths. It may be taken at any time of day, but preferably before meals and at bedtime.

### The Warm Bath (90° to 100° F.)

This is the appropriate bath for infants, and helps to prevent sleeplessness in adults when taken just before bedtime. It also is excellent after severe muscular exercise to relieve soreness and stiffness of joints and muscles. It should not be used after meals until two or three hours have elapsed, as blood may be drawn away from the stomach, with resulting digestive disturbances. It is unwise for the bather to venture into the cold air immediately after a warm bath.

The warm bath before retiring is essentially a cleansing one. The heat causes dilation of the skin blood vessels with resulting redness of the skin and increase in perspiration.

No one should remain in the tub bath, be it tepid, hot or warm, longer than half an hour. In most instances ten minutes is enough.

### The Hot Bath (100° to 110° F.)

The hot bath is unsuitable in general, except for the strong or the young, as it is depressing to the circulation. It should be used only at night, or when the bather is to stay in a warm atmosphere, and not after meals. At bedtime the hot bath may, however, cause insomnia unless a cold cloth is kept on the head during the bath. The hot bath is valuable in preventing colds after exposure and chilling, and to produce sweating in many disorders.

The hot bath should not be taken without express permission of a physician.

### Foot Baths

The objects of a foot bath are to increase the circulation in the foot or legs or to relieve congestion in another part of the body; to stimulate general blood circulation; to relax general nervous tension.

### How to Give a Foot Bath

Place the patient's feet gently in the tub. Hot water may be added after the feet are in the tub, to bring the water up to the temperature suggested by the physician. Placc a blanket over the tub so that the patient's feet are covered. At the end of the foot bath (ten to thirty minutes) lift the feet out of the tub; dry them and wrap them in a blanket.

### How to Give a Mustard Foot Bath

The proportion is one tablespoonful of mustard to one gallon of water. Dissolve the requisite amount of dry mustard in a small amount of tepid water. Stir the dissolved mustard into the full tub of water (105°F.).

## BEDSORES

The test of good nursing is in the prevention of bedsores. These may occur in any form of chronic invalidism when patients are bedridden.

Those who are ill from disturbances of the nervous system are the most likely to develop bedsores as a result of prolonged pressure on the skin over certain areas. These areas most particularly are the base of the spine, the buttocks, the shoulders and the heels.

***Prevention of Bedsores.***

1. Always remember to change the position of the chronically ill frequently.

2. Wash the back at least twice daily with a mild soap and warm water. This should also be done to any part of the body where there is pressure. Follow with an alcohol rub. Dust with a simple powder such as powdered starch or zinc stearate. Massage the soap well into the part with a circular movement.

Use only a mild soap. The alcohol should be gently massaged into the part. Cleanliness and massaging of the patient's back are of great importance. A good rub brings fresh blood to the back, thus stimulating circulation, and relieves numbness or irritation. The patient should lie on his side, and the gown should be raised to expose the whole back. If the room is cold, the back rub may be given under the blanket. Start at the neck and shoulders and move the hands down to the lower spine and buttocks, and up again to the neck. Keep the hands on the body and use long, firm, gentle strokes. The hands should be well powdered, moistened with rubbing alcohol, or lubricated with cocoa butter or olive oil. *Give special attention to the base of the spine and the buttocks.* Be sure that the nightgown is smooth and the bedclothes are in place when you are through. A back rub is particularly comforting at bedtime.

3. Prevent friction from the undersheet. This will not occur when it is kept smooth and free from creases and from crumbs in the bed. The friction may be the result of irritation from a part being left improperly dried, or from harsh soaps used on tender skins, or from soaking when there is inability to hold urine.

4. When the patient cannot control urination, special attention must be given to the prevention of bedsores. Each time the patient requires a change of sheet, wash his back well and dry it carefully. Instead of using alcohol and powder, rub some ointment in with a circular movement, but do not dust with powder, as it is apt to cake into a hard mass on the ointment. Use lanolin or zinc ointment.

5. If the skin is reddened or is broken, consult your doctor about the treatment at once. Watchful expectancy should guide nursing in all such cases.

### Appliances for Relieving Pressure in Bed

In preventing bedsores, rubber rings and pillows, cotton rings and pads, or soft and hard pillows may be used to relieve pressure. The rubber rings are on sale at drugstores.

Select a rubber ring of the proper size for the patient, as it must fit comfortably. Inflate the ring until it is hard enough to stand the pressure from the body and yet not so hard that it will itself cause pressure. Cover the ring with a bandage, pillowcase, or wide strips of old muslin, so that the flesh never comes in contact with the rubber. Place it under the patient in such a way that the end of the spine, where the pressure is greatest, will come over the opening in the ring. Keep the covering of the ring clean and dry, changing it as often as necessary.

To make a cotton batting ring or pad, form pieces of cotton into rings and cover with a bandage or strips of muslin. Fasten end firmly by a few stitches. Cotton rings are used to relieve pressure on small parts such as the heels, ankles, elbows, etc., and the opening should be made larger than the part to be relieved.

Pillows can be used to relieve pressure by placing them under the shoulders, hips and elbows, in the hollow of the back, and between the knees. They are also helpful for elevating an inflamed limb. Two to four are usually required, depending on the degree of elevation desired. Place the pillows lengthwise, one upon another, in "step fashion" and arranged so as to form an incline up to the thigh or armpit. If there are dressings or wet compresses on the leg, protect the pillowcase by a small rubber sheet covered with a towel.

## HOW TO GIVE AN ENEMA

***Enemas for Infants and Children.*** During some illnesses of infants, as of older children and adults, it is safer to give an enema than a cathartic by mouth. However, in the case of abdominal pains, an enema should be used only on the advice of a physician.

For an infant or small child it is best to use a rubber ear syringe with a soft rubber tip. The bulb should be completely filled so that no air remains within it. The tip should be covered with cold cream, soap, or vaseline, and inserted an inch or two. The injection should be carried out slowly. For older children an enema-bag or an enema-can is usable, with a rubber tube and a narrow, hard, rubber tip. The bag should be placed not more than one to two feet above the level of the buttocks.

***Enemas for Adults.*** The usual enema for adults with soapsuds consists of one to two quarts, given with the rectal tube inserted three to four inches. Open the stop-cock and let some water run through first to expel air bubbles. Never use force in inserting a rectal tube.

***Cleansing Enema.*** This is generally prescribed at the end of an attack of diarrhea. For a cleansing enema, use tap water or a mild salt solution—one pint for a child, three to four pints for an adult; temperature, 100° to 105°F. Allow solution to run slowly from can or rubber bag hung about sixteen inches above the patient's head, through a well-lubricated rectal tip or tube, inserted from three to five inches into the rectum. Stop flow occasionally, especially if patient complains of pain, to permit him to rest. Instruct him to retain enema solution from five to ten minutes, if possible, to insure good results.

***Emollient (Softening) Enema.*** A softening enema is used in constipation. All that is required is olive oil, six ounces, to be retained over night.

***Glycerin Enema.*** This is used to get a bowel movement directly. It consists of Epsom salts, one ounce; glycerin, two ounces; water, three ounces. Retain as long as possible; repeat if necessary. This enema will cause expulsion of most fecal matter. One may also use simple mixtures of glycerin and water without Epsom salts. This type of enema may be painful if hemorrhoids or other inflammatory conditions are present.

## HOW TO ADJUST A BED-PAN

Place a small pad of cotton or folded towel over the seat of the bed-pan if the patient is very thin or old. Always be gentle. Never push the pan roughly under the patient. For a stout person, or moist skin, powder both the patient and the pan. Do not leave the patient too long on the hard surface of the bed-pan or douche-pan. Always warm the pan before using.

## HOW TO USE A HOT WATER BOTTLE

Always press the air from the hot water bottle before starting to fill it. Then only *half fill* it with very hot, *not boiling,* water; fold over the upper half of the bottle to expel any remaining air, and cork quickly. Hold the bottle upside down to make sure it is tightly corked, dry it, and cover it before placing it next to the patient. Be very careful not to burn the patient. This can happen in chronic cases where the skin resistance is low.

## HOW TO USE HEATING PADS

Always keep the pad dry. It should not be used when there is excessive perspiration or other moisture, as it may cause a shock. Never stick safety pins in the pad to keep it in place. To keep the pad in good condition, do not pull it by the cord from one place to another, as the wire connections of the heating elements may thus be broken. Do not fold the pad, or hang it by the cord in a closet. It is best to keep it in the box. *And above all, never let the patient go to sleep with a heating pad still connected.*

## HOW TO APPLY DRESSINGS

A dressing is any covering which can be applied to an injured or diseased part of the body. Dressings may be used: (1) to cover a wound and prevent contamination from dirt or disease germs; (2) to prevent inflammation; (3) to relieve pain; (4) to reduce swelling; (5) to arrest bleeding by pressure on a wound.

***Wound Dressings.*** Good wound dressings are those that will dry-sterilize easily, and absorb wound discharges well. They prevent infection and harm from without, and help in keeping the patient quiet through limiting his motion.

Almost all wound dressings consist either solely of gauze or of a mixture of gauze and cotton, the gauze always coming directly next to, or on, the wound. Dressings may be plain, sterile, or antiseptically medicated. All dressings which go next to the wound are sterile, and as a rule, all such dressings should be sterile throughout. They can be purchased at any drugstore. They cannot be prepared in the home.

***Dry and Wet Dressings.*** Dressings may be applied dry or wet. Wet dressings include hot compresses which are used to relieve pain, to reduce inflammation and to prevent death of tissue; cold compresses also relieve pain, reduce swelling, and lessen bleeding. Saline dressings, as the name denotes, are made with salt in the proportion of one teaspoonful of salt to each pint of water. The lotion should be sterilized whenever possible before use. Antiseptic dressings are sometimes used in place of dry dressings to avoid having them stick to the skin. An effective dressing of this sort is made with sulfanilamide. Sometimes the powdered drug is dusted on the wound, but only by doctor's order.

## HOW TO APPLY HOT WET DRESSINGS

***Articles Needed for Hot Wet Dressing.*** Sheet wadding or absorbent cotton; oil-silk or light-weight oilcloth; towel; dressing towel; basin; solution; pitcher.

***Wet-Dressing Procedure.*** Fill pitcher with solution at required temperature. Place towel or stupe wringer over the basin with ends hanging over the edge. Place pad of gauze on towel. Pour solution over pad until saturated. Take ends of the towel and twist tightly in opposite directions, wringing as dry as possible. Open towel, remove pad, and place quickly on the affected area. Cover with sheet wadding and oil-silk to maintain heat and moisture. Cover with towel and fasten with safety pin. An abdominal binder (page 463) made of a broad piece of muslin will keep the dressing in place.

## HOW TO MAKE AND APPLY COMPRESSES (STUPES)

***Articles Needed for Making a Compress.*** Flannel, two- or three-fold thickness; basin; wringer (small clean towel will do); boiling water; oiled silk (or oiled muslin or lightweight oilcloth).

Fold flannel in wringer and place in basin, leaving ends hanging. Cover with boiling water. Wring as dry as possible, shake to free from steam, and apply gently to part. Cover quickly with wool cloth and either oiled silk, oiled muslin or oilcloth. This type of compress should be changed frequently. It does not have to be held in place.

### Turpentine Compress

This compress is used on direction of the physician. Sprinkle one-half to three-quarters teaspoonful of turpentine over a piece of flannel folded in a wringer. Pour on boiling water and wring as dry as possible. Shake, apply, cover with flannel. The edge must be lifted after five or ten minutes to note whether skin is reddening. After skin is red, remove. Watch carefully. Blistering easily occurs.

### How to Apply Cold Compresses

To apply a cold compress, use three layers of old linen or gauze, wrung out of water about 60° F., so that it is not dripping. Cover compress with thin piece of flannel. Change every hour. After compress is removed, warm the skin by gentle rubbing or by covering with flannel.

### Eye Compresses

On eyes that are discharging, use compress only once; discard in paper bag. Use firm but gentle touch. Avoid pressure on the eyeballs. Treatments should not last longer than twenty minutes—one hour apart. Have a tray covered with clean towel, six or more oval pads, 2 x 1½ inches; bowl for ice (cover ice with gauze); face towel; cotton balls; solution; paper bag; safety pin; small basin. Move patient to the edge of the bed and have him lie on his back. Remove all pillows but one, unless he has difficulty in breathing. Attach paper bag to

# Care of the Baby

A baby's well-being depends mostly on his mother. He needs love almost as much as food.

## COD-LIVER OIL

This oil, rich in vitamin D, helps bones grow. The amount to give depends on your baby's age.

## SOLID FOOD

Nowadays, solid food is introduced in the first half year. Cereals, easily digested, are a good starter, and some precooked ones are vitamin-enriched. Baby may rebel at his new food, so be patient with him.

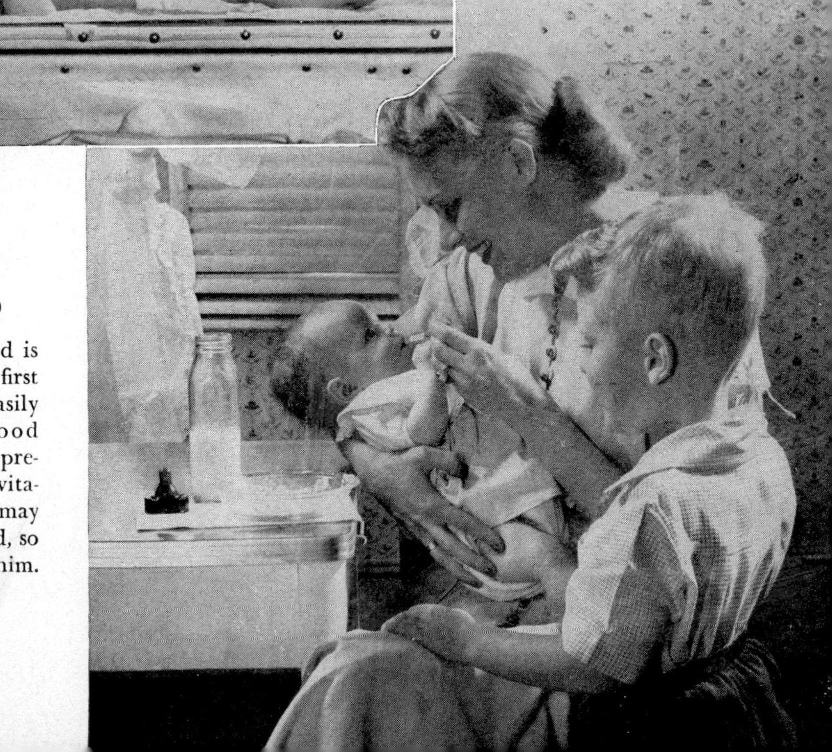

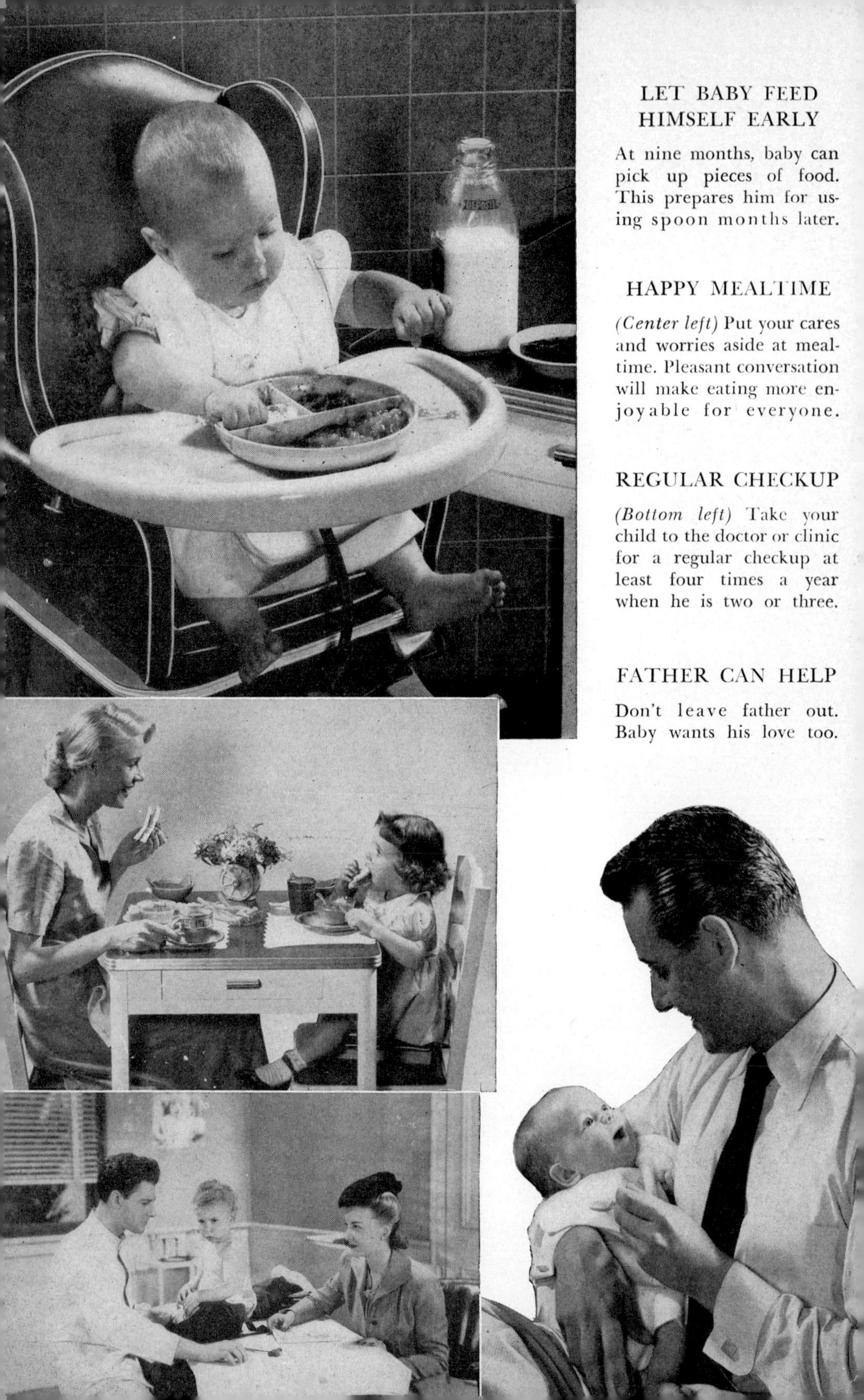

LET BABY FEED HIMSELF EARLY

At nine months, baby can pick up pieces of food. This prepares him for using spoon months later.

HAPPY MEALTIME

*(Center left)* Put your cares and worries aside at mealtime. Pleasant conversation will make eating more enjoyable for everyone.

REGULAR CHECKUP

*(Bottom left)* Take your child to the doctor or clinic for a regular checkup at least four times a year when he is two or three.

FATHER CAN HELP

Don't leave father out. Baby wants his love too.

bedside with safety pin. Place towel across patient's chest. With clean cotton moistened in the solution, remove any eye discharge, moving in the direction of the nose. Fold compress once, moisten with solution, place on ice; when thoroughly chilled, place on the eye. Change compresses every half minute and oftener if necessary. Dry the eye and face; be sure to leave the patient comfortable and the bedside in order.

## HOW TO USE AN ICE-BAG

Fill ice-bag half full with ice broken into small pieces. Drain the water off. Expel the air, screw the lid on firmly, and invert the bag to test for any leaks. Dry the outside of the bag, and place an outside cover on it. The ice must be renewed as soon as it is melted.

## HOW TO APPLY AN ABDOMINAL BINDER

The abdominal binder is utilized to hold pads, poultices, ice-caps, or stupes (compresses) in place, and to exert pressure after the birth of a child.

The binder is usually made of a straight, doubled piece of unbleached muslin, wide enough to extend from the waistline to the region of the pubic hair (private parts) and long enough to encircle the patient completely, leaving a margin in front for pinning.

The binder is first slipped under the hips, and brought down to the pubic region. The ends are adjusted, not too tightly, to fit the body. The fastening is begun at the bottom, working upward. The edge of the folds and the safety pins should make a straight line up the center of the abdomen.

## HOW TO GIVE A VAGINAL IRRIGATION OR DOUCHE

This is sometimes indicated in inflammatory conditions, or where there is pain or congestion; also, in the case of discharges. A vaginal irrigation should not be given when the patient is menstruating or pregnant; nor immediately after childbirth.

A general cleansing douche (about two quarts) should have a temperature of 100° F. For inflammatory conditions, the douche may consist of from two quarts to two gallons, at 100° F.

***Solutions for Vaginal Douche.*** Solutions which may be used are: sterile water; normal salt solution—teaspoonful to a quart; boric acid solution—five level teaspoonfuls of boric acid powder to one quart of water; bicarbonate of soda solution—2½ level teaspoonfuls of the powder to two quarts of water.

***Equipment for Vaginal Douche.*** Equipment should consist of: douche bag; douche nozzle; bath thermometer; large bath blanket; pitcher; cotton balls for wiping; small basin. For a cleansing douche, the equipment must be clean, but not necessarily sterile.

Hang the douche bag on the level of the vagina, never higher. Too much pressure may carry an infection up into the uterine cavity. The patient should lie on her back.

## HOW TO ARRANGE CROUP STEAMER AND A CROUP TENT

The treatment of croup is the same as that of a cold. Hot or cold wet compresses should be applied around the throat. (For an acute attack give syrup of ipecac.) Steam inhalations are given from a teakettle of water to which one-half teaspoonful compound tincture of benzoin, menthol or eucalyptus should be added. These must often be continued for many different hours, sometimes on successive days. Keep the child in a warm room—the smaller the better.

***Making the Croup Tent.*** The articles required are: a wooden frame; blankets; linen covering; electric hot plate; teakettle. Place the wooden frame around the head of the bed. Cover with blankets and place linen covering over the blankets. Leave side near bedside table open. Connect electric hot plate. Put water and medication in the croup kettle and place on hot plate. Extend spout of kettle into the opening at the side of the bed.

## HOW TO STERILIZE ARTICLES

Heat, in some form, is the most effective sterilizing agent. Boiling water is the most universally available form of utilizing heat, killing all varieties of germs. Allow water to boil for five minutes with the articles to be sterilized already in the container. The temperature should be 212° F.

## THE FAMILY MEDICINE CHEST

The family medicine chest should contain bandages, adhesive tape, vaseline, zinc oxide ointment, mercurochrome or tincture of metaphen, boric acid, aspirin, aromatic spirits of ammonia, hydrogen peroxide, thermometers (mouth and rectal), an electric pad, an ice-bag, and a first-aid kit.

### Rules Which Should Never Be Broken

1. Keep all medicines, lotions, liniments, etc., under lock and key.
2. Keep all poisons in a place separate from medicines.
3. Keep all poisons plainly labeled as such.
4. Keep all drugs intended for *external use only* in a separate place and have them labeled as such, in addition to any poison label they may have. If only one medicine cupboard is available, keep the drugs for external use on a separate shelf.
5. *Never* keep any drug without a proper label, and make sure the correct dose is marked on it.
6. *Never* give any medicine, or use any drug internally, without first re-reading the label, no matter how often you may use the bottle.
7. Never leave a medicine bottle uncorked. Evaporation of an essential ingredient may render the drug useless, or even turn it into a dangerous concentrate.
8. Never leave the medicine cupboard unlocked.

## POPULAR MEASURES AND THEIR EQUIVALENTS

| | | |
|---|---|---|
| 1 drop | 1 minim | 0.05 cc. |
| 1 teaspoonful | 1 fluid drachm | 4 cc. |
| 1 dessertspoonful | 2 fluid drachms | 8 cc. |
| 1 tablespoonful | 4 fluid drachms | 15 cc. |
| 1 wineglassful | 2 fluid ounces | 60 cc. |
| 1 teacupful | 4 fluid ounces | 125 cc. |
| 1 tumblerful | 8 fluid ounces | 200 cc. |
| 1 pint | 16 fluid ounces | 500 cc. |
| 1 quart | 32 fluid ounces (1 liter) | 1000 cc. |

4 teaspoonfuls = ½ ounce or 1 tablespoonful
2 tablespoonfuls = 1 ounce

## METRIC AND APOTHECARY MEASURES

| *Metric* | *Approximate Apothecary Equivalent* |
|---|---|
| 1 cc. | 15 minims |
| 2 cc. | 30 minims |
| 3 cc. | 45 minims |
| 4 cc. | 1 fluid drachm |
| 5 cc. | 1¼ fluid drachms |
| 8 cc. | 2 fluid drachms |
| 10 cc. | 2½ fluid drachms |
| 15 cc. | ½ fluid ounce |
| 30 cc. | 1 fluid ounce |
| 50 cc. | 1¾ fluid ounces |
| 100 cc. | 3½ fluid ounces |
| 200 cc. | 7 fluid ounces |
| 250 cc. | 8 fluid ounces |
| 500 cc. | 1 pint |
| 750 cc. | 1½ pints |
| 1000 cc. | 1 quart |

## HOW TO GIVE MEDICINE

Medicine given by mouth is in one or the other of the following forms: liquid, powder, pills, or tablets.

Note the label, shake the bottle, measure the dose accurately, give it to the patient, and see that it is swallowed. A small drink of water will take away an unpleasant taste, or the medicine may be taken through a glass tube or a straw.

Use measuring glass or spoon marked in drachms or ounces, or with the words "teaspoon," "dessertspoon," or "tablespoon," or spoons specified.

As in feeding, the patient's head and shoulders should be well raised before the dose is given. Powders may be mixed with water. Pills, tabloids, and tablets can be swallowed more easily if the patient is given some water at the same time.

## HOW TO MAKE VARIOUS SOLUTIONS

When a doctor orders a saturated solution of a dry drug, he means all the drug the water can hold without powder or crystals collecting at the bottom of the container.

***Baking Soda.*** Add two or three heaping tablespoonfuls of baking soda to one quart of warm water which has been boiled and cooled.

***Salt Solutions for Swelling.*** Add three heaping tablespoonfuls of table salt to one quart of hot water which has been boiled and cooled.

***Epsom Salts.*** Add six heaping tablespoonfuls of Epsom salts to one quart of hot boiled water.

CHAPTER 28

# FIRST AID

**How to Prevent Accidents . . . Accidents to the Aged . . . How to Treat Bruises and "Blood Tumor" . . . Various Kinds of Wounds and Their Routine Treatment . . . The Tourniquet and Its Uses . . . How to Treat Burns . . . Chemical Burns . . . Electricity Burns . . . Scalds . . . Strains . . . Sprains and Their Care . . . Dislocations . . . Fractures or Broken Bones . . . First Aid for All Fractures . . . Head Injuries . . . Different Types of Bandages and How to Apply Them . . . Heat Stroke . . . Electric Shock . . . How to Rescue a Person Shocked by Electricity . . . How to Give Artificial Respiration . . . Freezing . . . Frostbite . . . Chilblains . . . Poisons Taken by Mouth . . . Insect Bites . . . Animal Bites . . . Poisoning by Plants . . . Food Poisoning . . . "Ptomaine Poisoning" . . . Botulism . . . Mushroom Poisoning . . . Death Cup . . . Poison Sprays on Fruit (Arsenic and Lead), etc.**

*How to Prevent Accidents.* In the past several years, accidents have ranked fourth as the cause of incapacity and death. The number of accidental deaths in the United States has reached almost one hundred thousand a year. One-third of these fatalities occur in persons over sixty-five years of age. Nearly 50 per cent of all accidents occur within the home.

*Accident Hazards.* There are many accident hazards in the home. These include, for example, extra-length telephone cords, long extension wires, small scatter rugs on highly polished floors, too much furniture, and bath tubs that have no rubber mats to prevent slipping. With such hazards present, it is all too easy to catch the foot or heel in the wires, and bump against unnecessarily exposed objects. Then, too, there are in every home sharp household implements such as kitchen knives and can openers, which, if not handled carefully, can cause serious harm. The useful stepladder is a very great offender too. Numerous injuries occur as a result of falls from these when people are hanging draperies or are outside the home, trimming trees or cleaning drain pipes. Most of the accidents are due either to overconfidence or pure carelessness, and are entirely preventable.

*Accidents to the Aged.* These are more likely to happen because of the "slowing up" which comes with advancing years, such as impaired vision and hearing, decreased alertness and decrease in muscular activity. A mental quirk in many old people makes them stubbornly refuse to take advice, often to the point of doing exactly the opposite of what they should, and again the toll of accidents mounts.

Much can be done to prevent accidents among the aged and others.

## GENERAL PRINCIPLES OF FIRST AID

Keep cool.
Work fast, but carefully.
Keep the injured person quiet, warm, and comfortable.
Loosen tight clothing, collar, waistband, and belt.
Keep the crowd away, but, if necessary, select a capable person or two to help you.

Obtain medical aid quickly—phone the doctor, get someone to call him, or get the injured person to doctor or to hospital.

Avoid letting the injured person see his own injury, and in severe cases do not let him know how badly he is hurt.

Always treat the most dangerous condition first; for example, stop bleeding before attending to a fracture.

If the injured person vomits, lower his head and turn it to one side, so that the vomited material may not go into the lungs.

---

1. Don't allow bleeding to go unchecked.
2. Don't overlook shock.
3. Don't fail to give artificial respiration when needed.
4. Don't fail to remove false teeth, tobacco, and chewing gum from the mouth of an unconscious person.
5. Don't attempt to give an unconscious person anything to drink.
6. Don't touch a wound with your fingers.
7. Don't burn the injured person with an unwrapped hot-water bottle or other heated object.
8. Don't allow the injured person with a fracture or suspected fracture to be moved until splints have been applied.
9. Do not aggravate injury by unnecessary movements.

Do not leave extra-length wires exposed. Take up slippery rugs, and do not leave objects in the middle of the floor after dark. Be sure that your stair carpet has no holes and is not loose on any of the treads. Spread salt or gravel on icy walks and steps outside your house.

## BRUISES

***Causes of Bruises.*** Bruises are also called contusions. They are often caused by blows or the impact of blunt objects. Although the skin is not penetrated in contused wounds, there may be considerable crushing of the tissues beneath the skin.

***Blood Tumor.*** At times the muscle may be injured and a large "lump" will result. This is due to a swelling of the muscle fibres and infiltration of blood into the muscle. Then, again, one or more small blood vessels may be ruptured nearer the surface and produce a hemorrhage under the skin. This is called a hematoma or tumor of blood. It is, of course, not a real tumor (the word tumor means a swelling), but it may be so large that a doctor will have to make an incision to remove the clot.

***Treatment of Bruises.*** A severe contusion may incapacitate the person for days or even weeks, requiring complete rest in bed until the pain subsides. Application of heat by an electric pad or hot compresses will help. However, cold compresses may also be used if more agreeable to the patient. Never use massage, as it will do more harm than good.

## WOUNDS

***Kinds of Wounds.*** An open wound is one in which the skin is cut or torn, exposing the tissues beneath. According to its severity it is

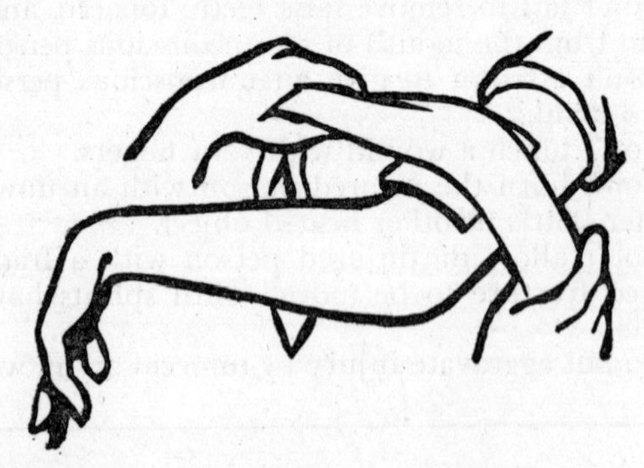

BANDAGING A MINOR WOUND

After applying an antiseptic, such as mercurochrome, place a piece of sterile gauze over the wound and bandage securely.

called (1) an abrasion, which is very superficial; (2) an incised wound, which may be of any depth and leaves a clean-cut, smooth edge; (3) lacerated, which means a wound with a jagged edge, such as may be caused by stepping on an upturned garden implement, or (4) a punctured wound, such as may be caused by running a nail into your foot or running the point of an ice pick into your hand.

***Gunshot Wounds.*** A gunshot wound is a penetrating wound made by a bullet or shell fragment striking a body at a high velocity. The point of entrance of such a bullet or fragment is much smaller than its area of exit when it passes through the body completely.

***How to Treat Gunshot Wounds.*** Tetanus toxoid is given, and the wound is covered with sterile dressings. The first-aider should not try to wash out deep wounds, lest bleeding be started again. Authorities differ as to the healing value of sulfonamides in wounds, but, if available, three to ten grams of sulfanilamide or sulfadiazine may be sprinkled on the wound at the direction of the physician; the precise amount is determined by the size of the wound.

***Blast Wounds.*** These wounds are caused by the detonation of high explosives near the body. No external wound is detected but the patient suffers from multiple hemorrhages from the lungs, as a result of the positive or negative pressure, depending upon the distance of the body from the explosion. The victim must be quickly hospitalized.

## ROUTINE TREATMENT OF WOUNDS

***Bleeding.*** The adequate control of bleeding is the first consideration. Any cut around the face or scalp will bleed profusely because of the rich blood supply of these areas. The bleeding is controlled by pressure with any clean cloth or gauze available. After the bleeding slows down—this can be determined by gently releasing the pressure—try to bring the two edges of the wound together temporarily with adhesive plaster and again make pressure.

If the gash is long and the bleeding profuse, a doctor should be called at once or, better still, the patient should go to a nearby hospital. It may be necessary to take stitches to close the cut. As long as pressure is continued, the bleeding cannot become serious—that is, there will not be enough blood lost to endanger life.

***Control of Severe Bleeding.*** Should you have no bandage available, you can control arterial bleeding in the limbs and in certain other parts of the body, if you know how and where to apply finger pressure. If, for example, the bleeding is from the right arm, stand on the person's injured side, facing as he does, and grasp his upper right arm with your left hand. Your fingers should sink into the space on the inner side of the arm between the muscle in the front and the muscle in the back of the arm. Your thumb presses against the outer

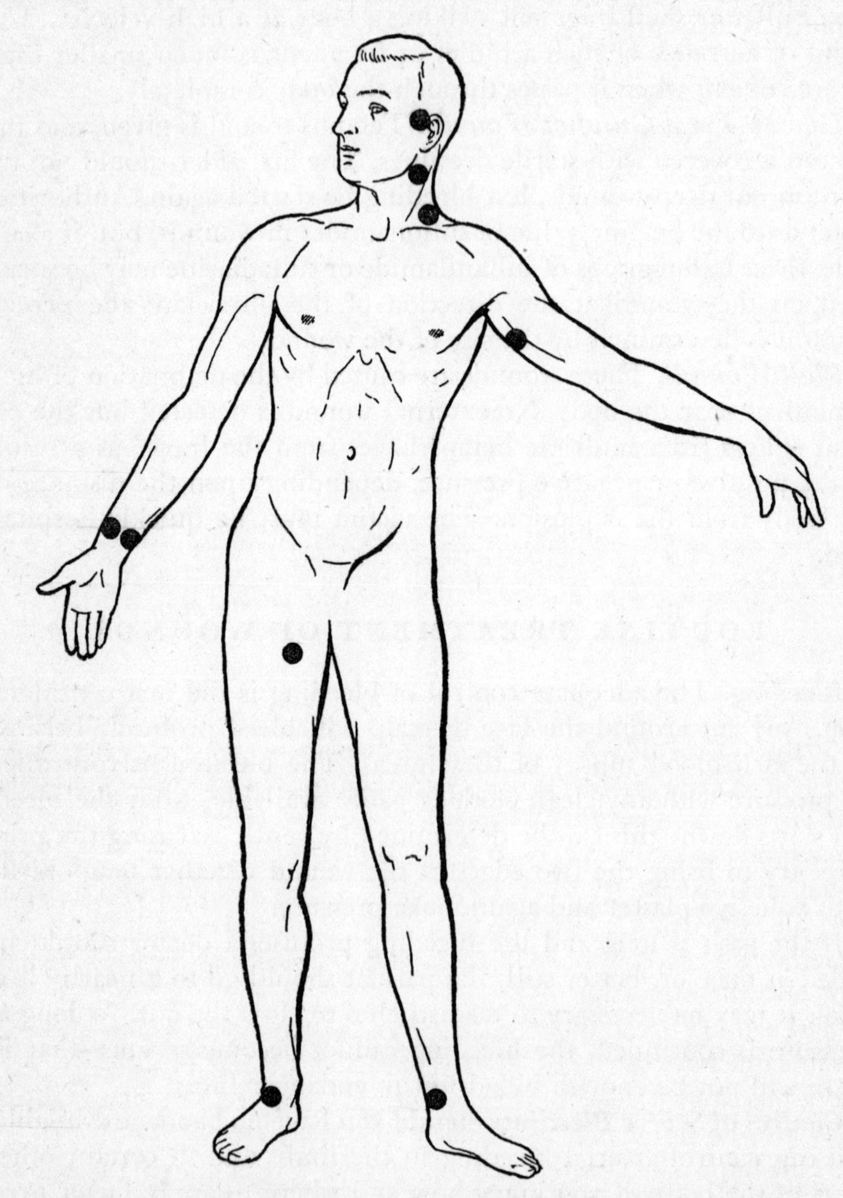

FINGER-PRESSURE AREAS TO STOP BLEEDING

Dots indicate areas for finger-pressure control of bleeding from some main arteries. The dot on the thigh is the exception—here apply a tourniquet, since the artery is too deeply situated beneath the muscles to be compressed.

side of the arm, the arm is tightly held between your fingers and thumb, compressing the artery against the bone.

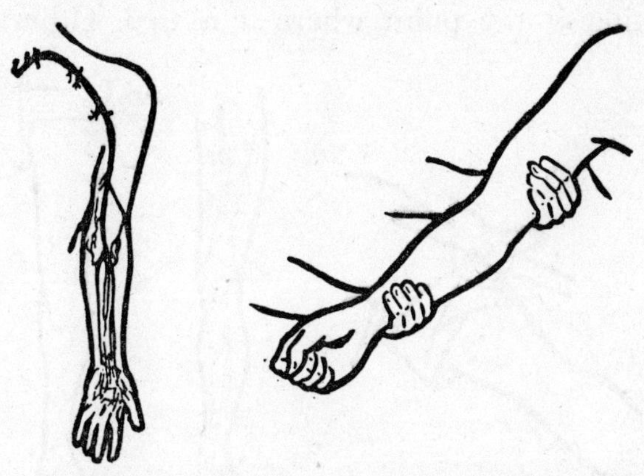

CONTROL OF ARM BLEEDING

(*Left*) Showing the course of the main arteries of the arm and shoulder. (*Right*) To control bleeding from the arm, press with your fingers the inner side of the arm below the armpit.

### The Tourniquet and Its Uses

If the cut involves one of the large arteries of the arm, wrist, finger, leg or foot, hemorrhage is best controlled by constricting the member just above the cut. This is what is called using the tourniquet. The tourniquet is necessary when the bleeding is taking place in spurts. That means an artery has been severed—if it is a large one the patient can bleed to death quickly. Arterial blood is bright red in color. Profuse oozing of dark blood means venous bleeding and can usually be controlled by pressure.

For a tourniquet, any cordlike contrivance will do. The most desirable one is a piece of small-calibre rubber tubing. However, a necktie, a piece of toweling or sheet torn into a strip will do. Tourniquets may also be purchased ready-made at a drugstore.

The improvised tourniquet should be long enough to take two turns around the arm before it is tied on the outer side of the limb. Use a square knot; it holds well and is easy to loosen. Through one of the knots thrust a stick or a pencil or any object that will make it possible for you to twist the knot till the bleeding comes under control: after this your fingers may be removed. Do not use a wire or rope for a tourniquet, as with these there is a great danger of seriously injuring the tissues. The use of a pad under the tourniquet adds greatly to its effectiveness.

A tourniquet must not be left in place longer than fifteen minutes without relaxing at the point where it is tied. Otherwise there is

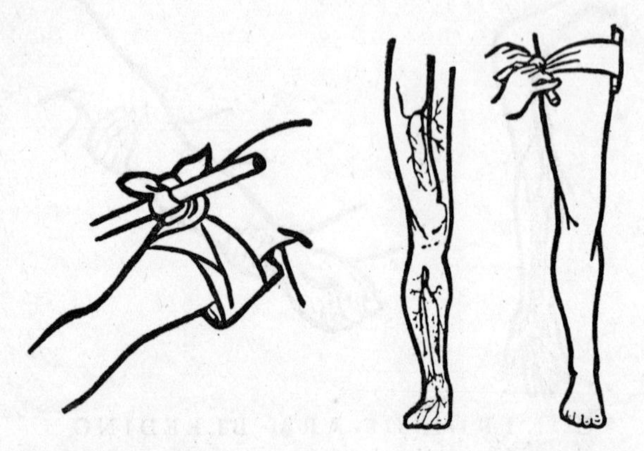

TOURNIQUET FOR ARM AND LEG

(*Left*) Showing a tourniquet for the upper arm. (*Right*) Course of the main arteries of the leg, and how to apply a tourniquet for the thigh.

danger of injury to the blood vessels blocked off. If the bleeding starts again, pull again on the constrictor. Get to a doctor as soon as possible so that he can quickly tie off the bleeding artery.

### Disinfection

After the bleeding is under control, the next thought should be directed toward disinfection. The best all-around antiseptic that is usually available in every household is rubbing alcohol. Pour this generously over any cut. There is only one exception to this—if the cut is on a young child. Alcohol stings very markedly, so as a substitute use solution of mercurochrome. It has only one objection: it is messy and permanently stains whatever it comes in contact with.

Never use any antiseptic powder or ointment. Either will seal up the wound and cause a scab formation which is a perfect invitation for infection.

### Anti-tetanic Serum

Last, but by no means of lesser importance, is the administration of anti-tetanic serum. This is to prevent lockjaw, which is usually

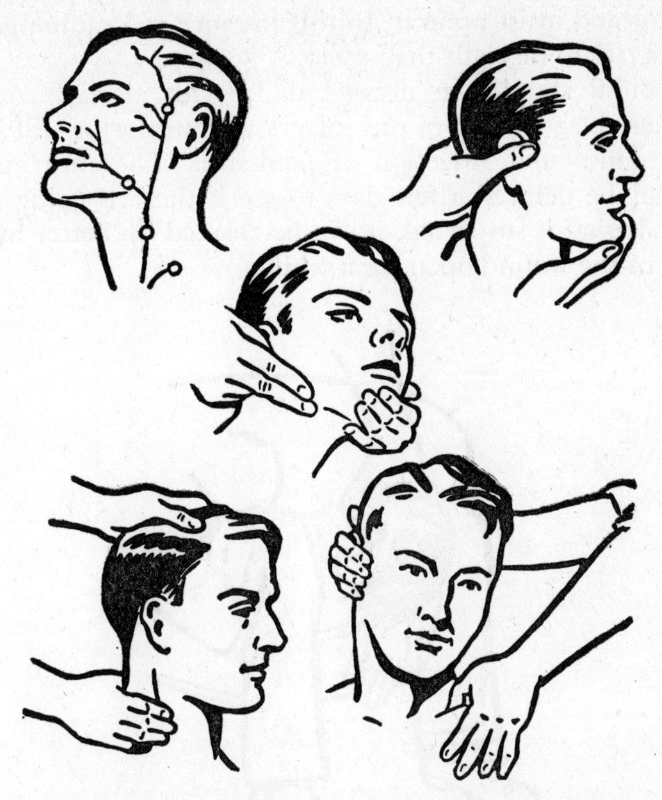

HOW TO CONTROL BLEEDING FROM THE HEAD, NECK, AND SHOULDERS

(*Top Left*) Showing the points at which to control bleeding by finger pressure. (*Top Right*) To control bleeding from the scalp or forehead, press your thumb in front of the opening of the ear on the side of bleeding. (*Center*) For bleeding from the face, press the side of the lower jaw in front of the angle of the jaw bone. (*Bottom Left*) In case of bleeding from the neck or a cut throat, place your fingers on the neck beside the windpipe and press toward the backbone. (*Bottom Right*) For bleeding from the shoulder or armpit, tip the head toward the injured side and press down with your thumb at the side of the neck.

fatal. Anti-tetanic serum cannot be given by anyone except a physician. It has to be given in broken doses in order to avoid the possibility of an allergic reaction. The use of a serum is vital in all cases of wounds from implements that may be contaminated by dirt, especially manure. Manure and dirt harbor the tetanus spores and bacilli. If your doctor does not suggest giving the serum, you suggest it to your doctor and insist upon it. In this instance you cannot go wrong, and it is better to be right than sorry.

The wound should be dressed daily with alcohol compresses. Should there be any signs of pus infection, your doctor will probably advise intramuscular injection of penicillin. The suturing of the wound may be delayed a few days to see if there is going to be an infection. If that is suspected, it can be cleaned up better by leaving the edges of the wound open for a while.

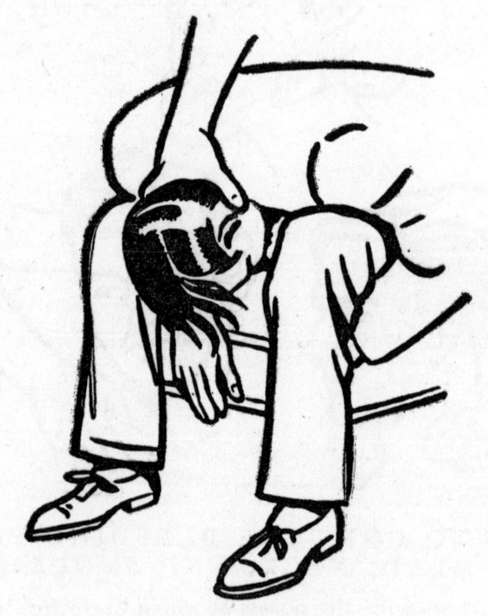

HOW TO PREVENT FAINTING

To prevent fainting, bend the head between the knees till the feeling of giddiness goes away.

## BURNS

It is estimated that there are annually in the United States six thousand deaths from accidental burns and scalds. Forty per cent of these are in persons under fifteen years of age. The rate is lower in the summer months because children spend more time out of doors. In winter children are exposed to such accidents as are encountered in connection with stoves, hot water and matches.

Scalds are the principal cause of accidental burns. To prevent these burns, babies and young children should be kept away from contact with boiling water, hot radiators and other potential danger spots such as open grate fireplaces.

***Degrees of Severity of Burns.*** *First degree*—the surface of the skin is scorched, but there is no actual destruction of tissues. The burn appears red and inflamed.

*Second degree*—the two main layers of the skin are separated and fluid collects between them, producing a blister.

*Third degree*—there is injury to the deeper layers of the skin.

*Fourth degree*—the whole thickness of the skin is destroyed, and the underlying tissue, for example, fat and muscle, becomes visible.

*Fifth and sixth degrees*—These comprise all subsequent degrees of severity, including burning of the muscles and bone.

### Treatment of Burns

In extensive burns every effort should be made to get professional medical attention. The special reason for this is the urgency of treating the most serious symptom of shock which always accompanies extensive burns. Unless there is rapid administration of blood plasma by intravenous injection, the patient will die very quickly. Pending the arrival of a physician, the body should be kept warm. If the patient is conscious, give copiously of strong hot coffee. Should there be any delay in getting a physician, get the patient to a hospital quickly.

A picric acid gauze such as can be had in the drugstore may be used to cover the wound and prevent contact with the air, which is painful. Moisten the gauze with warm water and apply it to the burn several layers thick.

If the burn occurs at home, soak sterile gauze in a warm solution of baking soda, made by adding two or three heaping tablespoonfuls of baking powder to a quart of water. (Do not use *hot* water, for that will change the baking soda into washing soda, which is not an antiseptic and will not do the burn any good.) The burned area should be bandaged with thick layers of gauze soaked in the soda solution and the person covered with blankets to keep him warm until the physician arrives.

There is only one kind of burn that you can safely treat alone—a small first or second degree burn which does not destroy much of the body tissue. This kind of burn is seldom accompanied by shock.

In the case of small surface burns it is important to relieve pain. Immerse the burned part in cool water, or apply cold wet compresses for quick relief. Next the first cleansing should be done, if advisable. Fine mesh gauze with some bland ointment on it can be applied. A firm secure dressing should be put on and changed from time to time.

There are, of course, many other ways of treating burns. For example, the burned area may be thoroughly cleansed, and the burned surface covered with a sterile dressing of vaseline gauze. Over the dressing, a large fluff dressing of gauze or cotton waste is applied, and a pressure bandage is placed over it, ordinarily one of the all-cotton elastic bandages. This dressing is left in place for ten days to two weeks, unless the temperature rises to over one hundred degrees Fahrenheit.

## CHEMICAL BURNS

Chemical burns resemble heat burns in most respects. As a first step in treatment, remove the chemical with a large amount of water. The water may be applied by a shower, hose or any other means that will supply it in quantity. It must be sufficient for its cooling effect to overcome the heat of dilution of the chemical. Otherwise a thermal burn may be produced.

### Phosphorus Burns

For phosphorus burns, use about one teaspoonful of sodium bicarbonate to a pint of water and 2 per cent copper sulphate solution. Just before using, mix the solution in a bowl in roughly equal quantities.

### Burns Caused by Strong Mineral Acids or by Alkalies

If acids are the cause, the skin should not be washed at first, but either chalk, whiting, or some mild alkali, as baking soda, should be strewn over the burn. Then, after the effect of the acid is neutralized, wash off the soda with stream of warm water. Dry gently with gauze. Apply Carron oil or paste of boric acid and vaseline, equal parts. These can be had at the drugstore. If strong alkalies have been spilled on the skin, as ammonia, potash, or quicklime, vinegar is the proper substance to employ, followed by washing. Dry gently. Vaseline or cold cream is usually sufficient as after-treatment. Limewater or castor oil is useful in counteracting the effect of acids spattered in the eye. In the case of alkalies in the eye, the vinegar used should be diluted with three parts of water.

### Pitch Burns

If a burn is caused by pitch, do not attempt to dislodge the hot pitch. Apply an oily dressing until it separates away in a day or two.

### Electricity Burns

In the case of burns caused by electricity, ointments and salt solution applications are effective. Treat the victim for shock. Large amounts of fluid should be given with table salt.

## SCALDS

There is likely to be shock in the case of a severe scald. Coffee or another stimulant should be given, and the patient should be kept warm. Apply bicarbonate solution or the dry powder to the scalded area. A gauze dressing can be placed over vaseline and the part bandaged loosely if the patient is to be transported to a hospital. Give plenty of fluids.

In scalds of the throat, the services of a physician must be quickly obtained. While awaiting the physician, hold small pieces of ice in the mouth. Sip cod-liver oil or a mixture of cod-liver oil and lime water in equal parts.

## STRAINS

A strain is a slight pull or a wrench on the structures of the arms or legs. It may involve the shoulder, the wrist, one or more fingers, the hip, knee, ankle, foot or toes. Except for a short period of pain, strains usually clear up without any treatment.

## SPRAINS

***Causes and Symptoms of Sprains.*** Sprains may occur from the same causes as strains, but involve the deeper structures such as the tendons, as well as the muscles. The pain is more severe, and swelling usually occurs promptly, although it may not occur for several hours or even before the following day. Recovery of use of the injured joint or muscles may require many days. Usually an area of "black and blue" remains for some days. This discoloration, which is under the skin, is due to the accumulation of blood which has oozed from a tiny blood vessel at the point of injury. It should not cause any worry, as it will disappear eventually.

***Treatment of Sprains.*** There is a difference of opinion as to the treatment. Some do better by the careful use of the limb, others by more or less rest. Moist heat by means of hot towels is always helpful. A hot bath is even better, for fifteen minutes, several times a day.

If the pain is severe, an aspirin or an empirin tablet taken every three to four hours will bring a measure of relief.

If the pain persists over a period of days without any improvement, there may be a torn ligament. It is then advisable to consult a physician, who may find it necessary to apply a plaster cast or a light steel splint to immobilize the affected part. In these protracted cases, it is always advisable to have an X-ray picture taken in order to establish an accurate diagnosis.

## SPRAINED BACK

***Causes and Symptoms of Sprained Back.*** Back sprain is caused by overstretching the ligaments which connect the bones of the spinal column, or twisting the muscles of the back (the kidney regions). Back sprains are usually low down. There is pain, particularly on movement, and it may persist for several days.

Back sprains commonly involve the sacrum. This is called sacro-iliac joint sprain. If the muscles of the kidney (lumbar) regions are involved, it is called "lumbago."

A great deal of confusion can exist here. Continued low backache following a wrench or twist may have nothing to do with the original sprain. The pain or discomfort may be due to other conditions which may have existed, but were not recognized, before the sprain. The two most common of these conditions are fallen arches and what is called a silent kidney stone.

***Treatment of Back Sprain.*** In the acute stage it is usually necessary to remain in bed. Opiates may at times be necessary to relieve the pain. Continued heat is called for, and a hot electric pad is the best source of this. The pain on movement may persist for many days. A good osteopath who is gentle can many times produce dramatic relief.

## SPRAINED NECK

***Causes and Symptoms of Sprained Neck.*** Sprained neck is of common occurrence and may result from a sudden turning of the head. The pain may be very severe. The muscles may stiffen for several days, and it may be impossible to turn the head. This is called torticollis or wry neck. There are other ways torticollis is produced. Acute infections in the deep structures of the neck muscles, abscess of a molar tooth, and exposure to cold are its principal causes.

***Treatment of Sprained Neck.*** In the acute stage, rest in bed may be necessary. The head should be propped up high on pillows so that there is no pull on the neck muscles. The electric pad should be used continuously. Aspirin or empirin should be taken to relieve the pain.

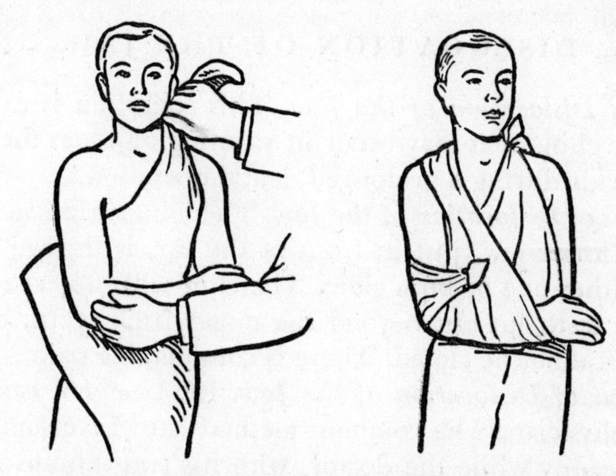

HOW TO MAKE AN ARM SLING

You can easily make the broad arm sling shown at the right by following these steps: (1) Take a triangular bandage and hold it with its long side vertical. (2) Bring the central point or apex behind the elbow of the injured arm and pass the upper end behind the neck, as shown at the left. (3) Bring up the lower end of the triangle and tie it to the upper one with a secure knot. Pin the loose end to the front of the sling.

## DISLOCATIONS

***Causes of Dislocations.*** A dislocation occurs when one bone slips out of adjustment with its neighboring bone. This may be caused by an exaggerated wrench or twist of a joint. The joints of the shoulder, wrist, hip, fingers, and toes are the joints most frequently dislocated. Dislocations are more common in young children and the aged because their joint ligaments are not sufficiently strong to withstand extra strain.

***Symptoms of Dislocations.*** A dislocation can usually be diagnosed by the protrusion of the bone involved and the severe pain, which is continuous.

***Treatment of Dislocations.*** Do *not* attempt to replace the dislocated bone. You may cause great harm. Call a doctor, preferably a bone specialist (orthopedic surgeon).

If medical assistance is not readily obtainable, place the injured part in the most comfortable position. If the injury is of the upper extremity, place the arm in a sling. If it is of the lower limb, support the leg on a pillow.

## DISLOCATION OF THE JAW

***Causes of Dislocation of the Jaw.*** This condition is caused by a blow on the chin, or it may occur in yawning or when the mouth is kept open wide during a prolonged dental operation.

***Symptoms of Dislocation of the Jaw.*** The joint surface at the upper part of the lower jaw, just in front of the ear, is thrown out of its socket on either one or both sides. The chin will project so that the lower front teeth jut out beyond the upper front teeth; the mouth is open and cannot be closed. There is considerable pain.

***Treatment of Dislocation of the Jaw.*** Replacement can be made only by a physician. The common method is to have someone hold the head steadily while the doctor, with his two thumbs in the patient's mouth, presses downward and backward, grasping under the chin with the forefingers of each hand and raising it up. When the jaw slips back into its socket, it is held there by a properly fitting bandage. The bandage is usually left on for about a week. In the meantime the patient is fed liquids through a drinking tube.

## DISLOCATION OF THE SHOULDER

***Causes of Dislocation of the Shoulder.*** This is the most common dislocation in adults. It is caused by a fall or blow on the upper arm or shoulder or by falling upon the elbow or outstretched hand.

***Symptoms of Dislocation of the Shoulder.*** The upper part of the upper bone of the arm slips downward out of the socket, or inward and forward. The shoulder of the injured side loses its fullness and looks flatter in front and on the side. The arm is held with the elbow a few inches away from the side, and the line of the arm slopes inward toward the shoulder. The arm cannot be moved by the patient although it can be lifted up by another person. Any manipulation causes great pain.

*Treatment of Dislocation of the Shoulder.* Only a physician should attempt replacing the shoulder into its socket. The ligaments can be easily torn or overstretched if an incompetent person attempts the replacement. The patient is made to lie down on the injured side, with the arm hanging downward toward the floor. A gentle pull is then made on the arm, which is carefully rotated outward, then carried upward to the opposite shoulder and held in that position until the correct (spica) bandage is applied.

## DISLOCATION OF THE BACK

*Causes of Dislocation of the Back.* This dislocation is due to falls from heights, either directly upon the back or upon the buttocks. The injury may be at any location along the spinal column. The higher up the injury, the more serious the result.

*Symptoms of Dislocation of the Back.* If the spinal cord is injured either directly by the fall or by pressure on the cord by the displaced vertebra, there will be symptoms of paralysis of the legs or arms. Otherwise a sort of shock in a mild degree will be present.

*Treatment of Dislocation of the Back.* Great harm can be done by careless or improper handling of the patient. The danger is that the spinal cord may be injured. Unless the patient is exposed to the weather, it is better to let him lie in the position he is found in. If he is to be moved, then there should, if possible, be three persons to do this properly. One places his hands under the shoulders, and one under the abdomen or back, according to which position he is in. The third person carries the legs at the level of the knees. The patient is gently put on a stretcher. The doctor will attempt correction only in a hospital, where the necessary equipment is at hand. Anesthesia is usually necessary.

## DISLOCATION OF THE ELBOW

*Causes of Dislocation of the Elbow.* This dislocation is more frequent in children. It is commonly produced by a fall with the hand outstretched.

*Symptoms of Dislocation of the Elbow.* The forearm is displaced backward on the arm. The elbow joint rapidly swells and is held in a slightly bent position. No movement is possible without great pain.

*Treatment of Dislocation of Elbow.* This can be carried out only in a hospital under a doctor's care. The injury must first be X-rayed to make sure there is no break in the bones. Anesthesia is used, and the displaced bones are brought back into position. The joint is bandaged and held in a sling.

## DISLOCATION OF THE WRIST

***Causes of Dislocation of the Wrist.*** This type of injury is always caused by a fall with the hand outstretched.

***Symptoms of Dislocation of the Wrist.*** The displaced bone may protrude either forward or backward, and either one or both of the wrist bones may be involved.

***Treatment of Dislocation of the Wrist.*** An X-ray should be taken at once. Fractures of this joint are more common than dislocations. The bones are placed back into their socket by gentle pulling downward. A light anesthesia may be necessary to get the necessary relaxation of the ligaments.

## DISLOCATION OF THE THUMB

This injury is caused by a fall with the thumb outstretched. A prominent symptom besides pain, is that the dislocated end protrudes either backwards or forwards. Replacement is usually easy if done soon after the injury. A light steel splint is applied and has to be worn from two to three weeks.

## DISLOCATION OF THE HIP

***Causes of Dislocation of the Hip.*** This occurs more often in adult men. It is always due to external violence.

***Symptoms of Dislocation of the Hip.*** When the patient is standing, the injured joint will be readily seen to cause a shortening of the leg on the side of the dislocation. The toes will be turned inward, so much so that the foot crosses over the instep of the uninjured foot. Pain is very marked.

***Treatment of Dislocation of the Hip.*** Great care must be taken to determine if there is any fracture; this is diagnosed by the X-ray. Fracture of the hip is very common in the aged, and dislocations are very uncommon. It is always necessary to give an anaesthetic in order to relax the ligaments sufficiently to get the displaced bones into the normal socket.

## DISLOCATION OF THE KNEE

This injury rarely happens. When it does, it is due to a fall upon the knee. One symptom is that there is usually some part of the ligaments torn, which causes a protrusion of the bone, now displaced backward. The patient cannot walk. An X-ray is needed since there may be a small chip off the bone. A plaster cast may have to be worn as long as three months.

## DISLOCATION OF THE KNEECAP

Since the ligaments of the kneecap are so firmly fixed, this is an extremely rare injury. Any injury of the knee is usually a fracture of the kneecap. In treatment a plaster cast is applied and kept on several months.

## DISLOCATION OF THE ANKLE

***Causes of Dislocation of the Ankle.*** Since the entire body weight is carried by the ankles, it is not to be wondered at that this joint is so frequently dislocated. The injury is usually the result of sudden turning in or turning out of the foot when tripping upon an irregular surface or stepping off some elevation unknowingly.

***Symptoms of Dislocation of the Ankle.*** Pain is present. Forward dislocations are usually accompanied by fracture, and an X-ray must be immediately taken. There is danger of pressure upon the large blood vessel of the foot if the damage to the joint is not promptly corrected.

***Treatment of Dislocation of the Ankle.*** Replacement of a simple dislocation is not difficult. Care must always be observed following a dislocation of this joint. The ankle becomes weakened after an injury, and the dislocation is therefore likely to repeat itself. Orthopedists (bone specialists) disagree as to whether the ankle should be immobilized or only a light bandage placed on it and use of the foot not delayed too long. The question of stiffening of the joint is also involved.

## DISLOCATION OF THE TOE

It is rare for any toe other than the big one to be dislocated. The dislocation is caused practically always by stubbing the toe. In this injury the farthest end of the toe protrudes upward. It is usually very painful. Replacement is made without any difficulty. A light bandage is applied, and the patient has to remain off his feet for a few days. If there is any swelling, it is helpful to place the foot in a hot water bath.

## FRACTURES OR BROKEN BONES

*Causes of Fractures.* In and about the home, fractures are much more common than they should be. In almost every instance, pure carelessness is responsible. Falls and dropping heavy weights on the feet and hands cause a great number of fractures. Falls in the bath tub and tripping over long electric cords, slipping on small rugs placed on highly polished floors, bumping into misplaced pieces of furniture in the dark and falling off step ladders—these accidents often result in fractures, and yet practically all are avoidable if care is exercised.

Fractures resulting from either direct or indirect violence may be partly due to defective bone strength, particularly in advanced age, when the bone calcium is reduced. Other bone involvement such as cysts and tumors may give first evidence of their existence when a spontaneous fracture occurs, even though the person is stepping down only lightly, or merely twisting a limb. This kind of injury is known as a pathological fracture.

*Kinds of Fractures.* For our purpose here, we shall consider only simple and compound fractures. The simple fracture is a break in the bone leaving the two ends not too greatly separated from each other. The compound fracture is one in which an end of the broken bone penetrates through the skin. This is by far the more serious break. Fractures in the home in the order of their frequency are: thigh bone (femur), ribs, wrist, fingers, and toes. Rarely do we find a skull fracture, which, of course, is the most serious. Occasionally there is a fracture of the nose.

### First Aid for All Fractures

***How to Treat Shock.*** Shock is treated by placing the patient in a recumbent position, carefully raising the buttocks higher than the head. The reason for this is to help the flow of blood to the heart and head. Apply heat to the body and cover with blankets. Give brandy or strong coffee if the patient can swallow. If the patient is unconscious, do not pour the coffee or liquor down into the mouth. If you do, the fluids may go down the windpipe instead of into the stomach, causing a very undesirable irritation in the bronchial tubes.

In old persons there may be considerable shock associated with a fracture, usually of the thigh bone.

***Altering the Patient's Position.*** If the fracture is compound, it is best to leave the patient lying flat, provided he is not exposed to cold or drafts. Since many fractures occur in the bath tub, of course the patient should be lifted out of the tub. This should be done by three persons, one placing the hands under the broken limb in the effort to avoid any further injury, particularly if the fracture is compound.

***Preliminary Splint.*** This is essential in order to reduce further injury to a minimum. A simple temporary splint is a large pillow. Place it under the two broken ends of the bone lengthwise and tie around the leg with pieces of bandage.

***Hemorrhage.*** This usually occurs in compound fractures. An artery may be severed. If so, red blood will spurt through the torn skin. This is controlled by use of a tourniquet (page 473).

*Now call a doctor. Never attempt to set any bone. Only an experienced physician can do this correctly.*

***Care of the Aged.*** If an aged patient has a broken thigh bone, he should be transported to a hospital at once. In the past few years these patients have been treated surgically very soon after the break. The new method of bringing the two ends together and fixing with a wooden peg gives far better results than the former procedure of simply putting the leg in a cast and extending the leg with weights. The convalescence is much more rapid and therefore there is less danger of pneumonia from lying on the back for so long a time.

## FRACTURE OF THE BREAST BONE

The patient should be kept lying on his back, a firm pillow between his shoulders. Loosen tight or constrictive clothing around his chest. Give him treatment for shock, if present. A stretcher should be used to transport the patient.

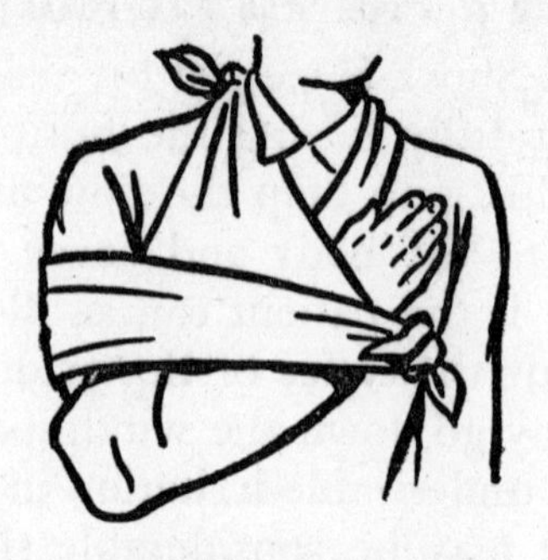

TRIANGULAR SLING AND BANDAGE

The triangular sling and bandage shown above are recommended for a fractured arm and collar-bone. The fractured arm should be firmly held in a splint. Do not attempt to set a broken bone by yourself. Secure the aid of a doctor.

## FRACTURE OF THE COLLAR-BONE

Place a pad in the patient's armpit. Push his arm upward. Support the arm with a sling. Tie the arm to the side of the body with a strong bandage. Now secure a physician's help.

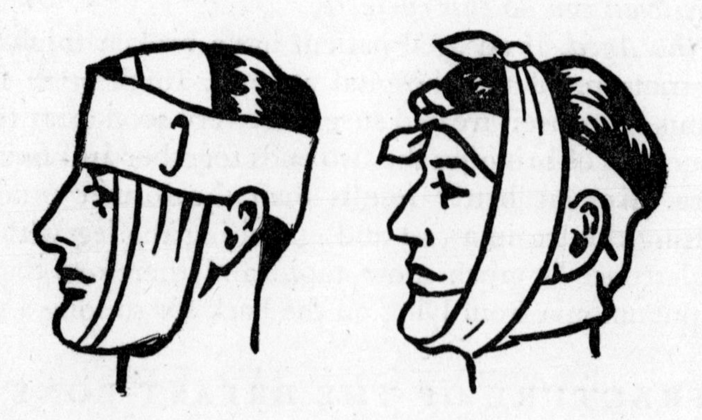

BANDAGES FOR HEAD, JAW, AND CHIN INJURIES

These simple bandages can be quickly made, even by the beginner. (*Left*) Roller bandage for head or jaw. (*Right*) Application of cravat bandages for the chin.

## FRACTURE OF THE LOWER JAW

Bring lower jaw to upper and, while thus supported, apply triangular bandage running from around the chin to the top of the head.

## FRACTURE OF THE NOSE

Nose fractures and dislocations are among the most common of all bodily injuries. With young people particularly, sports such as hockey, football, basketball, baseball, wrestling, etc., contribute to this high percentage.

***Symptoms of Nose Fracture.*** In many nose fractures, the fragments are firmly held together. Fractures may be simple or compound. Nose fractures may be recognized by the following symptoms: (1) pain, usually not severe; (2) bleeding; (3) nasal obstruction; (4) black and blue discoloration; (5) air in the tissues (this is definite evidence that the nasal sinuses are involved); (6) external deformity; (7) internal deformities; (8) sometimes complications inside the skull.

***Treatment of Nose Fracture.*** Usually little treatment is required for simple nose fractures without deformity. It is important, however, to treat fractures promptly, if possible, before the swelling of the soft parts obscures the shape of the nose. Unfortunately, in many instances, a surgeon is not consulted until long after the injury, and it is then better to wait until the swelling has subsided completely.

All nose fractures should receive the immediate attention of a physician or plastic surgeon. Many fractures of the bones of the nose remain unrecognized and neglected because of the large amount of swelling and black and blue discoloration resulting from the injury. The patient thinks he has merely had a "bump on the nose." If there is noticeable displacement to the side, or a depressed bridge of the nose, the fracture can easily be recognized. X-ray diagnosis is usually necessary.

## FRACTURE OF THE RIBS

There is often a possibility that the lungs have been injured, and a danger of driving the broken ends of the ribs still farther into the lungs. Loosen the clothing, and place the patient on the uninjured side. The physician will care for him further.

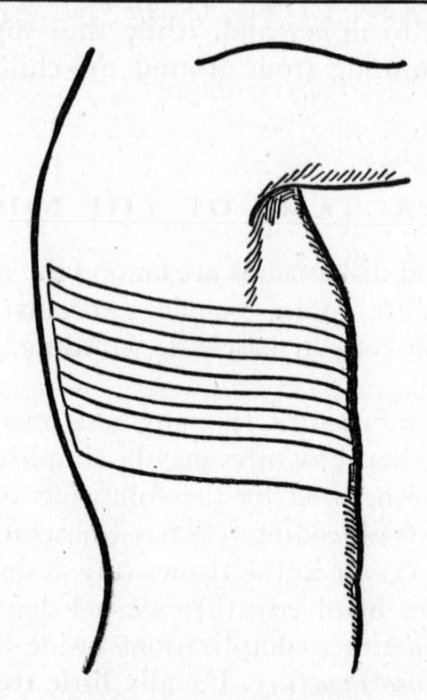

STRAPPED CHEST

In case of a fractured rib, the rib is immobilized with strips of adhesive plaster which begin at the spinal column and are carried forward. This procedure, however, can be followed only by the intensively trained first-aider. With rib injuries, there is possibility of damage to the lung, and the only safe thing is to leave the patient resting on his uninjured side while you bring a doctor to him.

## FRACTURE OF THE SHOULDER BLADE

Use a broad bandage. Place the center of the upper edge of the bandage under the armpit on the injured side, allowing the width to extend down the side of the body; carry the ends upwards across the front and back of the chest, in turn. The lower end of the bandage extends to directly below the broken shoulder blade. On the shoulder of the uninjured side, cross the ends of the bandage and pull them tightly. Carry the ends into the armpit of the sound side and tie them tightly in this situation. Be careful not to make pressure on the blood vessels. Place the arm on the affected side in a sling.

## FRACTURE OF THE HIP

The patient is placed on his back, with the lower limbs either straight or bent according to which position the patient finds more comfortable. The upper part of the body is to be either raised or lowered as the patient desires. A broad fold bandage is passed around the pelvis and tightened just enough to afford support. The center of the bandage is placed in the middle of the back and the knot in the middle of the body in front. All movement must be prevented. A blanket is placed beneath the patient, with the least disturbance possible, so that he can be carried on it. Remove him to a hospital.

## FRACTURE OF THE LEG

If the proper emergency treatment is given when fractures of the leg occur, there will be little or no damage to the limb while waiting for professional treatment. Correct emergency measures will lessen pain and shock to the patient.

A side-splint should be used. Straighten the limb with care. Both feet and ankles should be tied together by a figure-of-eight bandage. This is begun behind the ankles. The ends are brought upward and crossed over the instep. They are then carried under the soles of the feet and tied in this position. In a certain definite order, pass a series of seven folded bandages under the patient's body. Fold each bandage over a splint, and pass it from the injured side, under the patient's body, and then pull one end of the bandage through the sound side. In this way all the bandages are placed under the patient without any need to move his body. Use the natural hollows of the body whenever possible in carrying out this technique. The bandages should lie under the chest, just below the armpits; under the hips; under both ankles; under both thighs; above the level of the fracture; under both thighs below the level of the fracture; under both legs; under both knees.

The long splint may be padded. It should be placed along the injured side of the patient, extending from the armpit to the foot. The splint is secured in position by tying the bandages in the same order they were passed in.

## FRACTURE OF THE KNEECAP

Keep the leg high so that the heel is at least a foot from the ground. Raise the patient's head and shoulders; keep them in position with a back-rest such as may be made by tipping a chair over on its back. Along the back of the limb place a splint extending from the top of the thigh to well below the level of the foot. See that the splint is padded where there are natural hollows under the knee and under the ankle. Fasten the splint to the leg by three bandages made as follows: First bandage—twice around the thigh and tie on top of the limb. Second bandage—twice around the leg and tie in line with the first knot. Third bandage—a double figure-of-eight around the foot and ankle. Tie a figure-of-eight bandage around the knee to support the fragments by following this procedure: Take a narrow bandage and place its center just above the upper fragment; next, carry the ends to the back of the splint, cross them, and pull them as tight as possible so as to draw the upper fragment downwards. Now carry the ends to the front of the knee and tie below the lower fragment.

## FRACTURE OF THE FOOT

Take the shoe and sock off the injured foot. Apply to the sole a well-padded splint reaching from the heel to the toes. Secure it in position by a bandage.

## FRACTURE OF THE UPPER ARM

Secure the upper arm to the side by a broad bandage. No splint is needed; bend the forearm to a right angle and support it in a small arm sling.

## FRACTURE OF THE LOWER ARM

The patient is made to sit or lie down comfortably with his elbow bent. You should never try to set the arm back to its original position —this takes more skill than the first-aider ordinarily possesses. Procure two cravat bandages and two well-padded splints. The first splint should be long enough to extend from a few inches beyond the elbow to beyond the fingertips. This is for the outside of the arm. The other splint, to be placed on the inner side of the arm, should be long enough to reach from the elbow to a distance a few inches short of the fingertips. Place the first cravat bandage over the splints in the area of the hand and tie it on the back of the arm over the wrist. Place the second bandage at the upper part of the forearm and tie.

## FRACTURE OF THE ELBOW

Fractures directly above the joint commonly occur after a fall on the hand, particularly in children. The diagnosis is usually obvious from the history, deformity, pain, loss of use, swelling, and black and blue discoloration. An X-ray examination should never be omitted

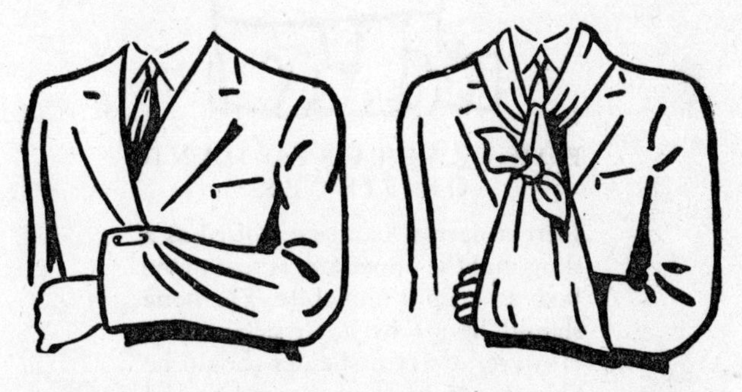

HOW TO MAKE EMERGENCY SLINGS

(*Left*) How to make an emergency sling with the sleeve of the patient's coat. This sling may be used in case of a fractured elbow. (*Right*) Sling made with handkerchiefs.

before or after the fracture is set. Correction, carried out only by a physician, should be prompt and under an anesthetic. Meanwhile, a splint or sling is used to keep the elbow immobile, bent almost at right angles.

## FRACTURE OF THE WRIST

A well-padded shingle or a few layers of cardboard may be used for a splint. In putting splints on a fracture of the lower forearm, the thumb should be pointing upward. In this position, the two bones in the forearm are in correct line with each other. It is while the forearm is in this position that the splints are applied.

## FRACTURE OF THE HAND

Use a well-padded splint if available. Apply it to the patient's forearm. It should extend beyond his fingers. Around the hand and wrist tie a figure-of-eight bandage. Be sure to keep the thumb inside the bandage. Fasten the splint to the forearm by a narrow bandage wrapped twice around the arm and tied on the back of the arm. A large arm sling is used.

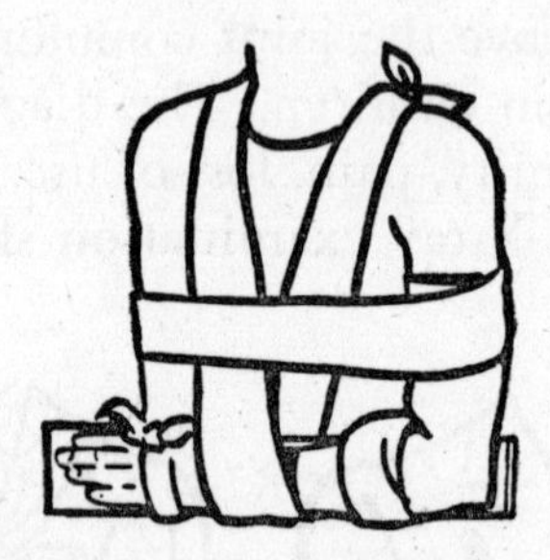

FOR FRACTURED HAND OR FINGER

Here a narrow bandage is used as a sling, and the upper arm is tied to the body to keep it immobile. The bone should be set by a physician only. However, every first-aider should be able to prepare a proper splint and sling, so that the patient can be brought to the physician without further injury.

## FRACTURE OF THE FINGER

The fractured finger is held at the tip and pulled gently until it seems normally aligned. On the inner side of the fractured finger, place a well-padded wooden tongue depressor with one end reaching a bit beyond the fingertip and the other end over the palm. Make the splint immobile with an ascending spiral bandage, that is, one starting from the bottom. Fasten the splint with a descending spiral bandage and secure the ends at the wrist with several figure-of-eight turns of the bandage.

## FRACTURE OF THE NECK

When fracture occurs in the middle of the neck, the patient usually suffers paralysis of his arms and legs. He cannot control his bladder

# How to Treat a Snakebite

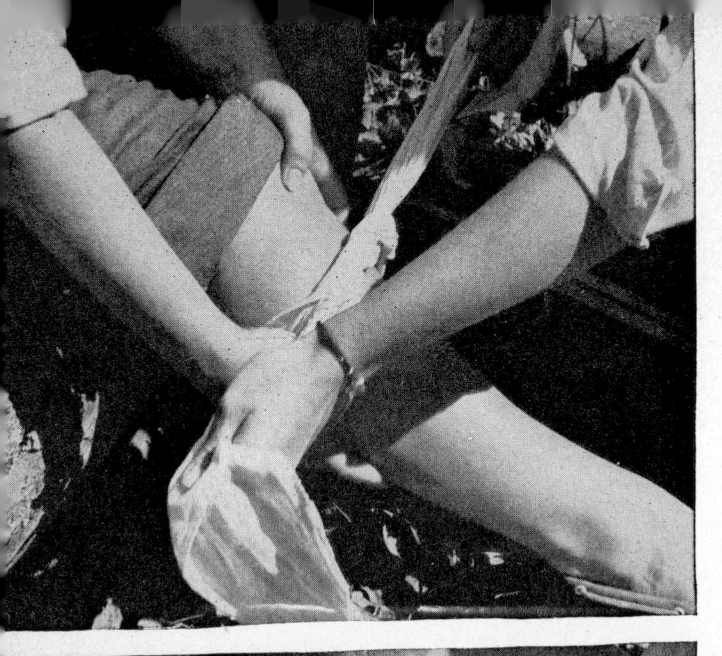

### STEP ONE

Apply a restricting bandage or tourniquet above bite. Wash skin around bite and paint with iodine. (Bandage should not be too tight, should be kept on about two hours, loosened for a moment every thirty minutes.)

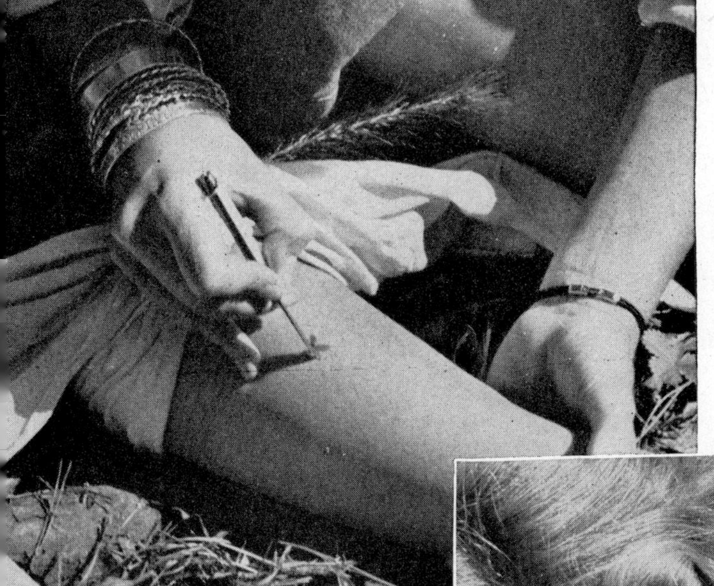

### STEP TWO

With sharp sterile blade, make crosscut incision across fang marks. This should serve to bring on profuse bleeding, start outward flow of blood that has been infected with poison from snake's bite.

American Red Cross Photos by Doris Wallace

### STEP THREE

First-aider places mouth to wound, sucks out poisoned blood. If suction cup is available, it should be used instead. Patient should have rest, get large doses of antivenin from doctor.

# Safety in the Home

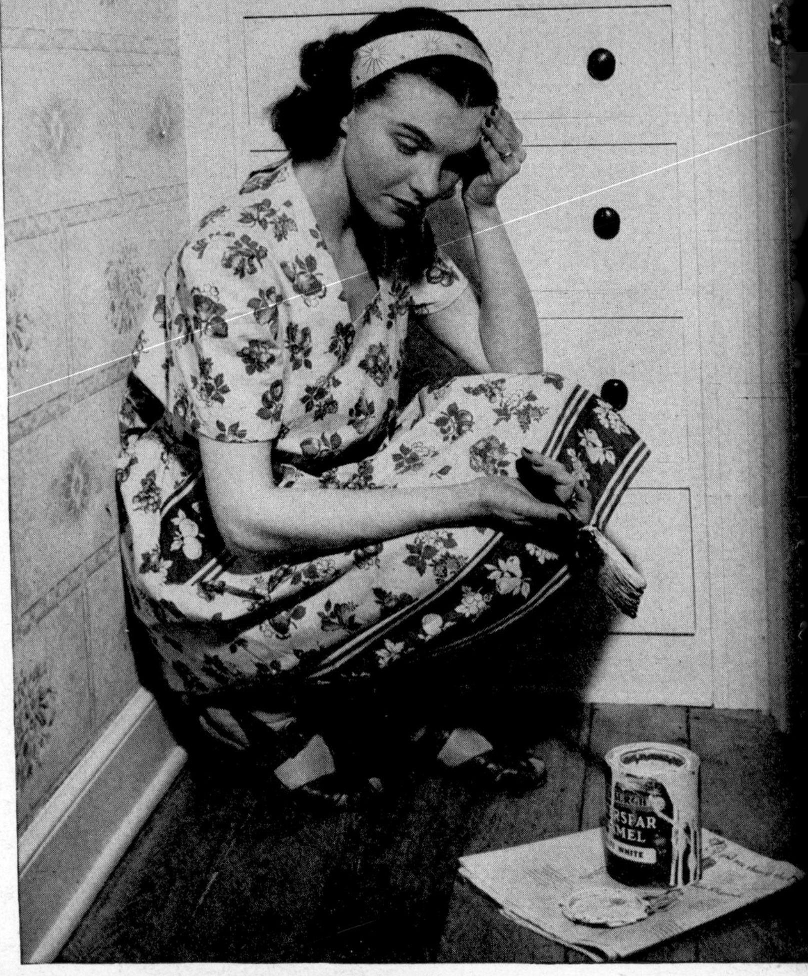

## PAINT FUMES

When you paint indoors, open a window or a door to make certain you will get plenty of fresh air. Fumes of paint can be toxic if ventilation is inadequate.

National Safety Council

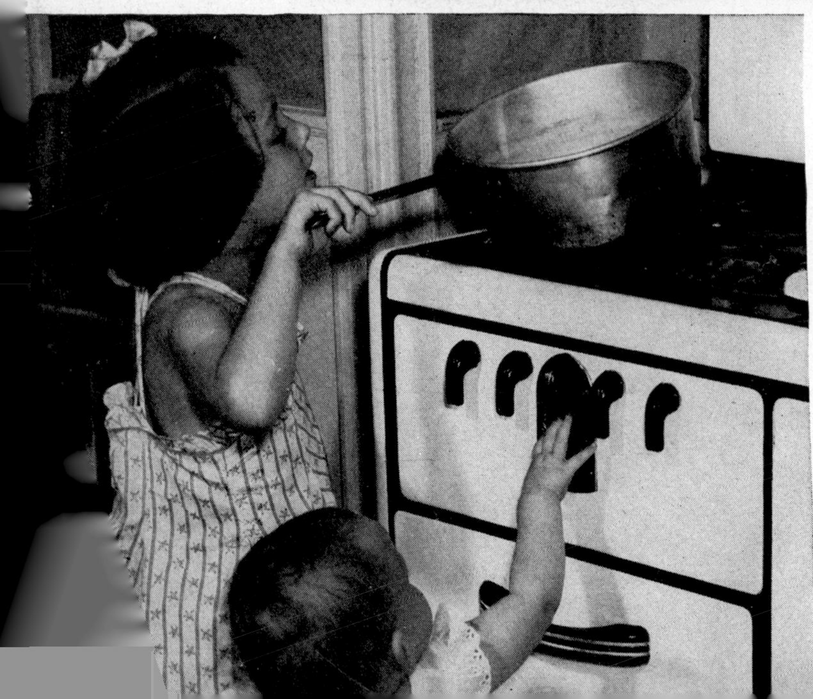

## CHILDREN IN THE KITCHEN

For safety's sake, whenever possible keep children out of the kitchen while cooking. Always turn pot handles in, away from edge of stove, to avoid possibility of scalds.

and finds it hard to breathe. Artificial respiration is required if such is the case.

It is dangerous to bend the patient's head forward. A board is placed next to him, and it should reach about four inches beyond his head. One assistant takes hold of the patient at the shoulder and the hip, placing his own foot against the board to keep it from slipping. Another assistant steadies the patient's head and neck between his own hands. In one movement, the patient is slid onto the board. Now his arms are folded and his coat sleeves pinned together. To prevent the patient from falling off, he is strapped to the board. The board is lifted at both ends to move the patient.

## FRACTURE OF THE BACK

In fracture of the back, if there has been no displacement of the vertebrae and no injury of the cord, the only symptom may be pain in the back. However, if there is some displacement, one observes an irregularity in the shape of the spinal column. In addition, the patient will be paralyzed below the point of injury. If his soles are tickled he will not be able to draw up his legs. The higher up in the spinal column the fracture has occurred, the greater will be the degree of paralysis. If the injury is in the area of the neck, the victim may die instantaneously.

Thus, injuries to the spinal column may, for convenience, be divided into those associated with paralysis and those in which no paralysis is present. If the victim's condition is suggestive of a fracture of one or more of the vertebrae, the spinal column should not be bent, and under no circumstances should the patient be lifted by the shoulders and the legs. Instead, place a blanket, folded lengthwise, next to the patient. He should be grasped at the shoulder and hip. Then without twisting the spinal column in any manner, he should be slowly and gently rolled over onto the blanket so as to lie face down with the head turned to one side. When two men carry the patient, one stands at one end and grasps the blanket just above the level of the patient's shoulders. The second man stands at the other end and grasps the blanket at the level of the injured person's knee. Then they both lift the victim at the same time.

The patient should be moved by first-aiders only in an extreme emergency. It is far better to have the doctor supervise his moving.

## HEAD INJURIES

*Concussion.* Head injuries happen as a result of direct or indirect violence. A common form of unconsciousnes produced by a fall or blow on the head is that accompanying concussion of the brain. In such a case the insensibility may be short, the patient may be pale and confused, and have nausea or vomiting on recovery. In the severer form, the patient is unconscious but may reply in monosyllables if he is shouted at. If the victim can move his limbs there is no paralysis, but there may be convulsions, occasionally. Recovery of consciousness usually occurs within twenty-four hours, but headache, dizziness, and incapacity for mental work may persist for a considerable time. In all head injuries, the care of a physician is urgently required.

*Fracture of the Skull.* In the more dangerous head injuries, resulting in bleeding and clots upon, or in the substance of, the brain, in fracture or breaking of the bones of the skull, or in damage to the covers of the brain, with pressure on the brain, the following symptoms are usually present: complete unconsciousness, so that the patient shows no response to any effort to arouse him; noisy, snoring breathing; slow pulse; and wide pupils. In fracture, one often sees no outward sign, although there may be a depression in the skull, or the broken bones may be felt grating together when the skull is manipulated. A continuous flow of blood, or watery fluid (spinal) from the ear or nose is usually a sign of fracture; also the appearance of bloodstaining of the white of the eye or lid soon after the accident. Sometimes there is bleeding into the neck muscles.

## BANDAGES AND BANDAGING

Bandages are usually applied for the following purposes: to create pressure to prevent bleeding, to hold dressings in place, to increase the temperature of the part bandaged, and to anchor splints.

It is a common error when putting on the average bandage to place it too loosely. It is just as much an error to apply it too tightly.

Apply a bandage with the limb held in the position in which it is to be carried. Wherever possible, the tips of the fingers and toes should be left exposed so that you can observe any color changes indicating interference with the circulation. If a bandage is too tight, a limb may become numb.

There are a few basic turns for bandaging. The circular turn is most suitable for round parts. A spiral bandage is applied in a spiral manner. When the part to be bandaged is slightly cone-shaped—like the forearm—the spiral reverse bandage is of special value.

## RULES FOR BANDAGING

You should stand in front of the patient on the same side as the part you are bandaging, looking over the patient's shoulder. (The

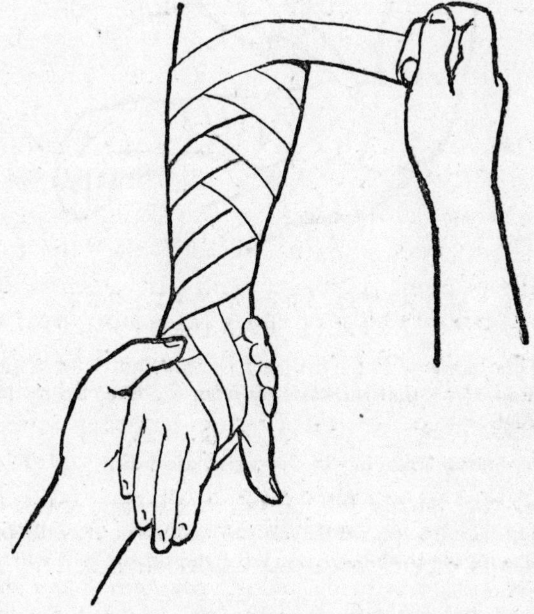

HOW TO APPLY SPIRAL BANDAGE

This bandage is best adapted for use on the trunk or limbs, and not directly over a joint.

one exception to this is eye bandaging. Eye bandages are applied standing behind the patient.) Hold the part you are bandaging in the position it is to remain in. If you are using the roller bandage, hold it in the right hand, keeping the roll up and unrolling it from the bottom. Do not unroll over an inch or so of the bandage at one time.

Begin with an oblique or slanting turn downwards. You should unroll the bandage on the part; it is wrong to unroll it first and then put it on. Work from within outwards on the limbs. On the head and trunk, make equal use of both hands in bandaging. Work from the side of the injury across the front. (An exception is made in the case of a fractured clavicle.) Work from below upwards. Each new turn should cover two-thirds of the previous turn. The turns should be kept parallel with one another. Make the pattern lie on the outer side of the limb and keep it in one line.

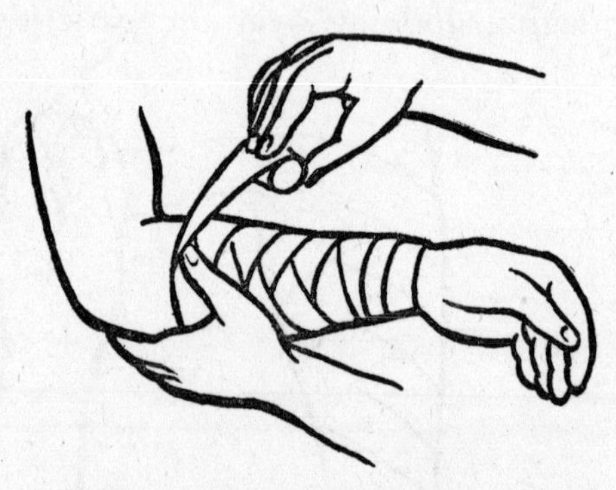

HOW TO APPLY REVERSE SPIRAL BANDAGE

This bandage is particularly recommended for a circumference that increases, as from the knee up to the thigh, etc.

(1) Start bandaging at the wrist, ascending.

(2) After the first few turns of the bandage, reverse it by turning it on itself. You can do this most easily by placing the thumb of your left hand on the spot where you wish to make the reverse; now turn your right hand, holding the roll of bandage, so that the palm faces downward. By doing this, you have turned the bandage. The reverse turn should be pulled tight.

(3) Make each reverse turn directly above and overlapping the lower one.

A bandage should be finished off securely with a safety pin or adhesive plaster. Care must be taken to avoid placing a knot or pin over a bone or wound or where it will cause discomfort or pressure if the patient leans on it. A wet bandage should not be tied tightly as it may shrink and become too constricting. However, a bandage may be made tight to prevent swelling and provide support in case of sprains.

It is important to use a bandage of suitable width: one inch for thumb and fingers; one and one-half to two inches for the head, foot and forearm; three to four inches for the leg, thigh and upper arm; four inches for breast and spica (see page 501) for shoulder; six inches for armpit and trunk bandages.

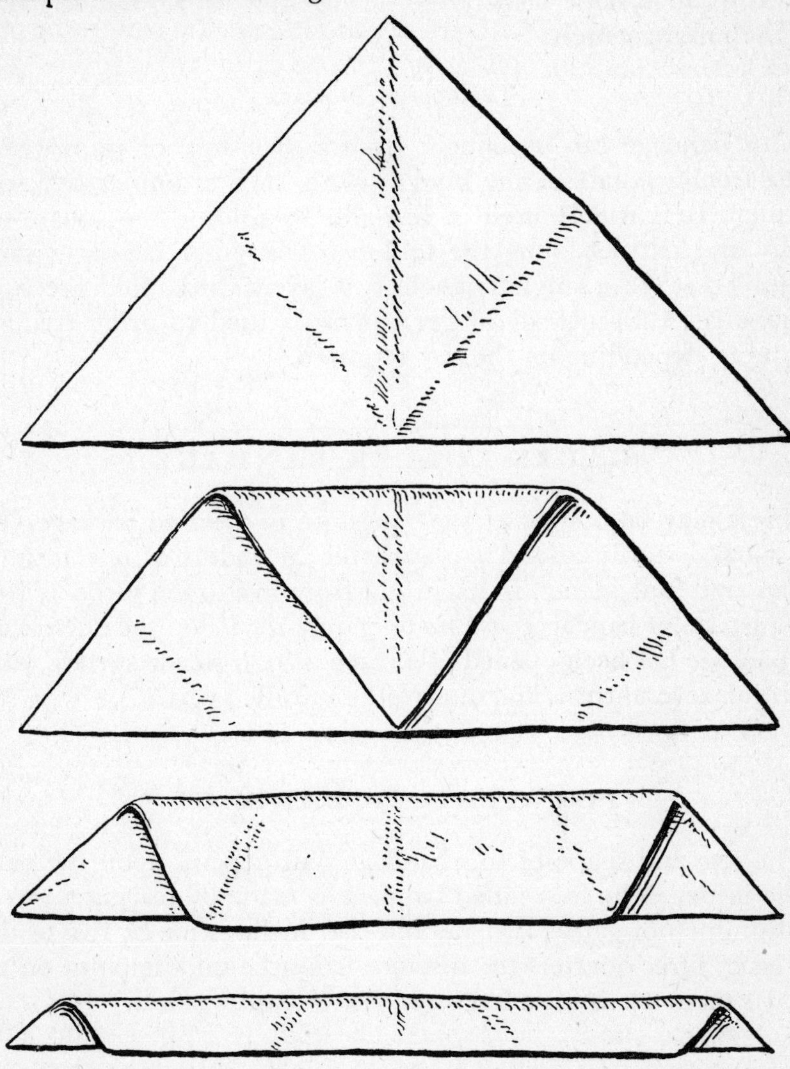

HOW TO MAKE A CRAVAT BANDAGE

A triangular bandage is what you start with. Bring the peak of the triangle down to the base, as shown in the second drawing. Now fold the top half down over the bottom one, as in the third drawing. Continue folding down this way till you achieve the desired width. The cravat bandage may be used in tying splints, as a sling, or over many different parts of the body.

### Spiral Bandage

This bandage is applied so that it slopes upward a bit. It should fit snugly. When you have made one or two turns of the simple spiral on a limb, begin in the opposite direction after the part is increased in size; change slope of bandage, bringing it up across the front of the limb more acutely.

### Triangular Bandage

This bandage can be bought from a drugstore or improvised at home from a square of any kind of cloth, such as unbleached cotton or linen. It is widely used in first-aid. By folding the square diagonally and cutting along the fold two triangular bandages can be made. To make a single triangle two layers thick, fold the square diagonally. A 24-inch or longer square is used to make triangular bandages, depending on the size required.

## GAUZE ROLLER BANDAGE

These may be bought at the drugstore in a sealed package. They are marked sterilized and are available in widths of one inch, two inches, and four inches, in lengths of from five to ten yards.

Gauze roller bandages will *no longer be sterile* on the outside after the package has been opened. To reach a fresh sterile surface, unroll the roller several turns and discard the unrolled part.

## FOUR-TAILED BANDAGE

The size and shape of this bandage will depend upon the nature of the injury. The four-tailed bandage is made by tearing a piece of muslin, linen or gauze, two and one-half inches wide by two or three feet long, three-quarters the distance from the middle point on each end. Its main use is for a fractured jaw or chin wounds.

## FIGURE-OF-EIGHT BANDAGE

This consists of several slanting turns that cross one another and thus assume a form resembling a figure of eight. This type of bandage is particularly good for bandaging the elbow, knee or ankle joints.

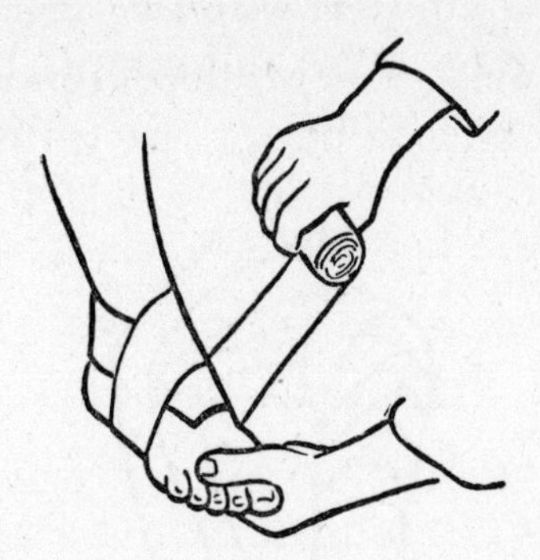

FIGURE-OF-EIGHT BANDAGE

(1) Place the beginning of the bandage over the front of the foot.

(2) Pass the bandage behind the ankle joint and forward over the previous turn.

(3) Make several oblique turns, alternately ascending and descending, so as to cross each other, thus forming the figure eight. This type of bandage is most effective for an injured ankle, elbow, or knee.

## SPICA BANDAGE

This is similar to a figure-of-eight, but differs in that one loop is much smaller than the other. The bandage is suitable in case of injury to the shoulder, hip or thumb. The small loop is wound around the thigh, arm or thumb, as the case may be. The large loop is wound around the waist, chest or wrist. It may be used either as an ascending or descending spica.

To place an ascending spica for the shoulder, start with an oblique turn downwards. Working from within outwards, carry the bandage around the arm and then up over the shoulder, across the back and under the opposite armpit. Next carry it across the front of the chest, over the shoulder and around the arm again, one-third of the width of the bandage higher up the arm than the first turn. Next, carry the bandage up over the shoulder and across back to the opposite armpit, then back over the front of the chest, over the shoulder and around the arm again, one-third of the width of the bandage higher up. Continue with alternate arm and chest turns until the dressing is covered.

For the descending spica, start with the turns high up in the armpit, or high on the shoulder. Work downwards, one-third of the width of the bandage lower, each time.

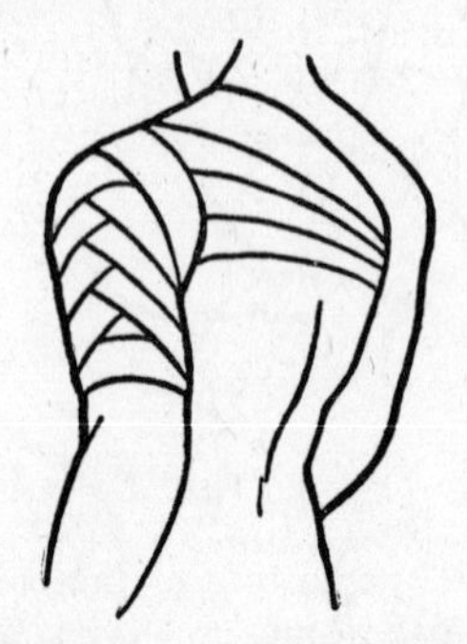

ASCENDING SPICA BANDAGE

This bandage closely resembles the figure-of-eight bandage. It is important that it be firmly applied. Begin bandaging at the upper arm. The crossing of the first turn should go as high upon the shoulder as the bandage will lie. The turns of the bandage should be made oblique, and they should overlap. Each turn crosses the previous one, making an angle with it.

## BANDAGING THE HEAD

To prepare a head bandage take two roller bandages and sew or pin the ends together smoothly. Place that part where the two bandages join, in the center of the forehead, and bring the bandages around the greatest circumference of the head above the ears to the lower part of the back of the head. Here cross the bandages. Then turn one and carry it up over the center of the top of the head to the forehead. Next carry the other straight on around the head immediately over the previous turn and bring it over the other turn at the forehead.

Turn the first bandage back again over the top of the head slightly to one side of the center line of the lower part of the head, and again carry the other end around the head and over it at the back. Again turn the first bandage and carry it back over the top of the head slightly to the opposite side of the middle line. Catch it by the other bandage at the forehead. Continue in the same manner, always using the same bandage to go backwards and forwards over the head, and working outwards, leaving a third of the previous turn uncovered.

Carry the bandage around and around the head to catch and hold down the backward and forward turns. Work on until the bandages overlap well at the sides.

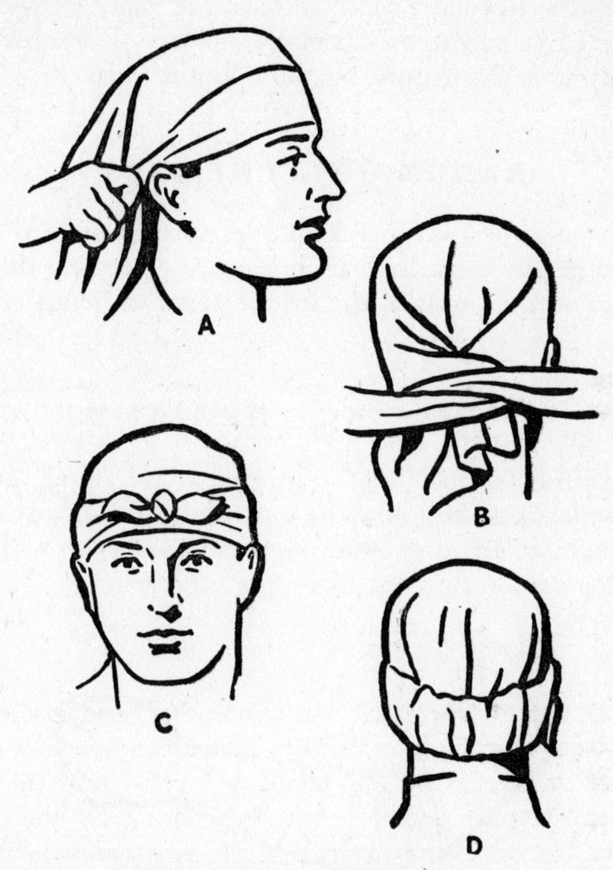


AN EASY HEAD BANDAGE

Place a triangular bandage on the head as shown in the first drawing, and turn and tie the ends as the following pictures suggest.

## BANDAGING THE SHOULDER

For keeping a shoulder dressing in place, you may need both a triangular bandage and a narrow fold bandage. Turn up the base of the first bandage and apply it to the arm. Cross the ends behind the arm, then bring them to the front. Tie the bandage in front of the arm with a reef (square) knot. Place the forearm of the injured shoulder in a small sling. Slip the point of the bandage under the sling and turn it back and pin it to the bandage on the shoulder. If the shoulder is unable to bear the weight of the arm in a sling, fold a second narrow bandage, place it over the point of the shoulder bandage, carry one end across the chest and the other across the back, and tie in front of the armpit on the opposite side.

## BANDAGING THE RIBS

Take two or three four-inch bandages, placed one on top of the other, and bind the chest with them, securely keeping the center of the bandages on the point of the injury. Knot the ends at the opposite side.

## BANDAGING THE WRIST

Place a pad on the back of the injured wrist. Carry the end of a two-inch bandage around the wrist until the pad is firmly fixed, then cross them behind. Bring the ends forward and fasten with adhesive. A broad sling should be used to support the arm.

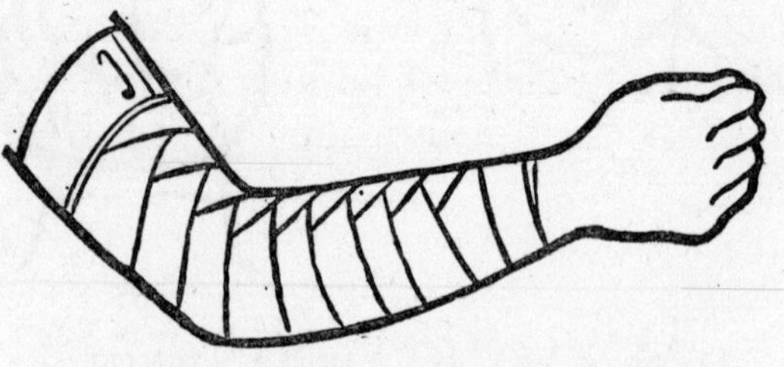

BANDAGE FOR ELBOW AND FOREARM

A roller bandage is tied in spiral fashion starting at the wrist and fastened on the upper arm with a safety pin.

## BANDAGING THE ELBOW

The joint must be bent in order to allow a certain amount of movement. Use the figure-of-eight method until the joint is completely covered. Tie in front or, better still, fasten with adhesive tape. Use a narrow sling for support.

## BANDAGE FOR ARM WOUNDS

After the wound has been dressed, take a two or three-inch bandage, place the center of it over the wound, carry the ends around the arm and bring them back again to the side where the wound is. Tie the ends, taking care that the knot does not press directly on the wound. The arm should be supported in a sling.

## BANDAGING THE COLLAR-BONE

A firm pad, about two inches by four inches, should be placed well up under the armpit on the injured side. Gently push up the elbow and place the forearm diagonally across the chest. Fold a broad triangular bandage, place the center on the elbow, take the ends around the chest and tie on the opposite side, in front. A sling should be used.

## BANDAGING THE NECK

With a thick pad of sterile gauze, cover the wound. Make a simple circular bandage over the compress. Bring the bandage down under one armpit and back to the neck and tie. Be careful that there is no pull in the armpit as it will impair the circulation of the large vessels of the arm.

## BANDAGING THE KNEE

Fold a narrow hem along the base of a triangular bandage. Place its center under the kneecap with the point toward the thigh. Carry the bandage behind the knee, then bring the ends forward and tie above the knee.

## BANDAGING THE LEG OR THIGH

While applying the bandage, rest the foot on a support, such as a chair. Fold a triangular bandage, broad, and place the center of it over the pad on the wound. Carry around the limb and cross behind. Bring forward and tie in front.

## BANDAGING THE FOOT

To bandage the foot, a full-sized triangular bandage is needed. Place the base of the bandage well up the ankle so that it will fit well. Set the foot in the center of the unfolded bandage with the toes to-

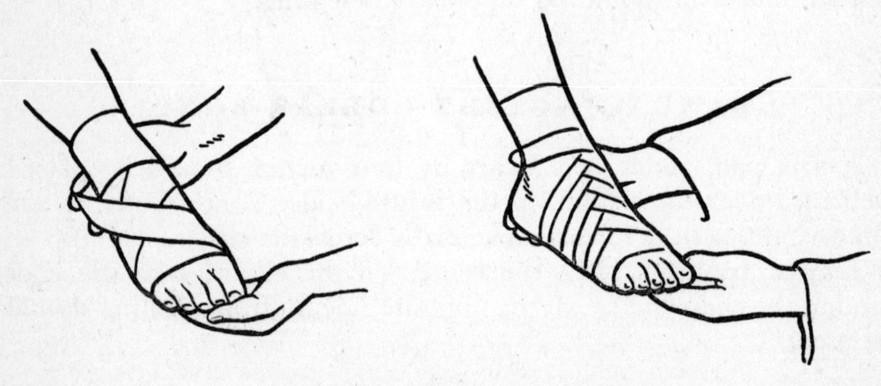

A SECURE FOOT BANDAGE

*(Left)* Start the bandage over the front of the foot, directly above the toes, and bring it around the sole of the foot. Now pass the bandage obliquely upward around the back of the ankle and downward obliquely toward the toes, over the first turn. Bring it around the sole of the foot again and upward obliquely to behind ankle. *(Right)* Continue downward, making turns over front of ankle and sole of foot. Each turn obliquely overlaps the previous one, basket-weave fashion.

wards the point. Bring the point backwards over the foot. Gather up the ends fairly close to the foot. Cross the ends over. Carry the ends round the ankle and cross them behind, taking in the lower border. Bring the ends forward and tie them in front. Pull down the point over the knot and pin it.

## BANDAGING THE EYE

First place a pad on the injured eye. Fold a narrow triangular bandage. Arrange the center of the bandage over the eye, carry upwards over the forehead and then downwards under the ear. Cross behind the head, continue around the head and tie over the pad. Start by placing the bandage on the bridge of the nose when bandaging both eyes.

## BANDAGING THE CHIN AND EARS

Place a pad on the wounded part. Fold a narrow triangular bandage and place the center on the chin and carry the ends upwards. Tie the ends on top of the head.

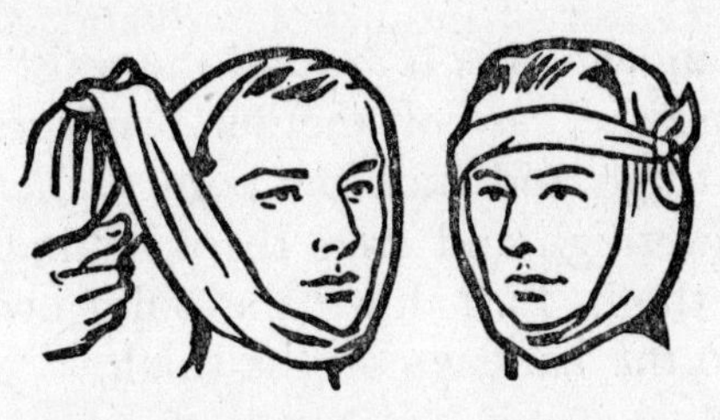

BANDAGE FOR CHIN OR SIDE OF FACE

Here is another application of the cravat bandage. As shown in the illustration at the left, the bandage is brought vertically around the head, crossed at the temple, and wrapped around the upper part of the head. A firm knot keeps it secure. (The basic method of making a cravat bandage is explained in detail on page 499.)

## BANDAGING THE NOSE

Make a four-tailed bandage by dividing the tails of a large sterile bandage compress. Place the pad of a compress on the wound, cross the tails, carry them above and below the ears on each side, to the back of the head. Tie the tails.

## BANDAGING THE SCALP

Fold a hem, one and one-half inches wide, on the base of a triangular bandage. Arrange the middle of the hem on the forehead, just above the eyebrows, with the point hanging down over the back of the head. Pull down the point at the back to make the bandage fit snugly over the head. Tie on the forehead with a double knot. Bring the point up to the top of the head and pin it.

## BANDAGING THE LOWER JAW

Use a bandage, two or three inches wide, folded. Place the center under the chin and take the ends upwards and tie on top of the head.

Fold a second bandage, place the center under the lower lip, bring the ends backwards and tie at the base of the skull.

## BANDAGING THE HIP

Fold a narrow bandage. Tie it around the waist like a girdle. Fold a narrow hem along the base of another bandage, apply the center of the base to the thigh and tuck the point under the girdle; carry the ends around the thigh and cross them behind. Tie the ends on the outside of the thigh. Pull down the point over the knot of the girdle and pin it to the bandage on the thigh.

## BANDAGING THE SIDE OF THE CHEST

A broad bandage is applied folded over the pad on the wound. The ends are brought around the chest and tied on the opposite side.

## BANDAGING THE ABDOMEN

Fold a four-inch bandage; apply the center to the pad on the wound and tie on the opposite side.

## BANDAGING THE HAND

Place an unfolded bandage on the table. Place the injured hand palm downwards on the bandage with the wrist on the center of the lower border and the fingers directed towards the point of the bandage. Next fold the bandage over the fingers and the back of the hand and carry the point up the forearm. Now take the ends and, crossing them on the back of the hand, carry them to the front of the wrist. Cross the bandage here once more. Bring the ends to the back of the wrist, knot them, covering the knot by folding down the point and fixing it with a safety pin.

## BANDAGING THE FINGER

A reverse bandage is applied. It should be one inch wide and four yards long. Take the bandage once over the middle of the finger, holding it on each side. Make two more turns over the finger, one on each side of the middle finger. Finish off with a figure-of-eight around the wrist. Pin or tie.

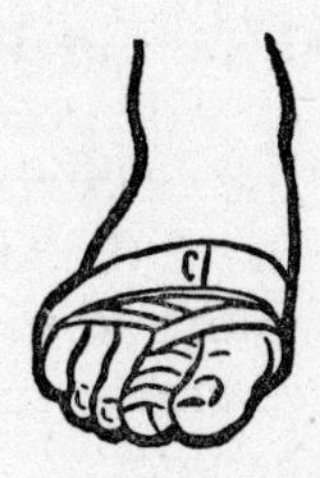

AN EASY WAY TO MAKE A ROLLER BANDAGE FOR THE TOE

The toe is securely wrapped in the roller bandage, which is then brought around the foot several times, as shown. (Basic facts about roller bandages are presented on page 500. You should also familiarize yourself with the rules for bandaging in general, which you will find on pages 497 and 498.)

## BANDAGING THE PALM

Fold a bandage, narrow. Place the center of it on the palm. Carry the two ends over to the back of the hand, cross them there and bring them around to the front of the wrist. Cross them once more, and carry them to the back of the wrist. Knot them there.

## HEAT STROKE

***Causes of Heat Stroke.*** This is about the same as heat exhaustion. It is caused by loss of fluid and salt from the body through excessive perspiration. The condition may also be brought about by prolonged activity in overheated and poorly ventilated areas where humidity is high.

***How to Avoid Heat Stroke.*** If much water is lost through perspiration, more salt and water should be taken into the body. The salt can be added to the drinking water. Exertion should be avoided when it is very hot.

***Symptoms of Heat Stroke.*** Common symptoms are faintness and dizziness, nausea, cold clammy skin, dilated pupils, subnormal temperature, severe muscular cramps, profuse sweating, pulse that is rapid, weak and thready.

***Treatment of Heat Stroke.*** The patient should be placed in the shade. Lower his head and apply an ice-cap to it. Loosen his clothing and give him large quantities of cool drinks. Add to the drinks one-quarter teaspoonful of table salt. If the patient has fainted and his temperature is below normal, he should be wrapped in a blanket. A hot water bottle at his feet will prove helpful. Intravenous salt solution should be given by the physician.

Heat stroke and sun stroke have the same effect on the body. Heat stroke is the result of the exposure to intense heat indoors, and sun-stroke is the result of prolonged exposure to the direct rays of the sun. The treatment of both is the same.

## ELECTRIC SHOCK

***How to Avoid Electric Shock.*** With only elementary precautions, electric shock can be avoided. If there are any exposed wires in the home, replace them or cover them. Electric equipment that is not working properly should not be used. Electric outlets not in use should be plugged up so children cannot get at them.

Electric cords require special care. Do not run them over pipes or radiators, or in places where they are subject to any particular wear and tear. Avoid touching a switch when your hands are wet, for water is a good conductor. Keep all electric appliances dry.

Outdoors, keep away from trees during an electric storm. Do not use a steel shaft umbrella.

## HOW TO RESCUE A PERSON SHOCKED BY ELECTRICITY

It is important to shut off the current or break the contact with the live wire at once. If the power cannot be shut off, cut the wire with an ax having a wooden handle. Metal cutting objects may be used if you are wearing rubber gloves. You must not touch the victim if you are not completely insulated against shock.

Your hands should be protected with silk, a rubber coat or some thicknesses of dry cloth. Stand on a dry plant or a pile of dry paper. If the floor is not wet you may pull the person off the wire with bare hands *if* you make sure to touch nothing but his clothing, which must be dry. Above all, take care not to touch the wire yourself.

In case the wire is on the person, push it off him with a dry stick.

Artificial respiration should be begun as quickly as possible. Often persons suffering from electric shock are alive but unconscious. Timely use of artificial respiration revives them.

## ARTIFICIAL RESPIRATION

When respiration has temporarily ceased, as occurs in drowning, gas poisoning, or electric shock, artificial ventilation of the lungs should be promptly applied. By this means oxygen is supplied to the tissues until spontaneous respiration again takes place, when the paralyzed respiratory center in the brain recovers its function. As long as the heart beats, recovery is possible. This may happen after even eight or more hours of artificial respiration.

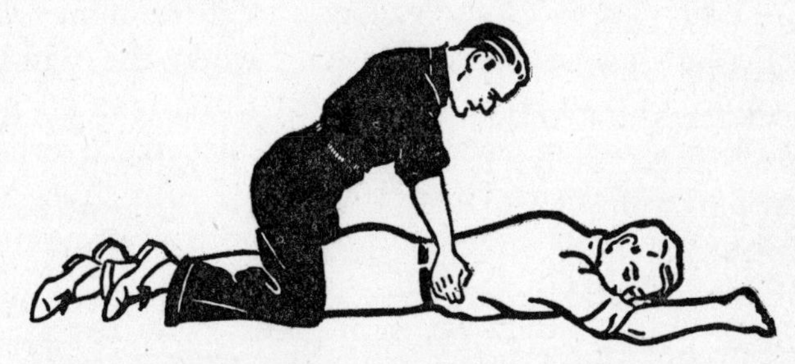

SCHAEFER OR PRONE METHOD OF ARTIFICIAL RESPIRATION

Showing the position in which artificial respiration is started. If the first-aider becomes fatigued—it may be necessary to continue for hours—another person should replace him without breaking the rhythm. Several persons may spell each other off in doing this work. If the patient has to be moved, artificial respiration is continued en route. Nothing should be given him by mouth until he is fully recovered, at which time stimulants such as hot tea or coffee are recommended.

***Schaefer Technique.*** Among the simple methods of artificial respiration, the Schaefer technique is the most adequate and should be used until a mechanical device is available. First loosen all clothing about the chest, abdomen, and neck. Clear the mouth of water and mucus; remove artificial teeth. Hold the tongue forward. Place the patient face downward, his chest resting on the floor; one of his arms is stretched overhead, and the head, turned to one side, rests on the other, so that air may pass freely through his mouth and nose. The operator straddles one of the thighs. The hands are placed over the lowermost ribs with the palms down and the thumbs separated and parallel near the spine. With arms fixed in a straight position, the operator swings forward, applying pressure firmly on the lower ribs for two seconds, forcing the air out of the lungs. The pressure is then released for a period of three seconds, allowing the lungs to recoil and take in air. Alternate pressure (two seconds) and release (three seconds) is continuously performed. The procedure is not to be stopped until normal respiration is established or the victim is pronounced dead.

## FREEZING

***How to Avoid Freezing.*** Above all, it is essential to be properly dressed when outdoors in cold weather. Your clothing should be warm and not fit you too loosely. Keep in movement when out-of-doors, and do not stay exposed too long when the wind is strong. When you come indoors, even for a short time, take off heavy outer clothing and overshoes so that you do not become overheated. It is dangerous to go outdoors when overheated. If your shoes or stockings get wet, they should be changed. Do not go out when your hands are wet or when you do not feel well.

If you are spending much time out-of-doors in the cold weather, see to it that you eat regularly of well-balanced nourishing foods that will keep your resistance high.

### Frostbite

***Symptoms of Frostbite.*** The nose, chin, ears, fingers, and toes are the parts usually frozen. Severe results ending in death of the frozen part occur more often owing to low vitality of the patient than to the cold itself. In the milder degree of frostbite there is stiffness, numbness, and tingling of the frozen member. The skin is of a pale, bluish hue and somewhat shrunken. Recovery ensues with burning pain, tingling, redness, swelling and peeling of the outer skin as after slight burns. The skin is icy cold, white, and insensitive in severe forms of frostbite. If not skillfully treated, it later becomes either swollen and discolored, or shriveled, dry, and black. In either event, the frozen part dies and is separated from the living tissue after the establishment of a sharp line of inflammation which results in ulceration and formation of pus. The dead part sloughs off. It is, however, possible for a part thoroughly frozen to regain its vitality.

***Treatment of Frostbite.*** The essential element in the treatment is to secure a very gradual return of blood to the frozen tissues, and so avoid violent inflammation. To obtain this result the patient should be cared for in a cold room. The frozen parts are rubbed gently with soft snow, or cloth wet with ice water, until they resume their usual warmth. Then it is well to rub them with a mixture of equal parts of alcohol and water for a time, and expose them to the usual temperature of a dwelling room. Warm drinks are now administered to the patient. The frozen member, if hand or foot, is raised high on pillows and covered well with absorbent cotton and bandage. If much redness, swelling, and pain result, this dressing is removed and the part is wrapped in a single thickness of cotton cloth kept continuously wet with alcohol and water. The patient should make active movements of the damaged part, which is kept elevated. As an alternative procedure, the frozen part may be immersed in a water bath of about 50° F., in which the patient carries out active movements.

For a frozen part of the face, cold irrigations or compresses can be used.

When the blood circulation in the damaged part is restored, cleansing should be the next step, which is then followed by exposure to gentle heat.

If medical help is not forthcoming, subsequent treatment consists in keeping the damaged parts covered with vaseline or cold cream, absorbent cotton, and bandage. If blisters and sores result, the care is similar to that described for like conditions under burns.

## CHILBLAINS AND MILD FROSTBITES

***Symptoms of Chilblains.*** The effects of severe cold on the body are very similar to those of intense heat, though they are very much slower in making their appearance. After a person has frozen a finger or toe, he may not notice much inconvenience for days. Then, suddenly, violent inflammation may set in. The fingers, ears, nose, and toes are the members which suffer most frequently from the effects of cold. Symptoms of inflammation also result from cold, that is, redness and swelling of the skin, blisters with more severe and deeper inflammatory involvement, or, in case the parts are thoroughly frozen, local death and destruction of the tissues. But it is not essential that the body be exposed to the freezing temperature or be frozen at all, in order that some harm may result, for chilblains often follow when the temperature has not been lower than 40° F., or thereabouts.

The effect of cold is to contract the blood vessels, with the production of numbness, pallor, and tingling of the skin. When the cold no longer acts, then the blood vessels dilate to more than their usual and normal state, and more or less inflammation results. The more sudden the return to warmth, the greater the inflammation that follows.

Chilblains represent the mildest morbid effect of cold on the body. They are present as bluish-red swellings of the skin, usually on the feet or hands. They may attack the nose or ears, and are attended by burning, itching, and smarting. This condition is caused by dilation of the vessels following exposure to cold. It is more apt to happen in young, anemic women. Chilblains usually disappear during the warm weather. Scratching, friction, or the severity of the attack may lead to the appearance of blisters and sores. In severe conditions the fingers and toes present a sausage-like appearance, owing to swelling.

***Treatment of Chilblains.*** Susceptible persons should wear thick, warm (not rough) stockings and warm gloves. The chilled members must never be suddenly warmed. Regular exercise and cold shower baths are good to strengthen the circulation. However, the feet and hands must be washed in warm water only, and thoroughly aired. If sweating of these parts is a common occurrence, starch or zinc oxide should be dusted on freely, night and morning. Cod-liver oil is an efficacious remedy in these cases.

The affected parts are bathed twice daily in a solution of zinc acetate (one dram to one pint of water), and followed by the application, on soft linen or cotton, of zinc-oxide ointment containing 2 per cent of carbolic acid. If this is not curative, iodine ointment mixed with an equal quantity of lard may be tried. Exposure to cold will immediately bring on a recurrence of the trouble. If the affection of the feet is severe, the patient must rest in bed. If the parts become blistered and open sores appear, then the same treatment as for burns should be followed.

## POISONS TAKEN BY MOUTH

There are two kinds of poisons: those which are prescribed for medicinal purposes and become poisonous when taken in overdoses, and those which come under the heading of chemicals which are either corrosive or highly toxic.

***Fundamental Treatment.*** There are four important steps in treatment: to send for a doctor, dilute the poison, empty the stomach by emesis (vomiting), and give special treatment as indicated.

When calling a doctor, tell him if possible what the poison is that has been taken. Saving a few minutes may mean saving a life—the doctor can tell you what to do while he is en route to you.

***Diluting the Poison.*** Diluting the poison means taking certain solutions into the stomach that will both dilute the poison and cause vomiting. The special diluents will be given under the accompanying table of special treatment. A demulcent is a special substance used to dilute corrosive poisons such as carbolic acid or lysol. The best demulcents are milk, white of eggs, and oatmeal gruel. If none of these is available, force the index finger as far back in the patient's throat as possible. This will often cause vomiting.

***Emetics to Use.*** An emetic is a fluid or a drug that will cause vomiting. Vomiting is called emesis. The commonest emetic and the easiest to prepare is warm soapsuds water, two or three glasses. Warm mustard water, half a teaspoonful to the glass, is also a good emetic. Syrup of ipecac, which can be purchased at the drugstore, will surely cause the patient to vomit. Give a tablespoonful. It will not be necessary to repeat, as it will surely work—the only difficulty may be in getting it quickly enough. It is most important to remember that if the poison taken is a strong acid or alkali, you should not give an emetic, as the vomiting may rupture the already damaged walls of the stomach and gullet. In such cases, wait for the doctor to arrive. If the patient is unconscious there is nothing that can be done until the doctor comes. He will immediately put in a stomach tube and wash out the stomach.

## POISONING FROM INSECT BITES

As a rule, insect bites and stings are not serious, although they often cause intense pain for a while. Certain spider bites, like that of the black-widow, are an exception. The bites that result when a person is attacked by a swarm of hornets or some other stinging insects may also be dangerous.

***Bee Sting.*** Some bees leave their sting in the victim's body. The sting is removable by pressing or pushing sideways with the fingers. It can usually be seen. Do not try to pull the sting with the thumb and forefinger or you may squeeze any residual venom into the wound. In contrast to bees, wasps retain their stings. Prompt application of ammonia often relieves the pain of stings.

***Chiggers.*** Chiggers do their damage by burrowing into the skin. As they are digging their way in, it is possible many times to pick them out. A drop of iodine or kerosene on a chigger bite will give relief. To prevent bites, rub kerosene or a salve containing menthol about the ankles, wrists and waist.

## TABLE OF COMMON POISONS—SYMPTOMS AND TREATMENT

| *Poison* | *Symptoms* | *Treatment* | *Special Antidote* |
|---|---|---|---|
| Advertised headache remedies: Acentanilid, Antipyrin, Phenacetin | Blueness of the nails and lips, shallow breathing, weakness, profuse sweating, collapse | Emetic, large amounts of milk, oatmeal, liquids, coffee, heat to body | None |
| Ammonia | Pain in throat, gullet, and stomach; vomiting, collapse | Milk, albumin, water, gruels, emetic | Diluted vinegar, lemon and orange juice |
| Arsenic, Paris green (rat poison) | Burning pain in the throat, stomach cramps, diarrhea and collapse | Large amounts of milk, thin starch solution, albumin, water, thin gruels. Produce profuse emesis | There is a standard antidote for arsenic. It is principally iron chloride. Any drugstore clerk will know how to prepare it. Tablespoonful given every half hour. Also give emetic |
| Alcohol (wood, methyl) | Headache, nausea and vomiting, stupor and collapse | Give an emetic as quickly as possible as alcohol rapidly passes out of the stomach. Keep warm. Give copiously of strong coffee | Large doses of baking soda given frequently |
| Carbona, cleaning fluid | Nausea and vomiting, pain on swallowing, drowsiness, collapse | If taken in any quantity it will soon prove fatal unless the stomach can be rapidly emptied. Give large amounts of strong coffee and apply heat to the body | None |
| Carbon monoxide or cooking gas | Blueness of lips, fingernails; collapse, unconsciousness. | Fresh air; try to keep on feet; artificial respiration. Send for pulmotor | Fresh air |

| Poison | Symptoms | Treatment | Special Antidote |
|---|---|---|---|
| Hypnotics (sleeping pills, also known as barbiturates) | Unconsciousness, blueness (cyanosis), collapse, thready pulse, shallow breathing | Empty the stomach; give stimulants of whiskey or strong coffee | None |
| Iodine | Brown stain in the mouth, painful swallowing, collapse | Make a thin paste of household starch, have patient drink copiously of it; oatmeal gruel or mashed potatoes and water | Have doctor wash stomach with large quantities of starch solution |
| Lysol, carbolic acid, cresol | Vomiting of brownish fluid; odor of typical corrosive fluid like carbolic; severe pain all along the digestive tract | Large amounts of milk, butter, olive oil; stimulate with coffee | Several tablespoonfuls of diluted pure alcohol, several glasses of wine, then emetic |
| Mercury bichloride (corrosive sublimate) | White discoloration of the mouth mucous membrane. Metallic taste, vomiting, watery and bloody stools, unconsciousness | Several eggs beaten up in milk; follow with an emetic. Repeat several times | The doctor will wash out the stomach with calcium sulphate solution |
| Opium:<br>Morphine<br>Codeine<br>Laudanum<br>Paregoric | Drowsiness deepening into unconsciousness, shallow breathing, slow pulse | If conscious, give emetic quickly. Give copiously of strong coffee. Keep awake by constant slapping of the body. Artificial respiration may be needed | None |
| Phosphorus (rat poison) | Vomiting that has an odor like garlic, intense pain in stomach. Jaundice develops in several days. Death is common | Secure profuse vomiting with an emetic. Give prompt treatment, even in absence of vomiting | Give quarter glass of hydrogen peroxide diluted four times in water |

***Flea Bite.*** Camphor water, alcohol, or calamine lotion should be applied to the wound.

***Hornet Sting.*** Soda bicarbonate solution, a slice of onion, or dilute ammonia water should be applied to the wound. Apply ice in case of swelling.

***Mosquito Bite.*** When bitten, apply theophorin ointment (5 per cent). To prevent bites, apply a formula your druggist can prepare for you: 33 per cent pyrethrum extract, 52 per cent mineral or castor oil, and 15 per cent oil of pennyroyal. Smear this on your face and hands.

***Spider Bite.*** The bites of the black-widow spider and tarantula are dangerous. In either case, send for a doctor at once. For a tarantula bite, before the physician arrives, wash or suck the wound clean. There is no first-aid treatment for the bite of the black-widow spider.

***Woodtick Bite.*** Cracked ice should be applied to the wound. Dip cloths in cold lead water and alcohol; wring out and apply.

## POISONING FROM ANIMAL BITES

***Cat Bite.*** The bite of any animal may transmit rabies to the victim. Rabies vaccine should be administered immediately. The cat's mouth, incidentally, contains germs that are more dangerous to human beings than the germs found in a dog's mouth. The area of the bite should be washed carefully and an antiseptic and a sterile dressing applied. A physician should be summoned.

***Dog Bite.*** The prevention of hydrophobia is extremely important. A bite by a healthy dog that is known to you is likely to be just a slight injury. The treatment consists of applying an antiseptic and a protective dressing. The dog should be watched for several days by a veterinarian to find out whether any symptoms of rabies develop. However, if a stray dog is responsible for the bite, the doctor must determine whether or not the dog was carrying the germs of rabies. If such is the case, it is essential to cauterize at once and give the Pasteur treatment. The same consideration must be given rat or squirrel bites. In first aid, wash the wound thoroughly at once. Apply a strong antiseptic—excellent for practical purposes are strong tincture of iodine or commercial formalin. Consult a physician at once.

***Human Bite.*** It is important to cleanse the wound carefully since these bites are often a cause of infection. Tincture of iodine, a wet dressing of salt solution, or alcohol should be applied to the wound.

***Snake Bite.*** The United States has four varieties of poisonous snakes—the cotton-mouth moccasin, the copper-head moccasin, the rattlesnake and the coral snake. They are unlikely to bite provided they are not directly molested.

Sterilize the skin with alcohol. Sterilize a sharp knife or razor blade with an antiseptic or by passing it through a flame. Make a criss-cross incision about one-half inch by one-half inch through each fang mark, avoiding as far as possible superficial veins and arteries. Each incision should go well through the skin to allow free bleeding. Apply suction for at least half an hour by mouth. As the swelling spreads, a ring of incisions about one-quarter inch by one-quarter inch may be made directly in the swollen area about two inches from the primary incisions, and suction applied to each incision for fifteen minutes out of each hour, for ten to fifteen hours.

Before slashing open the wound it is best to be sure that the bite has been made by a snake of a poisonous species. After the head of the snake has been severed, if it can be done quickly and safely, pry the mouth of the snake wide open and examine its teeth. If some of them are hollow or there are grooved fangs exuding a fluid on pressure, the snake is poisonous. The fangs are relatively long in comparison with the other teeth and are located in the upper jaw. Do not forget that muscular reflexes may result in the quick closing of a snake's jaw even after the head has been severed from the body and that venom from the head may be absorbed through cuts or scratches on the hands. Therefore be careful in handling the head of even a dead snake.

The patient should be kept warm and quiet until a physician can reach him. Anti-venin is exceedingly valuable in the treatment when it is available and can be given at once. Contrary to popular belief, whiskey is of no value in the treatment.

Only the very large black-fanged snakes, as a general rule, constitute a serious danger to sportsmen. Seek advance information regarding them in the area in which you intend to travel. In hot, dry localities snakes usually hide during the day and come out at night to hunt.

## POISONING BY PLANTS

The best way to protect yourself against poisonous plants is to avoid contact with them. When going into places where there are poisonous plants, wear gloves and long trousers. You can also obtain 5 per cent solution of ferric chloride or a strong solution of sodium hyposulphite and apply this to your hands and feet. Wash yourself with strong soap and water on any areas of the body you believe have been exposed to poisonous plants.

Poisoning by plants may result not only from contact with them but by swallowing. Poisonous plant matter that has been swallowed is treated by giving an emetic and calling a doctor.

***Black Nightshade (Deadly).*** Emetics, cathartic and stimulants are used as treatment.

***Hemlock.*** Give an emetic, tea, stimulants, warmth to the limbs and artificial respiration.

***Henbane.*** Use emetics, give strong tea, tannic acid or infusion of oak bark. Apply artificial respiration.

***Ivy.*** See Index.

***Jamestown or Jimson Weed.*** This is an extremely dangerous plant. Use the same remedies as for henbane.

***Oak.*** See Index.

## FOOD POISONING

Food poisoning is usually caused by bacteria. Its main symptoms are upset of the stomach and intestines. The upset may range from mild dyspepsia to severe diarrhea and collapse.

In general, if food is insufficiently cooked, bacteria find a favorable medium for growth. When foods are removed from cans and kept for any length of time, they should be refrigerated and recooked before use. Any food which is to be eaten raw should be fresh, free from any abnormal odor or spoiled areas. It should be washed thoroughly in clean water. Above all, it is important never to taste any food to determine if it is spoiled or not, because even a minute quantity is sometimes sufficient to cause serious illness.

## "PTOMAINE" POISONING

Severe disturbances of the digestive tract accompanied by nausea, vomiting, and diarrhea are often mistakenly called "ptomaine" poisoning.

The disturbances which popularly go by this name really belong to one of several groups: first, they may be caused by poisonous substances in the food; second, they may be attributable to disease-producing germs consumed with the food; and third, they may be due to an individual sensitivity which causes an abnormal reaction to foods in themselves perfectly wholesome.

Scientifically speaking, ptomaines are a class of organic bases produced by putrefactive bacteria acting on matter that is nitrogenous in nature. Most ptomaines cause no harm. In any event, the poisoning generally attributed to them is not caused by them, but by specific bacterial poisons.

***Treatment of Food Poisoning.*** This should be in the hands of a physician. It is important to clean out the stomach. If the patient is not vomiting, the physician may bring it on by having him drink several glasses of warm water; otherwise a saline laxative or a high colonic irrigation is given. All foods should be prohibited. Two hours after the cathartic has been administered, milk of bismuth in tablespoonful doses, or bismuth subcarbonate in one-gram doses are given every few hours, if necessary. However, the precise treatment is up to the physician, Hot applications to the abdomen may afford relief, and the first-aider should provide these while awaiting the physician's arrival.

### Botulism

Botulism is an acute poisoning, caused by germs. It is exceedingly dangerous. Meat products are most frequently contaminated. Many home-canned vegetables or fruits served cold are responsible for this kind of poisoning. To avoid botulism, cook food thoroughly to destroy spores of bacteria.

Symptoms of botulism are weakness, subnormal temperature, and a sensation of dizziness. It may be hard to swallow.

Treatment should be only by a physician, who will administer botulinus toxin.

## MUSHROOM POISONING

Only a few varieties of mushrooms contain deadly poison. It is unwise for the average person to pick and eat his own mushrooms unless he is well trained in their identification. The best course, otherwise, is to use only mushrooms that are commercially grown.

***Death Cup (Amanita phalloides).*** The most frequent cause of fungus poisoning and the most deadly species known, this mushroom is pleasant to the taste. It is not rendered harmless by cooking or digestive processes. (There is a popular belief to the effect that a test shows it to blacken silver. It does not.) Safety depends on recognizing the plant at sight. The death cup has white gills readily seen, a cap marked with faint, dark green stripes and a large bulbous stem.

Treatment consists in the elimination of the toxin and restoration of fluid balance. A physician must be consulted early.

## POISON SPRAYS ON FRUIT

The widespread spraying of fruit trees and vegetables with insecticides containing arsenic and lead has introduced a new hazard in connection with certain foods. It is best to take the precaution of thoroughly washing vegetables and of discarding the skins and cores of fruits which have been sprayed.

Most of the chemical poisoning of food sources is accidental. It is usually owing to carelessness in the handling of insecticides, disinfectants, rodent poisons and other chemicals. A physician must be consulted in all cases of suspected poisoning. He is the only one qualified to make an accurate diagnosis.

CHAPTER 29

# PROTECTING YOURSELF AGAINST AN ATOMIC BOMB

**Air Bursts and How They Damage Surrounding Areas . . . Ground and Water Bursts and the Danger from Them . . . What to Do in an Air Raid . . . Sneak Attack . . . Air Raid Warnings . . . When You Hear the Alert . . . After an Air Burst . . . After a Ground or Water Burst . . . What You Should and Should Not Do . . . How Atomic Radiation Affects the Body . . . First Aid for Radiation Sickness . . . What to Do in Case of Fire . . . Simple Rules to Follow in Caring for Burns . . . How to Check Bleeding . . . Using a Tourniquet . . . What to Do for Fractures or Broken Bones, etc.**

WE HOPE that your closest acquaintance with an atomic bomb will be in reading this chapter. But if you are to understand what to do if an A-bomb should fall on your city, you must first know what an A-bomb does.

An atomic bomb set off in mid-air, about 2,000 feet from ground level, is more destructive than either a water or ground burst, so we must consider this kind of attack as the most likely.

***Air Burst.*** Here is what happens in an air burst: at the instant of the explosion, a brilliant fireball appears in the sky and quickly grows to about 900 feet in diameter. It could probably be seen for 50 miles in daylight, 200 miles at night. From this fireball, brighter than 100 suns, deadly heat and radiation burst out in all directions. The heat flash is dangerous up to 2 miles, but the radiation intensity falls off rapidly after 4,000 feet. In the first second, half of the radiation has already passed. In three seconds heat and most of harmful radiation are over.

Following the heat flash, a tremendous shock wave caused by the expansion of hot gases from the explosion sweeps over the area. Winds of 800 mph accompany the shock wave in its early stages but fall off rapidly in intensity, dropping to 100 mph within a mile and a half. Several seconds later, another wind roars in toward the center of the explosion with about half the force of the outrushing blast. At the end of 10 seconds, the immediate danger from the explosion itself has passed.

If you are above ground anywhere within three quarters of a mile from the air burst, you will have less than a 50-50 chance of survival.

If you are underground within this area, you will have a good chance of coming through, unless you are almost directly under the point where the bomb explodes.

*Here are some estimates of how an atomic explosion would damage the area around it:*

*Within one-half mile.* Complete devastation. Little chance of survival if above ground.

*From one-half to one mile.* All buildings, except those of concrete and heavy steel frame, will be gutted or destroyed. The heat flash will be intense, but radiation will be reduced.

*From one mile to a mile and a half.* Most old-style brick and frame buildings will be destroyed. Modern buildings will be seriously damaged. There will be great danger from flying debris. Radiation will no longer be a hazard. The heat flash will still be dangerous, but not lethal.

Hundreds of scattered fires will break out, many of them caused by broken gas mains, oil lines and tanks or shorted electric circuits. All utilities will be destroyed or seriously damaged.

*At two miles.* Damage here will almost all be due to blast and secondary fires. Public utilities will be badly damaged. Only moderate burns, if any, will be caused by the heat flash.

*At four miles.* There will still be some blast damage, especially to frame and old-style wooden buildings, and scattered secondary fires. Rubble will block the streets.

*Beyond four miles.* In some instances blast damage might extend to a distance of six miles, depending upon the wind, weather and the terrain. Glass and plaster breakage might occur up to a distance of 8 miles. Utilities might be disrupted from damage in the central blast area.

About a half hour after the explosion a strong wind will blow in toward the center of the damaged area, spreading the fires that have already been started.

## GROUND AND WATER BURSTS

While it is likely that an enemy will prefer an air burst because of the greater damage it does, he may deliberately or accidentally explode an atomic bomb on the ground or in a harbor.

In ground or water bursts the effects of the blast, heat and direct radiation do not extend nearly as far as in an air burst. In the case of a water burst, heat and direct radiation are negligible, and damage from the shock wave does not extend beyond one mile.

However, both ground and water bursts have a particular danger of their own which is almost completely lacking in air bursts. The clouds of spray or dust thrown into the air by these bursts become highly radioactive. As they drift with the wind over the surrounding area, they contaminate all objects in their path and poison people who are exposed to them too long.

## WHAT TO DO IN AN AIR RAID

A radar network and a force of volunteer airplane spotters will detect an enemy attack. If enemy raiders are sighted, air raid sirens will be sounded. But we must also consider the possibility that the enemy will be able to evade our defenses and deliver a bomb before a warning can be sounded.

### Sneak Attack

In case of a sneak attack there are several things you can do to protect yourself, even though you may not be able to reach shelter.

The blinding flash of the explosion will be your first warning. If you are in the open, immediately fall to the ground face down next to a building wall, if possible, so you will be shielded from falling brick and stones. Close your eyes and cover your face, neck and arms. This will give you some protection against the deadly radiation and scorching heat.

If you are on the street, dodge into a doorway if it is not more than a step or two away. Stand to one side under the arch of the door. Turn away from the flash and cover your face and other exposed areas of the body.

If you are in the house, crawl under a bed or table or drop behind a sofa or any other large object which can protect you from flying glass. Keep out of line with windows. *Cover up.*

### Air Raid Warnings

When enemy planes are spotted coming toward your city, the sirens will blow a signal.

*An attacking plane may fly over many towns before reaching its target. All these towns will be warned.* The air raid warning does not necessarily mean that your city is the target. But remember that the signal means *trouble is at hand. Take cover.*

Unless announced in advance that tests will be held, an air raid warning *means business.*

### When You Hear the Alert

Know your designated shelter. Get down into it or into the basement, as fast as you can without pushing people around. Take cover, but be sensible. *Do not panic.*

Blast is most destructive to the upper portion of buildings. If you can't get downstairs, get into the center hall, the core of the structure.

***If You Cannot Get Out of Your Office or Apartment in Time.*** Get under a desk or table if possible or lie close to the wall where you are not in line with the windows. Cover your neck, head and arms with your coat. Close your eyes tightly. These precautions will help protect you from flying glass or debris, as well as the heat and radiation from the explosion.

***If You Are on the Street.*** Get to the nearest shelter, basement or subway.

If no air-raid shelter is available, step into the nearest doorway or, better yet, into the lobby of a concrete building. Face away from the street and from windows. Pull your coat over your head or if you are without a coat shield your head with your arms.

***If You Are Driving a Car.*** Park at the curb as quickly as you can. Do not park where you will block a street or a corner. Leave your keys in the car. Get out and seek shelter at once. If you are riding in a taxi or bus, get out and take cover.

***If You Live in a Frame House.*** Shut off at the source all oil, gas, light and water. Put out fires. Close all doors and windows. Draw curtains and blinds.

Get into the basement if you have one. Take a flashlight and, if it is winter, a supply of warm clothing. After all fires have been extinguished, close fuel lines and draft doors of coal furnaces or stoves.

Have several buckets of sand and water and a complete first aid kit handy.

### The All Clear

When the enemy plane has been shot down or has passed by without attack or has made its attack and departed, the sirens will blow an "All Clear."

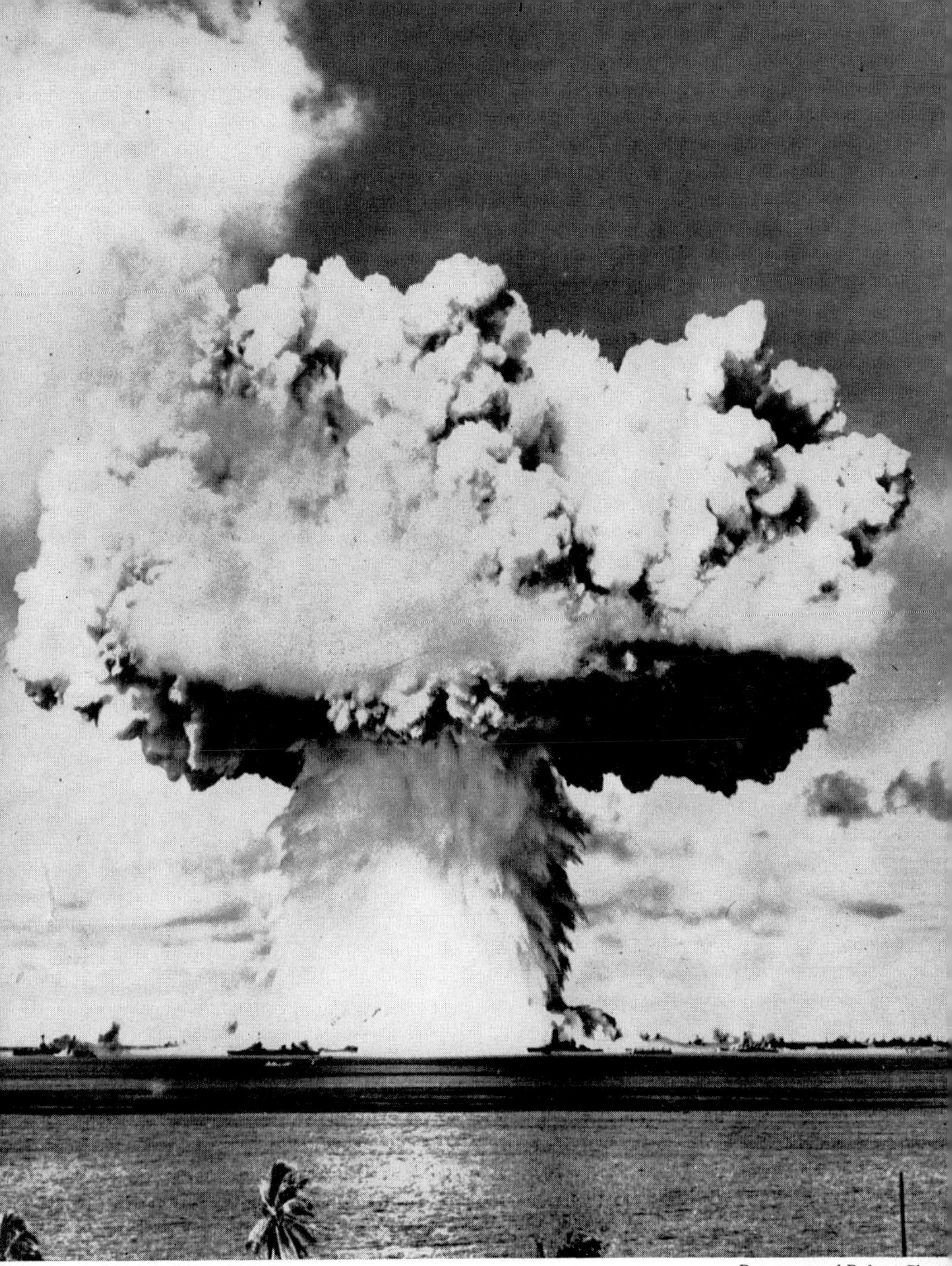

Department of Defense Photo

# You Can Beat the Atomic Bomb

Your chances of escaping alive if you are in the area where an atomic bomb explodes are better than is commonly believed. A person one-half to one mile away has a fifty-fifty chance. Beyond two miles, the explosion will cause almost no deaths. Much depends on whether or not your shelter is adequate. Concrete buildings, with heavy steel frames, are much safer than frame houses. Over half of all bomb injuries are the result of being tossed about or struck by flying and falling objects. See Chapter 29 for basic precautions.

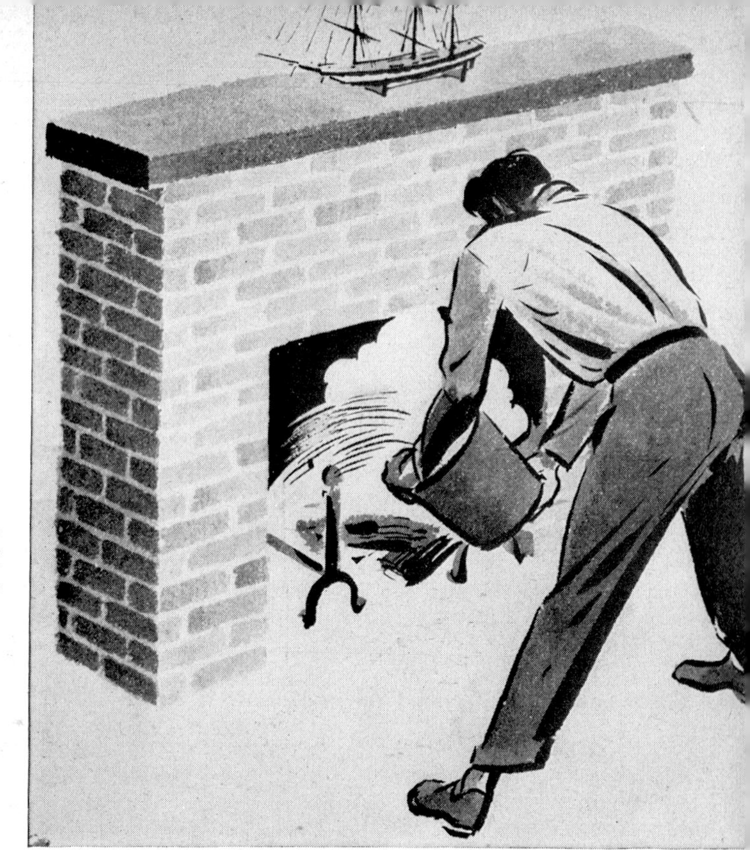

PUT OUT FIRES

When you hear an alert, extinguish all fires, to prevent the spread of flames in case your house should be damaged.

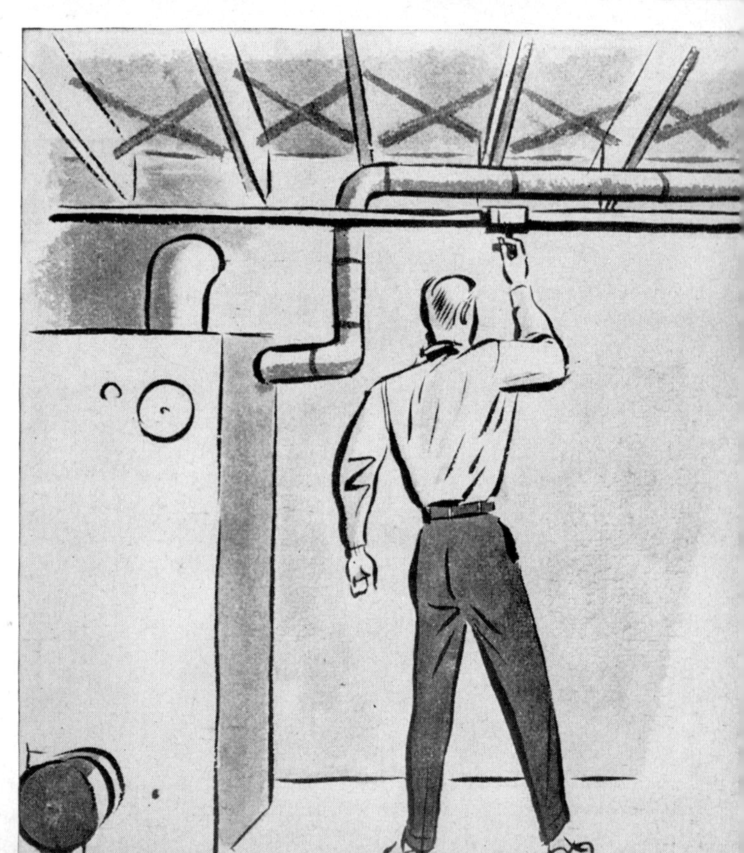

TURN OFF WATER

A blast may damage water system. Turn off water supply at main valve when you hear the alert. This way, you conserve water for vital needs later.

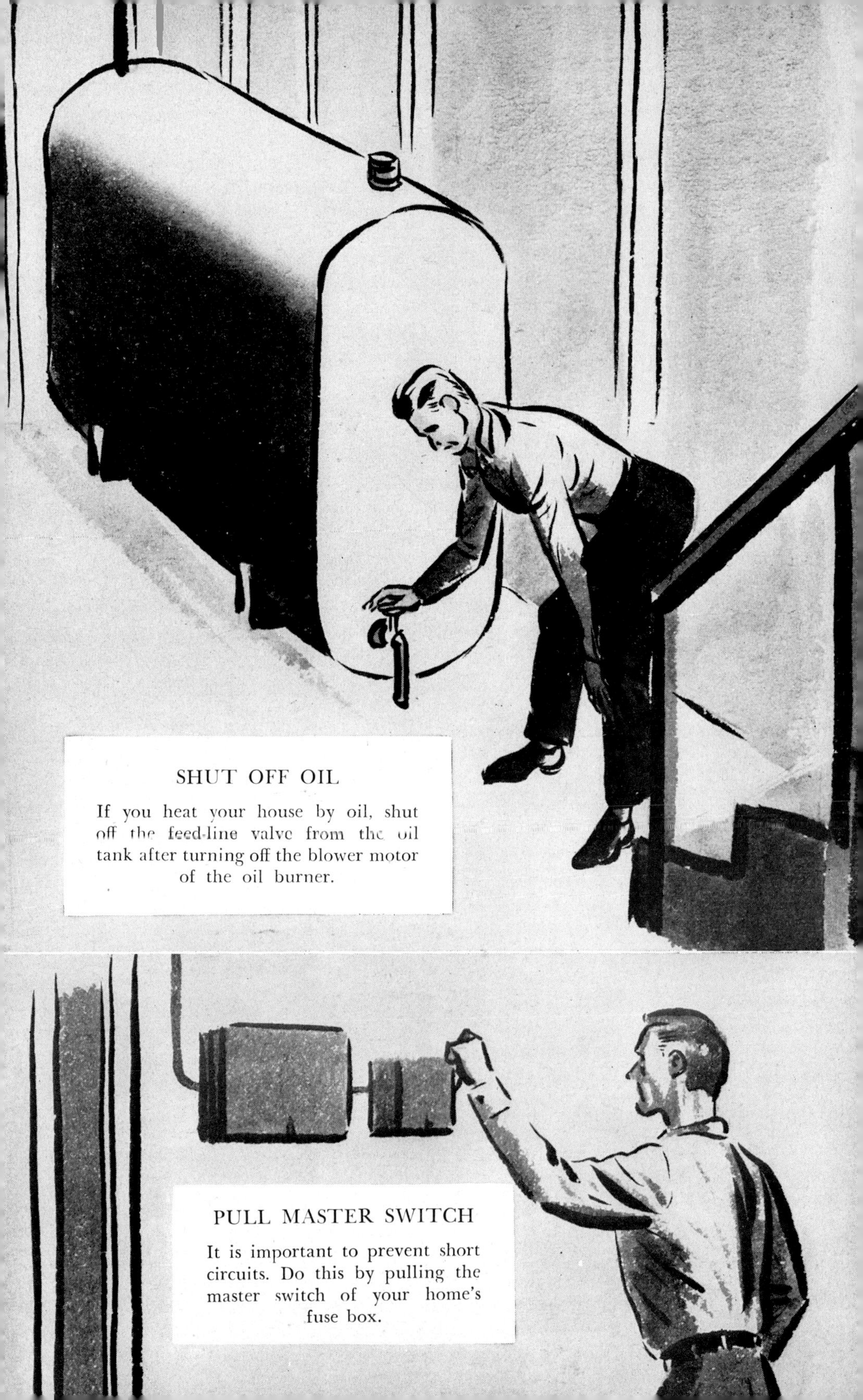

SHUT OFF OIL

If you heat your house by oil, shut off the feed-line valve from the oil tank after turning off the blower motor of the oil burner.

PULL MASTER SWITCH

It is important to prevent short circuits. Do this by pulling the master switch of your home's fuse box.

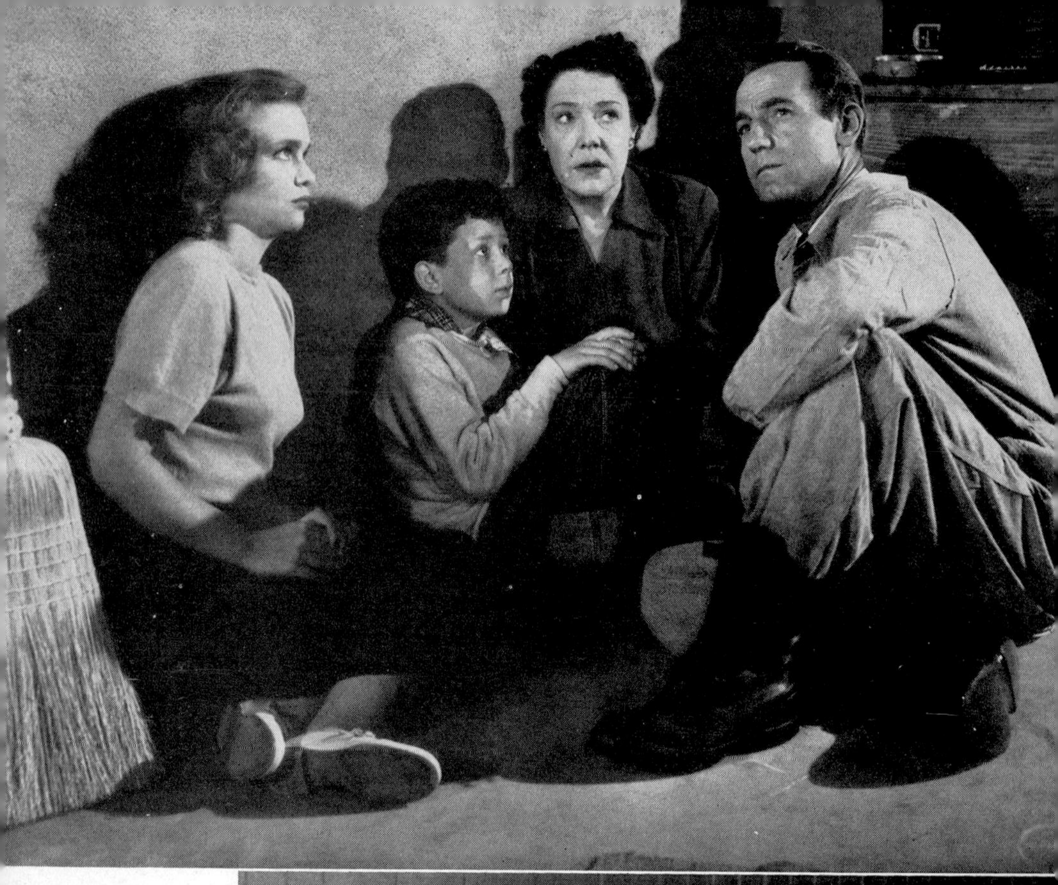

IN THE BASEMENT

When siren sounds, turn off all utilities, close doors and windows, draw curtains and blinds, and take shelter in your basement.

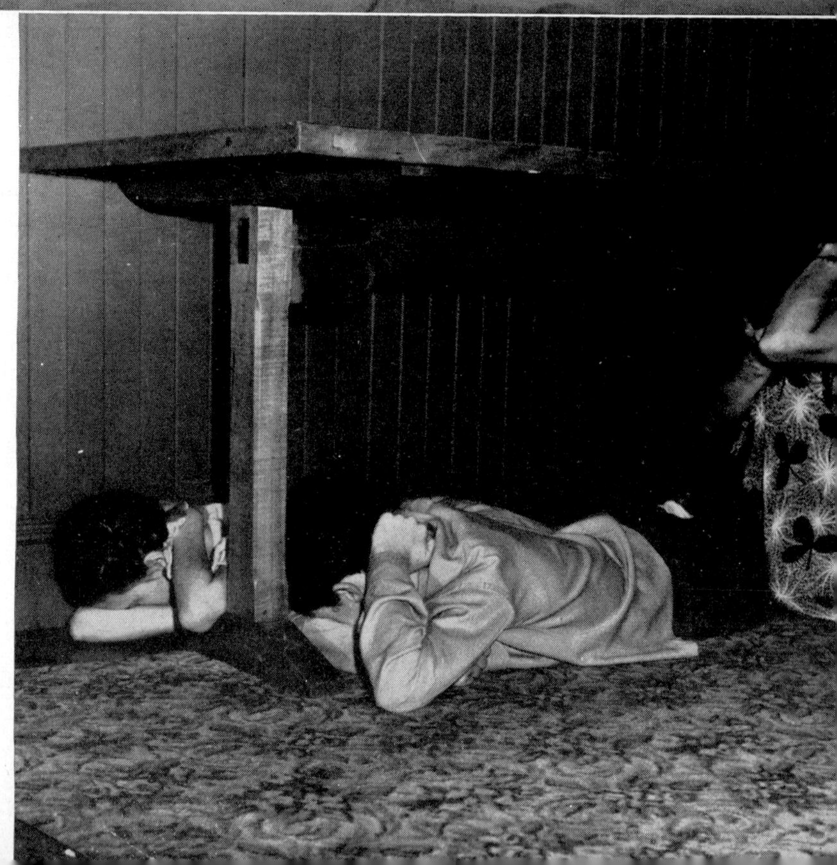

GET UNDER THE TABLE

Hide under a table to protect yourself against falling plaster and flying objects. Bury your face in arms.

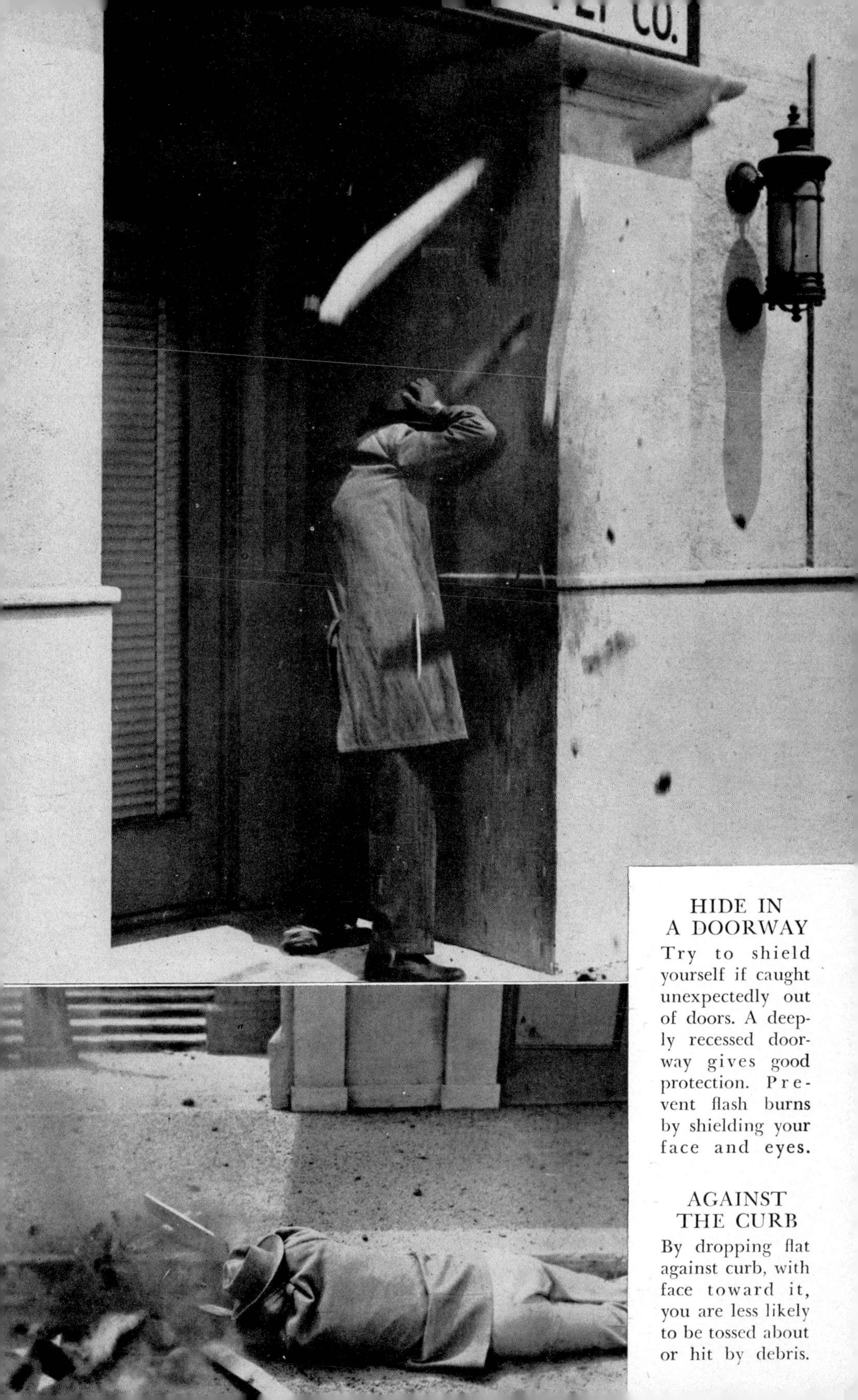


HIDE IN A DOORWAY

Try to shield yourself if caught unexpectedly out of doors. A deeply recessed doorway gives good protection. Prevent flash burns by shielding your face and eyes.

AGAINST THE CURB

By dropping flat against curb, with face toward it, you are less likely to be tossed about or hit by debris.

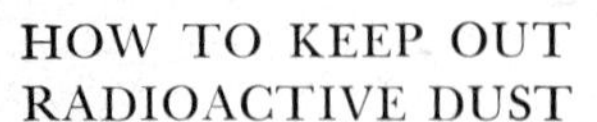

## HOW TO KEEP OUT RADIOACTIVE DUST

After a blast, you must take precautions to keep out radioactive dust or fog. Doors and windows should be kept closed. Cover over your fireplace. If your windows are broken, it is a good idea to nail drapes or other cloth over them.

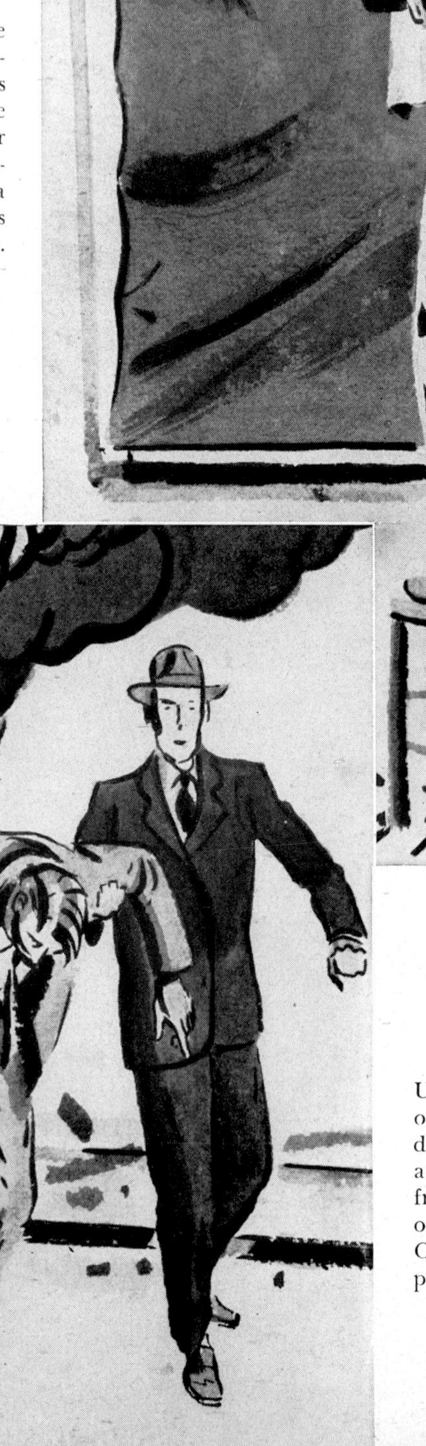

## CARE OF INJURED

Unskilled handling of injured persons is dangerous. Remove an injured person from scene of fire only to save his life. Otherwise wait for a physician to arrive.

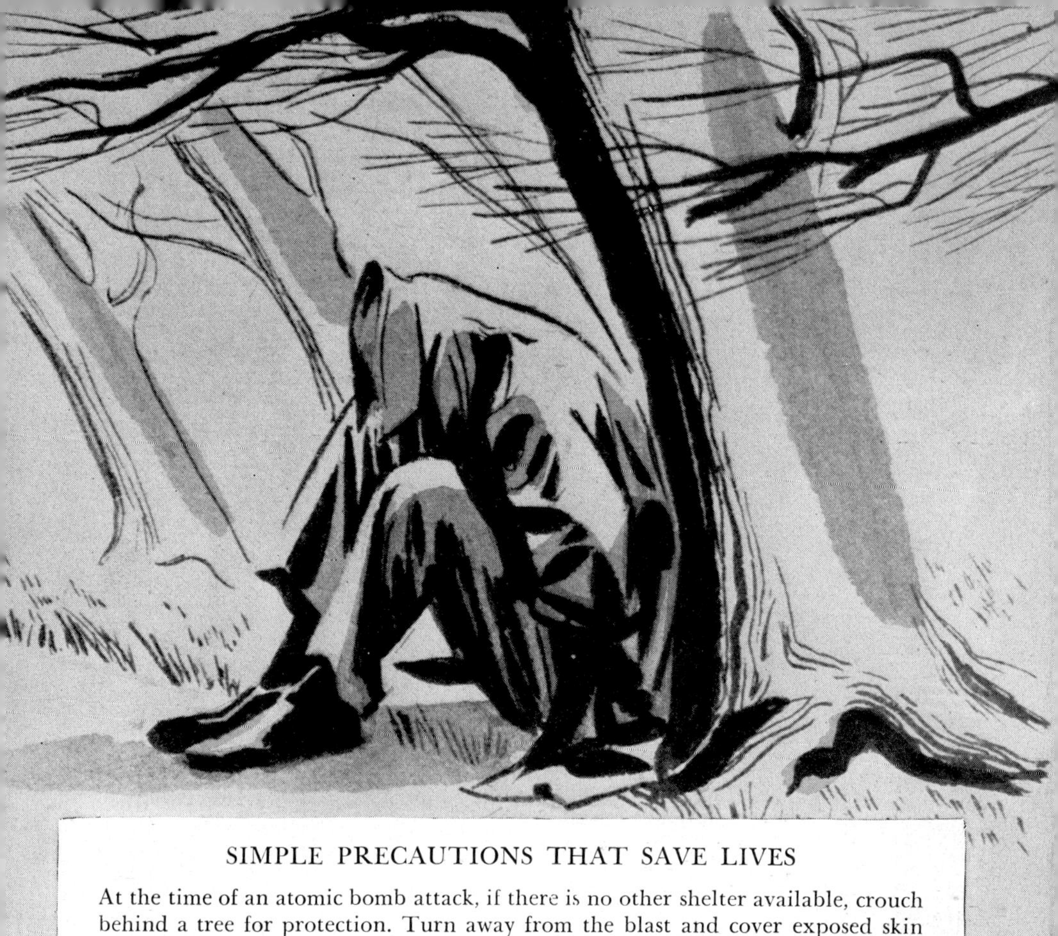

## SIMPLE PRECAUTIONS THAT SAVE LIVES

At the time of an atomic bomb attack, if there is no other shelter available, crouch behind a tree for protection. Turn away from the blast and cover exposed skin by pulling your coat over your head. *(Below)* Mother caught out of doors with baby carriage should dash into doorway, cover herself and baby with blanket.

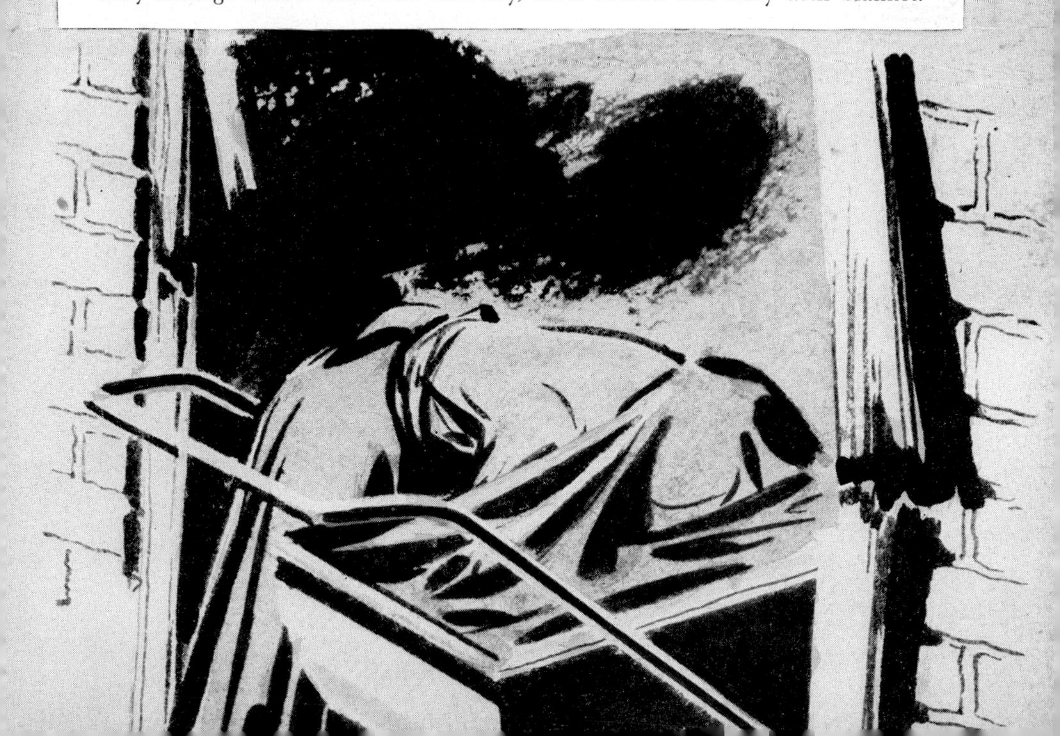

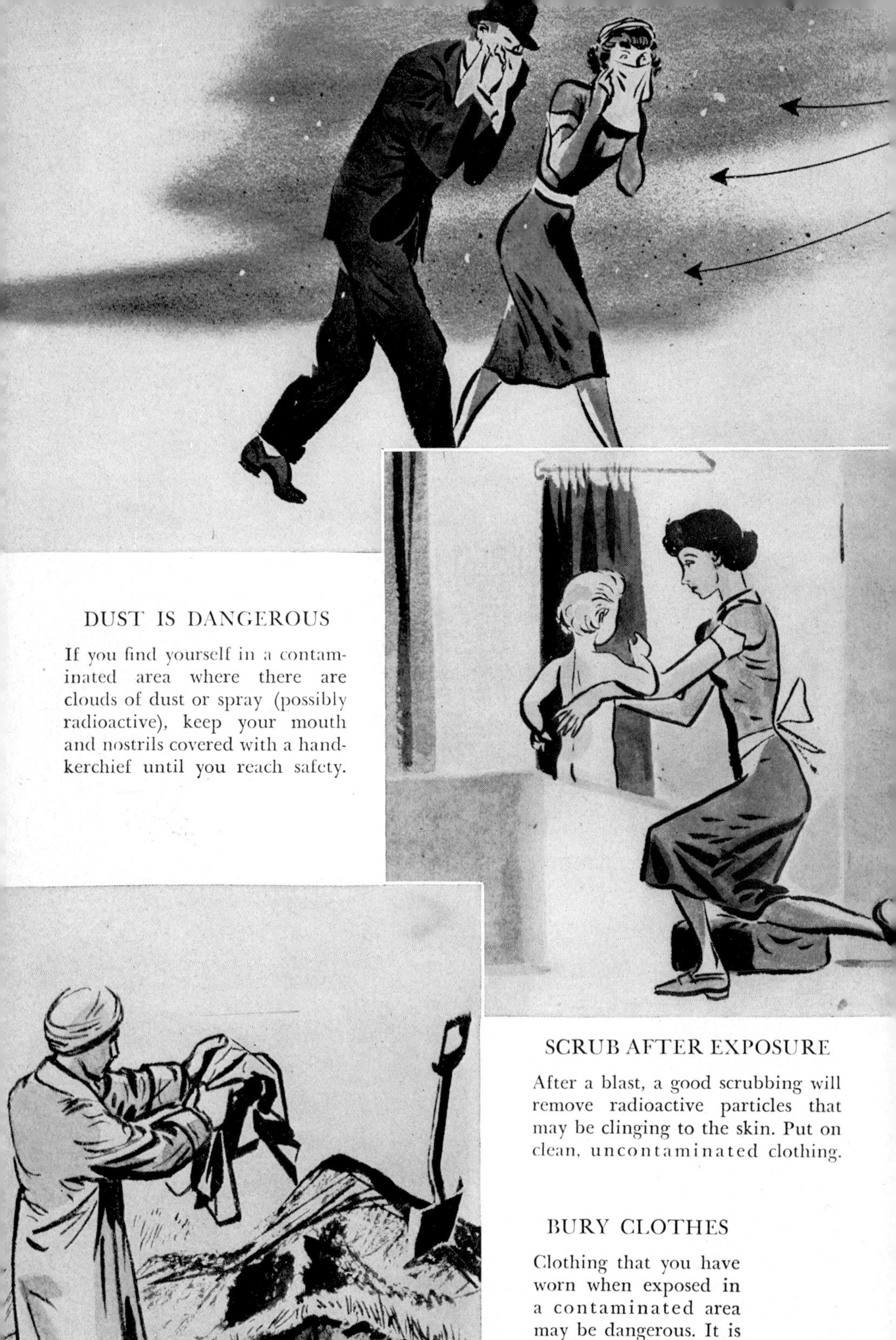

## DUST IS DANGEROUS

If you find yourself in a contaminated area where there are clouds of dust or spray (possibly radioactive), keep your mouth and nostrils covered with a handkerchief until you reach safety.

## SCRUB AFTER EXPOSURE

After a blast, a good scrubbing will remove radioactive particles that may be clinging to the skin. Put on clean, uncontaminated clothing.

## BURY CLOTHES

Clothing that you have worn when exposed in a contaminated area may be dangerous. It is best to bury it—taking adequate precautions while you do so.

## After an Air Burst

The immediate effect of the explosion will be over in a few seconds, but before you leave cover look out for falling wreckage. The greatest danger after the attack is from fires set by the heat of the explosion or resulting from broken gas and oil lines and short circuits. Use your head. Don't let yourself get trapped by big fires. But don't run off and let a small fire burn your house down if it can be controlled with a fire extinguisher or sand.

If, because of fire or damage, you must leave the building you are in and there are clouds of dust or spray outside, cover your mouth and nose with your handkerchief. (The dust probably is from the wreckage and may be harmless, but be careful; a ground or water burst may have spread radioactive dirt or fog through the air.)

If you are not in the area of serious damage, stay indoors and close the windows.

Once the enemy raiders are clear of the area, change your clothes the first opportunity. Bathe or shower; scrub hard and use plenty of soap. Be particularly careful to get your hair and fingernails entirely clean.

## After a Ground or Water Burst

If you have been officially notified that the explosion was a ground or water burst and you are near the damage area, do not use any food or drink which has been exposed. It may be contaminated.

As soon as possible after a water or ground burst, specially trained teams with detecting instruments will determine the areas which are seriously contaminated. You will be told if you must leave the area. Bathe and change to uncontaminated clothes.

Against the radioactive fog created by a water burst there is no certain protection, but obviously it is wise to take cover in as well sealed a place as possible since the fog can seep through broken windows or small cracks. Until you are out of the contaminated area, try to keep your mouth and nostrils covered to avoid inhaling radioactive dust or spray.

Do not pick up objects on your way out of a contaminated area; you will be carrying contamination with you.

*Here is a summary of the most important things to remember in case of an atomic attack.*

**What You Should Do**

Keep calm.

If there is time, get to shelter at once.

If no underground shelter is close by, get into the ground floor of a nearby building or even stand in a doorway if nothing better is available.

If you see the bomb flash and there is no cover of any kind within a step or two, drop to the street or gutter, turn away from flash, and close eyes tightly. Cover your head, face, neck, arms and other exposed areas of the body.

If you are indoors, turn off gas, electricity, water and oil at first warning and hang drapes over windows. Get into the core of your building and under a desk or table if there isn't time to get to the basement. Lie face downward and out of line with windows. After the burst tie handkerchief over mouth if area is contaminated.

**What You Should Not Do**

Don't telephone.

Don't turn on water after blast, unless to fight fire.

Don't eat or drink in a contaminated area.

Don't use metal goods in a contaminated zone.

Don't touch things after ground or water burst.

Don't try to drive your car.

Don't get excited or excite others.

## RADIATION

You need not worry about lingering radioactivity after an air burst. It is now known that there is much less residual radiation from an atomic air burst than was at first feared.

But a ground or water burst leaves a great amount of deadly radioactivity behind in the spray or dirt that spreads contamination as it falls to earth. Radiation, even if you have absorbed a considerable amount of it, is not always fatal, however.

There is no immediate way of knowing when you have been exposed to radiation during or after the atomic burst. You will not feel anything if radiation hits you. Signs of radiation sickness show up later. How much later depends upon how much radiation you have absorbed.

If you have absorbed a large amount, you will know it within a few hours. The first signs are nausea and shock.

In the first day or two, the shock will be followed by vomiting, diarrhea and fever. There will be no pain, but you will suffer discomfort, depression and fatigue.

The symptoms will disappear, then return for two or three days. In the *worst* and *untreated* cases, death follows.

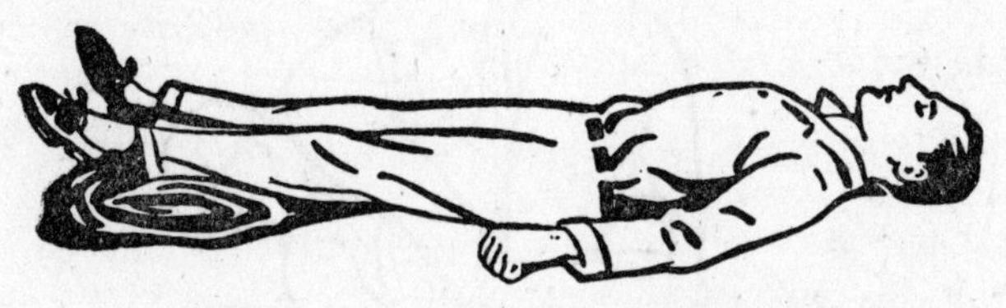

HOW TO TREAT FOR SHOCK

Shock is present in many injuries, and may be severe. The patient's face is pale, his pulse weak or rapid, he breathes irregularly, and he may be nauseous or unconscious. The legs should be raised, the head low. Absolute rest and warmth are essential. Stimulants should be given if the patient is conscious, and a physician called at once.

In moderate cases these symptoms will appear only after several days—in some cases two or three weeks. During this time the mouth and gums will bleed, and there will be internal bleeding. All bleeding, even from small cuts, will be difficult to stop. Loss of appetite and falling hair also may indicate radiation sickness.

### Medical Attention Important

In many cases radiation sickness symptoms disappear entirely for a time. This does not mean you are out of danger. The symptoms may return at a later time.

If you show any signs of radiation sickness or have reason to believe the area you have been in is radioactive, go to a medical station at once.

Conditions after the bombing, however, may not permit you to get proper medical treatment immediately. In this case follow these simple rules until help comes: Keep warm. Get complete rest; stay in bed if possible. Drink warm, nourishing liquids and eat foods rich in sugar and protein, but do not eat or drink foods or liquids that have been exposed in a contaminated area.

## FIRE

You may ask why you need concern yourself with fire when there is a fire department nearby. The answer is that no fire department system, even with the help of its auxiliary services, can deal with the multitude of fires which would result from enemy attack.

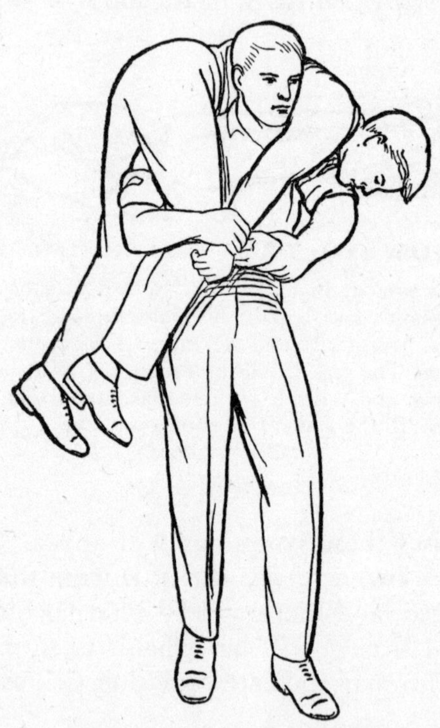

HOW TO CARRY AN INJURED PERSON

The across-the-shoulder carry provides a convenient way of transporting an injured person if his condition permits him to be moved.

If the area in which you live is attacked, the first responsibility for providing fire protection (especially in case your house is set afire) rests directly upon you.

This responsibility involves the provision of the necessary fire fighting equipment and the knowledge of how to use it.

A single attack may start hundreds of fires, and probably so much water would be used by the fire department that there would be little or no water pressure in homes. Also, any special fire fighting equipment which operates by electricity should not be counted on, since power lines may be broken.

But a great deal can be done with individual fire fighting appliances if they are used properly and promptly. If you act fast, you can help reduce losses from small fires and leave the regular fire departments free to go to work on the big blazes. They will come to your aid as soon as possible.

*Here are some things for you to do and not to do:*

**What to Do**

1. Close doors and windows to prevent draft.
2. To force a door, break panel near lock.
3. Crawl, don't walk when in thick smoke.
4. Keep near walls where floors are strongest.
5. Attack fire at closest possible range.
6. Use sand or foam to quench oil fires.
7. Keep buckets of water and sand in the house and be sure extinguishers are filled and in order.
8. When searching a house for fires start at top.

**What Not to Do**

1. Don't enter a smoke-filled room alone, except to save a life.
2. Don't enter burning building or room without fire-fighting appliances, except to save life.
3. Don't play water on electric wiring.

*If your attic is full of odds and ends get rid of them. They are a fire hazard.*

## FIRST AID

First aid, particularly in the case of serious injuries and burns, is delicate work—for experts only. If medical aid is available, it is better to remain calm and let qualified medical people handle the situation. Otherwise you will do more harm than good.

But you might find yourself in a situation where help is not at hand and injuries are such that they need immediate attention.

### Burns

If medical aid can possibly be secured, do not touch or treat any severe burn. Remember that infection may reduce chances of recovery by 50%. Any handling will increase the danger of infection.

***A Few Simple Rules:***

1. Exclude air from the burned area with clean gauze, soft, clean cloths, or absorbent cotton, then bandage gently.

2. Unless absolutely necessary, do not remove clothing. If garments must be taken off, cut the cloth around the burn. If material sticks to the flesh, *do not remove it*. If blisters have formed, they should not be broken or punctured.

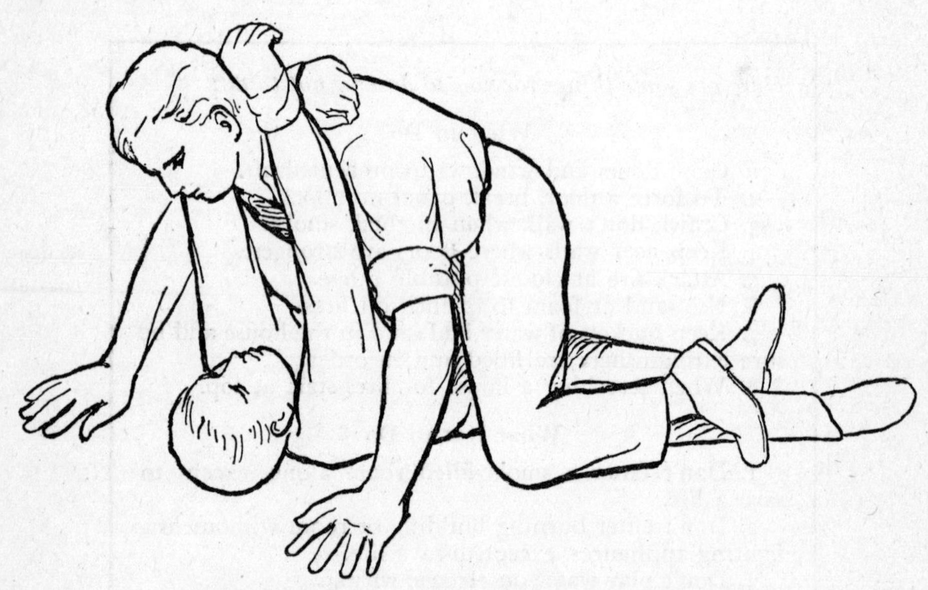

RESCUE IN A BURNING BUILDING

It is best to stay close to the floor, since there is more air there. If the person to be rescued is injured or unconscious, his hands should be tied together (not too tightly) at the wrists and placed over the neck of the rescuer, who straddles the prostrate body and draws it with him as he crawls to safety.

3. Dressings may be soaked in a lotion made by stirring baking soda in clean water (about two teaspoonsful to the pint). Keep strips wet by repeatedly pouring the lotion over them. Do not remove the dressings.

4. If pain is unbearable and no medical aid can be secured, smear clean gauze with petroleum jelly (vaseline), and apply to the burned area.

5. Dressings should overlap each other. Overtight bandages may lead to serious injury. The patient should be kept warm; give hot, sweet drinks if he is conscious.

### Hemorrhage

1. If bleeding is slight or there is only a small amount of oozing, it is best to ignore it. Remember, touching or handling a wound will increase the risk of infection. If there has been a ground or water burst, cover the patient with some garment to keep out contaminated water and dirt.

2. Bleeding may be checked by the use of a compress of gauze or cloth held by a moderately tight bandage. A tourniquet should be used only when there is excessive bleeding. A tourniquet or pressure bandage must be loosened momentarily at half hour intervals to prevent serious damage.

### Fractures

1. Do not try to set a broken bone.

2. Do not move the patient unless he is in danger from fire or falling debris.

3. If necessary to move the patient, bind the limb tightly to a pillow, a padded board or other improvised support. When possible lay the patient on a door or other flat surface before moving him.

4. Keep the patient warm; give hot, sweet drinks if he is conscious.

(The subject of first aid is presented in full detail in the preceding chapter. )

CHAPTER 30

# DICTIONARY OF COMMON MEDICAL TERMS

The following pages present a concise dictionary of medical terms the average person is likely to encounter in everyday life. It includes expressions from surgery, anatomy, physiology, nutrition, and other branches of the study of the human body. For further information or additional definitions, the reader is invited to consult the Index at the end of this book.

## *A*

*ABDOMEN*. Belly.

*ABORTION*. The spontaneous or induced expulsion of the unborn child in early pregnancy.

*ABRASION*. Injury to skin of any part of the body.

*ABSCESS*. Collection of pus surrounded by a wall of inflamed tissue.

*ACCOMMODATION*. Focusing the eye on a near object.

*ACNE*. Condition of skin of face occurring in adolescents.

*ACROMEGALY*. Enlargement of hands and extremities.

*ACUTE*. Abrupt or brief onset (beginning) and duration of disease.

*ADDISON'S DISEASE*. A disease of the adrenal glands. Usually fatal.

*ADDUCTORS*. A group of muscles which run on the inner side of the thigh.

*ADENITIS*. Inflammation of the lymph glands.

*ADIPOSE*. Fatty (tissue).

*ADRENALIN*. The internal secretion of the medulla of the adrenal glands.

*AFFERENT NERVES*. Nerves that convey impulses toward the brain.

*AGGLUTINATION*. Clumping in the blood.

*ALBUMEN (ALBUMIN)*. A protein found in blood and egg-white, etc.

*ALBUMINURIA*. Presence of albumen in the urine.

*ALIMENTARY TRACT*. Same as digestive organs.

*ALVEOLI*. The small air sacs of the lung.

*AMENORRHEA*. Abnormal interruption or absence of menstrual flow.
*AMNESIA*. Lack or loss of memory.
*AMYLASE*. An enzyme which splits starch and sugars.
*ANABOLIC*. Building-up processes of metabolism.
*ANALGESIC*. A pain-killer.
*ANEMIA*. Deficiency in quality or quantity of red blood corpuscles.
*ANGINA PECTORIS*. Sudden sharp pain in region of the heart.
*ANKYLOSIS*. Stiff joint following some form of injury.
*ANTHRAX*. A disease named after the bacillus of this name.
*ANTIBIOTIC*. Any drug that has the property of destroying germs.
*ANTIDOTE*. Any substance used to counteract effect of a poison.
*ANTI-HORMONES*. Substances which act against hormones.
*ANTI-RACHITIC*. Refers to diet to cure or prevent rickets.
*ANTI-SCORBUTIC*. Refers to diet to cure or prevent scurvy.
*ANTISEPTIC*. Any chemical which will prevent the growth of bacteria.
*ANTITOXIN*. An antibody which neutralizes toxin.
*ANURIA*. Cessation of secretion of the urine.
*ANUS*. The opening of the bowel on the surface.
*AORTA*. The main blood vessel of the body, arising from the heart.
*AQUEOUS HUMOR*. Watery substance in the front chamber of the eye.
*ARTERIOLES*. Small arteries.
*ARTERIOSCLEROSIS*. Hardening of the arteries.
*ASCENDING COLON*. Part of large bowel on right side of body.
*ASCORBIC ACID*. Vitamin C.
*ASPHYXIA*. Suffocation.
*ASPIRATION*. A breath, or act of breathing.
*ATHLETE'S FOOT*. Fungus infection of the skin of the feet.
*ATLAS VERTEBRA*. The first cervical vertebra.
*AURICLE*. A thin-walled chamber of the heart.
*AXILLARY ARTERY*. Artery that runs across the armpit.

## *B*

*BACILLI*. Rod-shaped bacteria.
*BACTERIA*. Germs.
*BARBER'S ITCH*. Infection of the hair follicles of the beard.
*BARBITURATES*. Drugs which form the basis of most sleeping pills.
*BENIGN*. Mild in character (said of a tumor).

*BERIBERI*. Disease due to deficiency of vitamin B.
*BILE*. Digestive fluid secreted by the liver.
*BOIL (FURUNCLE)*. Localized infection of the skin.
*BOTULISM*. Type of food poisoning.
*BRACHIAL ARTERY*. Main artery of the arm.
*BRIGHT'S DISEASE*. Acute or chronic disease of the kidneys.
*BRONCHI*. Main air tubes of the lung.
*BRONCHIOLES*. Small air tubes.
*BRONCHITIS*. Inflammation of the bronchial tubes.
*BUNION*. Inflammation and enlargement of first joint of the big toes.

## C

*CAESARIAN SECTION*. Delivery of a child through incision made in the skin, abdominal wall, and womb.
*CAFFEIN*. A drug found in coffee.
*CALCULUS*. Stony mass of variable size and shape formed in gall bladder, kidneys, or urinary bladder.
*CALORIE*. A unit of heat, the amount of which raises the temperature of 1 c.c. of water 1° C.
*CANCER*. Any malignant growth anywhere in the body.
*CAPILLARY*. Smallest blood vessel.
*CARBOHYDRATE*. Substance containing carbon and hydrogen and oxygen in the same proportions as water.
*CARDIAC*. Pertaining to the heart.
*CARIES*. Disease of the teeth causing cavities.
*CAROTENE*. A pigment contained in carrots and related to vitamin A.
*CAROTID ARTERIES*. Arteries of the neck.
*CATARACT*. Opacity of the lens of the eye.
*CATHARTIC*. Any medicine that will relieve constipation.
*CECUM*. A blind sac at the beginning of the colon.
*CELLULOSE*. A tough, starchy material in plant cells.
*CEREBELLUM*. Part of the brain.
*CEREBRAL CORTEX*. Outer layer of the brain.
*CEREBRUM*. The main part of the brain.
*CERVICAL REGION*. Neck region.
*CERVIX*. Neck of the uterus.
*CHANCRE*. Primary sore of syphilis.
*CHILBLAINS*. Painful swelling and blueness of skin, usually of hands and feet, due to exposure to cold.

*CHLOROPHYLL*. Green pigment of plants.
*CHOLESTEROL*. A fatty substance of the body deposited on the wall of the arteries.
*CHRONIC*. In reference to diseases: prolonged (opposite of acute).
*CHYME*. Soft mass of digested material.
*CILIA*. Whiplike processes from cells.
*CLAVICLE*. Collar-bone.
*CLIMACTERIC*. Change of life in women and in men.
*COCCI*. Round bacteria.
*COCCYGEAL REGION*. Near coccyx and on tip of spine.
*COCCYX*. Last bone of the spine.
*COCHLEA*. The bony, hearing part of the ear.
*COITUS*. Sexual intercourse.
*COLITIS*. Inflammation of the large bowel.
*COLLOID*. Suspension of microscopic particles in solution.
*COMA*. Deep unconsciousness.
*CONCUSSION*. In reference to brain injury.
*CONGENITAL*. Said of an abnormal condition or disease existing at birth.
*CONGESTION*. Abnormal accumulation of excess blood, etc., in any organ.
*CONJUNCTIVA*. Membrane lining the lids and front of eyeball.
*CONTAGION*. Spread of infectious disease from one person to another.
*CONTUSION*. A bruise, an injury to any part of the body in which the skin is not broken.
*CORNEA*. The clear front of eye.
*CORONARY ARTERIES*. Arteries of the heart muscle itself.
*CORPUS LUTEUM*. A formation in the ovary which matures and discharges its contents when pregnancy takes place.
*CORTEX*. Outer layer.
*CORYZA*. Acute cold.
*CRETIN*. Dwarfism due to deficiency of thyroid gland.
*CYANOSIS*. Blueness of skin, lips, and nail-beds.
*CYST*. Saclike cavity filled with fluid.
*CYSTITIS*. Inflammation of the bladder.

## *D*

*DEBILITY*. Weakness, lack of strength.
*DEFECATION*. Moving the bowels.
*DELTOID MUSCLES*. Muscles covering front of the shoulder.

*DENDRITES*. Short processes of a nerve cell.
*DESCENDING COLON*. Colon on left passing down to rectum.
*DIABETES INSIPIDUS*. Chronic disease characterized by passing of large amount of urine which does not contain any sugar.
*DIABETES MELLITUS*. Disease of pancreas characterized by thirst, hunger, sugar in urine, and loss of weight.
*DIAPHRAGM*. Midriff sheet of muscle between thorax and abdomen.
*DIARRHEA*. Frequent watery stools.
*DIASTOLE*. Interval between heartbeats.
*DIURETIC*. A drug which induces increased passage of urine.
*DUODENUM*. Beginning of small intestine.
*DYSMENORRHEA*. Painful menstruation.
*DYSPAREUNIA*. Painful sexual intercourse; of the female.
*DYSPEPSIA*. Indigestion.
*DYSURIA*. Painful urination.

### *E*

*EDEMA*. Excess of lymph fluid in the tissues, causing swelling.
*EFFERENT SYSTEM*. Nerves which carry impulses away from brain.
*ELECTROCARDIOGRAPH*. Instrument for detecting changes in the heart.
*EMBRYO*. Product of conception up to third month of pregnancy.
*EMBRYOLOGY*. Study of development of the body from the egg-cell upwards.
*EMETIC*. A drug which produces vomiting.
*ENDOCARDITIS*. Infection or disease of the inner heart lining.
*ENDOCRINE*. Refers to glands of internal secretion.
*ENDOMETRITIS*. Inflammation of the lining of the womb.
*ENURESIS*. Failure to have bladder control.
*ENZYME*. A catalyst made in the body.
*EPIDERMIS*. Outer layer of skin.
*EPIGLOTTIS*. Protective structure at top of larynx.
*ERYSIPELAS*. Infectious disease of the skin, usually the face.
*ESOPHAGUS*. The gullet.
*ESTRONE*. Hormone from the ovary.
*EUGENICS*. Science of improvement of human race.
*EUSTACHIAN TUBE*. Tube from ear to pharynx.
*EXOPHTHALMIC GOITRE*. Also called Graves' disease and toxic goitre. It is a disease of the thyroid gland.

*EXTERNAL AUDITORY MEATUS*. Tube from outside to ear-drum.

*F*

*FAINTING*. State of temporary unconsciousness.
*FALLOPIAN TUBE*. Tube from ovary to uterus.
*FECES*. Excretion from the bowel.
*FEMORA*. Thigh bones.
*FETUS*. Product of conception from end of third month to birth.
*FIBRIN*. One of the substances which form blood clots.
*FIBRINOGEN*. The substance from which fibrin is formed.
*FILTERABLE VIRUS*. A virus which passes through special filters.
*FLEXION*. Bending of any part of the body.
*FOMENTATION*. Application of warm, moist compresses to the body to allay pain.
*FONTANELLES*. Gaps between the bones of the infant's skull.
*FRONTAL BONES*. Bones of the forehead.
*FRUCTOSE*. Fruit sugar.

*G*

*GALL BLADDER*. Bag containing bile, lying beneath the liver.
*GANGLION*. A collection of nerve cells.
*GANGRENE*. Rotting of tissue due to an infection.
*GASTRIC*. Pertaining to the stomach.
*GENES*. Characteristics grouped in chromosomes.
*GENITALIA*. The sexual organs.
*GINGIVITIS*. Inflammation of the gums.
*GLOMERULUS*. The essential filtering organ of the kidney.
*GLOTTIS*. Upper end of voice-box.
*GLUCOSE*. The simplest sugar.
*GLYCOGEN*. The storage form of glucose.
*GOITRE*. Swelling of the thyroid gland.
*GONADS*. The testicles or ovaries.
*GONORRHEA*. A venereal disease characterized by pus discharge from the urinary canal.
*GYNECOLOGY*. Study of diseases of women.

*H*

*HEARTBURN*. Indigestion.
*HEMATEMESIS*. Vomiting blood.
*HEMATIN*. Iron containing pigment.

*HEMATURIA*. Blood in the urine.

*HEMOGLOBIN*. Hematin and globin (protein); hemoglobin of the blood.

*HEMOLYSIS*. Destruction of red blood cells.

*HEMOPHILIA*. Bleeding disease.

*HEMOPTYSIS*. Expectorating of blood.

*HEREDITARY*. Refers to a disease or characteristic inherited from one or both of the parents.

*HIVES*. Blotchy, red itching eruption of skin.

*HODGKIN'S DISEASE*. Progressive enlarging of lymph glands, especially those in neck and chest.

*HORMONE*. A chemical substance secreted by an endocrine gland.

*HUMERUS*. Main bone of arm.

*HYDROCEPHALUS*. Water on the brain.

*HYPOCHONDRIAC*. Person afflicted with imaginary diseases.

*HYPODERMIC*. Beneath the skin.

*HYSTERECTOMY*. The surgical removal of the womb (uterus).

## *I*

*ILIUM*. Bone of the hip.

*INCUBATION*. The length of time from the exposure to the development of a disease.

*INFERIOR VENA CAVA*. Main vein collecting blood from both lower limbs.

*INHIBITION*. Sub-conscious self-restraint.

*INSIDIOUS*. Having an effect more serious than appears at first.

*INSOMNIA*. Sleeplessness.

*INSPIRATION* (of breathing). Breathing in.

*INSULIN*. The internal secretion of the pancreas.

*INTRAMUSCULAR*. Refers to any medication that is injected into the muscles of the body.

*IRIS*. The curtain which surrounds the pupil of the eye.

*IRRIGATION*. The cleansing of a wound or cavity of the body by the use of copious amounts of different kinds of fluids.

*ISLETS OF LANGERHANS*. The dotted collections of cells which produce insulin (in the pancreas).

## *J*

*JAUNDICE*. Yellow discoloration of skin and mucous membranes due to absorption of the bile by the circulation.

## *K*

*KETONE BODIES.* Poisonous, acid bodies formed in the body fat.

## *L*

*LACHRYMAL GLAND.* Tear gland.
*LACTATION.* Suckling period of supplying human milk.
*LACTEAL.* Small lymphatic which carries fat from the villus of the intestine.
*LARYNGOSCOPE.* Instrument for viewing vocal cords.
*LARYNX.* Voice-box.
*LEUCOCYTOSIS.* Increase in number of white blood corpuscles in acute inflammation.
*LEUCORRHOEA.* Mucous vaginal discharge, at times very profuse.
*LEUKEMIA.* Disease of bone marrow and spleen characterized by tremendous increase of the white corpuscles.
*LIPASE.* A fat-splitting enzyme.
*LUMBAR REGION.* The loins.
*LYMPH.* The fluid round the tissue cells.
*LYMPHOCYTES.* White blood cells—forming 25 per cent of the total.

## *M*

*MALNUTRITION.* Ill health with loss of weight due to improper eating.
*MAMMARY GLANDS.* The breasts.
*MANDIBLE.* Lower jawbone.
*MASTOID.* Knobby protuberance behind the ear.
*MEDULLA OBLONGATA.* Small portion of brain at top end of spinal cord where the nerve centers are found.
*MEMBRANA TYMPANI.* Eardrum.
*MENINGES.* Wrappings of brain and spinal cord.
*MENOPAUSE.* Change in life of the female. Also called climacteric.
*METABOLISM.* The total chemical changes of the body.
*MIDRIFF.* See Diaphragm.
*MISCARRIAGE.* Loss of fetus from the womb. Also called abortion.
*MITRAL VALVE.* Heart valve between left auricle and ventricle.
*MUCOUS MEMBRANE.* The lining of any of the cavities of the body.
*MULTIPLE SCLEROSIS.* A progressive disease of the spinal cord which may go on for many years.
*MYOCARDITIS.* Inflammation of the heart muscle.

## *N*

*NEPHRECTOMY*. Surgical removal of the kidney.
*NEURITIS*. Inflammation of one or more nerves.
*NEURONE*. Nerve cell.
*NUCLEUS*. Vital, central part of a cell.

## *O*

*OBESITY*. Overweight.
*ORCHITIS*. Inflammation of the testicles.
*OSSIFICATION*. Bone formation.
*OSTEOMYELITIS*. Infection of the marrow of the bones
*OTITIS*. Inflammation of the middle-ear.
*OVARECTOMY*. Surgical removal of an ovary.
*OVARIAN FOLLICLE*. Small blister of fluid on the ovary.
*OVARY*. Female sex organ.
*OVUM*. The egg cell which is shed from the follicle in the ovary.

## *P*

*PANCREAS*. Gland that forms digestive juices and insulin.
*PARATHYROID GLAND*. Glands lying near or embedded in the thyroid.
*PAROTID*. Salivary gland in cheek.
*PAROTITIS*. Inflammation of the parotid gland. In epidemic form it is called mumps.
*PATELLA*. Kneecap.
*PATHOGENIC*. Causing disease.
*PATHOLOGY*. Anything not normal about the body.
*PECTORAL MUSCLES*. Muscles of chest.
*PEDICULOSIS*. Infestation with lice.
*PENIS*. Male sex organ.
*PEPSIN*. Digestive enzyme of stomach, splitting proteins.
*PERICARDIUM*. Fibrous sheath round the heart.
*PERIOSTEUM*. Fibrous sheath round bone.
*PERISTALSIS*. Movement of gut and stomach.
*PERITONEUM*. Lining membrane of abdominal cavity.
*PHAGOCYTES*. White blood cells which devour bacteria.
*PHARYNX*. Back of throat.
*PHRENIC NERVES*. Nerves to the diaphragm.
*PHYSIOLOGY*. The study of the functioning of the normal body.
*PINNA*. The outer ear.

*PITUITARY GLAND*. Endocrine gland located on the floor of the brain.
*PLACENTA*. Afterbirth.
*PLASMA*. The fluid part of blood.
*PLATELETS*. Smallest bodies in blood.
*PLEURA*. Lining of chest wall and lungs.
*PORTAL SYSTEM*. Veins draining the intestines, so carrying food in blood, to the liver.
*PROGNOSIS*. Prediction of the ultimate result of a disease.
*PROPHYLAXIS*. Measures used to prevent a disease.
*PROSTATE GLAND*. Gland which plays a part in man's sex life.
*PROTEINS*. Complex chemical substances containing nitrogen, carbon, hydrogen and oxygen; sometimes other elements.
*PROTHROMBIN*. An essential part of the clotting process of blood.
*PROTOPLASM*. Essential living substance of body cells.
*PSYCHOSIS*. An acute mental illness.
*PSYCHOSOMATIC*. Illness involving both the body and the mind, in which the mind dominates the condition.
*PTYALIN*. Enzyme in saliva.
*PUBERTY*. Period between childhood and adolescence.
*PUERPERIUM*. Refers to the period after a birth, before the organs return to normal. This is about six weeks.
*PULMONARY*. Pertaining to the lung.
*PURPURA*. Spontaneous bleeding.
*PYLORUS*. Portion of stomach.

## *Q*

*QUINSY*. An abscess formation behind one of the tonsils.

## *R*

*RABIES*. Hydrophobia.
*RADIAL ARTERY*. Artery of the forearm, felt as the pulse.
*RADIUM*. A rare metal that has healing qualities, but prolonged exposure to it will also produce serious burns.
*RECTUM*. Last part of colon.
*REFRACTION*. Bending of light in glass, etc.
*RENAL ARTERIES*. Arteries of the kidney.
*RETINA*. Sensitive part of the eye where light is detected.
*RHINITIS*. An acute catarrhal inflammation of the nasal cavity, a cold.
*RINGWORM*. Contagious infection of the skin and scalp.

## S

*SACRAL REGION.* Round the sacrum; lower vertebrae of the spine.

*SACRUM.* Lower vertebrae between lumbar vertebrae and coccyx.

*SALINE.* Refers to any salty substance; the most common variety is ordinary table salt.

*SALPINGITIS.* Inflammation of the Fallopian tube.

*SCAPULA.* Shoulder blade.

*SCLERA.* Thick white coat of the eyeball.

*SCROTUM.* Bag holding the testicles.

*SCURVY.* A nutritional disease due to absence of certain vitamins.

*SEBACEOUS GLANDS.* Glands which secret sebum. In the ear they secrete the wax.

*SEBUM.* The fatty matter which the sebaceous glands secrete.

*SECRETIN.* Internal secretion of the duodenum which stimulates the pancreas to secrete its digestive juices.

*SEDATIVE.* A quieting drug.

*SEPTICEMIA.* Blood poisoning, with the germs present in the blood stream.

*SERUM.* Blood plasma minus fibrin.

*SEXUAL IMPOTENCY.* The inability of the male to have satisfactory sexual intercourse.

*SIGMOID COLON.* Last coil of colon.

*SOLAR PLEXUS.* Ganglia of sympathetic cells in the belly.

*SOMATIC.* Bodily.

*SPERMATOZOA.* Male sex cells.

*SPIROCHETES.* Finely coiled microscopic organisms (bacteria), including those which cause syphilis.

*SPRAIN.* Injury to a joint which may involve tearing of a ligament.

*SPUTUM.* Spit or phlegm.

*STAPHYLOCOCCI.* Cocci in groups.

*STERILITY.* Inability to have children.

*STERNUM.* Breast bone.

*STILLBIRTH.* Birth of a dead infant.

*STREPTOCOCCI.* Cocci in chains.

*SUBLINGUAL GLAND.* Salivary gland beneath the tongue.

*SUBMAXILLARY.* Salivary gland beneath lower jaw.

*SUPERIOR VENA CAVA.* Main vein from head and neck leading into heart.

*SUPRARENAL GLANDS.* Glands on top of the kidney which secrete adrenalin.

*SYNAPSES.* The junction of two neurones.
*SYNOVIAL MEMBRANE.* Layer of fibrous tissue inside a joint.
*SYNTHESIS.* Building up.
*SYSTEMIC.* Referring to the general systems of the body, for example, the urinary system or gastro-intestinal system.
*SYSTOLE.* Contraction of the heart.

## *T*

*TASTE BUDS.* Cells, shaped like buds, in the tongue.
*TESTES.* Male gonads or sex glands, which produce sperm.
*TESTOSTERONE.* Internal secretion of testes.
*TETANY.* Form of spasm.
*THERAPY.* Treatment.
*THORACIC REGION.* Chest region.
*THROMBIN.* Part of the substances essential to clotting of blood.
*THROMBOSIS.* Clotting of blood in the body.
*THROMBUS.* A clot in a living vessel.
*THYMUS.* A gland in the neck below the thyroid.
*THYROID.* A gland in the neck that secretes thyroxin.
*THYROXIN.* The hormone of the thyroid gland.
*TOXIC.* Poisonous or bacterial.
*TOXIN.* A poison secreted by bacteria.
*TRACHEA.* Windpipe.
*TRACTION.* The pulling either by hand or by mechanical means on a fractured or dislocated bone; it is done to align broken ends of a bone.
*TRANSVERSE COLON.* Part of colon which passes from right to left.
*TRICHINOSIS.* A disease caused by infected pork.
*TRYPSIN.* Digestive ferment of pancreas that acts on protein.

## *U*

*UMBILICAL CORD.* Cord connecting fetus and placenta.
*UREA.* Waste product formed from unused amino-acids by the liver.
*UREMIA.* Condition of poisoning from kidney failure.
*URETER.* Tube from kidney to bladder.
*URETHRA.* Tube from bladder to outside.
*URETHRITIS.* Inflammation of the canal which carries the urine from the bladder.
*UTERUS.* Womb.

## *V*

*VACCINE.* A substance which is injected to form antibodies and establish immunity to a disease.

*VAGINA.* Canal leading from womb to surface of the body.

*VAGUS NERVE.* The tenth cranial nerve which supplies most of the viscera.

*VAS DEFERENS.* Duct carrying sperm from testes to urethra.

*VERTIGO.* Dizziness.

*VILLUS.* Projection of small intestine mucosa which absorbs food.

*VISCERA.* Organs such as lung, kidneys, etc.

*VITAMIN.* A chemical necessary for life. Exists in all food.

*VOMITUS.* The material that comes from the stomach when vomiting occurs.

# INDEX